Current Concepts of Bone Fragility

Edited by Hans K. Uhthoff

Associate Editor Elvira Stahl

With 166 Figures

Springer-Verlag
Berlin Heidelberg New York
London Paris Tokyo

Editor:
HANS K. UHTHOFF, M.D., FRCS (C)
Chairman and Professor
Division of Orthopaedic Surgery
University of Ottawa
Ottawa General Hospital
501 Smyth Road
Ottawa, Ontario K1H 8L6, Canada

Associate Editor:
ELVIRA STAHL, BA, FAAAS, FAMWA
2021 Atwater, Suite 1610
Montréal, Qué. H3H 2P2, Canada

ISBN-13:978-3-642-70711-7 e-ISBN-13:978-3-642-70709-4
DOI: 10.1007/978-3-642-70709-4

Library of Congress Cataloging-in-Publication Data. Current concepts of bone fragility. Proceeding of the 12th Applied Basic Science Course, held in Ottawa, Ont., in 1985. Includes index. 1. Bones – Diseases – Congresses. 2. Osteoporosis – Congresses. I. Uhthoff, Hans K., 1925– . II. Stahl, Elvira. III. Applied Basic Science Course (12th : 1985 : Ottawa, Ont.) [DNLM: 1. Bone Diseases – congresses. WE 225 C976 1985]
RC930.C87 1986 616.7'16 86-13120

Softcover reprint of the hardcover 1st edition 1986

2124/3130-543210

Preface

"Physicians have always known, though often they are reluctant to admit it, that the quality of their daily practice depends on the results of research."

Irvine H. Page *

The 1985 Applied Basic Science Course distinguished itself for three important reasons. First, it showed clearly the extent to which biotechnology and biomechanics have become an integral part of orthopedics.

Second, it emphasized the increasingly important role the orthopedist will have to play in the treatment of the aging population. Projected Canadian statistics estimate that the population aged 65 years and older will increase from the current 9.7% to 13% by the year 2000. Based on the current total population of almost 25 million, the number of hip fractures caused by age-related bone loss will almost double and will reach approximately 28,000 per year in Canada. Extrapolation of these figures according to populations in other countries is easy. The costs in expenditures and human suffering are inestimable. This is an area where orthopedic research will have to redouble its efforts in the hope of finding better preventive measures. Furthermore, knowledge of the pathogenetic mechanisms of bone loss becomes increasingly important in osteoporosis associated with weightlessness.

The third impressive insight we derived from the presentations at this symposium was the revelations of the latest imaging techniques and monitoring devices. Nuclear medicine, computer assisted tomography, and nuclear-magnetic resonance are being applied to bone disease. Moreover, bone-specific biochemical markers and quantitative assessments of bone mass and turnover are elucidating many events that we had formerly based on empirical presumptions. Biomathematics, biomechanics and kinetic studies can now demonstrate to us precisely the cellular mechanism underlying bone structure, the dynamic turnover of bone, and adaptation of bone structure to function. The origins of malfunctions, metabolic deficiencies and ensuing deformation, disease and pain are becoming much clearer to us. No doubt, our therapeutic management can in future be based on much firmer grounds.

Bone is often compared to structural steel and reinforced concrete. Like architecture, we are experimenting and already using an even wider selection of materials for repair and replacement of bones and joints. We should never forget, however, that bone, unlike reinforced concrete, is a living material which responds to every action by a reaction.

Clinically, we've learned a great deal during this conference about how varied are the metabolic bone diseases that cause the osteoporoses and osteopenias. Whether disordered bone tissue synthesis or imbalanced metabolic processes of bone formation and resorption, the result is loss of bone mass, skeletal rarefaction and frequent fractures. No doubt, the longer man's life-span the more his musculoskeletal parts will become used up long before his death.

Fortunately, new diagnostics have cleared up many confusing assumptions and debates about the osteoporoses and their management. Black holes remain, however, and need further intensive exploring.

Finally, this symposium has not only focused on the great strides we have made in clinical and scientific orthopedics, but it has sought to bridge and to blend scientific and clinical experience instead of each going its own way.

I should like to express my gratitude to Dr. Z.F.G. Jaworski who worked untiringly to organize this meeting and to monitor the program. I also thank my associate editor and her team and, above all Dr. Götze, Mrs. Kalow, and the production staff of the Springer Verlag in Heidelberg for their invaluable cooperation in the publication of these Proceedings.

Hans K. Uhthoff
University of Ottawa
Ottawa, Canada

* Medical Research as I See It.
JAMA 194:13, 1965.

Table of Contents

Skeleton as an Organ of Physical Support

Diagnostic and Monitoring Tools

Loads versus Bone Strength

Disorganized Bone Structure

Reversible Osteopenias

Osteoporosis

List of Contributors

ADLER, C.-P.	Institute of Pathology, University of Freiburg, Albertstr. 19, D-7800 Freiburg, West Germany
ANDERSON, C.	4034 Health Sciences Centre, University of Western Ontario, London, Ontario N6A 5C1, Canada
BAYLINK, D.J.	Department of Medicine, Loma Linda University, Loma Linda, CA 92357, USA
BIRCH, J.G.	Division of Orthopedics, University of Texas Health Science Center of Dallas, 5323 Harry Hines Blvd., Dallas, Texas 75235, USA
BRUNET, J.A.	Division of Orthopedic Surgery, University of Ottawa, Ottawa, Ontario, Canada
BURR, D.B.	Departments of Anatomy and Orthopedic Surgery, West Virginia University Medical Center, Morgantown, WV 26506, USA
CORKAL, J.	Department of Surgery, University of Ottawa, Ottawa, Ontario, Canada
D'ASTOUS, J.	Children's Hospital of Eastern Ontario, 401 Smyth Road, Ottawa, Ontario K1H 8L1, Canada
DHEM, A.	Human Anatomy Research Unit, Faculty of Medicine, University of Louvain, Tour Vesale 5240, Avenue E. Mounier, 52, B-1200 Brussels, Belgium
ENKER, I.P.	Department of Orthopedic Surgery, Sir Mortimer B. Davis-Jewish General Hospital, 3755 Côte Ste. Catherine Road, Montréal, Québec H3T 1E2, Canada
FINNEGAN, M.	Division of Orthopedic Surgery, University of Ottawa, Ottawa General Hospital, 501 Smyth Road, Ottawa, Ontario K1H 8L6, Canada
FRANKLIN, N.	Department of Orthopedic Surgery, West Virginia University Medical Center, Morgantown, WV 26506, USA

FROST, H.M.	Southern Colorado Clinic, 2002 Lake Ave., Pueblo, CO 81004, USA
HADJIPAVLOU, A.G.	Department of Orthopedic Surgery, Sir Mortimer B. Davis-Jewish General Hospital, 3755 Côte Ste. Catherine Road, Montréal, Québec H3T 1E2, Canada
HANGARTNER, T.N.	Department of Applied Sciences in Medicine, University of Alberta, 10-102 Clinical Sciences Building, Edmonton, Alberta T6G 2G3, Canada
HAYES, W.C.	Department of Orthopedic Surgery, Charles A. Dana Research Institute, Beth Israel Hospital and Harvard Medical School, Boston, MA 02215, USA
HEALEY, J.H.	Division of Orthopedic Surgery, Memorial Sloan-Kettering Cancer Center, New York, NY 10021, USA
JAWORSKI, Z.F.G.	Department of Medicine, University of Ottawa, Ottawa General Hospital, 501 Smyth Road, Ottawa, Ontario K1H 8L6, Canada
JOHNSTON, C.C., Jr.	Indiana University School of Medicine, Indianapolis, Indiana 46223, USA
KAYE, M.	Division of Nephrology, Montreal General Hospital, 1650 Cedar Avenue, Montréal, Québec H3G 1A4 Canada
KRÖPELIN, T.	Institut für Röntgendiagnostik, Universitätsklinik, Hugstetterstrasse 55, D-7800 Freiburg, West Germany
LANDER, P.H.	Department of Orthopedic Surgery, Sir Mortimer B. Davis-Jewish General Hospital, 3755 Côte Ste. Catherine Road, Montréal, Québec H3T 1E2, Canada
LANE, J.M.	Division of Orthopedic Surgery, Memorial Sloan-Kettering Cancer Center, New York, NY 10021, USA
LANYON, L.E.	Department of Anatomy, Royal Veterinary College, Royal College Street, London NW1 0TU, England
LEFEVER, S.	Department of Orthopedic Surgery, West Virginia University Medical Center, Morgantown, WV 26506, USA
MANN, K.G.	Department of Biochemistry, University of Vermont, School of Medicine, Burlington, Vermont 05405, USA
MARTIN, R.B.	Department of Orthopedic Surgery, University of California, Davis, CA 92093, USA

McINTYRE, W.M.	Division of Orthopedic Surgery, University of Ottawa, Children's Hospital of Eastern Ontario, 401 Smyth Road, Ottawa, Ontario K1H 8L1, Canada
MELTON, L.J., III	Department of Medical Statistics and Epidemiology, Mayo Clinic, Rochester, MN 55905, USA
MURNAGHAN, J.P.	Division of Orthopedic Surgery, University of Ottawa, Department of Surgery, Ottawa Civic Hospital, 1053 Carling Avenue, Ottawa, Ontario K1Y 4E9, Canada
NAROD, S.	Department of Epidemiology and Community Medicine, University of Ottawa, Health Sciences Building, 451 Smyth Road, Ottawa, Ontario K1H 8M5, Canada
ODVINA, C.V.	Department of Medicine, Loma Linda University, Jerry L. Pettis Memorial VA Hospital, 11201 Benton Street, Loma Linda, CA 92357, USA
PARFITT, A.M.	Bone and Mineral Research Laboratory, Henry Ford Hospital, Detroit, MI 48202, USA
REINBOLD, W.D.	Institute für Röntgendiagnostik, Universitätsklinik, Hugstetterstrasse 55, D-7800 Freiburg, West Germany
RICHTER, G.	Institute für Röntgendiagnostik, Universitätsklinik, Hugstetterstrasse 55, D-7800 Freiburg, West Germany
RIGGS, B.L.	Division of Endocrinology, Department of Internal Medicine, Mayo Clinic and Mayo Foundation, Rochester, MN 55905, USA
ROBERT, V.	Human Anatomy Research Unit, Faculty of Medicine, University of Louvain, Tour Vesale 5240, Avenue E. Mounier, 52, B-1200 Brussels, Belgium.
ROSENTHALL, L.	Department of Radiology, McGill University, Division of Nuclear Medicine, Montreal General Hospital, 1650 Cedar Avenue, Montréal, Québec H3G 1A4, Canada
ROWE, D.W.	Department of Pediatrics, University of Connecticut Health, Farmington, Conn. 06032, USA
RUFF, C.B.	Department of Cell Biology and Anatomy, Johns Hopkins University School of Medicine, 225 North Wolfe Street, Baltimore, MD 21205, USA
SHAPIRO, J.R.	Department of Medicine, Tufts University, New England Medical Center, Boston, MA 02111, USA

SOLOMON, L.	Department of Orthopedic Surgery, University of the Witwatersrand, Johannesburg 2193, South Africa
SPASOFF, R.A.	Department of Epidemiology and Community Medicine, University of Ottawa, Health Sciences Building, 451 Smyth Road, Ottawa, Ontario K1H 8M5, Canada
THOMPSON, G.	Department of Orthopedic Surgery, West Virginia University Medical Center, Morgantown, WV 26506, USA
UHTHOFF, H.K.	Division of Orthopedic Surgery, University of Ottawa, Ottawa General Hospital, 501 Smyth Road, Ottawa, Ontario K1H 8L6, Canada
VIGORITA, V.J.	Department of Pathology, Lutheran Hospital, Hospital for Special Surgery, New York, NY 10021, USA
WENZ, W.	Institut für Röntgendiagnostik, Universitätsklinik, Hugstetterstrasse 55, D-7800 Freiburg, West Germany
WERGEDAL, J.E.	Department of Medicine, Loma Linda University, Loma Linda, CA 92357, USA
WERNTZ, J.R.	Metabolic Bone Disease Service, Hospital for Special Surgery, New York, NY 10021, USA
WILEY, J.J.	Division of Orthopedic Surgery, University of Ottawa, Children's Hospital of Eastern Ontario, 401 Smyth Road, Ottawa, Ontario K1H 8L1, Canada
WIMMER, B.	Institut für Röntgendiagnostik, Universitätsklinik, Hugstetterstrasse 55, D-7800 Freiburg, West Germany

IN MEMORIAM

We dedicate this volume to the memory of Professor H. I. Chu (1903 - 1984), Honorary President of Tianjin Medical College, People's Republic of China, and a pioneer in the field of metabolic bone diseases.

Skeleton as an Organ of Physical Support

Basic Biomechanics of the Skeleton

W. C. HAYES

Introduction

Bone is unique among structural materials in that it is self-repairing and can alter its properties and configuration in response to changes in mechanical demand (Hayes, 1979; Hayes and Snyder, 1981; Jowsey, 1977; Lane and Vigorita, 1983; Woo et al, 1981). Certain skeletal conditions such as osteoporosis can seriously compromise the structural integrity of the skeleton (Avioli, 1983; Jowsey, 1977). The associated reduction in bone mass gradually increases vulnerability to fracture, particularly of the femoral neck and vertebrae (Jowsey, 1977; Kelsey et al, 1978; Lane and Vigorita, 1983). The frequency of osteoporosis in the United States is well recognized, with 50% of women 45 years of age or older exhibiting radiographic evidence of osteoporosis of the lumbar spine (Kelsey et al, 1978). From 16-18 million women in the United States have a significant degree of vertebral atrophy and over 4 million women aged 50 years or older have osteoporosis severe enough to cause vertebral fractures. Epidemiologic studies suggest that from 15-30% of all white women in the United States develop symptomatic osteoporosis (Kelsey et al, 1978; Lane and Vigorita, 1983). Of approximately one million fractures experienced each year by women 45 years or older in the United States, about 700,000 are incurred by women with osteoporosis.

Noninvasive techniques (Cohn, 1981; Dequeker and Johnston, 1982; Mazess, 1983a; 1983b) for the identification of bone loss include the use of radiographic features such as the Singh index of femoral trabecular pattern (Singh et al, 1972). Such indices appear useful in identifying osteoporosis in general populations but correlate only moderately with bone density and fracture incidence. Radiographic morphometry (Meema and Meema, 1981) and radiographic photodensitometry (Colbert and Bachtell, 1981) both use quantitative measures of standardized skeletal sites. Their interpretation, however, may depend on bone geometric features which change with age (Ruff and Hayes, 1982; 1983a; 1983b) and for which population norms are not available. Single and dual-energy photon absorptiometry (Mazess, 1983a; Mazess et al, 1981a; 1981b; Peppler and Mazess, 1981) is currently widely used since it is both accurate and highly reproducible. However, the degree of correlation with osteoporosis depends on the anatomic site. Interpretation of the results must be made with care due to a sensitivity to changes in cross-sectional geometry. Other noninvasive techniques using radionuclide uptake, Compton scattering, and neutron activation are still considered experimental or are not widely available. Computerized tomography (CT) for diagnostic imaging provides a new method for the assessment of skeletal mineral with a

Current Concepts of Bone Fragility

number of advantages over other available techniques (Bradley et al, 1978; Genant and Boyd, 1977; Genant et al, 1981; Posner and Griffiths, 1977; Reich et al, 1976; Ruegsegger et al, 1976; 1984). These include: 1) display of cross-sectional geometry with separation of trabecular and cortical bone; and 2) determination (in the dual energy mode) of bone mineral in the presence of unknown fat and soft tissue content.

Osteoporosis is clearly a serious national health problem which can be expected to increase along with the average age of the population. Despite advances in understanding its pathophysiology and major efforts to develop improved diagnostic tools, the identification of individual patients exhibiting increased fracture risk remains an illusive goal. In fact, in many clinical settings, the occurrence of spontaneous vertebral fractures provides the only conclusive evidence of disease. Although such fractures are the major clinical sequelae of osteoporosis, the biomechanics of osteoporotic bone have received little attention, Thus, the structural consequences of known levels of bone loss are not well quantified.

Some background material on basic mechanical concepts can be used to describe the mechanical behavior of bone as a material and of bones as structures. No attempt is made to be comprehensive but to focus on a few simple loading cases which illustrate the required concepts.

Basic Concepts

Material vs structural behavior

When forces are applied to any solid object, the object will be deformed from its original dimensions. At the same time, internal forces will be produced within the object. The deformations created at any point are referred to as the strains at that point. The internal force intensities (force/area) are referred to as the stresses at that point. When a bone is subjected to forces, these stresses and strains are introduced throughout the structure and can vary in a complex manner. To avoid some of these complexities and demonstrate some important mechanical concepts, it is use-

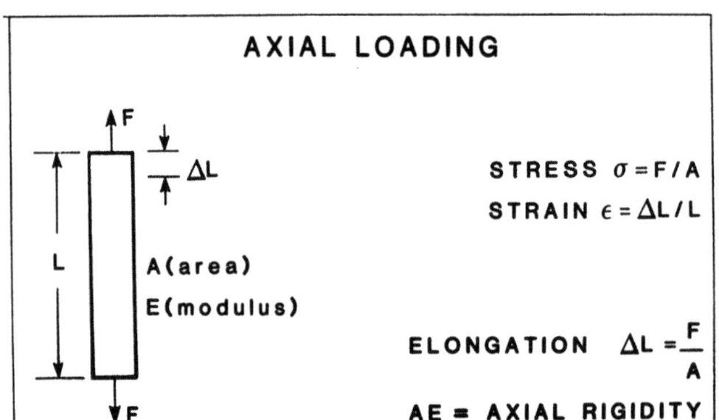

Fig. 1. Tensile loading of a cylindrical rod of uniform cross-sectional geometry. The elongation is inversely proportional to the axial rigidity, AE.

ful to focus on a regular structure loaded under well-defined conditions (Fig. 1). Similar specimens of regular geometry are used to determine the material properties of bone tissue. In Figure 1, a cylindrical bar of length L and a constant cross-sectional area (A) is shown subjected to pure tensile loading (F). As load is applied, the cylinder begins to stretch. The elongation of the cylinder is given by $L = FL/AE$ (1), where (L) is the elongation of the cylinder, L is the original unstretched length, A is the cross-sectional area, F is the force, and E is the stiffness (or modulus) of the material. From the simple relationship shown in (2), the elongation (L) is directly proportional to the applied force and to the original length and inversely proportional to the cross-sectional area and to the modulus of the material. Note particularly the combination of a geometric parameter (area, A) and a material parameter (modulus, E) in the denominator of this relationship. The combination AE occurs frequently and is referred to as the axial rigidity. Note also from Figure 1 that the total elongation depends both on the original length and on the cross-sectional area of the bar.

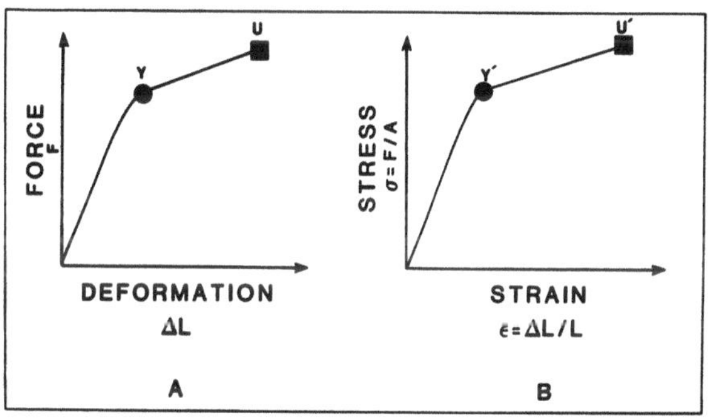

Fig. 2. Material versus structual behavior: a) a force-deformation curve describes structural behavior since it reflects both geometric characteristics and material properties; b) a stress-strain curve describes material behavior since the influences of geometric characteristics have been eliminated by normalizing for the cross-sectional area and the original length.

We can plot a force-deformation curve to represent the structural behavior of the cylindrical bar (Fig. 2A). A cylinder of bone tested in tension would yield a linear region (also known as the elastic region) from O-Y. At Y, yielding occurs and there is an internal rearrangement of the structure, often involving damage accumulation (Reilly and Burstein, 1974; Reilly et al, 1974). In the region Y-U, nonelastic deformation occurs until finally, at U, fracture results in the loss of load-bearing capacity of the bar. It is particularly important to note that a force-deformation curve expresses the mechanical behavior of the structure since the curve would differ for a cylindrical bar of a different cross-sectional area or different length (Eq. 2).

To provide a standardized representation of the mechanical behavior of the material (as opposed to the behavior of the structure), we plot a normalized curve known as a stress-strain curve (Fig. 2B). This normalizes the force-deformation relationship (ie, eliminates the influence of the geometry of the cylinder) by dividing the applied force (F) by the cross-sectional area (A) and the deformation (L) by the original length (L). We define this internal force intensity as stress. The units of stress are Newtons/m² or Pascals (Pa). (1 Newton = 0.225 pounds force; 1 Pa = 6895 psi). We often express stresses in terms of megapascals (MPa) (1 MPa = 1 x 10^6 Pa), or gigapascals (GPa)(1 GPa = 1 x 10^9 Pa).

The ratio of the elongation to the original length is defined as the strain. Note that strain is a nondimensional quantity. In a stress-strain curve (Fig. 2B), the slope of the linear elastic region is referred to as the modulus. Since the modulus is defined as the slope of the stress-strain curve in the elastic region and since the units of stress are MPa and strain is nondimensional, the units of modulus are the same as those of stress, MPa or GPa. In the stress-strain curve at Y´, the material yields at a stress level known as the yield strength (again with units of MPa). At U´ the material fractures at a stress level known as the fracture strength or ultimate tensile strength (units of MPa). Note that the stress-strain representation allows us to compare different materials, both in terms of the slope of the stress strain curve and these strength parameters. From such stress-strain curves, the modulus of steel is approximately 10 times that of cortical bone. The ultimate tensile strength of steel is approximately five times that of cortical bone.

Loading pattern in whole bones

Bones of the appendicular skeleton are long, slender, slightly curved elements which are loaded primarily by compressive forces applied at the joints. Because of this gentle curvature, bones are subjected to a combination of axial compressive forces and bending forces. It is therefore instructive to focus first on these two loading cases separately and then to examine how these load cases can combine to produce the general loading patterns of whole bones. We have already discussed the axial loading case for tension (Fig. 1). Compressive loading is analogous except that the deformation L is now a shortening of the bar. The magnitude of this shortening is still given by L = FL/AE with the associated compressive stress being given by F/A. By convention, compressive stresses are assumed negative, and tensile stresses are positive.

In engineering, long slender structures which are designed to resist transverse or bending loads are referred to as beams. Examples are the I-beams commonly used in civil engineering structures. Such beams are usually long in comparison to their cross-sectional dimensions and, for this reason, are similar to the long bones of the appendicular skeleton. A beam can be subjected to bending loads by applying two sets of forces near the beam ends (Fig. 3). To make this loading situation clearer, imagine grasping a yardstick near its ends in such a way that it is flexed into a bowed shape. The deflection of the midpoint of the beam is a relatively complex relationship involving the geometric characteristics of the beam and the location of the applied forces (as expressed by L and a), the magnitude of applied forces, the modulus of the beam material (ie, as above, its stiffness), and a new quantity known as the moment of inertia. This geometric parameter expresses the characteristics of the distribution of the beam cross-sectional area in relation to a transverse axis. It reflects, for instance, the large differences in bending resistance of the yardstick bent when it is held flat versus when it is held on edge.

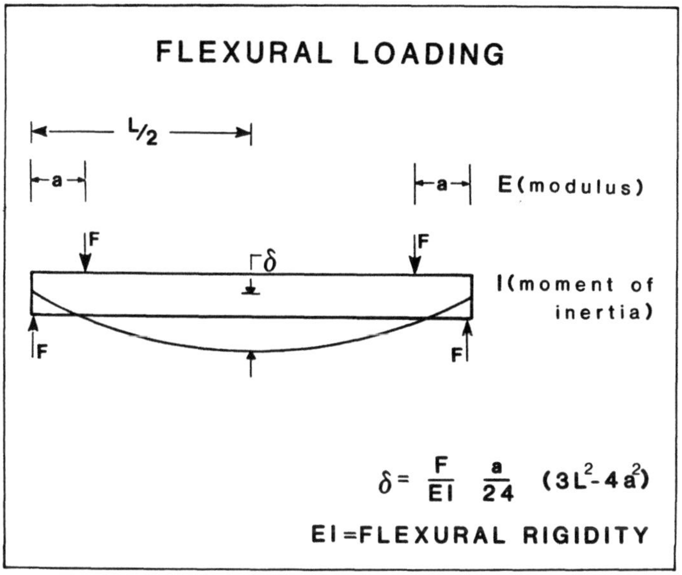

Fig. 3. Flexural (bending) loading of a beam. The mid-span deflection is inversely proportional to the flexural rigidity, EI.

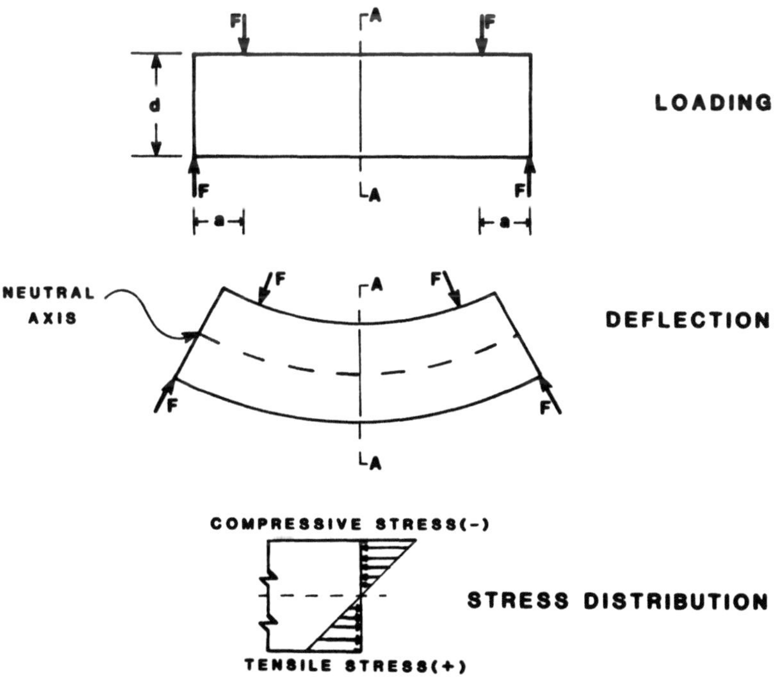

Fig. 4. Stresses associated with flexural loading of beams. Tensile stresses are generated on the convex surface and compressive stresses on the concave surface. The unstressed central region is referred to as the neutral axis.

There are similarities between the expressions used to characterize axial loading and flexural loadings (Fig. 1, 3). In both cases, the deformations are directly proportional to the applied forces and to certain geometric features of the structure. In both cases, the deformations are inversely proportional to a combination of parameters reflecting material stiffness E and a geometric feature of the cross section. In axial loading, we called this combination AE, the axial rigidity. In bending (or flexure) we call this combination EI, the flexural ridigity.

To visualize the internal forces or stresses which occur in a beam, imagine holding the ends of the yardstick and bending it so as to produce a convex surface on one side and a concave surface on the other side. It can be shown that the material on the convex side of the beam is subjected to tensile (or stretching) strains. The material on the concave side will be subjected to compressive strains. This suggests that at some point between the two surfaces, the strains are zero (ie, the original length of the beam is unchanged). This location is referred to as the neutral axis. The strains produced at any cross section of the beam also result in stresses at that cross section. The concave side of the beam is subjected to compressive stresses while the convex side experiences tensile stresses (Fig. 4). It should be noted that the maximum stresses are experienced by the material on the surface of the beam. If the bending forces are increased until the

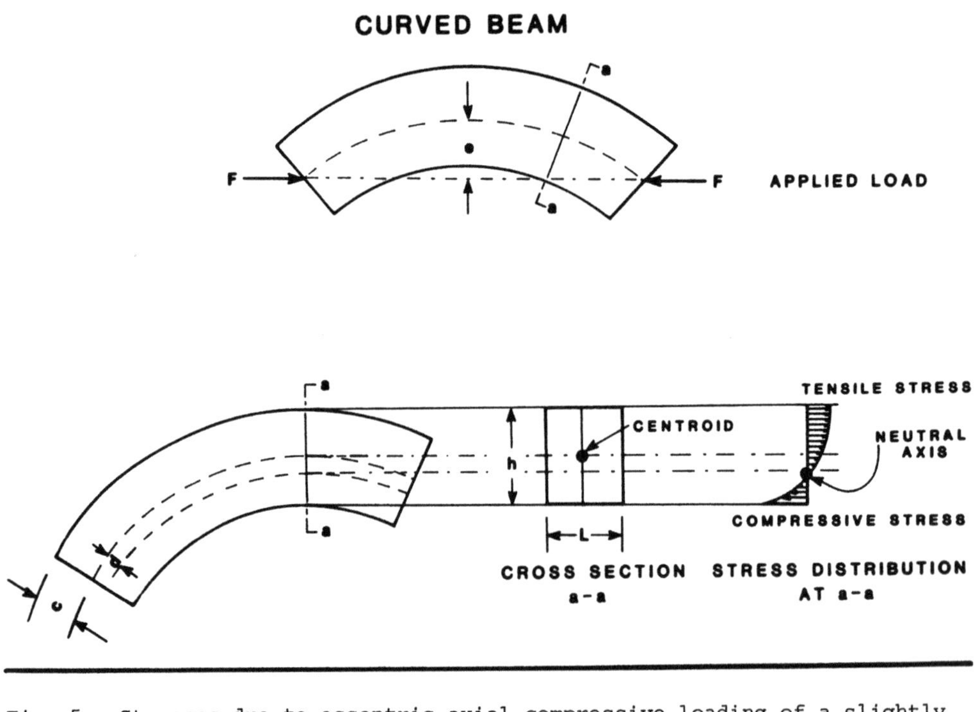

Fig. 5. Stresses due to eccentric axial compressive loading of a slightly curved beam. Due to the eccentricity of the applied load, stresses due to axial compression and bending are combined, resulting in reduced tensile stresses on the convex surface and increased compressive stresses on the concave surface.

bar begins to fracture, the fracture will be initiated at the surface of the beam where the stresses are highest.

Since bones are slightly curved and are subjected to compressive loads applied at the joint surfaces, the most common loading situation *in vivo* is a combination of compressive and bending loads. The resulting stresses on a transverse section through a slightly curved member can be found by summing the stresses caused by the compressive axial forces and by the bending stresses (Fig. 5). As a result of the addition of the compressive stresses from axial loading and the compressive stresses from bending, even higher compressive stresses will be created on the concave side of the bar, while the convex side will experience either reduced compressive stresses or even tensile stresses, depending on the magnitude of the axial force and its eccentricity. These stresses can be described with reasonable accuracy by simply combining the stresses due to axial compression with those from bending:

(combined stress) = (compressive stress) ± (bending stress)

The compressive stresses from axial loading and bending are of the same sign (additive) while the two contributions to stresses on the tensile surface are of opposite sign (Fig. 5). Similar situations occur in long bones and, in general, compressive stresses are higher than the tensile stresses throughout the appendicular skeleton.

Geometric features of long bones

The above discussion of loading patterns suggests that several aspects of bone cross-sectional geometry are important to the structural behavior of whole bones. These include the cross-sectional area A and the moment of inertia, I. The area, of course, reflects the size of the bone cross section. Subjected to axial compressive loads, a large bone is more resistant to fracture (Eq. 1) simply because it distributes the internal forces over a larger surface area (resulting in lower stresses).

The moment of inertia expresses the shape of the cross section and the particular distribution of the cross-sectional area with respect to the applied bending loads. This last statement is important because it suggests that the moment of inertia must always be expressed with relation to a particular axis. Expressions for the moments of inertia for several regular geometric cross sections (calculated with respect to a transverse axis through the centroid or center of the area) are shown in Figure 6. Methods for calculating moments of inertia can be found in any calculus text. The moment of inertia is highly sensitive to the distribution of area with respect to the axis. Area that is at a greater distance from the neutral axis (ie, the unstretched axis of the beam) is much more efficient in resisting bending with respect to that axis. These concepts demonstrate why a yardstick turned on edge is more efficient in resisting bending than a yardstick turned horizontally. This also explains why an I-beam (Fig. 6) is such an efficient section for resisting bending in one direction since most of the material is located at distance from the neutral axis.

If bones were subjected to bending loads in only one direction, their cross-sectional shapes would probably have evolved toward something like an I-beam. Instead, long bones are loaded, as suggested above, by axial compression, bending (in multiple directions), and torsion. Under these conditions, the most efficient cross-sectional shape is the cylindrical tube. A tubular

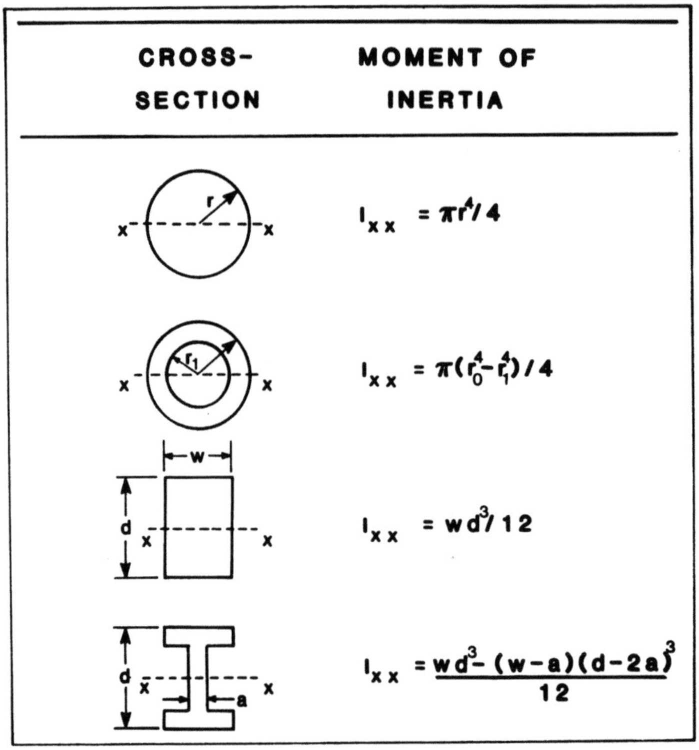

Fig. 6. Moments of inertia for some common structured cross sections.

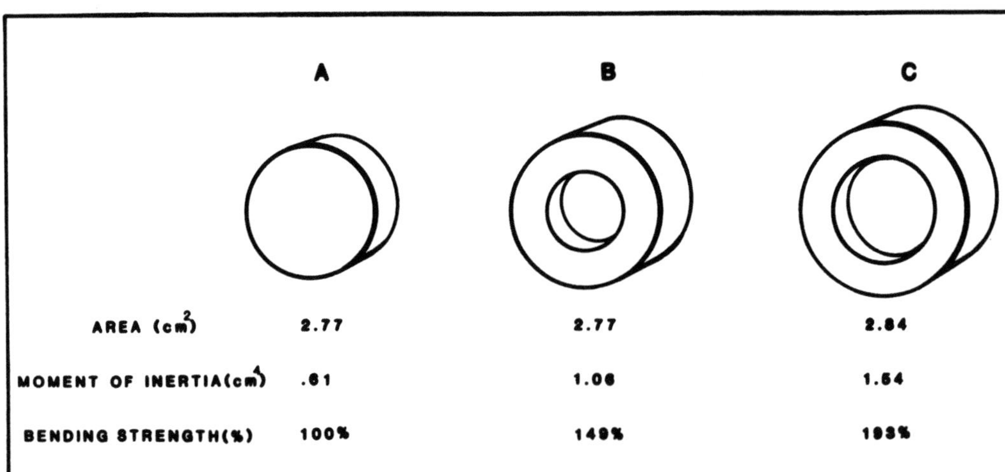

Fig. 7. Effects of change in distribution of cross-sectional area on the area, moments of inertia and bending strength of some regular cylindrical geometries. These idealized geometries reflect the approximate dimensions of the femoral midshaft in the Pecos Pueblo population (Ruff and Hayes, 1983a). The changes between B and C are thus comparable to the geometric remodeling that occurred with aging in that population.

structure can better distribute the stresses imposed by bending and torsional loading than can a solid bar of the same cross-sectional area since the material is distributed at a greater distance from the central axis. Figure 7 shows three cylindrical rods of different cross-sectional geometries. Bar A is a solid cylinder and has a radius of 0.94 cm. Bar B is a hollow tube of outer radius 1.09 cm and inner radius 0.53 cm. The areas of A and B are approximately the same. Bar C is again a hollow tube, but in this instance both the outer radius and the inner radius have been increased by 1.25 cm and 0.76 cm, respectively. The values for the cross-sectional areas and moments of inertia of these simple shapes are also shown in Figure 7. Since the tensile or compressive strengths are inversely proportional to the cross-sectional area (= - F/A), bars A and B exhibit similar strengths and bar C is increased in strength by about 3%. In bending loading, however, the more favorable distribution of the cross-sectional area results in increases in bending strengths by factors of 1.49 and 1.93 for bars B and C. In particular, the changes in inner and outer radii for tube C in comparison to B results in an increase in bending strength by a factor of about 1.29. These idealized cross-sectional geometries are based on the approximate dimensions of the human femoral midshaft in an archeologic sample (Ruff and Hayes, 1982; 1983a; 1983b) and approximately reflect the change in cross-sectional properties with age in that sample.

Obviously, bone cross-sectional geometries are not as regular as the simple geometric shapes discussed above. To calculate the geometric parameters needed to specify the structural behavior of whole bones and to provide increased precision in describing the effects of age, gender, cultural effects, and exercise, we have developed computer software which provides automated calculation of all the necessary geometric parameters (Nagurka and Hayes, 1980). The method requires that periosteal and endosteal boundaries of the cross section be traced on a digitizer and then provides values for area, centroid location and the moments of inertia. These methods have been used to characterize bone geometry changes with age in both modern and archeologic populations (Ruff and Hayes, 1982; 1983a; 1983b). The results are discussed below.

Mechanical Properties of Bone Tissue

Material properties of cortical bone

The fracture behavior of whole bones is strongly dependent on the material behavior of the bone tissues. To determine the mechanical properties of bone tissue we test small, uniform specimens which are loaded under well-defined conditions. Such testing conditions produce uniform, known stresses throughout the specimen (Fig. 1). Specimen deformation can then be measured and the strains calculated using the relationships we have described. The material properties of the tissue can thus be determined for the specific loading conditions imposed. This general approach to materials testing has allowed documentation of cortical bone material properties in tension, compression, bending, and torsion (Burstein et al, 1972a; 1972b; 1975; 1976; Evans, 1957; 1973; Hayes, 1978; Hayes and Carter, 1979; Reilly and Burstein, 1974; Reilly et al, 1974; Wright, 1980; Wright and Hayes, 1976).

Several factors influence the material properties of cortical bone. The properties are dependent on the rate at which the bone tissue is loaded. A specimen of cortical bone that is rapidly subjected to forces will have a greater elastic modulus and ultimate strength than bone tissue that is loaded more slowly. Materials such as bone whose stress-strain characteristics and strength properties are dependent on the applied strain rate are said to be viscoelastic (or time-dependent materials). However, this rate dependency is relatively weak (Wright and Hayes, 1976). The elastic modulus and ultimate strength of bone are approximately proportional to the strain rate raised to the 0.06 power. Thus, over a wide range of strain rates, the ultimate tensile strength increases by a factor of three and the modulus increases by about a factor of two.

The stress-strain behavior of cortical bone is also strongly dependent on the orientation of the bone microstructure with respect to the direction of loading. Several investigators have demonstrated that cortical bone is stronger and stiffer in the longitudinal direction (direction of osteon orientation) than in the transverse direction. In addition, bone specimens loaded in a direction perpendicular to the osteons tend to fail in a more brittle manner, with little nonelastic deformation after yielding. Long bones are therefore better able to resist stresses along the axis of the bone than across the bone axis. Material such as bone whose elastic and strength properties are dependent on the direction of applied loading are said to be anisotropic materials. The viscoelastic, anisotropic nature of cortical bone distinguishes it as a complex material. Because of these characteristics, one must specify the strain rate and the direction of applied loading when describing material behavior.

Table I. Strength of femoral cortical bone*

Loading mode	Ultimate strength (MPa)
Longitudinal	
Tension	133
Compression	193
Shear	68
Transverse	
Tension	51
Compression	133

* Mean values from Reilly and Burstein (1974).
Age span of population: 19-80 years.

Ultimate strengths of adult femoral cortical bone under various modes of loading in both longitudinal and transverse directions (Carter and Spengler, 1978; Reilly and Burstein, 1974; Reilly et al, 1974) are summarized in Table I. These results indicate that the material strength of bone tissue is dependent on the type of loading as well as on the loading direction. The compressive strength is greater than the tensile strength in both longitudinal and transverse directions. Transverse specimens are weaker than longitudinal specimens in both tension and compression. The shear properties (determined by torsion tests about the longitudinal axis and reflecting shear stresses along transverse and longitudinal planes) are about one-third of the compressive strength. The modulus values for adult femoral cortical bone are shown in Table II (Carter and Spengler, 1978; Reilly and Burstein,

Table II. Modulus of femoral cortical bone*

Longitudinal	17.0 GPa
Transverse	11.5 GPa
Shear	3.3 GPa

* Mean values from Reilly and Burstein (1974).
Age span of population: 19-80 years.
1 GPa (gigapascal) = 1000 MPa

1974; Reilly et al, 1974). The longitudinal elastic modulus is approximately 50% greater than the transverse elastic modulus. The shear modulus for torsion about the longitudinal axis is about one-fifth the longitudinal modulus.

The material properties of cortical bone also decline with age (Burstein et al, 1976). Both tensile strength (Fig. 8) and modulus (Fig. 9) decrease about 2% per decade over the age range 20-90. Thus, the ultimate tensile strength declines from 140 MPa in the third decade to 120 MPa in the ninth decade. Over the same period, the elastic modulus decreases from 17 GPa to 15.6 GPa (Burstein et al, 1976).

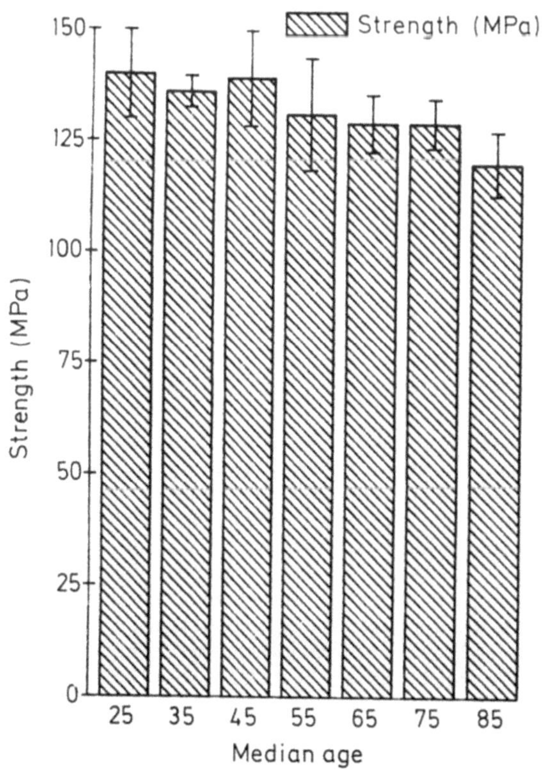

Fig. 8. Ultimate tensile strength versus age for human femoral cortical bone.

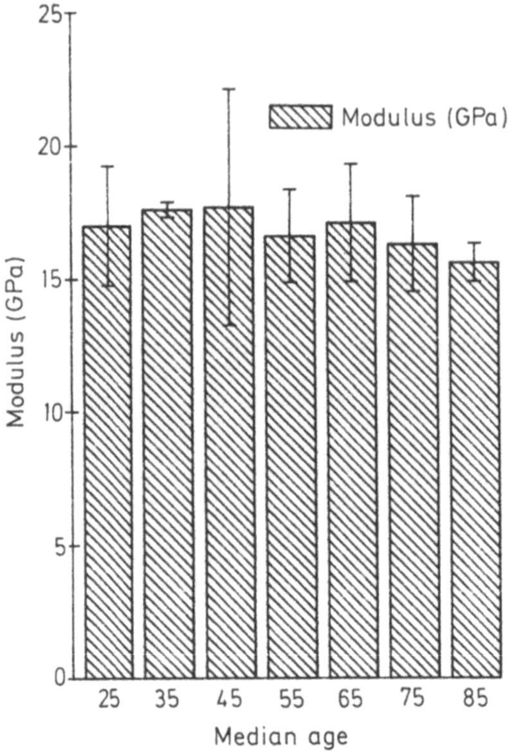

Fig. 9. Elastic modulus versus age for human femoral cortical bone.

Material properties of trabecular bone

The major physical difference between trabecular bone and cortical bone is the higher degree of porosity of trabecular bone. This porosity is reflected by measuring the apparent density (ie, the mass of bone tissue divided by the bulk volume of the test specimen, including mineralized bone and bone marrow spaces). In the human skeleton, the apparent density of trabecular bone ranges from approximately 0.1 g/cm^3 to 1.0 g/cm^3. The apparent density of cortical bone is about 1.8 g/cm^3. A specimen with an apparent density of 0.2 g/cm^3 has a porosity of approximately 90%.

Both the compressive strength and the compressive modulus of trabecular bone are markedly influenced by the apparent density of the tissue (Fig. 10). The data presented here include cortical bone with an apparent density of approximately 1.8 g/cm^3 as well as trabecular bone specimens representing a wide range of apparent densities. These relationships indicate that the compressive strength of all bone tissue in the skeleton is approximately proportional to the square of the apparent density (Carter and Hayes, 1976; 1977). The elastic modulus of all bone tissue is approximately proportional to the cube of the apparent density. Although these relationships were initially derived from compression tests, tensile tests of trabecular bone indicate that its strength in tension is approximately the same as that in compression (Carter et al, 1980). In addition, the elastic modulus of trabecular bone is approximately the same in both tensile and compressive loading.

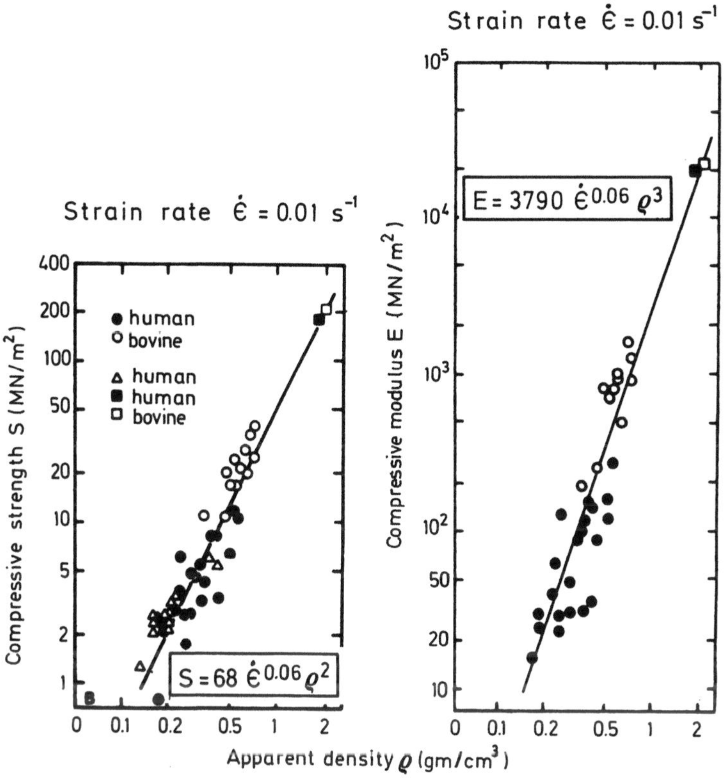

Fig. 10. Influence of apparent density on the compressive strength and modulus of trabecular bone. Filled circles represent human trabecular bone tested in compression. Empty circles and empty triangles represent bovine and human trabecular specimens tested in compression at strains of 0.01 and 0.1/sec, respectively. Filled and empty squares represent human and bovine compact bone, respectively.

These relationships between mechanical properties and the apparent density of bone tissue are of profound physiologic and biomechanical importance. First, they indicate that bone tissue can generate large changes in modulus and strength through small changes in bone apparent density. Conversely, subtle changes in bone apparent density result in large differences in strength and modulus. This is a sobering thought if we recall that bone density changes are usually not evident radiographically until the bone density has been reduced by 30-50%. The power-law relationships shown in Figure 10 indicate that such reductions in bone density result in nearly an order of magnitude reduction in bone stiffness and strength.

Summary

When the skeleton is exposed to trauma, regions of the skeleton are subjected to high forces. Fracture occurs when the local stresses exceed the ultimate strength of the bone in that region. Bone fracture can therefore be viewed as an event which is initiated at the material level and then effects the load-bearing capacity of the bone at the structural level. As indicated previously, the major difference between behavior at the material level and at the structural level relate to the inclusion of geometric features at the structural level and their exclusion at the material level. Thus, structural behavior includes both the effects of bone geometry and material properties, whereas material behavior basically eliminates the effects of complex bone geometries by testing specimens of simplified geometry. Any attempt to predict the structural behavior of a skeletal region must therefore reflect both the heterogeneous material properties of the region and the complex geometric arrangement of each type of bone.

References

1. Avioli, L.V.: The Osteoporotic Syndrome: Detection, Prevention, and Treatment. Grune and Stratton, New York, 1983.
2. Bradley, J.G., Huang, H.K., and Ledley, R.S.: Evaluation of calcium in bones from CT scans. Radiology 128, 103, 1978.
3. Burstein, A.H., Currey, J.D., Frankel, V.H., and Reilly, D.T.: The ultimate properties of bone tissue: the effects of yielding. J. Biomech. 5, 35, 1972a).
4. Burstein, A.H., Currey, J., Frankel, V.H., Heiple, K.G., Linseth, P., Vessely, J.C.: Bone strength: the effect of screw holes. J. Bone Joint Surg. 54A, 1143, 1972b.
5. Burstein, A.H., Zika, J.M., Heiple, K.G., and Klein, L.: Contribution of collagen and mineral to the elastic-plastic properties of bone. J. Bone Joint Surg. 57, 956, 1975.
6. Burstein, A.H., Reilly, D.T., and Martens, M.: Aging of bone tissue: mechanical properties. J. Bone Joint Surg. 58A, 82, 1976.
7. Carter, D.R. and Hayes, W.C.: Bone compressive strength: the influence of density and strain rate. Science 194, 1174, 1976.
8. Carter, D.R. and Hayes, W.C.: The compressive behavior of bone as a two-phase porous material. J. Bone Joint Surg. 49A, 954, 1977.
9. Carter, D.R. and Spengler, D.M.: Mechanical properties and composition of cortical bone. Clin. Orthop. 135, 192, 1978.
10. Carter, D.R., Schwab, G.H., and Spengler, D.M.: Tensile fracture of cancellous bone. Acta Orthop. Scand. 51, 733, 1980.
11. Cohn, S.H.: Non-Invasive Measurements of Bone Mass and Their Clinical Application. CRC Press, Boca Raton, FL, 1981.
12. Colbert, C. and Bachtell, R.S.: Radiographic absorptiometry (photodensitometry). In, Non-Invasive Measurements of Bone Mass and Their Clinical Application. Ed: Cohn, S.H., CRC Press, Boca Raton, FL, 1981, pp 51-84.
13. Dequeker, J. and Johnston, C.C., Jr.: In, Non-Invasive Measurements: Histological Problems. Radiogrammetry, Single and Dual Photon Absorptiometry, Neutron Activation and C.T. Densitometry. IRL Press, Washington, D.C., 1982.
14. Evans, F.G.: Stress and Strain in Bones. Chas.C. Thomas, Co., Springfield, IL, 1957.

15. Evans, F.G.: Mechanical Properties of Bone. Chas. C. Thomas Co., Springfield, IL., 1973.

16. Genant, H.K. and Boyd, D.: Quantitative bone mineral analysis using dual energy computed tomography. Invest. Radiol. 12, 545, 1977.

17. Genant, H.K., Boyd, D., Rosenfeld, D., Abols, Y., and Cann, C.E.: Computed tomography. In, Non-Invasive Measurements of Bone Mass and Their Clinical Application. Ed: Cohn, S.H., CRC Press, Boca Raton, FL., 1981. pp 121-149.

18. Hayes, W.C.: Biomechanical measurements of bone. In, CRC Handbook of Engineering in Medicine and Biology: Section B. Instruments and Measurements. Vol. 1. Eds: Burstein, A., Bahniuk, E., CRC Press, Cleveland, OH, 1978. pp 333-372.

19. Hayes, W.C.: Biomechanics of fracture treatment. In, Fracture Healing and Treatment. Ed: Heppenstall, R.B., W.B. Saunders, Philadelphia, 1979. pp 124-172.

20. Hayes, W.C. and Carter, D.R.: Biomechanics of bone. In, Skeletal Research: An Experimental Approach. Eds: Simmons, D.J., Kunin, A.S., Academic Press, New York, 1979. pp 263-300.

21. Hayes, W.C. and Snyder, B.D.: Toward a quantitative formulation of Wolff's Law in trabecular bone. In, Symposium on the Mechanical Properties of Bone. Am. Soc. Mech. Engineers, Boulder, CO, 1981, pp 43-68.

22. Jowsey, J.: In, Metabolic Diseases of Bone. W.B. Saunders Co., Philadelphia, 1977.

23. Kelsey, J.L., Harris, P., and Gerald, B.E., Jr.: Musculoskeletal Disorders: Their Frequency of Occurrence and Their Impact on the Population of the United States. Prodist, New York, 1978.

24. Lane, J.M. and Vigorita, V.J.: Osteoporosis: Current concepts review. J. Bone Joint Surg. 65A, 274, 1983

25. Mazess, R.B.: Noninvasive methods for quantitating trabecular bone. In, The Osteoporotic Syndrome: Detection Prevention and Treatment. Ed: Avioli, L.V., Grune & Stratton, New York, 1983a, pp 85-114.

26. Mazess, R.B.: The non-invasive measurement of skeletal mass. In, Bone and Mineral Research, Annual II. Excerpta Medica, 1983b, pp 223-279.

27. Mazess, R.B., Peppler, W.W., Chesnut, C.H., III, Nelp, W.B., Cohn, S.H., and Zanzi, I.: Total body bone mineral and lean body mass by dual-photon absorptiometry. II. Comparison with total body calcium by neutron activation analysis. Calcif. Tiss. Int. 33, 361, 1981a.

28. Mazess, R.B., Peppler, W.W., Harrison, J.E., and McNeill, K.G.: Total body bone mineral and lean body mass by dual-photon absorptiometry. III. Comparison with trunk calcium by neutron activation analysis. Calcif. Tiss. Int. 33, 365, 1981b.

29. Meema, H.E. and Meema, S.: Radiogrammetry. In, Non-Invasive Measurements of Bone Mass and Their Clinical Applications. Ed: Cohn, S.H., CRC Press, Boca Raton, FL, 1981. pp 5-50.

30. Nagurka, M.L. and Hayes, W.C.: Technical note: An interactive graphics package for calculating cross-sectional properties of complex shapes. J.Biomech. 13, 59, 1980.

31. Peppler, W.W. and Mazess, R.B.: Total body bone mineral and lean body mass by dual-photon absorptiometry. I. Theory and measurement procedure. Calcif. Tiss. Int. 33, 353, 1981.

32. Posner, I. and Griffiths, H.J.: Comparison of CT Scanning with Photon Absorptiometric Measurements of Bone Mineral Content in the Appendicular Skeleton. Invest. Radiol. 12, 542, 1977.

33. Reich, N.E., Seidelmann, F.E., and Tubbs, R.R.: Determination of bone mineral content using CT scanning. Am. J. Roentgenol. 127, 595, 1976.

34. Reilly, D.T. and Burstein, A.H.: The mechanical properties of cortical bone. J. Bone Joint Surg. 56A, 1001, 1974.

35. Reilly, D.T., Burstein, A.H., and Frankel, V.H.: The elastic modulus for bone. J. Biomech. 7, 271, 1974.

36. Ruegsegger, P., Dambacher, M.A., Ruegsegger, E., Fischer, J.A., and Anliker, M.: Bone loss in premenopausal and postmenopausal women. J. Bone Joint Surg. 66A, 1015, 1984.

37. Ruegsegger, R., Elsasser, V., and Anliker, M.: Quantification of bone mineralization using computed tomography. Radiology 121, 93, 1976.

38. Ruff, C.B. and Hayes, W.C.: Subperiosteal expansion and cortical remodeling of the human femur and tibia with aging. Science 217, 945, 1982.

39. Ruff, C.B. and Hayes, W.C.: Cross-sectional geometry of Pecos Pueblo femora and tibiae: A biomechanical investigation. I. Method and general patterns of variation. Am. J. Phys.Anthrop. 60, 359, 1983a.

40. Ruff, C.B. and Hayes, W.C.: Cross-sectional geometry of Pecos Pueblo femora and tibiae: A biomechanical investigation. II. Sex, age and size differences. Am. J. Phys.Anthrop. 60, 383, 1983b.

41. Singh, M., Riggs, L., Beabout, J.W., and Jowsey, J.: Femoral trabecular pattern index for evaluation of spinal osteoporosis. Ann. Intern. Med. 77, 63, 1972.

42. Woo, S.L.Y., Kuei, S.C., Amiel, D., Hayes, W.C., White, F.C., and Akeson, W.H.: The effect of prolonged physical training on the properties of long bone. J. Bone Joint Surg. 63A, 780, 1981.

43. Wright, T.M.: Mechanics of fracture and fracture propagation. In, Scientific Foundations of Orthopaedics. Eds: Goodfellow, O., Bullough, P., William Heinemann Medical Books, Ltd., London, 1980. pp 252-258.

44. Wright, T.M. and Hayes, W.C.: Tensile testing of bone over a wide range of strain rates: Effects of strain rate, microstructure and density. Med. Biol. Eng. 14, 671, 1976.

Biomechanical Factors in Adaptation of Bone Structure to Function

L. E. LANYON

Introduction

The general form of each bone, its attachments, and its anatomical relationships are all genetically determined and will develop in the absence of functional influences. However, the particular features on which each bone's load-bearing competence depends (ie, its mass, girth, cortical thickness, curvature, and the density and arrangement of its cancellous bone) are all achieved, and will only persist in the presence of continued functional load bearing. Normality of skeletal structure, and the load-bearing competence it reflects, is therefore not a predetermined state but rather the cumulative achievement of local adaptation to load bearing throughout the skeleton. Skeletal fragility may be viewed as a failure or insufficiency in the process which normally matches skeletal structure to its load-bearing requirements.

Under normal circumstances, the skeleton's adaptive response matches its structure to its load-bearing requirements by ensuring an adequate amount of bone tissue with suitable material properties arranged appropriately to withstand such load bearing without undue damage. Exercise-related differences in bone mass confirm the skeleton's potential to respond to the challenge of increased load bearing (Dalen and Olsson, 1974; Goodship et al, 1979; Jones et al, 1977; Krolner et al, 1983; Smith et al, 1981; Woo et al, 1981). Disuse-related bone loss indicates that any functionally appropriate level of bone mass is only maintained as a result of a continued load-bearing stimulus (Chantraine et al, 1979; Donaldson et al, 1970; Krolner and Toft, 1983; Uhthoff and Jaworski, 1978; Wronski and Morey, 1983; Young et al, 1983).

The processes responsible for effecting the functionally adaptive response are the familiar ones of coordinated osteoblastic and osteoclastic activity. These processes are subject to a number of influences in addition to those derived from weight bearing. These influences include systemic hormones primarily concerned with mineral metabolism and regulated by feedback from serum calcium, and local factors such as matrix-bound coupling factor (Drivdahl et al, 1982). There is no biochemical requirement for the skeleton to have any particular shape, and in general skeletal mass is so large compared with the daily calcium requirement that there is similarly no biochemical requirement for any particular mass of bone tissue. The only requirements for these variables are therefore those necessary for functional load-bearing. This being the case, it is logical that the only stimulus which is capable of organizing bone architecture, or stimulating a sustained

Current Concepts of Bone Fragility

increase in bone mass, is that provided by load bearing itself. The mechanism is not known whereby the loads supported by the bone matrix are transduced into signals recognizable by the cells responsible for remodelling control. However, since the result of load, mass, material properties, and architecture is strain, this is obviously one of the most important variables to regulate.

In one series of experiments (Rubin and Lanyon, 1984) we attached strain gauges to a number of skeletal sites in a variety of species to determine the peak strains engendered during any coordinated physical activity. The data from these experiments suggested that the peak principal physiologic strain is of the order of 0.002-0.003. This is of particular interest since Carter and Caler (1985) have shown that the damage caused in bone tissue by intermittent strains above this level is increasingly accounted for by creep rather than fatigue. It appears, therefore, that one of the prime objectives of functionally adaptive bone remodelling is to maintain customary strains below the level where creep is a factor.

Not only is strain one of the most important load-related variables to control but strain itself, or one of its immediate consequences such as intralacunar pressure, fluid flow, or streaming potentials, is a variable which can directly influence resident bone cells. A number of experiments have been conducted to determine the active principle of a bone's mechanical regimen responsible for influencing cell behavior to appropriately adjust bone architecture *in vivo*. One of the most productive experimental models involves using a procedure in which a bone is deprived of normal functional load bearing and instead is subjected to an artifical load-bearing regimen imposed from an external device (Lanyon and Rubin, 1984; Rubin and Lanyon, 1984).

This functionally isolated, externally loadable preparation is made by making proximal and distal metaphyseal osteotomies in the ulna of skeletally mature male turkeys. The cut ends of the diaphysis are then covered with stainless steel caps. These caps and the bone they enclose are transfixed by steel pins, the ends of which emerge through the skin on the dorsal and ventral surfaces of the wing. By using bone-bonded rosette strain gauges *in vivo*, the strains engendered in the midshaft of the bone are measured (Lanyon, 1976). During wing flapping in the intact bone these strains reached a maximum of 0.003 in compression, whereas those engendered at the same site by wing movement in the functionally isolated preparation were only 0.0002 (Lanyon and Rubin 1984). This preparation thus allows us to preserve for long periods the anatomic and nutritive connections of a large piece of living bone which remains exposed to all its normal systemic influences but is deprived of its normal load bearing. By applying loads through the transfixing pins, normal functional load bearing can be replaced by a controllable artificial load regimen. Examination of sections from bones treated in this way enables us to monitor the effect of various strain regimens on remodelling activity.

Artificial Loading Experiments

A number of experiments have been performed using this preparation. These experiments and their implications will be briefly discussed.

1. The effect of static versus dynamic strains.

Frost (1973) suggested and Hert et al (1971) first demonstrated that it was dynamic and not static strains which influenced bone remodelling activity. We confirmed this finding using the externally loadable avian ulna preparation (Lanyon and Rubin, 1984). Two load regimens were applied to the ends of the transfixing pins. In the first regimen, a static load was imposed by two helical springs (Fig. 1) which together engendered a peak compressive strain at the bone's midshaft of 0.002. These springs were left in place for 24 hours a day for 8 weeks. In the second regimen, the same load was applied but intermittently for 100 consecutive cycles daily at a frequency of 1.0 Hz. In each case the remodelling in the experimental ulna was compared with that in its intact contralateral control. The results from the two loading situations were then compared with those from another series of animals where the ulna preparation was subjected to no load at all.

In the disuse situation, the remodelling state was transformed from quiescence into considerable activity. The remodelling balance was predominantly

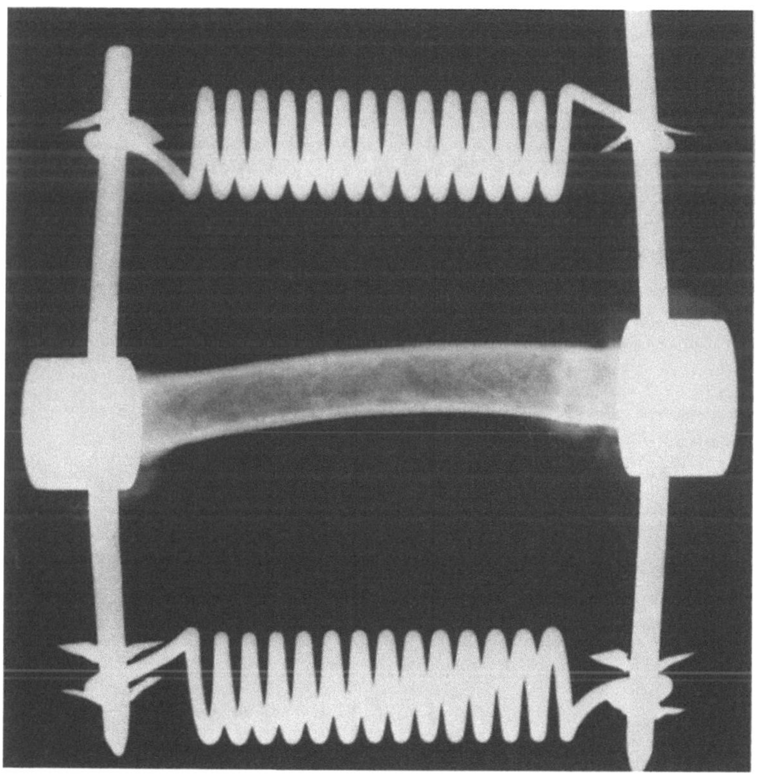

Fig. 1. Radiograph of the turkey ulna preparation, taken postmortem, showing the 110 mm portion of the bone's diaphysis with caps and transfixing pins in place. The ends of the pins, to which loads can be applied, penetrate the skin of the dorsal and ventral surfaces of the wing. In this case a static load is being applied by two helical springs. (Lanyon and Rubin, 1984)

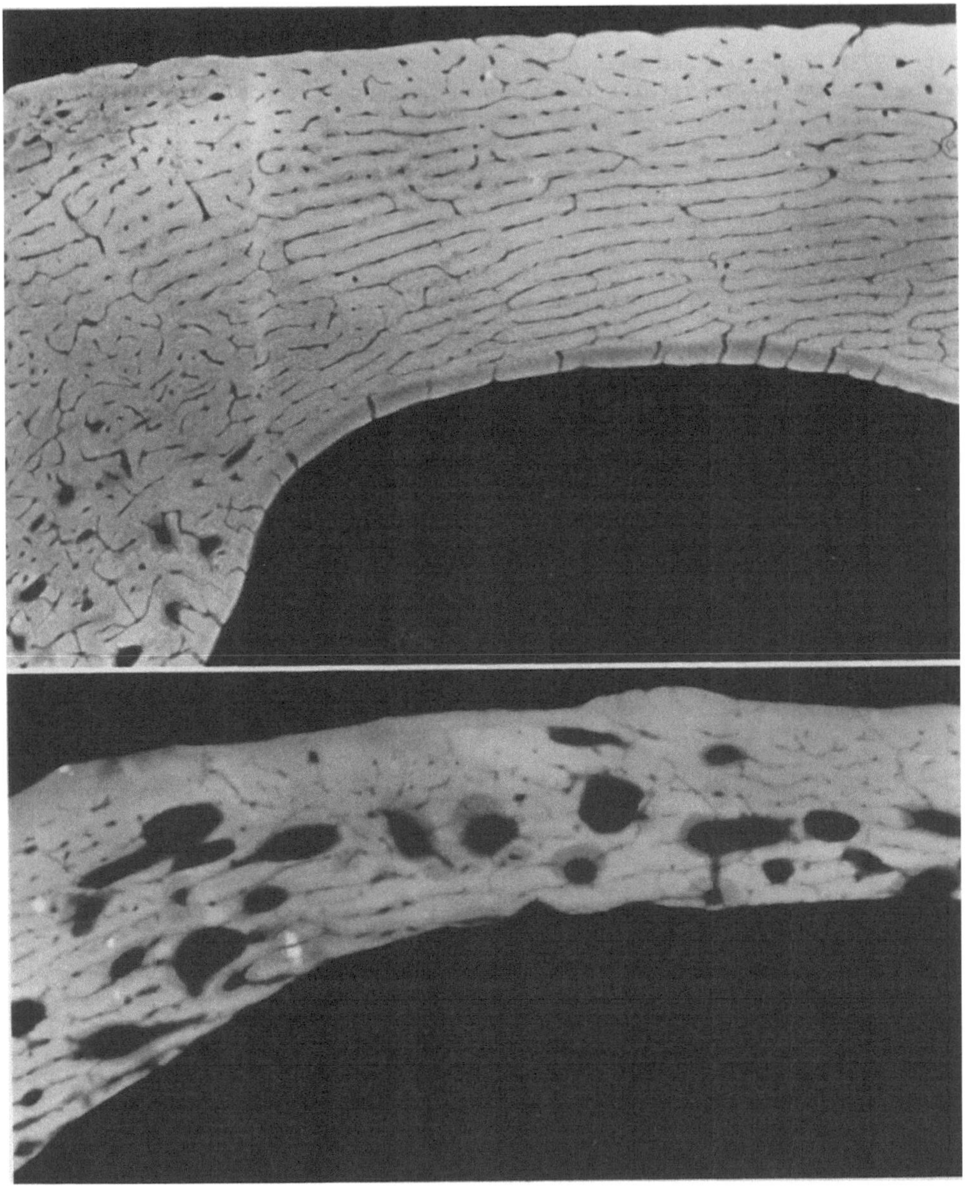

a

b

Fig. 2. a Microradiograph of a 100 micron thick transverse section of a mature male turkey's ulna. The bone is predominantly primary although there is some evidence of localized secondary osteonal activity. There is no activity on either the periosteal or endosteal surface. This is the normal remodelling situation in quiescent bones in this species when structure is appropriately matched to load bearing. b A microradiograph similar to that in a from a bone which for eight weeks had been isolated from load bearing. The cortex is thinned from endosteal resorption, and porotic from widespread incompletely infilled secondary osteonal remodelling. (Lanyon and Rubin, 1984)

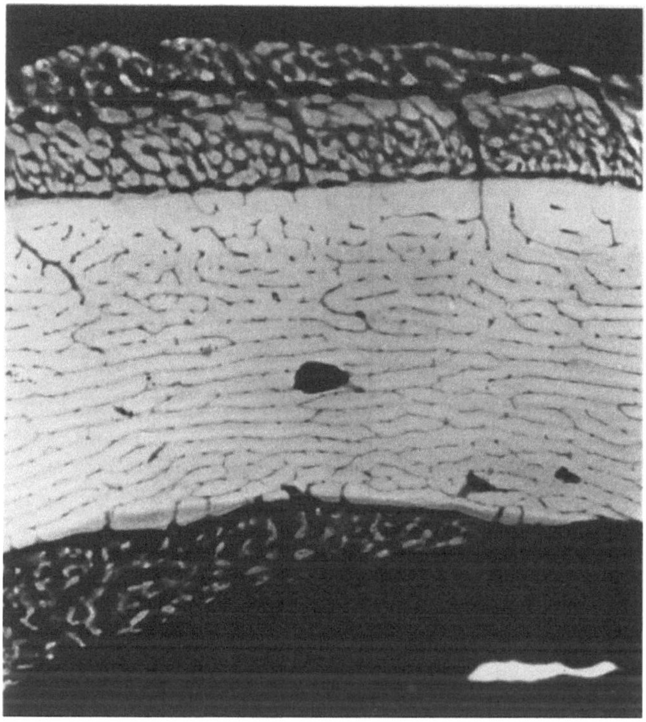

Fig. 2c. A microradiograph similar to those in a and b from a bone which for eight weeks had been isolated from natural load bearing but subjected to 100 consecutive 1 Hz cycles per day of an externally applied intermittent load producing peak strains of 0.003 around the circumference. New bone formation has been induced on both periosteal and endosteal surfaces. There is no evidence that this process is accompanied or preceded by surface resorption, and there is little remodelling intracortically. (Lanyon and Rubin, 1984)

negative, resulting in cortical thinning by endosteal resorption and intracortical porosis by incompletely infilled haversian remodelling (Figs. 2a, 2b). This conforms to the classical picture of disuse osteoporosis, and in this experiment was associated with a 15-20% reduction in bone cross-sectional area. Static loads maintained for 24 h/day appeared to have no modulating effect on this osteoporotic response. However, less than two minutes per day of intermittent loading, producing a similar peak strain as that in the static case, was associated with a 24% increase in cross-sectional area. This resulted from deposition of new bone predominantly but not exclusively, on the periosteal surface (Fig. 2c).

It seems that the cells responsible for perceiving the bones' mechanical situation are sensitive to dynamic but not static events.

2. The effect of graded dynamic loads

The same ulnar preparation was used to assess the effect of short periods of graded dynamic loads (Rubin and Lanyon, 1983). These loads were applied once daily as a strain of 100 consecutive cycles at 1.0 Hz. The load magnitude was adjusted to produce maximum compressive strains at the bone's midshaft of 0.0005, 0.001, 0.002, 0.003, or 0.004. The results showed that whereas the disuse response to lack of loading was associated with a 15-20% loss of bone tissue, peak strains of only 0.001 prevented this bone loss. Strains above 0.001 were associated with a proportional increase in cross-sectional area of up to 40% (Fig. 3). Thus, strains both above and below 0.001 were associated with increased remodelling activity. Below this strain level, the remodelling was negatively balanced and resulted in bone

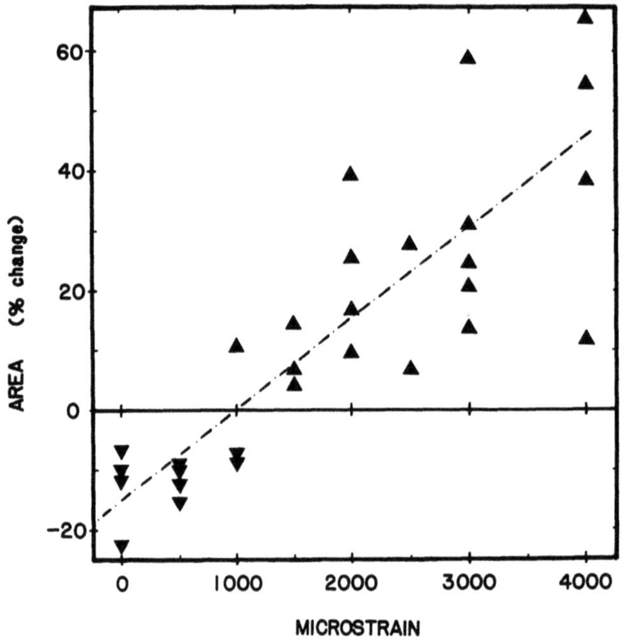

Fig. 3. Graph of the change in cross-sectional area of the ulna midshaft of bones similar to those in Figs. 1 and 2. The percentage change in area is based on the postmortem comparison between the area of left (experimental) and right (intact) bones after an eight week period subjected to a load regimen selected to produce different peak strains. Strains below 0.001 were associated with reduction in cross-sectional area (disuse osteoporosis), those between 0.001 and 0.004 with a progressive increase (functional hypertrophy). (Rubin and Lanyon, 1983)

loss. Above this level, it was positively balanced and resulted in bone gain. The increase in bone mass was achieved principally by periosteal new bone formation and was accompanied by little or no activity intracortically.

It appears that control of bone mass is directly influenced by characteristics of the bone's dynamic strain environment, one of the controlling variables of which is the peak strain magnitude.

3. The effect of the number of load cycles

The first variable investigated using the avian ulnar preparation was the effect of the number of load cycles (Rubin and Lanyon, 1984). Roosters, rather than turkeys, were used in this study and the ulna was subjected to 0, 4, 36, 360 or 1,800 consecutive loading cycles imposed at 0.5 Hz. Data from these experiments showed the expected response to absence of loading, namely an increase in remodelling activity characterized by endosteal absorption and negatively balanced intracortical remodelling. Remarkably, however, only four loading cycles per day (occupying 8 sec) were necessary

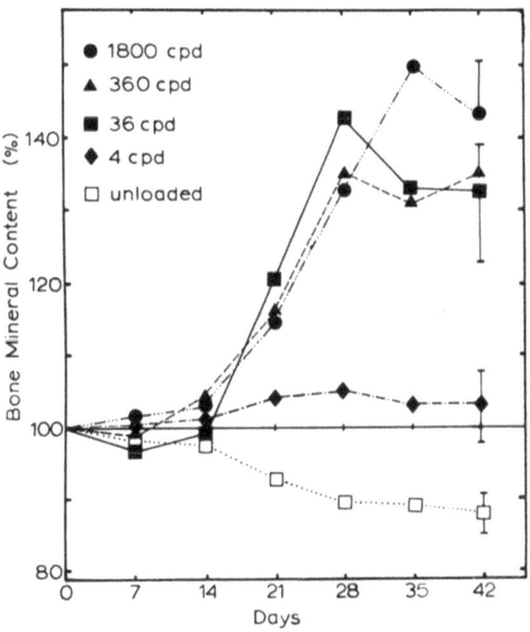

Fig. 4. Change in the bone mineral content (assessed by photon absorptiometry) at the midshaft of rooster ulna preparations over a six week experimental period in which the bones were subjected to 0, 4, 36, 360, or 1800 consecutive 0.5 Hz cycles per day of an identical load regimen. The vertical lines for the six-week values indicate standard deviations. Whereas disuse resulted in bone loss, only four cycles per day of a potentially osteogenic load regimen were sufficient to prevent this response. Thirty-six cycles per day resulted in a substantial increase in bone mass, which was not exeeded by exposure to 360 or 1800 cycles. (Rubin and Lanyon, 1984)

to prevent this remodelling response and to maintain the status quo. Thirty-six loading cycles per day (occupying 72 sec) were associated with substantial periosteal, and some endosteal, new bone formation, increasing the bone's cross-sectional area by between 30 and 40%. No additional increase in bone formation was achieved by 360 or 1,800 load cycles per day (Fig. 4).

It is unlikely that a remodelling response such as this could be produced by a nonspecific stimulus such as better perfusion. It is more likely that dynamic strain change provides a specific stimulus to which a strain-sensitive population of cells responds. In this experiment it appears that two strain-related effects are produced in sequence, and perhaps a dose-related response to a single strain-generated phenomenon. The first effect is that produced by the first four loading cycles and involves inhibition of resorption. The second effect is associated with continued exposure to the strain-related stimulus (the next 32 cycles) and results in substantial new bone formation. Since this osteogenic stimulus is a strain - related phenomenon, it is presumably self - limiting. Once bone mass has been modified sufficiently to restore the strains to their "appropriate" level this stimulus disappears.

4. The effect of disuse and artifical loading on bone remodelling during calcium deprivation.

In this experiment, female turkeys were made calcium deficient by inducing them to lay eggs while on a diet insufficient in calcium (Lanyon, 1984). The ulna on one side was exposed either to disuse or disuse modulated by a short daily period of artificial loading. Postmortem examination of the intact ulnas showed that calcium deprivation was associated with an increase in remodelling activity causing substantial endosteal and intracortical resorption. The degree of bone loss was 17% in six weeks. In

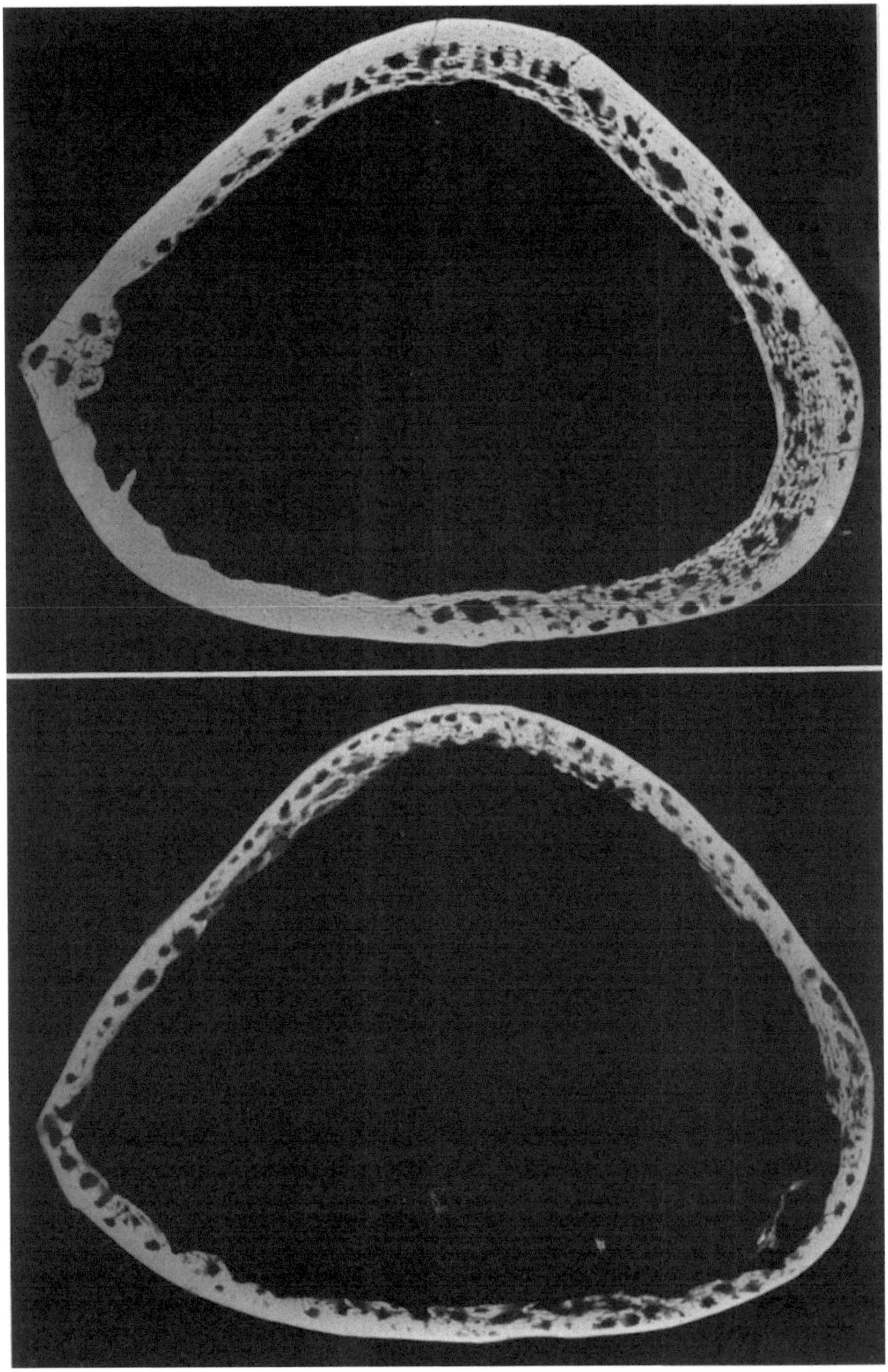

b

a

Fig. 5a,b (caption see opposite page)

ulnas which were also deprived of functional loading, the remodelling response was much more severe, and the loss of bone tissue totalled 37% (Fig. 5, 6). Substantial protection from resorption could be provided by short daily periods of artificial loading. However, a strain regimen which in males on a calcium-sufficient diet was osteogenic, in females on a calcium-insufficient diet was unable to provide complete protection from even the disuse component of the total bone loss.

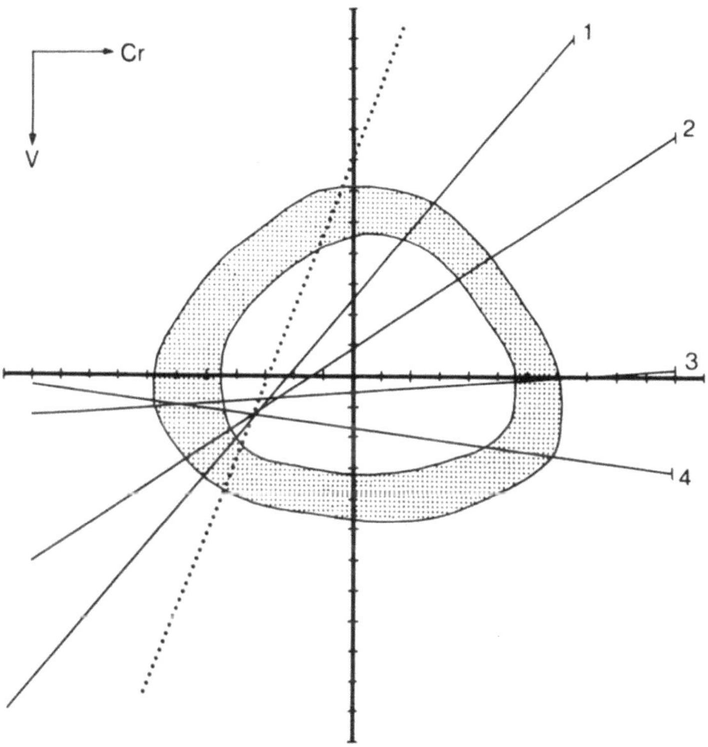

Fig. 6. The changing position of the neutral axis in the turkey ulna taken at different times during a single wing flapping cycle (solid lines) compared with the single constant position (dotted line) during artificial loading. The solid line labelled 3 indicates the position of the neutral axis at the time of peak strain during wing flapping. The directions v and cr are ventral and cranial respectively. The region of the cortex under compression is cranial to the neutral axis during artifical loading in the preparation, and dorsal to it in the intact bone during wing flapping.

Fig. 5. a Microradiograph of a whole cross-section of a female turkey's intact ulna taken after six weeks laying eggs on a calcium insufficient diet. The degree of resorptive remodelling is substantial both endosteally and intracortically. The degree of bone loss is approximately 17%. b Similar microradiograph to that in a taken from the contralateral ulna which was also deprived of mechanical load bearing. The degree of bone loss is much more substantial, indicating the protective effect of load bearing even during periods of hormonally-induced bone loss.

Discussion

We propose the hypothesis that the structural objective of bone remodelling is to maintain or modify bone architecture and adjust bone mass sufficiently to produce, at each location throughout the skeleton, a strain regimen which coincides with that coded genetically. The artificial loading experiments lead us to presume that at least two categories of strain variable are important in relation to bone remodelling: i) related to the strain wave form; and ii) related to the strain distribution.

i) Strain wave form.

It is apparent that substantial changes in bone mass can be achieved by exposing bone to short periods of dynamic strain change. Using the manner of loading applied in the avian experiments just described, it appears that strains below a certain peak magnitude were unable to provide sufficient protection from hormonal demands for resorption, resulting in disuse osteoporosis. Strains above that level not only protected the existing bone tissue from hormonally-engendered resorption, but also provided an osteogenic stimulus resulting in deposition of an amount of new bone proportional to the overstrain engendered.

We are as yet far from understanding the manner in which dynamic strain change influences bone cell behavior to produce structurally appropriate bone remodelling. At present, in addition to the experiments outlined here, we have used an artificial loading regimen on the sheep radius (O'Connor et al, 1982) to show that the osteogenic potential of a strain-related stimulus is also profoundly affected by the rate at which the strain changes. Further experiments may reveal other aspects of the strain wave form, such as frequency, intermittency, etc, which influence the size or nature of the strain-related stimulus. These experiments, while permitting us to define the stimulus in terms of the strain which engenders it, may also allow us to identify the actual strain-related variable which is perceived by the mechanically receptive cell population. At present, even the identity of these cells is unknown. They seem, however, to be sensitive to at least two components of the strain change wave form, namely, peak strain magnitude and strain rate.

ii) Strain distribution.

In the artificial loading experiments described above, the peak strains engendered by the applied loads were no larger than the peak strains that could have been engendered in the intact bone by wing flapping. If the objective of mechanically-related remodelling were only to regulate peak strain magnitude, then the question would arise why applying physiologic strains at physiologic strain rates should require an adaptive response at all. Presumably, had we been able to replicate exactly the strain distribution normally engendered during wing flapping, no new bone would have been stimulated unless, or until, we had exceeded the peak strain magnitudes or rates involved. In fact, the strain distribution engendered by artificial loading was quite different from that engendered naturally by wing flapping (Fig. 6). We therefore conjecture that it is the inappropriateness of the new strain situation which is the basis of the remodelling stimulus. Thus, in the avian ulna experiments, the nature of the remodelling stimulus could have been provided by the discrepancy between strain distribution in the normal and new loading situations and its strength determined by the characteristics of the strain wave form, such as the peak strain magnitude, or maximum strain rate.

The conclusion that strain distribution is an important determinant of remodelling behavior is supported by two series of experiments in sheep. In the first of these, an ulna osteotomy was used to cause a slight reorganization of strains in the adjacent radius (Lanyon et al, 1982). Loading was imposed naturally by the sheep walking, and an adaptive remodelling response was elicited which continued for a year. At the end of this time, some of the strains around the bone were actually lower than they were before the osteotomy was performed. Nevertheless, the new bone continued to be deposited on the radius until an area equal to that of the removed ulna was restored. In the second experiment artificial bending or compressive loads were applied to the metacarpus (Churches and Howlett, 1981). Whereas compressive loading caused an increase in bone mass, bending elicited no such response.

One of the consequences of assuming that the strain distribution is an important controlling variable for functional adaptation in bone tissue is that it implies that inappropriate strain situations, as well as excessive strain magnitudes, will generate adaptive remodelling responses. If each loading situation requires or stimulates a particular mass or arrangement of bone tissue, then an individual's bone mass at any time will reflect the diversity of their activities as well as the wave form produced during each of them.

If true, the conclusion that bone can respond to changes in strain distribution alone has implications as to the mechanism whereby strain-related remodelling must be controlled. To account for remodelling sensitivity to strain distribution,either each skeletal location must have a unique, previously determined, appropriate strain level (in which case remodelling can be controlled by locally independent responses to the strain situation in the immediate vicinity of the strain sensitive cells), or else there is an integrative step whereby the appreciation of strain distribution is formed by the relative strains throughout the structure. This latter hypothesis seems to us the more likely. The integrated assessment of strain distribution could be achieved either by extensive communication between strain-sensitive cells distributed throughout or around the load carrying matrix, or by some extracellular mechanism such as the pattern of electrical events produced as a consequence of mechanical strain throughout the structure.

At present, we consider it likely that the osteocytes form a strain-sensitive network which is capable of forming the necessary appreciation of strain distribution. The osteocytes themselves are hardly involved in the actual remodelling processes of the bone; we must therefore suppose that their influence on remodelling occurs following communication with cells on or near the bone's surfaces.

The level of this control process at which the consequences of mechanical strain interact with those from circulating hormones is unknown, but it could be that it is at the level of stem cell or surface cell activation. When considering strain-related and hormonally-engendered stimuli, the following relationships must be considered.

Removal of functional load bearing is associated with a disuse osteoporotic response. This response is not caused by change in the level of PTH or CT

(Chantraine et al, 1979). Nevertheless, the remodelling changes are indistinguishable from those produced by the increased levels of PTH associated with calcium deprivation. In parathyroidectomized animals, this disuse osteoporotic response does not occur (Burkhart and Jowsey, 1967). Furthermore, in nonparathyroidectomized animals, calcium deprivation combined with disuse results in the degree of osteoporosis being even more severe than in either condition alone (Lanyon, 1984).

These findings can be explained by supposing that exposure to an appropriate intermittent mechanical strain reduces bone cells' sensitivity to parathyroid hormont (PTH). Naturally, the higher the circulating PTH level the less effective this desensitization will be in preventing bone loss. Nevertheless, regardless of the actual level of PTH, only a reduction in mechanically-related stimulation is necessary at any time to permit this loss to be increased.

We propose that the remodelling balance at any time is maintained by an equilibrium between these competing and complementary influences tending to push the balance positive or negative. A scheme illustrating the possible contributors to this balance is illustrated in Fig. 7.

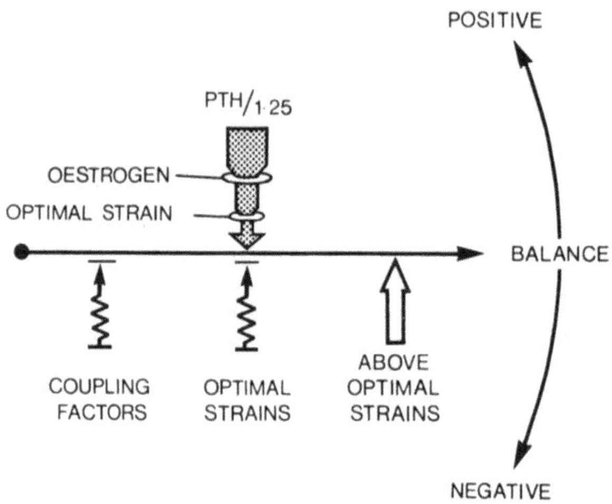

Fig. 7. A schema to illustrate the proposed interaction of hormonal and mechanical influences on remodelling. The PTH/1,25D axis provides a stimulus towards resorption whose effectiveness is reduced by both estrogen and by the local strain situation in each bone. When resorption does occur, restitution of bone is encouraged by the release of matrix-bound coupling factors and an osteogenic effect of mechanical strain. The only natural influence capable of producing a sustained increase in bone mass which is not subsequently negated by resorption is that derived by high, or inappropriate, strains.

On one side of the equilibrium is the PTH/1,25(OH)D axis tending to push the balance negatively by encouraging the generation of resorptive remodelling units. This effect appears to be reduced by estrogen, and we propose also by physical activity involving appropriate (or optimal) strains. When stimulation of resorptive remodelling units does occur, one of the influences normally tending to maintain the remodelling balance is the release of matrix-bound coupling factors which stimulate osteoblastic activity. Naturally, there is a deficit between the amount of bone that these factors stimulate and the amount of bone originally removed; otherwise bone mass could never be reduced. We propose that this deficit is normally made up by an osteogenic stimulus also generated by mechanical strains.

Thus, removal of functional strains leads to disuse osteoporosis as a result of two effects: 1) increased sensitivity to PTH which causes generation of a greater number of initially resorptive remodelling events, and 2) deficiency in the mechanically-related stimulus which by supplementing the effect of coupling factors would have ensured restoration of a similar amount of bone to that removed by the initial resorption involved in that remodelling event. Increased PTH stimulation, as in calcium deficiency, is sufficient to throw the remodelling balance negative by both these means despite exposure to appropriate strains. Withdrawal of estrogen also permits the stimulation of more initially resorptive remodelling units so that if mechanical strain cannot provide sufficient osteogenic stimulation to ensure complete restitution of bone tissue, then progressive bone loss will occur.

This is the scenario most likely to be involved in postmenopausal and senile osteoporosis. Our experiments have indicated that the osteogenic potential of a bone's strain regimen is dependent on the peak strains, the maximum strain rate, and the strain distributions involved. The decreasing diversity, vigor, and magnitude of load bearing characteristic of the middle-aged and elderly means that for each remodelling event the strain-generated osteogenic stimulus required for complete restitution of bone is deficient and thus bone loss occurs. Naturally, bone can only be lost as a result of remodelling, and so bone loss may be reduced by down-regulating the rate of generation of remodelling events by both estrogen and calcium therapy. However, provided that sufficient calcium is available, appropriate physical activity should be able to contribute towards a positive or neutral balance regardless of the level of remodelling activity.

The schema in Fig. 7 shows the two strain-related effects just outlined. The first is that due to optimal or appropriate strains which both down-regulate generation of initially resorptive remodelling events and stimulate complete restitution of bone when such events occur; the second is that produced by inappropriate or higher than optimal strains. This stimulus can actually cause an increase in bone mass by stimulation of intially osteogenic remodelling units. Indeed, we propose that, under normal circumstances in adults, this strain-generated stimulus is the only one which can stimulate an increase in bone mass not subsequently negated by resorption. Such a stimulus caused by high, or inappropriate, strains is of course self-regulating since once bone mass has increased, or adapted sufficiently to eliminate the high or inappropriate strain, the stimulus itself disappears.

Summary

A bone will be fragile (incapable of withstanding normal functional load bearing) unless it has modified its minimum (genetically determined) mass and architecture in response to functional load bearing. The influence derived from such load bearing is the only one specifically directed to maintaining structural competence.

A bone which has already achieved structural competence will become fragile should this functional input be discontinued. However, even during normal use this mechanically derived effect competes with others for influence over the remodelling process. Thus, the extent to which structurally appropriate bone architecture can be maintained is determined by the relative strengths which these influences possess. The characteristics of an appropriate strain environment will vary from one location to another. However, it appears that the strength of the mechanically-related stimulus is determined by a number of dynamic strain variables including the peak strain magnitude, the maximum strain rate, and the strain distribution. The mechanism by which variation in these variables exerts a controlling influence on bone remodelling is not known.

Acknowledgements

The author's experiments referred to in this article were performed in the Department of Anatomy, University of Bristol, the Department of Anatomy and Cellular Biology, Tufts University, Boston, and the Department of Anatomy, Royal Veterinary College, London. Support has been received from the MRC (UK), the Wellcome Trust, the Arthritis and Rheumatism Council, NIH, the US Army, and NASA. To these organizations, and for the collaboration of my colleagues, I am most grateful.

References

1. Burkhart, J.M., and Jowsey, J.: Parathyroid and thyroid hormone in the development of immobilisation osteoporosis. Endocrinology 81, 1053, 1967.

2. Carter, D.R., and Caler, W.E.: A cumulative damage model of bone fracture, J.Orthop.Res. 3, 84, 1985.

3. Chantraine, A., Heynen, G., and Franchimont, P.: Bone metabolism, parathyroid hormone, and calcitonin in paraplegia. Calcif.Tissue Int. 27, 199, 1979.

4. Churches, A.E., and Howlett, C.R.: The response of mature cortical bone to controlled time-varying loading. In, Mechanical Properties of Bone. Ed: Cowin, S.C., ASME publication AMD 45, 69, 1981.

5. Dalen, N., and Olsson, K.E.: Bone density in athletes. Clin.Orthop. Rel.Res. 77, 179, 1974.

6. Donaldson, C.L., Hulley, S.B., Vogel, J.M., Hattner, R.S., Bayers, J.H., and McMillan, D.E.: Effect of prolonged bedrest on bone mineral. Metabolism 19, 1071, 1970.

7. Drivdahl, R.H., Howard, G.A., and Baylink, D.J.: Extracts of bone contain a potent regulator of bone formation. Biochem.Biophys.Acta 714, 23, 1982.

8. Frost, H.M.: Bone Modelling and Skeletal Modelling Errors. Charles C. Thomas, Illinois, 1973.

9. Goodship, A.E., Lanyon, L.E., and MacFie, H.: Functional adaptation of bone to increased stress. J.Bone Joint Surg. 61A, 539, 1979.

10. Hert, J., Liskova, M., and Landa, J.: Reaction of bone to mechanical stimuli. Part 1: Continuous and intermittent loading of tibia in rabbit. Folia Morph. (Praha) 19, 290, 1971.

11. Jones, H.H., Priest, J.D., Hayes, W.C., Tichenor, C.C., and Nagel, D.A.: Humeral hypertrophy in response to exercise. J.Bone Joint Surg. 59A, 204, 1977.

12. Krolner, B. and Toft, B.: Vertebral bone loss: an unheeded side effect of therapeutic bed rest. Clin.Sc. 64, 537, 1983.

13. Krołner, B., Toft, B., Nielsen, S.P., and Tondevold, E.: Physical exercise as prophylaxis against involutional bone loss: a controlled trial. Clin.Sc. 64, 541, 1983.

14. Lanyon, L.E.: The measurement of bone strain *in vivo*. Acta Orthopaed. Belg. 42(Suppl.1), 98, 1976.

15. Lanyon, L.E.: Functional strain as a determinant for bone remodelling. Calcif.Tis.Int. 36, S56, 1984.

16. Lanyon, L.E., Goodship, A.E., Pye, C.J., and MacFie, H.: Mechanically adaptive bone remodelling. A quantitative study on functional adaptation in the radius following ulna osteotomy in sheep. J.Biomech. 15, 141, 1982.

17. Lanyon, L.E., and Rubin C.T.: Static versus dynamic loads as an influence on bone remodelling. J.Biomech. 17, 897, 1984.

18. O'Connor, J.A., Lanyon, L.E., and MacFie, H.: The influence of strain rate on adaptive bone remodelling. J.Biomech. 15, 767, 1982

19. Rubin, C.T., and Lanyon, L.E.: Regulation of bone mass by peak strain magnitude. Trans.Orthopaed.Res.Soc., 1983.

20. Rubin, C.T., and Lanyon, L.E.: Regulation of bone formation by applied dynamic loads. J.Bone Joint Surg. 66A, 397, 1984.

21. Rubin, C.T., and Lanyon, L.E.: Dynamic strain similarity in vertebrates: An alternative to allometric limbo bone scaling. J.Theor.Biol. 107, 321, 1984.

22. Smith, E.L., Reddan, W., and Smith, P.E.: Physical activity and calcium modalities for bone mineral increase in aged women. Med.Sc.Sports Exerc. 13, 60, 1981.

23. Uhthoff, H.K. and Jaworski, Z.F.G.: Bone loss in response to long-term immobilisation. J.Bone Joint.Surg. 60B, 420, 1978.

24. Woo, S.L-Y., Kuei, S.C., Amiel, D., Gomez, M.A., Hayes, W.C., White, F.C., and Akeson, W.H.: The effect of prolonged physical training on the properties of long bone: A study of Wolff's Law. J.Bone Joint. Surg. 63A, 780, 1981.

25. Wronski, T.J., and Morey, E.R.: Inhibition of cortical and trabecular bone formation in the long bones of immobilised monkeys. Clin.Orthopaed. 181, 269, 1983.

26. Young, D.R., Niklowitz, W.J., and Steel, C.R.: Tibial changes in experimental disuse osteoporosis in the monkey. Calcif.Tis.Int. 35, 304, 1983.

Cellular Mechanisms Underlying the Skeleton's Supportive Function

Z. F. G. JAWORSKI

Introduction

Regardless of etiology or type of structural alterations, metabolic bone diseases manifest clinically as a failure of the skeleton's supportive function, ie, bone pain, deformities, and fractures in strategic locations.

It is now apparent that all aspects of the skeleton's mechanical competence (MCSk) (Table I) depend, in the final analysis, on osteoblasts and osteoclasts. Osteoblasts provide the basic material from which the bones are made, ie, lamellar bone; osteoclasts, by resorbing bone in selective areas, contribute further to bone structuring.

Table I. Structural components of skeleton's mechanical competence (MCSk)

1.	Basic material: bone matrix and mineral
2.	Shape and architecture of bones
3.	Microscopic organization (grain) and mean age of bone tissue
4.	Bone volume

Characteristically, bones develop during growth in predetermined sequences. Similarly, they subsequently turn over at multiple sites via the resorption and formation of bone tissue in discrete areas by local, transient, self-renewing populations of osteoclasts and osteoblasts. Thus, the resulting cavities and packets of lamellar bone acquire a proper size, shape and orientation in bone space, and appear in a proper location and a proper time, proper from the point of view of establishing and maintaining the MCSk.

Under normal circumstances, therefore, the osteoblast and osteoclast populations work in concert; regardless of how they associate in space and time, they participate conjointly in various processes which the skeleton undergoes throughout life and which transcend the specific activity of each. No aspect of the resulting bone structure can therefore be understood in

Current Concepts of Bone Fragility

terms of one cell population alone. For that reason, they may be viewed conjointly as the effector organ of lamellar bone turnover system or EO LBTS (Jaworski, 1984a).

It would be difficult, however, to consider the mechanisms integrating into common function these two opposite cell populations as to their activity and asymmetric kinetics, without prior knowledge of the mode of individual cell assembly into the local populations. Moreover, without this knowledge, the pathogenesis of structural alterations responsible for bone fragility in various metabolic bone diseases cannot be effectively studied.

We propose, therefore, to review briefly first what is known about the mode of individual cell assembly in the local osteoblast or osteoclast populations; second, to consider the various ways the osteoblast and osteoclast populations associate in processes that establish and maintain mechanical skeletal competence (MCSk); and third, to conjecture how various etiologic factors, by interfering with the cellular processes in question, may produce structural alterations accounting for bone fragility in metabolic bone diseases.

Skeletal Development and Renewal

A. Embryonic stage

During this stage, basic anatomic relationships emerge that are characteristic of a given species (pattern development) along with the mechanisms for their subsequent growth (Wolpert, 1969). Thus, the development of bone structure is closely associated with that of the whole locomotor system, including the sites of tendon and muscle insertions on bone surfaces and of the bone marrow cavity within. These anatomic relations inscribed in the genome determine the mechanical loads to which the skeleton becomes subjected when assuming weight bearing and physical activity against gravity. In that sense, therefore, the structure of bones which evolved during phylogeny of a given species is predetermined.

The basic bone structure emerges sequentially: elaboration of the cartilaginous bone model first (primary modeling), replaced subsequently by woven and then lamellar bone. In the future spongy parts of the skeleton, such as the short bones and epiphyses of long bones, this is related to the appearance of the ossification centers -- formation of the primary and secondary spongiosa -- which, as the cartilaginous bone model expands at the periphery, replace it from within. On the other hand, formation of diaphyses of long bones has two components. The first is the piecemeal transformation of the growing cartilage in the metaphyseal growth plate into spongiosa. While resorbed at the periphery (metaphyseal collar) and in the bone center (bone marrow cavity), spongiosa undergoes compaction in-between to form the core of the future diaphyseal cortex. The second component is the apposition of bone on the external diaphyseal surface where the original perichondrium is replaced by the periosteum.

During the substitution of woven and lamellar bone for the cartilaginous model, the shape and architecture of bones, including the trabecular pattern in the spongy parts of the skeleton, assume their final structure (secondary modeling).

B. Bone growth

The increase in bone size is basically due to the growth of the cartilaginous model (primary modeling) with its continuous sequential replacement by woven and lamellar bone as initiated during the embryonic stage (Frost, 1979).

C. Maintenance of shape and architecture of bone during growth

The maintenance of bone's basic shape and architecture, including the trabecular pattern in the spongy parts of the skeleton as they increase in size or pattern growth (Wolpert, 1969), has to be clearly distinguished from the preceding process. It is the result of the piecemeal removals and/or additions of lamellar bone, mainly on periosteal and endosteal surfaces, referred to as the formation and resorption drifts (Frost, 1973a). All skeletons are subjected to it.

Drifts are of two types: macrodrifts and microdrifts. Macrodrifts consist of extensive areas of bone resorption or formation, occurring in separate locations, ie, resorption on one bone surface and formation on the opposite one, implying the independent activation of these two processes in space. This can be expressed as follows:

$$\text{Abl} \longrightarrow \text{F} \qquad \text{and} \qquad \text{Acl} \longrightarrow \text{R}$$

where Abl refers to the appearance (activation) of osteblast populations producing a packet of lamellar bone (F), and Acl to the appearance (activation) of osteoclast populations, in separate locations, where bone is removed (R).

Microdrifts consist of smaller, microscopic areas of bone resorption, followed *in situ* by bone formation. They occur mainly on the endosteal trabecular surfaces where they are instrumental in the maintenance of the trabecular pattern in the spongy areas of the growing skeleton. When viewed three-dimensionally, such turnover sites or BMUs (basic multicellular units of bone turnover) begin with the appearance of osteoclasts (Acl), which during their limited life-span erode a cavity (or a negative quantum of bone tissue) (R), followed by the appearance of osteoblasts (Abl) refilling the cavity with new bone (or a positive quantum) (F). Consequently, a new structural unit of lamellar bone (BSU) is left behind. Such a sequence can be represented schematically as:

$$\text{Acl} \longrightarrow \text{R} \longrightarrow \text{Abl} \longrightarrow \text{F} \longrightarrow \text{BSU}$$

These local sites of bone turnover, in addition to establishing and maintaining the trabecular pattern within growing bones, also promote expansion of the bone marrow cavity, accommodating the growing bone marrow. This implies a negative bone balance within the microdrifts, basically due to the excess of erosive depth (MDE) over the thickness of deposited bone (MWT). The steady increase in bone size reflects the longitudinal and transverse bone growth exceeding the loss of bone from the endosteal envelope. After the cessation of growth, the continuous, uncompensated expansion of the bone marrow cavity accounts for the universal, age-related bone loss further accentuated in postmenopausal women.

D. Haversian turnover in the diaphyseal compacta

In larger, long living mammals, including man, a special form of BMU-based turnover, evolved in the diaphyseal compacta, produces haversian systems. It appears during the first year of postnatal growth in man (Amprino and Bairati, 1966; Johnson, L.C., 1964) and remains essentially unchanged throughout life as to form and presumably function.

E. Maturity

With the cessation of growth, the established shape and the architecture of bones as well as the trabecular pattern in the spongy parts of the skeleton remain essentially unchanged. While the internal or haversian turnover in the diaphyseal compacta continues, however, on the periosteal and endosteal surfaces drifts and microdrifts subside to assume the characteristics and probably function of the haversian turnover, ie, of the internal restructuring. Thus, the quanta of lamellar bone replace locally the quanta removed, although the net balance within the periosteal sites remains slightly positive and negative on the endosteal cortical and trabecular surfaces (Frost, 1973b).

Cellular Mechanisms

A. Origin and differentiation of bone cells

Osteoblasts originate from the stroma cell line and osteoclasts from the monocytic series of the bone marrow which also give rise to macrophages (Owen, 1980).

During embryogenesis, rapidly proliferating cells of the fertilized ovum first differentiate into the three basic layers: the endoderm, the mesoderm and the ectoderm. Subsequently, cells of each layer, as they divide, differentiate further until they reach the stage of the committed progenitors. They provide the functional cells which constitute the tissues composing the organs and systems. The committed progenitor cells, by dividing, may either replicate themselves and thus maintain their pool or give rise to the fully differentiated functional cells, both during the organism's growth and maturity. The fully differentiated cells on the other hand generally lose the potential to divide.

B. Types of cell populations

Two main types of cell populations exist: the static and the self-renewing (Leblond, 1964). The former, for example the nerve cells, once created may last as long as the organism, their size subsequently depending on their original number and cell life-span (Jaworski, 1984a). The life-span of the self-renewing cell populations is limited; recruited from the dividing progenitors, they replace those that are lost. During the embryonic stage, both the static and self-renewing cell populations expand, the latter because the rate of their recruitment is faster than their attrition.

C. Osteoblasts and osteoclasts: A special type of self-renewing cell populations

These cells differ from other self-renewing cell populations in two important ways. First, in contrast to skin or gut epithelium, they operate as cohorts of discrete in-space (circumscribed) and time (transient) cell populations. This reflects two separate aspects of the committed progenitor cells' activities: a discrete location of their assembly (activation), and the subsequent rate and duration of their divisions.

The appearance in a given location of a discrete population of osteoblasts or osteoclasts implies a local recruitment and assembly of functional cells from the dividing committed progenitors. The activation, therefore, constitutes the basic determinant of lamellar bone turnover, suggesting some specific local conditions on bone surfaces required for activation. The number of such activated sites, that is the activation frequency (Frost, 1969), implies that such local conditions, whatever they may be, although discrete, are distributed in a characteristic and recurring pattern (Amprino and Marotti, 1964). This represents, as it were, a spatial horizontal aspect of committed progenitor cell activity. Activation constitutes a separate event from the subsequent rate and duration of committed progenitor cells' division which, along with the life-span and the fate of the differentiated functional cells, will determine the size and the life-span of the local osteoblast or osteoclast population (Jaworski, 1984a), presumably representing a spatial, vertical aspect of their activity.

Second, osteoblast and osteoclast populations differ from other cells or tissues by the nature of their product, ie, a properly structured extracellular material forming a rigid core of the locomotor system. Thus, the establishment of, and changes in, bone structure have two aspects: lamellar bone turnover as such and its mirror image, for example, its underlying cellular mechanisms. Methods of study relying on bone mineral content, such as radiographs, or on constituents of bone matrix, such as GLA or hydroxyproline measured in plasma or urine, must ignore the latter.

D. The effector organ of lamellar bone turnover (EO LBTS)

1. Sources of information

Information concerning the mode of individual cells assembling into local osteoblast and osteoclast populations is derived mainly from the study of cell kinetics in the evolving secondary haversian systems (Jaworski and Hooper, 1980; Jaworski et al, 1981). In such sites, the osteoclast and osteoblast populations are clearly separated, the former constituting the leading cutting cone and the latter, following it, the closing cone (Johnson, 1964) as shown in Figure 1. In the external two-thirds of diaphyseal compacta these systems are in balance, the rate of bone resorption and formation as well as the volumes of bone resorbed and produced being equal (Fig. 2). Consequently, the study of osteoclast and osteoblast kinetics may reveal how the net balance in such systems is achieved.

Such studies rely on their two-dimensional aspects, provided by cross or longitudinal sections (a usual study method). To interpret them correctly, however, one has to view the evolving haversian systems three-dimensionally and throughout their whole transit through bone tissue space.

2. Osteoclasts

The appearance of osteoclasts in a given location is termed activation (Frost, 1973b). Although the newly recruited mononuclear osteoclasts may derive from locally-dividing progenitors or may migrate from elsewhere to

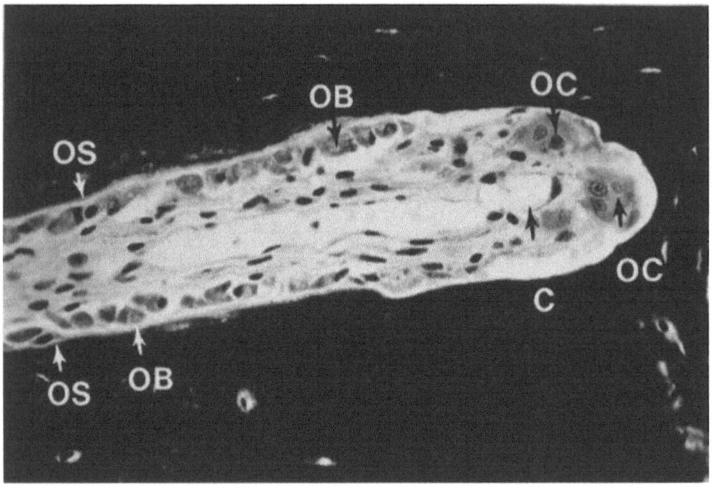

Fig. 1. This longitudinal section through the evolving secondary haversian system shows the osteoclast front (OC) and the monolayers of osteoblasts (OB) perpendicularly to the walls of the eroded cavity. Behind the osteoclasts, capillaries (C) and supporting tissue can be identified. The whole unit moves across the bone (to the right) at 40 to 50 µ per day. (Photomicrograph courtesy of Dr. R.K. Schenk, Bern University, Switzerland)

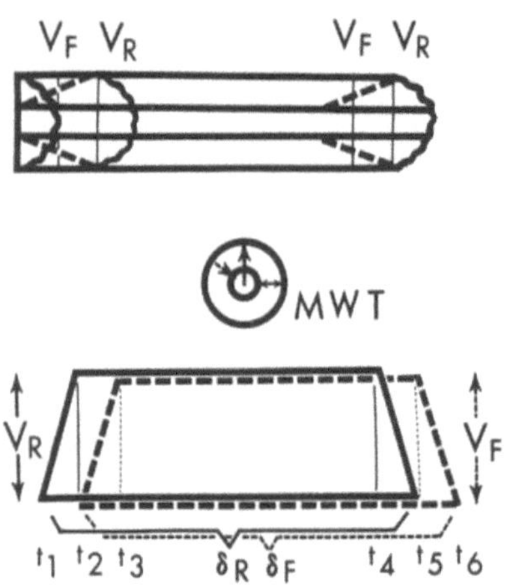

Fig. 2. Schematic representation of an evolving secondary osteon. Top: the cutting cone; following it, closing cone (moving from left to right). Middle: cross-section (MWT-mean wall thickness). Bottom: graphic representation of bone resorption rate by the cutting cone (Vr) and bone formation by the closing cone (Vf) at various stages of osteon's evolution. T_1: onset of cutting cone formation; T_2: completion of cutting cone formation and onset of closing cone formation; T_3: completion of closing cone formation; T_3-T_4: rates of bone resorption by the cutting cone (Vr) and of bone formation in the closing cone (Vf) in the constituted, evolving system are equal; T_4, completion of the new haversian system. (Jaworski et al, 1981).

the site of activation, the multinuclear osteoclasts (osteoclasts) are formed by fusion of mononuclear cells. They then continue to shed old and to co-opt new mononuclear cells during their life-span. Each osteoclast represents, therefore, a subdivision of the total mononuclear population that, due to the osteoclasts' motility, can provide a flexible spatially-oriented resorption process leaving cavities of varied shapes and orientations in bone space.

As shown in Figure 2, the rate of resorption by the cutting cone where the osteoclasts are tightly packed (Vr) is a product of cell efficiency (E), ie, resorption rate per nucleus, of which the linear resorption rate of about 50 microns per day provides an index (Jaworski et al, 1975) and the number of nuclei in the osteoclast population; in turn, the latter in a steady state is the product of nucleus mean life-span and of the number of new nuclei entering the population in a unit time (recruitment rate).

Once created, the size of the osteoclast population remains steady (evolving haversian systems) because the recruitment of new mononuclear cells equals the exit of the older cells from the population. Given also a particular efficiency of bone resorption per typical osteoclast nucleus, the rate of resorption by the cutting cone, as shown in Figure 2, would remain constant throughout the life-span of the cell population. However, the total volume of bone resorbed in making a completed osteon (Vol R) will depend also on the duration of the resorption front advance (T_1-T_2), ie, a period during which the new mononuclear cells continue to enter the population to replace others leaving it, which will be equal to the life-span of the whole osteoclast population. Consequently, assuming constant osteoclast efficiency and nuclei life-span, the total volume removed (Vol R) will be determined mainly by the rate and duration of the precursor cells' divisions.

The total volume of bone removed (Vol R) depends, in the haversian system, on the length of the tunnel resorbed (the length of the cutting cone advance) and its cross-sectional area. The latter depends on the radius or the depth of the erosion (MDE) which varies with the number of osteoclasts forming the cutting cone. In the paramedullary systems, the MDE is larger than in more peripheral systems. In the turnover sites on the endosteal and periosteal surfaces in adults, the MDE seems to vary less and the Vol R may depend more on the cavity surface area which may vary more with the number of osteoclasts in the resorption front. The standard MDE may be due to the osteoclastic front passing parallel to the bone surface, the osteoclast thus removing the layer of lamellar bone, 60-80 microns thick.

Consequently, the time required to resorb the whole thickness of bone tissue by the passing osteclastic front may be, in reality, very short (3-6 days), compared with the time required to form the whole thickness of the lamellar bone by osteoblasts (2-3 months) (Frost, 1969). In fact, the time required to erode the MDE equals the time the cutting cone takes to move its whole length from its tip to the base as shown in Figures 1 and 2 (Jaworski et al, 1975).

On the other hand, the size and configuration of the osteoclast front as well as the direction of its advance will determine the shape and orientation of the eroded cavity.

It appears that the number of cells in the population, the rate of the bone resorption (Vr) by the constituted cutting cone, the duration of the resorption process (T_1-T_2) and, finally, the volume and configuration of the resorbed cavity (Vol R) are all derivative of both fixed and flexible properties and are amenable to inherent controls of this cell system (Jaworski et al, 1981).

3. Osteoblasts

Osteoblasts derive from the committed progenitors dividing behind the advancing cutting cone within the so-called transitional zone (Baron et al,

1981). As soon as they are differentiated, they begin to deposit parallel to the bone surface lamellae of osteoid which then mineralize after about eight days' lag, referred to as maturation period. Thus, the evolving secondary haversian systems show longitudinal initiation of osteoid deposition and mineralization which advance at the speed of the osteoclastic fronts -- about 50 microns per day (Jaworski et al, 1975) -- as well as bone apposition perpendicularly to the bone surface at about 1-2 microns per day. Since the osteoblasts themselves do not move, a given osteoblast becomes progressively more distant from the advancing cutting cone separated from it by the newly recruited osteoblasts in front and from the original resorption surface by the layers of lamellar bone which they have deposited in the meantime (Fig. 1). Thus, while osteoblasts do not move themselves, the whole osteoblast population constituting the closing cone moves en block behind the cutting cone. The closing cone maintains the same configuration as well as the rate of bone formation (Vf) because the newly recruited osteoblasts in front replace cells that are lost from the population as osteocytes and finally lining cells (Fig. 2).

For reasons better understood than in the case of osteoclasts, one dimension of the packet of lamellar bone so produced remains relatively constant, namely the unit's wall thickness (MWT), because it is limited by a potential maximum. Thus, as in the case of the cavity, the volume of bone produced (Vol F) depends mainly on the site's formation surface area.

The wall thickness (MWT) cannot exceed 60-80 microns because it is produced by the original monolayer of osteoblasts. When fully differentiated they have a surface density of about 4000 per mm^2 (Jaworski and Wieczorek, 1985). Their density decreases, however, as the osteoblasts are lost from the original population as osteocyes at a rate proportional to the lamellar bone apposition (Frost, 1960). Since fewer osteoblasts remain on the osteoid surface and they are connected by the gap junctions, they progressively flatten to become lining cells (Marotti, 1976) with the terminal surface density of about 2000 per mm^2.

As mentioned, the life-span of the whole osteoblast population of the closing cone, as seen in three dimensions, is much longer than the life-span of the osteoblasts within the original monolayer reaching the bone surface as a lining cell, ie, the time to produce the whole wall thickness (MWT). Furthermore, it will last as long as the new osteoblasts continue to be recruited behind the cutting cone. The total volume of lamellar bone produced by such a cell population in a completed osteon (Vol F) will depend, therefore, on the life-span of the whole population. Contrary to the life-span of the osteoblast, therefore, limited by its recruitment and operation mode, the life-span of the whole population depends on the duration of the osteoblasts precursors' local division (T_1-T_2). In other words, assuming constant cell efficiency and life-span, the total volume of a packet of lamellar bone produced (Vol F) will depend mainly on the rate and duration of the precursor cells' divisions. The MWT, on the other hand, depends on the rate of osteoblast recruitment, ie, the precursors' division rate, allowing for their optimum surface density (about 4000 per mm^2).

Consequently, the number of cells in the population, the rate of bone formation (Vf) by the whole closing cone, the duration of bone formation and, finally, the volume (Vol F) and the configuration of a packet or quantum of bone formed derive from both the inherently fixed and flexible properties of the osteoblasts, the latter presumably amenable to control, ie, control variables (Jaworski, 1984a).

As to the activation in the BMU-based haversian turnover, in particular, the osteoblasts locally follow osteoclasts and bone resorption (local coupling).

4. Asymmetry of osteoblast and osteoclast populations

Comparison of these two cell populations reveals their inherent asymmetry. First, their efficiency per cell or nucleus differ, osteoclasts being 20 to 40 times as efficient per nucleus as the osteoblasts (Jaworski et al, 1981). Assuming, therefore, a standard efficiency and life-span, 20 to 40 times as many osteoblasts as osteoclasts (osteoclast nuclei) will be required to maintain local equilibrium (Fig. 2). The actual cell counts agree with that estimate: 80 osteoclastic nuclei per cutting cone and approximately 2000-4000 osteoblasts in the closing cone (Jaworski et al, 1981). Thus, to achieve any given bone balance in a given evolving turnover site, assuming unchanging efficiency and cells' life-span, a conjoint regulation of their respective precursor cells' division rates and durations is required.

The motility of osteoclasts and immobility of osteoblasts represent another important difference between these two types of cells bearing on the behavior of their respective cell populations, as discussed in the previous section.

The different fate and life-span of cells within each population, to a large extent determined genetically, are equally important. Thus, the transformation of osteoblasts into osteocytes in the process of bone apposition imposes a limit to the wall thickness (MWT). On the other hand, the depth of erosion (MDE) is presumably due to a single passage of osteoclasts forming the resorption front, parallel to the bone surface (in the direction opposite to the lamellar bone apposition), both in the haversian turnover sites, where the radius represents the depth of erosion (MDE), and in such sites on the endosteal and periosteal surfaces.

5. Sites of intervention (or interference) within the EO LBTS

The committed progenitors of osteoclasts and osteoblasts, and the functional cells of each population to which they give rise, inherently fixed and flexible, are amenable to control properties (control variables) and constitute, therefore, the effector organ of lamellar turnover system (EO LBTS).

The following control variables can be identified:

i. Location of new sites activation and activation frequency of osteoblast populations (primary lamellar bone formation during growth) and of osteoclasts. Thus, resorption and formation drifts imply separate sites of osteoblast and osteoclast activation. In the BMU-based turnover, however, as in microdrifts and haversian systems, the activation of osteoclast and osteoblast populations is locally linked or coupled, osteoblasts following osteoclasts.

ii. Local rate (determining the population size) and duration of osteoclast progenitors division (determining the volume of the cavity).

iii. The spatial organization of osteoclasts in the resorption front and direction of its movement, determining the shape of the BSU (the surface area of cavity varying more than the MDE).

iv. Local rate (determining the MWT) and the duration of osteoblast progenitors' division (determining along with the MDE the volume of the packet of lamellar bone produced).

Presumably, under normal circumstances, all these variables are simultaneously controlled but to a varied degree. Actually, the location of the activation sites, activation frequency (their spatially horizontal aspect), and the evolution of created functional cell populations (their spatially vertical aspects) may be controlled by different factors.

In abnormal situations, however, pathogenic factors may affect these sites of the EO LBTS control, the efficiency, and the life-span of the cells. As to the osteoblasts' functions, they may further interfere with osteoid synthesis (appositional rate) and the rate of its mineralization (Mineralization defect or lag time).

Afferent Loop (Feedback Mechanisms)

A. Nature and origin of signals

Theoretically, cell populations constituting the effector organ of LBTS could be so programmed genetically that all phases and forms of bone turnover could evolve automatically. Convincing evidence has shown, however, that the growing and the adult skeleton can adjust the structure to meet the actual mechanical demands. Therefore, as shown in Figure 3, osteoclast and osteoblast populations would represent conjointly an organ through which both the genetic, or intrinsic, instructions and the extrinsic, or environmental, factors could express themselves in bone structure.

It follows from the foregoing analysis that the opposite activities of osteoclasts and osteoblasts, ie, bone resorption and formation in all the processes which the skeleton undergoes, are integrated by a conjoint regulation of the respective control variables.

This implies the existence, on the one hand, of signals or stimuli distributed throughout the bone tissue and, presumably, generated by strains related to mechanical loading (Bassett, 1971). On the other hand, it implies the inherent specific, genetically determined cell responsiveness or sensitivity. It is a specific mode of interaction between the committed progenitor and/or functional cells and the pattern of signals and stimuli paralleling the strains, referred to as morphogenetic fields (Jaworski, 1984a). Thus, the space-oriented and structure-producing activity of EO LBTS cannot be regulated simply by growth factors or hormones. The latter can regulate the rate of cell proliferation or their function but not their spatial supracellular organization. Although the nature of the signals is not yet known, it may consist of electric streaming potentials (Eriksson, 1976) or of biochemical gradients related to changes in local hemodynamics produced by strain patterns under the condition of mechanical loading. One could conjecture that osteoblasts and osteoclasts, according to their respective inherent responsiveness, cluster according to such electric or biochemical gradients, and appear respectively in areas which biomechanically would be appropriate for the skeleton's supportive function (Bassett, 1971; Roberts et al, 1982).

B. Implications of osteoblast and osteoclast asymmetry

To achieve a given structural objective, the asymmetry of these two types of cells requires a complex balance act. As indicated in the preceding section, to achieve a balance within the evolving turnover site, due to different efficiencies and life-spans, a conjoint but differential regulation is required of the respective precursor cells' division rates and durations. Similarly, during growth, the maintenance of bone shape and architecture by means of resorption and formation of macro- and microdrifts in modeling and gross remodeling, requires an appropriate differential control of the respective populations' activition, and within sites, of respective cells' recruitment rates and durations. Presumably, the cells of each population respond specifically to a type or intensity of signals generated by strains, related to intrinsic or extrinsic mechanical loading. The first is related to growth of the whole locomotor system, and the second to the actual weight bearing and physical activity.

C. EO LBTS and processes which the skeleton undergoes

1. Preadaptation of bone structure

During the enbryonic stage the skeleton develops with the whole locomotor system, including the joints, tendons, muscles with their neurologic control, and the bone marrow. During the parallel growth of each element of the locomotor system, the genetically determined anatomic relations, such as the location of tendon and muscle insertions on bone surfaces, grossly remain the same. They determine the type of strains to which bones are submitted with actual mechanical usage, ie, weight bearing and physical exertion.

Apparently the structure of bone, considering the material they are made of, adapt during phylogenesis to the actual mechanical usage beginning during the postnatal period. In other words, their structure is such that on actual loading the strains remain within an optimal range.

2. Bone growth and adaptation

As all parts of the organism grow at approximately the same rate and the anatomic relations within the locomotor system remain the same, the structure of the growing bones, ie, their growth pattern, should also change at the same rate (Wolpert, 1969).

Increase of bone size (basically due to growth of the cartilaginous model), however, creates, until the arrest of growth, an imbalance between the bone structure trailing behind and the anatomic relations within the whole locomotor system. The actual weight bearing and physical exertion against gravity may reinforce the bending strains on bone surfaces (Frost, 1982; Lanyon, 1982) to which the EO LBTS responds appropriately, and intense translocations take place, such as drifts and microdrifts of lamellar bone tissue.

It appears, therefore, that the specific shape and architecture of bones evolve in a given species to optimize the strains resulting from the pattern of mechanical loading imposed by anatomic relations within the whole locomotor system. Such strains should remain strong enough to generate signals within bone tissue required for EO LBTS activity but below the range of mechanical fatigue (Frost, 1982).

As to the haversian turnover, since it is seen only in large, long-living mammals, its function from the beginning may consist in maintaining that quality of bone tissue which depends on its internal structure and grain as well as its mean age. With aging, bone tissue appears less resilient, being more susceptible to mechanical fatigue. Internal reconstruction and renewal would, therefore, on the one hand, reduce microdamage in areas of maximal strain and, on the other hand, prevent its accumulation.

3. LBTS in the mature skeleton

With the cessation of growth, bone shape, architecture and the pattern and intensity of mechanical loading finally equilibrate. Furthermore, with the surface strains diminishing, the macro- and microdrifts on the periosteal and endosteal surfaces, driven by growth of the cartilage, largely subside and assume the form and function of the haversian turnover in the diaphyseal compacta, ie, of internal reconstruction and renewal.

4. Effect of biomechanical factors on bone volume (strength)

Bones tend to be more massive in individuals who have been physically active during growth (Doyle et al, 1970); similarly, after the cessation of growth muscular activity appears to mitigate (but not to reverse) age-related bone loss or to balance the expansion of bone marrow cavity versus the periosteal gains (Hayes and Carter, 1979). This is reflected in the diaphyseal cortex thickness and thickness and number of trabeculae. Such an adjustment is mediated by the EO LBTS, ie, the depth of erosion (MDE) versus the mean wall thickness (MWT) in the drift areas and within the turnover sites on the periosteal, paramedullary haversian, and endosteal surfaces.

5. Components of skeleton mechanical competence

From the point of view of the skeleton as a whole, all the processes which it undergoes throughout life, especially those in which the EO LBTS participates -- the shaping of bone, their internal structuring with derivative bone renewal, and the adjustment of bone volume -- represent different functions of the same cell system. These functions are all geared towards the establishment and maintenance of the skeleton's competence and its supportive functions (MCSk), meaning its capacity to remain intact during customary mechanical usage.

All structural components of the skeleton's mechanical competence appear geared towards the optimization of strains produced by mechanical loading, strains sufficiently strong to generate signals to which EO LBTS may respond but below the level producing mechanical fatigue (Frost, 1982).

Permissive and Modulatory Factors

Although genetic factors, the inherent potential activities of EO LBTS cell populations, determine primarily the kind of their responses, biomechanical factors appear to regulate them further [specific feedback mechanism between the product and its cells (Fig. 3)]. They also require in their

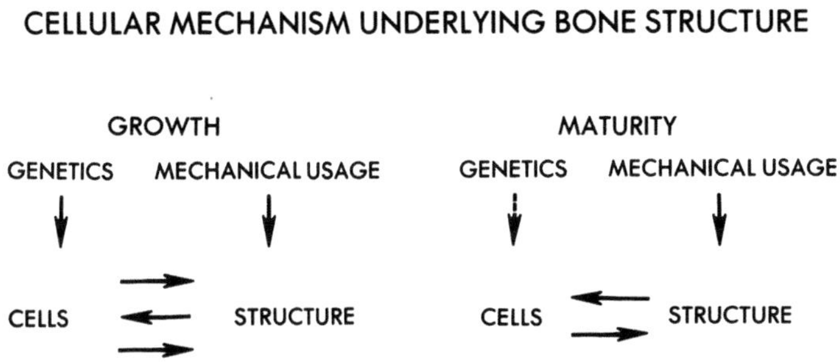

Fig. 3. During embryogenesis, the genetically determined potential of chondroblasts and EO LBTS accounts for the establishment and maintenance of bone structure (upper →) although the actual mechanical usage (weight bearing and physical exertion) via a specific feedback mechanism (middle ←) directs the EO LBTS activity towards further adjustment of bone structure to mechanical requirements (lower →). With cessation of growth during maturity, bone's mass, shape, and architecture are basically established and the MCSk is maintained by the EO LBTS activity referred to as remodeling.

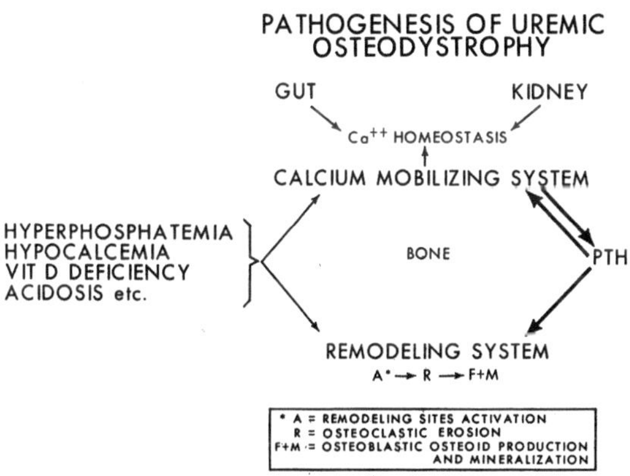

Fig. 4. Schematic representation of the linkage by parathyroid hormone (PTH) of calcium ion homeostasis in body fluids and the bone remodelling system. A = remodeling site activation; R = osteoclastic erosion; F+M = osteoid production and mineralization. Various disturbances in the biochemical milieu of bone cells, due to diseases of locomotor system and of extraskeletal tissues, organs, and systems constitute the clinical context of metabolic bone disease. (Jaworski, 1974)

microenvironment the presence of permissive factors related to the adequate function of several organs and systems (Table II). Nonspecific permissive factors include those necessary for the function of any body cells, such as a supply of oxygen and energy sources and removal of waste products. They also include specific factors on which the function of a given type of cell or tissue depends. The EO LBTS may be affected further, directly or indirectly, by modulatory factors, such as parathyroid hormone, vitamin D metabolites or estrogens, which link LBTS with the system maintaining calcium ion homeostasis in body fluids (Fig. 4).

Evidently, the lack or excess of the permissive or modulatory factors, due to disorders of a number of extraskeletal systems or organs or the presence of toxic substances in the cellular milieu (Table II), may interfere in various ways with the function of the EO LBTS, producing some characteristic, structural alterations of a given metabolic bone disease. Hence, the EO LBTS is not only important in establishing and maintaining the MCSk but also in the pathogenesis of structural alterations resulting in bone fragility.

Table II. Etiologic factors

I. INTRINSIC FACTORS (regulatory)

A. Withdrawal of the biomechanical stimuli (role of locomotor system: diseases of nervous sytem, muscles, joints, and bones)

B. Decline in inherent proliferation potential of bone cell precursors (age)*

II. EXTRINSIC FACTORS (modulatory and permissive)

A. Excess or lack of modulatory factors: disorders of calcium homeostasis or sex hormones (estrogens in women)

B. Excess or lack of permissive factors: dysfunction of almost all other systems:

1) endocrine (sex hormones, thyroid, adrenal)
2) gastrointestinal system (malabsorption)
3) nutrition (calcium, phosphate, vitamin D, proteins, vitamin C)
4) renal (parenchymal and tubular diseases)
5) hematologic and neoplastic disorders

C. Drugs and toxic factors (antacids, anticonvulsants, corticosteroids, alcohol, fluorides) not normally found internally.

* Decreased activation frequency as well as the rate and duration of differentiated cell recruitment.

Lining Cell - Osteocytic System and Calcium Ion Homeostasis

In addition to their structural role, bones constitute a vast reservoir of mineral in itself, a component of the system maintaining calcium ion homeostasis in body fluids. On a microscopic level, a huge surface consisting of the walls of osteocytic lacunae and canaliculae communicate with the surface beyond the lining cells on bone envelopes. Controlled mainly by the parathyroid hormone, calcium fluxes in and out of this compartment contribute to the short-term calcium ion homeostasis in body fluids (Matthews et al, 1977). Thus, the parathyroid hormone links the EO LBTS, both the osteoclasts and osteoblasts, with calcium ion homeostasis. Under normal circumstances, these two cell systems, while linked, do not interfere with each other's function but under pathologic conditions, as in a negative calcium balance, they may affect the EO LBTS functions and MCSk (Fig. 4).

Structural Causes of Bone Fragility

A. Pathology of bone cells' milieu

As mentioned above, lack or excess of permissive or modulatory factors in bone cell environment (Table II) or the presence of toxic materials may interfere with the primary function of EO LBTS.

It may be useful to distinguish between the pathogenesis of lack or excess of permissive or modulatory factors due to dysfunction of extraskeletal tissues, organs and systems (Table II) and the pathogenesis of various structural alterations causing bone fragility, such as EO LBTS dysfunctions (Table III).

Table III. Structural causes of bone fragility in metabolic bone disease

I. IRREVERSIBLE OSTEOPENIA (↓TBV): OSTEOPOROSIS

II. REVERSIBLE OSTEOPENIA (↑RMSp)

- A. Tissue level origin (↑ activation frequency)
- B. BMU level origin (↑sigma)
    - 1) Formation phase (sigma F)
        - a) ↓appositional rate (effective, actual)
        - b) intermittency (on and off)
        - c) mineralization lag (↑MOT)
            - delayed matrix maturation
            - inhibitor
            - mineral delivery
    - 2) Resorption phase (sigma R)
        - a) ↓resorption rate (?)
        - b) resorption block (osteitis fibrosa)
        - c) extension (MDE, ie, disuse osteoporosis, active phase)

III. ↑MEAN (BSU) BONE AGE

- A. ↓ Bone turnover rate (↓ activation frequency)
- B. ↓ BMU turnover rate (↑ sigma)
    - 1) Formation block (osteomalacia, osteoporosis)
    - 2) Resorption block (osteitis fibrosa)

IV. DISORGANIZED BONE STRUCTURE (PAGET'S DISEASE)

For example, there are several causes of hyperparathyroidism, but only one expression of associated bone disease, ie, osteitis fibrosa. Similarly, osteomalacia, characterized by the accumulation of wide osteoid seams, may be due to several etiologic factors such as hypophosphatemia or deficiency of vitamin D metabolites.

B. Pathogenesis of structural alterations in bone fragility

The type of structural alterations (Table III) depends, grossly, first, on a given process which the skeleton undergoes; second, on the type of cell within the EO LBTS affected by the pathogenic factor; and, third on whether it will affect the progenitor cells (activation and subsequent rate and duration of their divisions) or the differentiated cells (their function, life-span, etc). Depending on the severity and the rate of accumulation, such structural alterations will affect bone strength and eventually lead to fractures in strategic locations.

Although some of these cell activities or their morphologic outcomes -- for example, MDE and MWT -- can be measured, the intimate mechanisms by which a given pathogenic factor affects the MDE or MWT, and/or the time to produce them, cannot be easily determined. In this area the gaps in our knowledge of the pathogenesis of metabolic bone diseases, particularly osteoporosis, are still considerable.

C. Types of structural alterations

Grossly, as shown in Table III, structural alterations include: reversible and irreversible osteopenias (osteoporosis proper), increase in mean bone age (with the accumulation of microdamage), and disorganized bone structure.

As shown in Figure 5, bone fragility usually results from an overlap of various structural alterations.

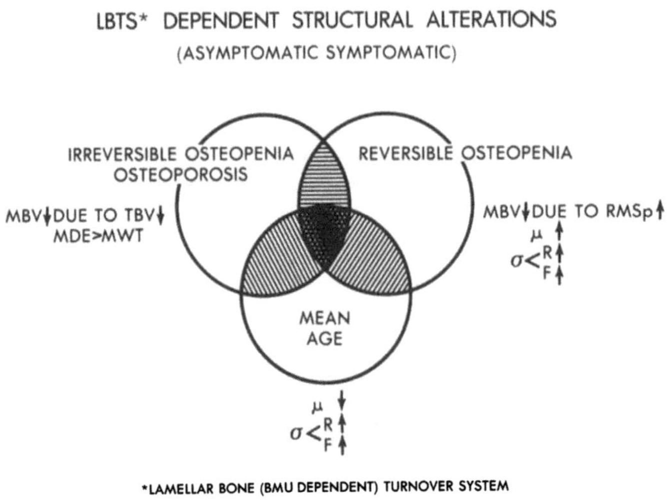

Fig. 5. Several structural alterations usually overlap in bone fragility syndromes. Accumulated microdamage may constitute their common final path leading to fractures in strategic locations. In Bone Fragility Syndrome of Aging (BFSA), the decrease in TBV combines with an increase in mean bone age, as a result of decrease in bone turnover (activation frequency (ν) and an increase in sigma (σ).

1. Osteopenias

Osteopenia, decreased bone density, radiographically visible, can be due to a decrease in mineral content or in amount of bone tissue. It may be further divided into reversible or irreversible types on morphologic grounds.

The piecemeal bone turnover that the skeleton undergoes underlies this classification. The total bone volume (TBV) represents the sum of mineralized bone volume (MBV) and of bone remodeling or turnover space (RMSp). The latter consists of the total volume of individual turnover sites in either the resorption or formation (osteoid) phase (Fig. 6). This may be expressed in the following equation:

$$TBV = MBV + RMSp$$

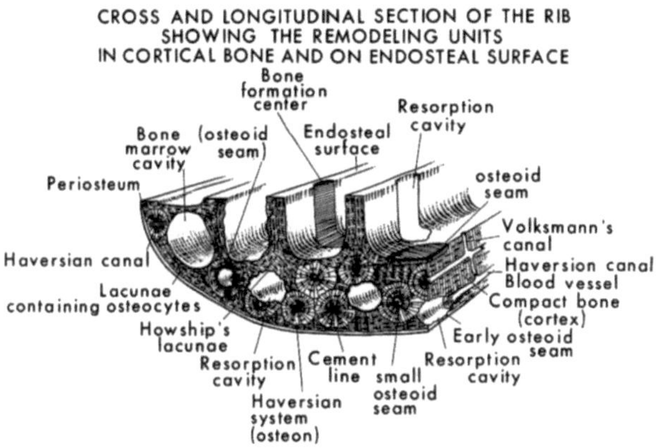

Fig. 6. Three-dimensional representation of a rib section showing cortical compacta and some trabeculae. Cement (reversal) line subdivides bone tissue into bone structural units (BSU), both in the compacta (the haversian systems) and on the endosteal-cortical and trabecular surface. BSUs are the outcome of local bone turnover sites, bone formation following the resorption of a cavity. In the compacta, such bone turnover units or BMUs (basic multicullular units of bone turnover) are represented by the evolving haversian systems; although morphology and dimensions differ, BMUs operate also on endosteal and periosteal bone surfaces. (Duncan and Jaworski, 1970)

a) Reversible osteopenias. Under normal circumstances, the RMSp represents a small proportion of TBV (Parfitt, 1980) and consequently MBV, paramount for supportive function, equals TBV (Fig. 7). In disease, however, the RMSp may expand considerably at the expense of MBV either because of increased activation frequency (bone turnover rate) or prolongation of the turnover time in individual sites (Fig. 7). For example, in severe osteitis fibrosa the RMSp expands because of increased activation frequency and the blockage of turnover sites in the resorption phase (bone marrow fibrosis). Similarly, in osteomalacia RMSp expands due to arrest of individual turnover sites in the bone formation phase. Consequently, mineralization defect or lag time causes osteoid accumulation at the expense of MBV. Furthermore, in both instances, the mean age of the MBV increases (Table III and Fig. 5).

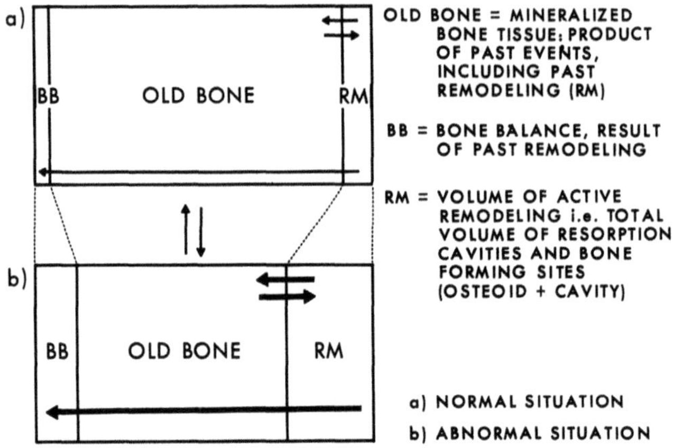

Fig. 7. Bone tissue compartments: old bone or MBV, remodeling space (RM), and bone balance (BB). Normally, [upper panel a)] RM represents a small fraction of TBV; TBV and MBV (old bone) differ little. Under steady state, new remodeling sites initiated within the preexisting old bone that enters the RM equal the number of remodeling sites completing their cycle and reentering the mineralized bone compartment as new structural units (BSUs) (short arrows in upper and lower panels). The BB on the left side of the rectangle represents the cumulative bone balance, positive or negative, resulting from the balances achieved in individual remodeling sites at the completion of the turnover cycles (in adults mainly on the endosteal bone envelope) (long arrow connecting the RM with the terminal or final BB). BB has to be distinguished clearly from the changes in MBV resulting from the change in the new remodeling sites' activation or in their life-span. When either one or both increase, the RM expands [lower panel b)] at the expense of old bone. This may have no effect on total BB, which is theoretically determined by the terminal BB at the BMU level. During the shift from one level of bone turnover to another [interrupted lines between panel a) and panel b)], which may be the result of a disease process [from a) to b)], change in MBV (old bone) may be due entirely to changes in RM, without the TBV being affected (reversible osteopenia). (Jaworski and Duncan, 1984)

The RMSp may expand also because of increased activation frequency, such as seen in thyrotoxicosis and early stages of hyperparathyroidism. In these cases, however, the mean bone age will decrease.

b) Irreversible osteopenia or osteoporosis proper. Irreversible osteopenia, on the other hand, means a decrease in MBV resulting from the decrease in TBV. This may be due to an inadequate buildup of bones during

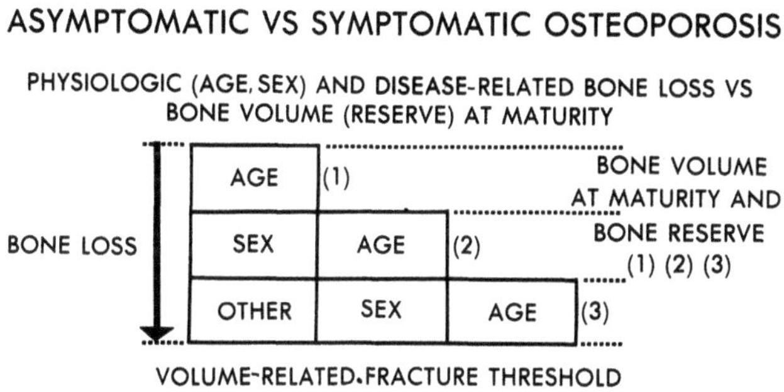

Fig. 8. Asymptomatic versus symptomatic osteoporosis (irreversible osteopenia). 1) In a person with adequate bone reserve, physiologic (age- and sex-related) bone loss alone is insufficient to produce osteoporosis. Additional reduction of mineralized bone volume or quality is required to cause fractures. 2) In those entering mature life with smaller bone reserve, the same physiologic (age- and sex-related) bone loss suffices to cause fractures sooner. 3) In women with an inadequate bone reserve, ordinary age-related bone loss will eventually result in fractures; they are also particularly vulnerable to any additional reduction in mineralized bone volume (irreversible or reversible) or impairment of its quality. (Jaworski and Duncan, 1984).

growth (developmental osteoporosis) or to bone losses, usually from the endosteal and paramedullary haversian surfaces, or as a result of a cumulative negative bone balance in the individual sites of turnover, MDE exceeding MWT (Fig. 8). Thus, the universal age-related bone loss on which all other specific causes of bone loss are superimposed (Table IV) is due to the continuous expansion of bone marrow cavity carried on from the growth period but no longer compensated by transverse bone growth (Jaworski, 1984b). MDE normally exceeds MWT in the haversian paramedullary systems. Since MWT is limited by a maximum (Jaworski and Wieczorek, 1985), the resulting increase in canal lumen, compared with osteons in the external two-thirds of the diaphyseal compacta, constitutes a morphologic substratum for the age-related bone loss in this area. Similarly, on the endosteal cortical and trabecular envelope, MDE exceeds consistently MWT throughout life, although the latter may decrease further with advancing age (Kragstrup et al, 1983; Lips et al, 1978) and even more so in specific osteoporoses (Darby and Meunier, 1981). Only during the reproductive life in women is this relationship apparently reversed (Garn, 1975).

The increase in MDE itself may be due to 1) the increased recruitment of osteoclasts, especially in the cutting cone of the haversian systems; 2) increased efficiency of osteoclasts; or 3) their increased life-span. On the other hand, the decrease in MWT below the potential maximum may be due to 1) the decreased recruitment rate of osteoblasts, producing the monolayer of cells with the surface density of less than 4000 per mm^2; 2) decreased efficiency per osteoblast; and 3) shortened life-span of osteoblasts (Jaworski, 1984b).

Table IV. Generalized osteoporoses (irreversible osteopenias)

I. DEVELOPMENTAL OSTEOPOROSES

- A. Osteogenesis imperfecta
- B. Disuse during growth

II. ADULT AGE-RELATED (physiologic)

III. INVOLUTIONAL

- A. Postmenopausal
- B. Senile

IV. RESIDUAL (post-high bone turnover)

- A. Disuse, phase III
- B. Corticosteroid, phase II
- C. Postthyrotoxicosis
- D. Posthyperparathyroidism

V. MISCELLANEOUS

- A. Myeloma
- B. Malnutrition (alcoholism)
- C. Heparin-induced
- D. Juvenile

Any bone loss due to an excess of MDE over MWT will be amplified on the paramedullary haversian and endosteal trabecular surfaces by increased activation frequency, ie, the bone turnover rate. This is due to the honeycomb structure in these areas. The thin plates connecting the horizontal and vertical trabeculae, as a result of the cumulative negative bone balance in individual turnover sites, will eventually sustain large irreversible perforations (Arnold, 1973).

Thus, osteoporoses can be broadly classified into two groups (Table IV). First, those due to the insufficient buildup during growth with normal age-related bone loss caused by the expansion of the bone marrow cavity. In this category one could also place osteogenesis imperfecta, where, in addition to an abnormal bone matrix, the development of bones is impaired. Second, osteoporoses due to the excessive bone loss regardless of bone volume accumulated at maturity, superimposed on universal age-related bone loss (Fig. 8).

2. Bone fragility syndrome of aging.

As shown in Figure 5, with aging several mechanisms lead to increased bone fragility, such as the bone fragility syndrome of aging (BFSA). The first is the reduction in MBV due to the decrease in TBV as a result of the expansion of bone marrow cavity (osteoporosis proper) and, the second, the increase in the bone mean age resulting in decrease in frequency activation and prolongation of bone turnover time (BMUs) (Frost, 1973b).

3. Disorganized structure.

The final category of structural causes of bone fragility could be the conditions of the disorganized bone structure such as Paget's disease of bone (Table III).

D. Strategic location of fractures in bone fragility syndromes

Interestingly, regardless of the specific structural alteration underlying bone fragility, the resulting fractures occur in the same preferred locations: in vertebrae, distal radius, proximal femur, ribs, or pelvic rami, contrary to fractures resulting from major trauma in normal bones which, depending on the circumstances, occur at the site of the impact. These preferred sites of fractures characterizing bone fragility indicate that within the skeleton, under normal circumstances, are biomechanically predetermined sites of potential weakness. Thus, the mechanical fatigue, ie, accumulation of microdamage, may constitute a final common path causing bone fragility and fractures for a variety of structural alterations (Fig. 5).

Acknowledgements

I wish to thank Mrs. Micheline Hoonaard for an expert preparation of the manuscript.

This paper is based on the studies supported by grants from the Medical Research Council of Canada from 1970 to 1983.

References

1. Amprino, R., and Bairati, A.: Processi di ricostruzione e di riassorbimento della sostanzea compatta delle ossa dell'uomo. Z. Zellforsch. 24, 439, 1966.

2. Amprino, R., and Marotti, G.: A topographic quantitative study of bone formation and reconstruction. In, Bone and Tooth Symposium. Ed., Blackwood, E.J.J. MacMillan Co., New York, 1964, pp 21-23.

3. Arnold, J.S.: Amount and quality of trabecular bone in osteoporotic vertebral fractures. Clin. Endocrinol. Metab. 2, 221, 1973.

4. Baron, R., Vignery, A., and Lang, R.: Reversal and osteopenia: defective coupling of resorption to formation in the pathogenesis of osteoporosis. In, Osteoporosis: Recent Advances in Pathogenesis and Treatment. Eds: DeLuca, H.F., Frost, H.M., Jee, W.S.S., Johnston, C.C. Jr., Parfitt, A.M. University Park Press, Baltimore, 1980. pp 311-320.

5. Bassett, C.A.L.: Biophysical principles affecting bone structure. In, The Biochemistry and Physiology of Bone. Vol. III (2nd edition). Ed: Bourne, G.H. Academic Press, New York and London, 1971, p. 1.

6. Darby, A.J., and Meunier, P.J.: Mean wall thickness and formation periods of trabecular bone packets in idiopathic osteoporosis. Calcif. Tissue Int. 33, 199, 1981.

7. Doyle, F., Brown, J., and Lachance, C.: Relation between bone mass and muscle weight. Lancet i, 391, 1970.

8. Duncan, H., and Jaworski, Z.F.G.: Osteoporosis. In, Tice's Practice of Medicine, Vol. V. Harper and Row, Hagerstown, Maryland, 1970, p. 1.

9. Eriksson, C.L.: Electrical properties of bone. In, The Biochemistry and Physiology of Bone. Vol. IV (2nd edition). Ed: Bourne, G.H. Academic Press, New York and London, 1976, p. 329.

10. Frost, H.M.: Measurement of osteocytes per unit volume and volume components of osteocytes and canaliculae in man. Henry Ford Hosp. Med. Bull. 8, 208, 1960.

11. Frost, H.M.: Tetracycline-based histologic analysis of bone remodeling. Calcif. Tissue Res. 3, 211, 1969.

12. Frost, H.M.: Bone Modeling and Skeletal Modeling Errors. Charles C. Thomas, Springfield, Ill., 1973a.

13. Frost, H.M.: Bone Remodeling and Its Relationship to Metabolic Bone Disease. Charles C. Thomas, Springfield, Ill., 1973b.

14. Frost, H.M.: A chondral modeling theory. Calcif. Tissue Int. 28, 181, 1979.

15. Frost, H.M.: Mechanical determinants of bone modeling. Metab. Bone Dis. Rel. Res. 4, 217, 1982.

16. Garn, S.M.: Bone loss and aging. In, Physiology and Pathology of Aging. Academic Press, New York, 1975. pp 39-57.

17. Hayes, W.C., and Carter, D.R.: Biomechanics of bone. In, Skeletal Research and Experimental Approach. Eds: Simmons, D.J. and Kunin, A. S. Academic Press, New York, 1979. pp 263-300.

18. Jaworski, Z.F.G.: Morphology and dynamics of bone remodeling in chronic renal failure. In, Proc., 5th Int. Congress of Nephrology. Ed.: Villard, H. S. Karger A.G., Basel, Switzerland, 1974. p. 149.

19. Jaworski, Z.F.G.: A lamellar bone turnover system and its effector organ. Calcif. Tissue Int. 36, S46, 1984a.

20. Jaworski, Z.F.G.: Coupling of bone formation to bone resorption: A broader view (Editorial). Calcif. Tissue Int. 36, 531, 1984b.

21. Jaworski, Z.F.G., and Duncan, H.: Osteoporosis. In, Clinical Medicine (Chapter 53). Ed: Spittell, J.A. Jr. Harper and Row, Philadelphia, 1984. pp 1-18.

22. Jaworski, Z.F.G., and Hooper, C.: Study of cell kinetics within evolving secondary haversian systems. J. Anat. 131, 91, 1980.

23. Jaworski, Z.F.G., and Wieczorek, D.: Constants in lamellar bone formation determined by osteoblast kinetics. Bone 6, 361, 1985.

24. Jaworski, Z.F.G., Duck, B., and Sekaly, G.: Kinetics of osteoclasts and their nuclei in evolving secondary haversian systems. J. Anat. 133, 397, 1981.

25. Jaworski, Z.F.G., Lok, E., and Wellington, J.L.: Impaired osteoclastic function and linear bone erosion rate in secondary hyperthyroidism associated with chronic renal failure. Clin. Orthop. 107, 298, 1975.

26. Johnson, L.C.: Morphologic analysis in pathology. In, Bone Biodynamics. Little, Brown and Company, Boston, 1964. pp. 543-654.

27. Kragstrup, J., Melsen, F., and Mosekilde, L.: Thickness of bone formed at remodeling sites in normal human live trabecular bone: Variations with age and sex. Metab. Bone Dis. Rel. Res. 5, 17, 1983.

28. Lanyon, L.E.: Mechanical function and bone remodeling. In, Bone in Clinical Orthopaedics. Ed: Summer-Smith, G. W.B. Saunders, Philadelphia, 1982. p. 273.

29. Leblond, C.P.: Classification of cell populations on the basis of their proliferative behaviour. Nat. Cancer Inst. Monographs. 14, 119, 1964.

30. Lips, P., Coupron, P., and Meunier, P.J.: Mean wall thickness of trabecular bone packets in human iliac crest: Changes with age. Calcif. Tissue Res. 26, 13, 1978.

31. Marotti, G.: Decrement in volume of osteoblasts during osteon formation and its effect on the size of the corresponding osteocytes. In, Bone Histomorphometry, 2nd International Workshop. Ed: Meunier, P.J. Armour Montagu, Paris, 1976, pp 385-397.

32. Matthews, L.J., Talmage, R.V., Martin, J.H., and Davis, W.L.: Osteoblasts, bone lining cells and the bone fluid compartment. In, Bone Histomorphometry. Ed: Meunier, P.J. Armour Montagu, Paris, 1977, pp. 239-247.

33. Owen, M.: The origin of bone cells in the postnatal organism. Arthritis Rheum. 23, 1073, 1980.

34. Parfitt, A.M.: Morphologic basis of bone mineral measurements: transient and steady state effects of treatment in osteoporosis mineral. Electrolytes Metab. 4, 273, 1980.

35. Roberts, W.E., Smith, R.K., and Cohen, J.A.: Change in electrical potential within periodontal ligament of a tooth subjected to osteogenic loading. In, Factors and Mechanisms Influencing Bone Growth. Eds: Dixon, A.D. and Sarnal, B.G. Allan R. Liss, New York, 1982.

36. Wolpert, L.: Positional information and the spatial pattern of cellular differentiation. J. Theor. Biol. 25, 1, 1969.

Diagnostic and Monitoring Tools

Diagnosis and Follow-up of Patients with Osteoporosis

C. C. JOHNSTON, JR.

It has been estimated that over 1.3 million fractures associated with osteoporosis occur each year in the U.S.A. alone, incurring costs over $3.8 billion a year (NIH Consensus on Osteoporosis, 1984).

The disease is characterized by low bone mass and fractures. Those fractures commonly associated with osteoporosis are of the vertebrae, distal radius, hip, proximal humerus and tibia, and the pelvis. For each type of these fractures, their incidence increases with age, predominantly in women. It has generally been considered that these fractures result from the same process of bone loss. Recently, however, it has been suggested that some of these fracture syndromes may differ pathogenetically (Riggs and Melton, 1983; Riggs et al, 1982).

Type I osteoporosis occurs primarily in women aged 51 to 65, and is associated with vertebral and distal radial fractures, probably caused by excessive loss of trabecular bone. Type II osteoporosis occurs in women and men over age 75, is associated with fractures of the hip, proximal humerus, proximal tibia and pelvis, and is due to loss of both cortical and trabecular bone.

We have recently had the opportunity to evaluate a group of women with vertebral crush fractures and hip fractures. Transiliac biopsies and bone mass measurements have confirmed that the two fracture syndromes apparently differ (Johnston et al, in press, (b)). The most striking differences were found in the iliac crest biopsies. Patients with crush fractures had significantly less trabecular bone measured as trabecular bone volume (TBV) than those with hip fractures ($12.0 \pm 4.4\%$ vs $14.8 \pm 3.6\%$, $p = .014$). Those with hip fractures had thinner cortices than those with crush fractures (436 ± 231 µm vs 823 ± 645 µm, $p < .01$). The TBV for crush fractures was significantly below that expected for age, but was significantly increased for age in the population with hip fractures. Surprisingly, radial cortical bone mass was not different between the two groups, perhaps indicating that the iliac crest cortices best reflect what is occurring at the femoral neck. We feel that these data are compatible with the hypothesis that crush fractures occur in a population of women with a significantly early deficit of trabecular bone.

It is not known, at present, whether these patients had a low trabecular mass at maturity or subsequently lost a greater amount. Hip fractures occur among a population that has lost both trabecular and cortical bone, but not

Current Concepts of Bone Fragility

an amount out of proportion to others of similar age who do not experience fractures. Of course, changes in bone mass at the femoral neck may not have been detected in this study; nevertheless, other factors, such as the presence of other diseases of bone (eg, osteomalacia or abnormalities in bone remodeling, and frequency and degree of trauma may be most important in predicting who among this group will have a fracture. We have, in fact, found documented osteomalacia in this population of patients with hip fractures who came from a retirement home for the elderly (Johnston et al, in press (b)). Unfortunately, we do not know the prevalence of this condition, but it certainly could be one remediable factor in hip fracture pathogenesis in the U.S.A.

Diagnosis of osteoporosis after the fracture occurs usually presents little problem. Most of the fractures of long bones are managed by orthopedists. Among these patients, especially the very old, other neuromuscular disease which may contribute to the frequency of trauma must be considered if repeated fractures are to be avoided. As noted above, osteomalacia must be considered, but we cannot estimate the magnitude of this problem. Bone biopsy may be necessary to establish the diagnosis, except in the most florid cases.

Vertebral osteoporosis, or crush fracture disease, is of principal concern to the primary physician. The patient, characteristically, is a postmenopausal caucasian woman, aged 50 to 65 years, who develops acute back pain with minimal trauma and is found to have a deformity of a vertebra on radiologic examination. Crush fractures may also develop asymptomatically (Gershon-Cohen et al, 1953), and it is difficult to judge the age of a deformity without previous films. Thus, a vertebral deformity may be seen, but the pain may be from another source.

When the diagnosis of spinal osteoporosis is considered, secondary causes of accelerated bone loss must be ruled out. These include excess serum levels of corticosteroids, either of endogenous or exogenous source; hyperthyroidism, and hyperparathyroidism (Table I). These diseases may have subtle clinical features, especially among the elderly, and great vigilance is required to detect these conditions.

Other diseases may masquerade as osteoporosis in the aging population, all of whom have lost bone and, thus, have a demineralized appearance on radio-

Table I. Conditions resembling osteoporosis

Secondary causes of bone loss
1) Excess glucocorticoids, endogenous or exogenous
2) Hyperthyroidism
3) Hyperparathyroidism
Differential diagnosis
1) Multiple myeloma
2) Metastatic disease
3) Osteomalacia

graphs. These other diseases include multiple myeloma, which may produce generalized demineralization and fracture, and metastatic disease with destruction of a vertebra (Table I).

Although the diagnosis of osteoporosis in a patient with a clinical fracture is seldom a problem, identification of the patient at risk of subsequent fractures at a time when effective preventive therapy can be undertaken is considerably more difficult. Many of our conclusions regarding risk factors are related to risk of developing low bone mass. A recent review of case-control studies of hip fractures (Cummings, 1985) concluded that low bone mass did not differ significantly between elderly subjects with fractures and without fractures. This finding would bring into question risk factors determined solely on bone mass. As noted by Cummings, however, a number of problems exist with all these studies, particularly inadequate measurement of bone mass at the site of the fracture. Nevertheless, these studies call for caution when interpreting the suggested risk factors.

As noted above, different fracture syndromes may have different pathogeneses and, thus, different risk factors may apply to each. A prospective study of a cohort followed from the menopause to time of fracture is needed but, at present, no such data are available.

Nevertheless, decisions must be made regarding prevention of bone loss, especially the use of estrogen replacement therapy, on the basis of the best available evidence. A review of the problem of prevention of age-related bone loss has been recently published (Johnston, 1984).

Table II. Principal risk factors for osteoporosis

Age
Female
Estrogen deficiency
Slender body habitus
Race - caucasian

Table II shows the principal risk factors in the development of osteoporosis as we now understand them. Since bone loss increases with age, and women have lower bone mass at maturity than men and experience accelerated bone loss after the menopause (Hui et al, 1982), postmenopausal women are at highest risk of low bone mass. Evidence also suggests that caucasian women are at higher risk of fractures than other races (Melton and Riggs, 1983), although few good epidemiologic studies are available on blacks, orientals, or hispanos. Estrogen deficiency is probably one of the leading risk factors for accelerated bone loss; thus, surgical oophorectomy or early menopause are important risks. A slender body build is also a risk factor, although the mechanism here is not clear. Perhaps body fat provides some protection, either because of its mechanical effect or, more likely, because of the increased production of estrone from androstenedione due to aromatase activity in the fat tissue (Johnston et al, in press (a)). Thus, slender, postmenopausal, caucasian women are the group at highest risk.

Other factors may add to the risk of low bone mass (Table III). Calcium deficiency, which is common in older women, may be responsible for acceler-

Table III. Secondary risk factors

Calcium deficiency
Immobilization or sedentary lifestyle
Family history
Alcohol or tobacco abuse
Disease
Glucocorticoid excess
Hyperthyroidism
Hyperparathyroidism
Chronic obstructive pulmonary disease (COPD)
Malabsorption
Liver disease

ated bone loss, and calcium supplementation may slow bone loss (Heaney et al, 1982). Immobilization is associated with increased bone loss, and the extremes of exercise can be associated with an increase in bone mass; however, the effect of exercise within the normal range of daily activity is not, as yet, clear (Johnston, 1984). No studies have been published on the genetic contribution to fractures, but there is a genetic determinant of peak bone mass (Smith et al, 1973) and, thus, a family history of osteoporosis may be important. Alcohol (Seeman et al, 1983) and tobacco abuse (Baron, 1984) may also contribute to the risk of low bone mass and osteoporotic fractures. A number of diseases are also associated with low bone mass and, thus, can contribute to fracture pathogenesis (Table III).

Recently, numerous methods have been reported which are useful in making precise and accurate assessment of bone mass, either at specific sites or for the skeleton as a whole (Mazess, 1983). These methods may be of value in determining risk of fracture and in following up patients, but their exact role has yet to be determined. It is apparent that bone at different sites in the skeleton behaves differently under different conditions (Seeman et al, 1983). This applies especially to differences between trabecular and cortical bone, but it is also possible that cortical or trabecular bone in different areas of the skeleton may behave differently. Thus, it may not be possible to draw conclusions concerning the area of interest unless that area is measured; eg, if the interest is in vertebral fracture, vertebrae should be measured.

These measurements probably play a small role in the assessment of patients with fractures unless therapy to increase bone mass is being evaluated; yet, they may be of value in assessing risk. However, sufficient information is not currently available to allow precise evaluation in a single patient. Low bone mass among the aging is a product of mass attained at maturity and subsequent rates of loss, and either or both factors, may play a dominant role in an individual (Johnston et al, 1981). Some investigators assume that mass at maturity is dominant. This would be true if subsequent rates of loss were linear and equal in different individuals, but rates vary considerably from one subject to another (Smith et al, 1976). If we assume that a 50-year old postmenopausal woman starts with a bone mass one standard deviation above normal and loses at a rate of one standard deviation above the average rate, then, by age 65, she would be one standard deviation below the expected average bone mass for that age (Hui and Berger, 1983). This illustration is hypothetical, but it is based on actual prospective measurements of bone mass and rate of change, and it does demonstrate that bone loss can be a dominant determinant of low bone mass in some individuals.

The available methods can accurately assess bone mass, and the precision of repeated measurements reported in the literature is good (Wahner et al, 1984); however, performance in the field is probably less precise than that reported from research laboratories, and the changes which occur in bone mass over time are quite small. Thus, it is very difficult to make precise measurements of rates in bone mass changes in individual patients without repeated measurements over long periods of time, and this probably is not clinically practical. These techniques, therefore, will best serve the clinician in determining bone mass at some point in time -- perhaps just after menopause -- rather than in measuring rates of change.

I would conclude that it is possible to make reasonable risk assessments for populations. Slender, estrogen-deficient caucasian women are at higher risk than those of other races. The further refinement of risk assessment for the individual within this group will require additional study. Other secondary risk factors may be important here, as well as judicious use of bone mass measurements.

Acknowledgement

This work was supported by Grant No. RR750 from the National Institute of Health.

References

1. Baron, J.A.: Smoking and estrogen-related disease. Am.J.Epidemiol. 119, 9, 1984.

2. Cummings, S.R.: Are patients with hip fractures more osteoporotic? Am.J.Med. 78, 487, 1985.

3. Gershon-Cohen, J., Rechtman, A.M., Scharer, H., and Blumberg, N.: Asymptomatic fractures in osteoporotic spines of the aged. JAMA 153, 625, 1953.

4. Heaney, R., Gallagher, J.C., Johnston, C.C. Jr., Neer, R., Parfitt, A.M., and Whedon, G.D.: Calcium nutrition in the elderly. Am.J.Clin. Nutrit. 36, 986, 1982.

5. Hui, S.L. and Berger, J.O.: Empirical Bayes estimation of rates in longitudinal studies. J.Am.Stat.Assn. 78, 753, 1983.

6. Hui, S.L., Wiske, P.S., Norton, J.A., and Johnston, C.C. Jr.: A prospective study of change in bone mass with age in postmenopausal women. J.Chron.Dis. 35, 715, 1982.

7. Johnston, C.C.: Studies in prevention of age-related bone loss. In, Bone and Mineral Research III, Ed: Peck, W.A., Elsevier, Amsterdam, 1984, pp 233-257.

8. Johnston, C.C. Jr., Hui, S.L., and Longcope, C.: Bone mass and sex steroid concentrations in postmenopausal caucasian diabetics. Metab. (in press, b).

9. Johnston, C.C. Jr., Hui, S.L., Wiske, P.S., Norton, J.A., and Epstein, S.: Bone mass at maturity and subsequent rates of loss as determinants of osteoporosis. In, Osteoporosis: Recent Advances in Pathogenesis and Treatment. Eds: DeLuca, H.F., Frost, H., Jee, W., Johnston, C.C. Jr., Parfitt, A.M. University Park Press, Baltimore, 1981; pp. 285-291.

10. Johnston, C.C. Jr., Norton, J.A., Khairi, M.R.A., Kernek, C., Edouard, C., Arlot, M., and Meunier, P.J.: Heterogeneity of fracture syndromes in postmenopausal women. J.Clin.Endocrinol.Metab. (in press, b).

11. Mazess, R.B.: The noninvasive measurement of skeletal mass. In, Bone and Mineral Research I, Ed: Peck, W.A.: Excerpta Medica, Amsterdam, 1983, pp. 223-279.

12. Melton, L.J. and Riggs, B.L.: Epidemiology of age-related fractures. In, The Osteoporotic Syndrome: Detection, Prevention, and Treatment, Ed: Avioli, L. Grune & Stratton, New York, 1983, pp 45-72.

13. NIH Consensus Conference: Osteoporosis. JAMA 252, 799, 1984.

14. Riggs, B.L. and Melton, L.J.: Heterogeneity of involutional osteoporosis: evidence for two osteoporotic syndromes. Am.J.Med. 75:899, 1983.

15. Riggs, B.L., Wahner, H.W., Seeman, E., Offord, K.P., Dunn, W.L., Mazess, R.B., Johnson, K.A., and Melton, L.J.: Changes in bone mineral density of the proximal femur. J.Clin.Invest. 70, 716, 1982.

16. Seeman, E., Melton, L.J., O'Fallon, W.M., and Riggs, B.L.: Risk factors for spinal osteoporosis in men. Am.J.Med. 75, 977, 1983.

17. Seeman, E., Wahner, H.W., Offord, K.P., Kumar, R., Johnson, W.J., and Riggs, B.L.: Differential effects of endocrine dysfunction on the axial and appendicular skeleton. J.Clin.Invest. 69, 1302, 1982.

18. Smith, D.M., Khairi, M.R.A., Norton, J.A., and Johnston, C.C. Jr.: Age and activity effects on rates of bone mineral loss. J.Clin.Invest. 58, 716, 1976.

19. Smith, D., Nance, W.E., Kang, K.W., Christian, J.C., and Johnston, C.C. Jr.: Genetic factors in determining bone mass. J.Clin.Invest. 52, 2800, 1973.

20. Wahner, H.W., Dunn, W.L., and Riggs, B.L.: Assessment of bone mineral, Part 2. J.Nucl.Med. 25, 1241, 1984.

Modern Imaging of Patients with Metabolic Bone Disease

W. WENZ, T. KRÖPELIN, B. WIMMER, W. D. REINBOLD, and G. RICHTER

On December 22, 1895 Conrad Whilhelm Roentgen took the first x-ray picture of the hand of his wife. Since that time, ordinary radiography has remained the basic examination in patients with skeletal disorders. Moreover, in metabolic bone disease, simple roentgen films permit determination of structural abnormalities and the differentiation between osteopenia and other conditions causing bone fragility.

Our purpose in this presentation is to demonstrate the use of imaging methods in the differentiation between osteoporosis and osteomalacia; to discuss the additional information obtained by computed tomography and magnetic resonance imaging; and finally to describe roentgen findings in other lesions associated with bone fragility.

Imaging Methods

Conventional radiographic techniques for the diagnosis of metabolic bone disease include:

- plain film radiography
- conventional tomography
- magnification techniques
- xeroradiography.

To compare the mineral content of bones in different locations, a maximum picture quality must be provided. Variations in exposure and processing techniques between serial examination may produce misleading findings.

Conventional tomography, either mono- or multidirectional, is of great value when superimposed effects must be eliminated.

Microradioscopy and other *magnification techniques* are helpful in detecting subperiosteal resorption earlier than by plain film technique alone.

Xeroradiography allows a better delineation between bone and soft tissue but has not been proved superior to the above-mentioned imaging techniques.

The introduction of computers in medical imaging made the following techniques possible:

Current Concepts of Bone Fragility

- digital radiography
- computed tomography
- magnetic resonance imaging.

Due to a very high reflection from bone structures, ultrasound does not play any role in this review.

Digital radiography today is routine in angiography, whereas conventional roentgen-films have not yet been replaced in the diagnosis of skeletal disorders. The so-called "topogram" starting a CT examination serves more for anatomic orientation than for structural analysis.

Computed tomography. Transverse sections through the bones and the possibility of density measurements are the most important advantages of computed tomography. Quantitative measurements have been greatly improved by this new imaging method.

Magnetic resonance imaging. This application is in its beginnings. There are no signals from the bony cortex and the spatial resolution is not as well-defined as in CT, up to now. However, recently we have found promising indications with a Bruker 0.23 T iron shielded magnet.

Osteopenia

Before discussing quantitative methods for evaluation of bone mineral content, we will review the radiologic features of osteopenia.

Osteoporosis results from deficient matrix formation. The primary radiologic sign, therefore, is diffuse decrease in bone density.

Thinning of cortices is usually marked, but the density of the remaining cortical bone is frequently normal. The weakened skeleton is naturally more subject to injury by slight trauma. Compression fractures of vertebral bodies, particularly in the midthoracic area, are especially common. Repair is very slow without significant demonstration of callus formation.

The formation of bone matrix depends on a number of factors that can rarely be identified by radiography alone.

Failure of mineralization of osteoid tissue results in *osteomalacia*. The lesion, therefore, shows inadequate osteoid mineralization in the adult, while the term "rickets" is still used when the disorder affects the immature skeleton.

The radiologic appearance consists of more or less excessive demineralization, and consequent reduction in bone strength, leading to secondary deformities. These changes are caused by the fragility of the impoverished bones, including:

- triradiate pelvis
- bowing of the lower limbs
- kyphosis of the thoracic cage
- basilar invagination of the skull
- hour-glass shape of the thoracic cage

Widespread radiolucency of the bony structures is observed and failure of mineralization of newly formed bone. In these weakened bone areas stress fractures may develop. The resultant osteoid seams, the site of occult fracture, are the Looser zones, lucent bands running transversely through the affected bone with little or no evidence of repair.

The stresses induced by normal activity tend to create these defects in constant and symmetrical sites:

- obturator rings of the pelvis
- lower ribs
- inferior angles of the scapula
- femoral necks and metatarsal shafts.

Quite frequently, displacements of the fragments contribute to the generalized deformities. With appropriate treatment, healing follows rapidly; but these anatomic abnormalities remain as permanent stigmata, representing a pathognomonic feature of osteomalacia in the adult skeleton.

In the growing skeleton, however, manifestations of rickets due to deficient mineralization of osteoid are even more extensive. They are apparent in the metaphysis where bands of radiolucency, with irregularity of metaphyseal margins, are constant features. In weight-bearing areas, the metaphyses become splayed by stress, and consequent bowleg deformities provide a classical clinical picture of the disease in severe cases.

Rarely are the severer forms of rickets in the western world the result of dietary or sunshine deficiency. Much more commonly, they reflect malabsorption syndromes, renal abnormalities or hypophosphatasia.

Bone fragility, similar to osteoporosis and osteomalacia, also occurs in *hyperparathyroidism*. Characteristic radiologic lesions are subperiosteal erosions, generally, or resorption in particular of the radial surfaces of the middle phalanges of the second and third fingers.

Other manifestations of subperiosteal resorption are:

- outer ends of the clavicula
- tibia and femur, medial surfaces
- radius and ulna, distal ends
- ischial tuberosity and sacroiliac joint
- pubis, ribs, and bony wall of sella turcica.

The lace-like pattern is followed by virtually complete cortical resorption of long bones, with a generalized increase in skeletal radiolucency.

Brown tumors in long bones generally present as well-defined, radiolucent defects, appearing as cystic lesions. Florid forms of the disorder with biconcave vertebral bodies, basilar impression, kyphoscoliosis and absence of the lamina dura around the teeth are associated with calcifications of arteries and other soft tissues around the joints. Renal calculi or nephrocalcinosis are observed in about one-third of individuals with hyperparathyroidism.

The skeletal changes, following removal of parathyroid adenoma, may be expected to revert toward normal. Brown tumors, however, usually develop an appearance comparable to fibrous dysplasia, or, rarely, become extremely dense.

Secondary hyperparathyroidism radiologic findings correspond to pathologic changes, including subperiosteal resorption, widening of the epiphyseal plates of long bones, generalized demineralization and Brown tumors. The skull may show a granular pattern, sometimes resembling Paget's disease. A classical rugger-jersey pattern in the spine or "sandwich-vertebrae is frequently encountered. Extraosseous calcification is a common feature.

Considering osteoporosis, osteomalacia and the radiologic features of hyperparathyroidism, the basic abnormality common to these three conditions is reduction of the mineral content of the skeleton, so that the bones become abnormally radiolucent. Osteopenia, therefore, may be a common denominator.

Differentiation between the three forms may be impossible, especially in earlier stages of osteopenia. Quantitative measuring techniques are consequently mandatory. Many of them have been described during the last decades, but only a few methods are of practical use.

Quantitative Assessment of the Mineral Content of Bone

Although the diagnostic value of roentgenography for osteopenia is great, in some cases a reduction of 30-50% of calcium may not be recognized by routine radiography. Therefore, several quantitative methods have been more or less successfully employed in the past:

- comparable structrual analysis
- photodensitometry
- radiographic morphometry
- photon absorptiometry

The appendicular bones are widely used for the noninvasive assessment of skeletal status. Bones, even in normal subjects of the same age and sex, differ highly from individual to individual.

Singh et al (1970) gave a classification of the trabecular bone pattern of the proximal femur; but Nilsson and Hagberg (1976) could not find an exact correlation between the grading of the trabecular loss and the fracture incidence.

Photodensitometry (Heuck, 1979) uses the comparison between the grey values of the film and a metallic phantom, such as aluminum, and allows recognition of differences of the mineral content between 3-4% in fingers and hand.

The bones in metabolic disease are reduced in osseous mass. With the aid of *radiographic morphometry*, the thickness of the cancellous bone indices can be measured for objective evaluation of the lesions. Hand radiographs, for example, enable the quantification of the metacarpal index.

Dual photon absorptiometry means the measurement of bone mineral content with a rectilinear scan of the region of interest with a ^{153}Gadolinium source-detector. Bone mineral content is obtained in units of grams hydroxyapatite. According to Wahner et al (1983), trabecular bone seems to have a higher remodeling rate and a higher rate of postmenopausal bone loss than cortical bone.

CT-tomometry (Genant, 1981) is performed using an oval region of interest to determine the mean number of Hounsfield units in a 4 cc volume within each vertebral body. The CT numbers derived from the calibration phantom scanned simultaneously with the patient are then used to calculate the mineral equivalent for each vertebra.

Finally, Bessler (1984) described a method for quantification of vertebral trabeculae by structural analysis with digital imaging. The method consists of digitalization of the roentgen-film followed by equalization of the grey values. Ninety-two patients with normal skeletal findings and 65 with osteoporosis have been successfully studied.

Our goal is the ability to quantitate the elements of bone. This is especially important for the control of therapy. It may be some time, however, before the systems are generally available. Until then, the visual analysis of the radiograph remains our standard approach to the diagnosis and grading of bone rarefaction.

Disorders Causing Bone Fragility

Among numerous disorders causing bone fragility, only a few will be discussed from the viewpoint of fast and noninvasive diagnostic procedures.

Little knowledge has been added since Sir James Paget gave the first description of *osteitis deformans* in 1877. Today, the disease still remains a mystery; the radiologic signs, however, are well known.

In the early stage of bone destruction, completely lytic skeletal areas are seen -- osteoporosis circumscripta-- sometimes very aggressive. This phase should be referred to as active Paget's disease. In long bones, such as the tibia, the radiolucent area ends in a "V", giving a flame-shaped appearance. We have observed healing under continuous application of calcitonin.

The second phase is that of new bone formation, obliterating demarcation between the cortex and spongiosa and increasing the actual size of the bone.

The roentgen-pattern in the third stage is dominated by a combination of bone replacement and new bone formation. Diffuse increase of density and residual bone formation indicate the inactive, sclerotic or amorphous form.

In contrast to Paget's disease, with a marked preponderance of elderly male adults, *osteogenesis imperfecta* is a problem of the very young. Considerable cortical thinning and diffuse demineralization are typical signs together with bowing deformities when the child begins walking. The long bones are slender and the ribs may become attenuated.

Similar to osteogenesis imperfecta, *hypophosphatasia* is a heritable disorder of bone metabolism characterized by defective skeletal mineralization resembling rickets. Radiologically, one observes large, irregular metaphyseal defects at the wrists, knees and osteochondral junctions.

- *Infantile form* (second week to sixth month): Cupping of the metaphyses of the long bones with widening of the cartilaginous growth plate. Fractures may heal with transient deformities. Premature craniosynostosis, short stature, bowed legs, abnormal teeth. Most of the children will survive; some die by the end of the first year.

- *Childhood form* (sixth month to two years): Rachitic stigmata.
- *Adult form:* Demineralization; osteoid seams or Looser zones; actual fractures representing typical osteomalacia.

Hypophosphatasia in its juvenile form is a classic example for demonstrating fragility in metabolic bone disease. A still more impressive form of congenital bone fragility is *thanatophoric dwarfism*. There are no neonatal survivors and fortunately it is rare. All radiologic signs discussed in the foregoing disorders can be demonstrated here in their extreme stages.

Summary

Modern imaging techniques are methods of choice for detection and localization of metabolic bone disease. Ordinary radiography allows a correct diagnosis in most of the cases. Digital radiography has contributed a better picture quality with lower radiation doses. Computed tomography permits transverse sections and a more exact technique for quantitative evaluation of the osseous structures. Therefore, it is most important for the earlier recognition of bone disorders and of the control of therapy. Magnetic resonance imaging, finally, gives information about the fatty content of the bone marrow as well as the surrounding soft tissue. Correlating histochemical results to imaging of the bony structures is expected for the near future.

References

1. Bessler, W.: Rarefizierende Osteopathien. Röntgenologische Strukturanalyse. Edition Medizin. Weinheim-Deerfield Beach, Florida-Basel, 1984.
2. Genant, H.K., Boyd, D., Rosenfeld, D., Abols, Y., and Cann, C.E.: Computed tomography. In, Non-Invasive Measurements of Bone Mass and Their Clinical Applications. Ed, Cohn, S.H. CRC Press, Boca Raton, Fla., 1981, pp 121-149.
3. Heuck, F.W.H.: Qualitative und quantitative radiologische Analyse des Knochens. In, Lehrbuch der Röntgendiagnostik. Bd.II, Teil 1 Skelett Hrsg., Schinze, H.R., Baensch, W.H., Frommhold, W., Glauner, R., Uehlinger, H., Wellauer, J. Thieme, Stuttgart, 1979.
4. Nilsson, B.E., and Hagberg, L.: Proceedings: Prediction of femoral neck fractures from a pelvic x-ray. Am. J. Roentgenol. 126, 1299, 1976.
5. Singh, M., Nagrath, A.R., Maini, P.S., and Haryana, R.: Changes in trabecular pattern of the upper end of the femur as an index of osteoporosis. J. Bone Joint Surg. 52A, 457, 1970.
6. Wahner, H.W., Dunn, W.L., and Riggs, B.L.: Noninvasive bone mineral measurements. Sem. Nucl. Med. 13, 282, 1983.

Selected Bibliography

1. Bradley, J.G., Huang, H.K., and Ledley, R.S.: Evaluation of calcium concentration in bones from CT scans. Radiology 128, 103, 1978.

2. Cann, C.E.: Low-dose CT scanning for quantitative spinal mineral analysis. Radiology 140, 813, 1981.

3. Cann, C.E., Genant, H.K., Ettinger, B., and Gordan, G.S.: Spinal mineral loss in oophorectomized women. JAMA 244, 2056, 1980.

4. Hesch, R.-D., Völker, W., and Schneider, H.P.G.: Prävention der Osteoporose. Dtsch. Ärztebl. 82, 485, 1985.

5. Heuck, F., and Vanselow, K.: In, Handbuch der Inneren Medizin. Klinische Osteologie A. Ed, Kuhlencordt, P. and Bartelheimer, H. Springer-Verlag, Berlin-Heidelberg-New York, 1980.

6. Krolner, B., Vesteral Jorgensen, J., and Pors Nielsen, S.: Spinal bone mineral content in myxoedema and thyrotoxicosis. Effects of thyroid hormones and antithyroid treatment. Clin. Endocrinol. 18, 439, 1983.

7. Krolner, B., and Pors Nielsen, S.: Bone mineral content of the lumbar spine in normal and osteoporotic women: Cross sectional and longitudinal studies. Clin. Sci. 62, 329, 1982.

8. Kuhlencordt, F., and Kruse, H.-P.: In, Handbuch der Inneren Medizin Klinische Osteologie B. Eds., Kuhlencordt, F., and Bartelheimer, H. Springer-Verlag, Berlin-Heidelberg-New York, 1980.

9. Laval-Jeantet, M., Laval-Jeantet, A.M., Lamarque, J.L., and Demoulin, B.: Evaluation de la minéralisation osseuse vertébrale par tomographie computerisée. J. Radiol. 60, 87, 1979.

10. Lee, K.T., Sagel, St. S., Stanley, R.J.: Computed Body Tomography. Raven Press, New York, 1983, pp 510-512.

11. Müller, K.-H.: Stoffwechselerkrankungen. In, Orthopädie in Praxis und Klinik. Ed., Witt, A.N., Rettig, H., Schlegel, K.F., Hackenbroch, M., and Hupfauer, W. Vol. III. Thieme, Stuttgart-New York, 1984.

12. Murray, R.O., and Jaconson, H.G.: The Radiology of Skeletal Disorders. Churchill Livingstone. Edinburgh-London-New York, 1977.

13. Posner, I., and Griffiths, H.J.: Comparison of CT scanning with photon absorptiometric measurement of bone mineral content in the appendicular skeleton. Invest. Radiol. 12, 542, 1977.

14. Revak, C.S.: Mineral content of cortical bone measured by conputed tomography. J. Comput. Assist. Tomogr. 4, 342, 1980.

15. Swoboda, W.: Das Skelet des Kindes. Thieme, Stuttgart, 1969.

16. Vetter, J.R., Perman, W.H., Calendar, W.A., Mazess, R.B., and Holden, J.E.: Evaluation of a prototype dual energy CT apparatus. II: Determination of vertebral bone mineral content. Presented at 70th Scientific Assembly and Annual Meeting of the RSNA, Washington, DC, 1984.

17. Weissberger, M.A., Zamenhoff, R. M., Aronow, S., and Neer, S.M.: Computed tomography scanning for the neasurement of bone mineral in the human spine. J. Comput. Assist. Tomogr. 2, 253, 1978.

Nuclear Medicine Applications to Metabolic Bone Disease

L. ROSENTHALL

Introduction

Metabolic bone disease provokes a generalized skeletal reaction which in the early stages of development usually produces normal radiophosphate images. As the disorder progresses, however, increased uptake of radiophosphate may become visually apparent. The sites with highest uptake are the periarticular bones, vertebral column, calvarium, mandible, anterior rib ends, and sternum. In severe disease, all these features are recognizable, and long bone involvement may also become obvious. The mechanism which facilitates this enhanced radiophosphate deposition is not precisely known. Changes in blood flow is one factor, but the details of extraction and binding sites at the molecular level are still debated (Charkes et al, 1978; 1979; Francis et al, 1980; Jones et al, 1976; Rosenthall and Kaye, 1976). It apparently occurs in the presence of increased osteoblastic activity, since a purely resorptive process is not associated with increased uptake of radiophosphate. Osteoblastic and osteoclastic activity are usually coupled, so that an increase or decrease in one is followed by an increase or decrease, respectively, in the other. It is the net difference in the two that determines whether the bones will become porotic or sclerotic. Therefore, the radiographic appearance or densitometric measurement of bone mineral content of bone does not necessarily correspond to the radionuclide results of metabolic activity.

Quantification of skeletal radiotracer uptake increases the sensitivity of bone scintigraphy in the disclosure of metabolic bone disease. Bone-to-soft tissue ratios at the distal end of the femur or lumbar spine determined by computer analysis have been used. They were found to be useful in separating the diseased population from normal as a group, but were too imprecise and inaccurate for the study of the individual patient. This was partly due to the fact that the area of interest chosen for computer analysis may not be the site of maximal uptake in a given patient. For example, in hyperparathyroidism the mandible may have a higher radiophosphate uptake than either the lumbar spine or distal femur (Fogelman et al, 1978; Holmes, 1978; Rosenthall and Kaye, 1975). The most accurate method is total body counting with a device specifically designed for the purpose, such as the shadow-shield whole-body monitor (Fogelman et al, 1978). Unfortunately, this instrument is available in only a few centers and not accessible for widespread patient diagnosis and monitoring. A satisfactory compromise is achieved with a simple thyroid probe and counting the patient at about a 15-foot crystal-subject distance. Total body counts are obtained at 5 min-

Current Concepts of Bone Fragility

utes and 24 hours after dosing, and the ratio of the latter to the former constitutes the 24-hour total body retention, the variable used for assessing metabolic bone disease (Rosenthall and Arzoumanian, 1983). The main disadvantage of the simple probe method vis à vis the shadow-shield whole-body counter is that it requires the usual scanning dose of about 20 mCi radiophosphate, whereas the latter is much more sensitive and employs about 1/300 of the dose. Since these patients are usually imaged to document the sites of increased uptake, the scanning dose is given in any event.

Primary Hyperparathyroidism

Primary hyperparathyroidism elicits an increased elaboration of parathormone, leading to hypophosphatemia and hypercalcemia. This results in recurrent nephrolithiasis, peptic ulcer, mental changes, pseudogout, and less frequently, excessive bone resorption. In over 80% of patients this is due to a neoplasm of a single parathyroid gland. Most of these are benign adenomas; the others include carcinoma, multiple adenomas, and hyperplasia of all four glands. Bone histologic examination shows an increase in both osteoclastic and osteoblastic activity, predominantly the former. The advent of multiphasic screening of blood calcium has led to the discovery of the disease much earlier in its evolution, antedating visible radiographic and radionuclide changes.

Qualitative radiophosphate images were compared with radiography in a small series of 14 patients. Abnormal concentrations of radiophosphate were found in seven patients (50%), whereas radiographic stigmata of hyperparathyroidism, such as osteopenia, brown tumors, cysts and subperiosteal bone resorption, occurred in only three (21%) patients (Fogelman and Carr, 1980). Another report of 20 patients with primary hyperparathyroidism related seven (35%) to radiographic evidence of subperiosteal cortical bone erosion and four (20%) to abnormal 5-hour bone/soft tissue ratios taken at the distal femurs (Wiegmann et al, 1977). On average, the 5-hour bone/soft tissue ratio was not significantly different from the control group. In another series of patients with primary hyperparathyroidism, the 4-hour bone/soft tissue ratios were also found to be statistically the same as controls, but the corresponding 24-hour whole-body retentions were different, attesting to the increased sensitivity of total body measurements. Using technitium-99m ethylene diphosphonate, the 24-hour retentions were $40.7 \pm 8.0\%$ and $19.4 \pm 3.4\%$ for primary hyperparathyroidism and controls, respectively. This was later expanded to a larger group where the mean 24-hour total body retention was $50 \pm 20.3\%$ and showed a coefficient of correlation of 0.86 with the plasma immunoreactive parathyroid hormone. In addition, 87% of the patients had normal radiographs (Fogelman et al, 1980a).

Following parathyroidectomy, one observes, first, normalization of the immunoreactive parathormone, then the alkaline phosphatase, and finally healing of bone and scintigraphically shown improvement (de Graaf et al, 1983). The radiophosphate bone scan may not return to normal for variable periods up to one year.

Metastatic calcification in the lung is a complication of primary hyperparathyroidism and is a cause of increased radiophosphate deposition. Excision of the hyperactive gland results in normalization of the lung concentration, preceding that of the bone scan portrayal (Cooper et al, 1978; Itoh and Furudate, 1979)(Fig. 1).

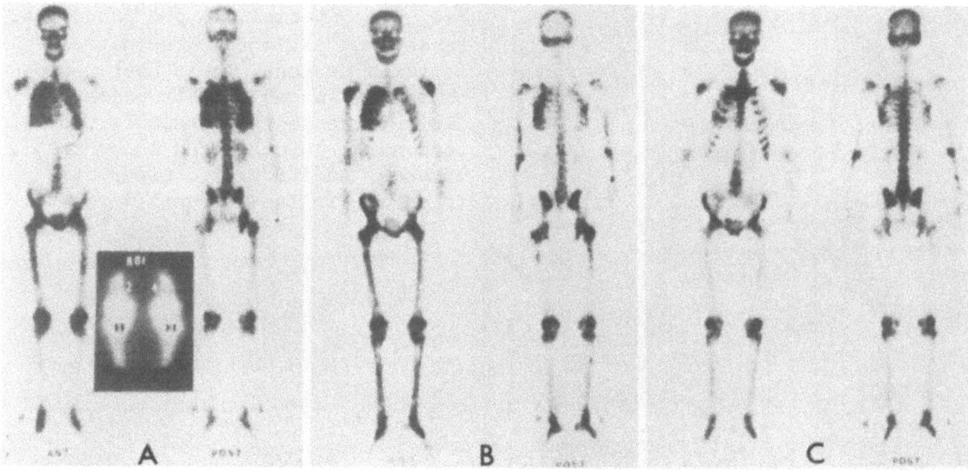

Fig. 1. Ectopic parathyroid adenoma causing hyperparathyroidism and metastatic lung calcification. A) Preoperative anterior and posterior Tc-99m-MDP total body images demonstrate increased skeletal uptake and a high concentration in both lungs. The bone/soft tissue ratio at the knee (inset scan) was 9.86 at 5 hours following radionuclide injection. B) Three weeks postoperative after removal of an ectopic adenoma in the left supraclavicular region. Some decrease in Tc-99m-MDP uptake in the lung is noted. C) Three months postoperative. Lung uptake of Tc-99m-MDP is barely perceptible. The skeletal concentration is still abnormally high, but less than the preoperative state.

Osteomalacia

Osteomalacia is a bone disorder caused by either an absolute or a relative deficiency of vitamin D. Before closure of the epiphyseal growth plates, this defect is called rickets. The deficit can be due to insufficient intake, reduced intestinal absorption following gastrectomy and small bowel bypass surgery, intestinal loss from various forms of malabsorption syndromes, decreased endogenous production of vitamin D due to insufficient exposure to ultraviolet light, excessive metabolism of vitamin D by anticonvulsant therapy, and vitamin D resistance caused by chronic renal failure, renal tubular disorders, and liver disease.

The radiographic signs of osteomalacia include osteopenia due to nonmineralized osteoid, a loss of longitudinal and transverse trabeculae with a coarsening of the remaining trabeculae and pseudofractures. Total body 24-hour retentions of radiophosphate are greatly elevated and the scans depict diffuse increased uptake, most prominent in the periarticular zones. Pseudofractures are reflected as focal concentrations of intense radioactivity. The consensus is that radiophosphate imaging is more sensitive than radiography in the disclosure of osteomalacia, although when the disease is advanced the radiographic signs are more specific just as they are in primary hyperparathyroidism (Fogelman et al, 1977b); MacFarlane et al, 1977; Singh et al, 1977). In one crossover study of 15 patients, radiophosphate detected

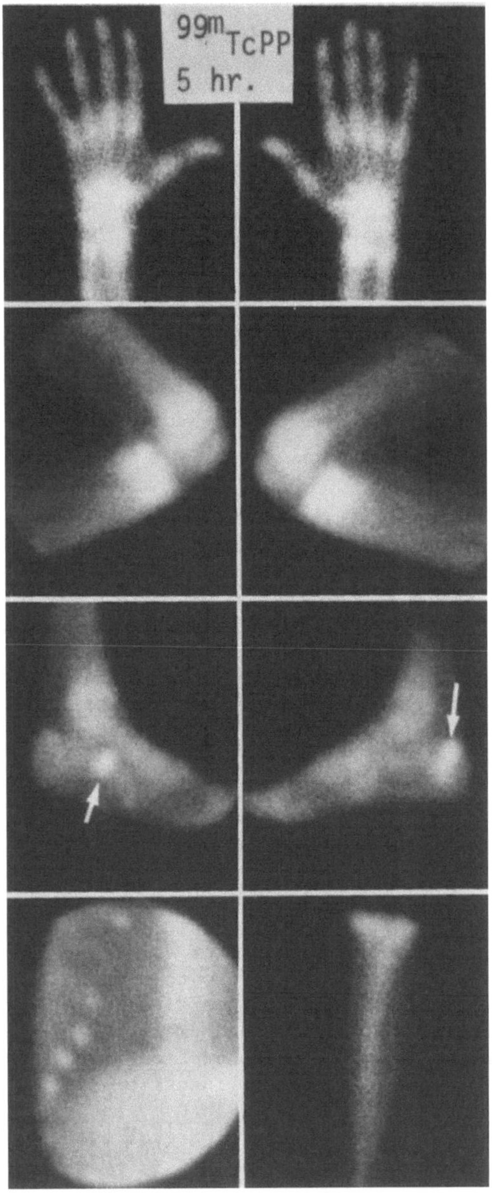

Fig. 2. Osteomalacia and pseudofractures in a patient suffering from anorexia nervosa. The 5 hour radiophosphate images exhibit characteristic increased periarticular, costochondral junction and long bone uptakes. Additionally, pseudofractures are in the calcanei (arrows).

osteomalacic changes in all patients, while only nine (60%) were diagnosed by radiography. Moreover, more pseudofractures were seen in the bone images than by radiography. In 11 elderly patients (70 to 95 years of age) with proven osteomalacia, all had radiophosphate scans showing diffuse generalized uptake, minimum visualization of the kidneys, and focal concentrations at the costochondral junctions. Some had pseudofractures and true fractures manifesting local accretions (Fig. 2). Treatment with calcium and vitamin D reversed these changes in the five patients who had repeat follow-up studies (Rai et al, 1981).

Renal Osteodystrophy

Renal osteodystrophy is a term applied to changes in bone metabolism resulting from prolonged chronic renal disease. The tubular forms of renal disease, such as vitamin D-resistant rickets, renal tubular acidosis, and Fanconi syndrome, cause osteomalacia. Rarely is associated secondary hyperparathyroidism observed. Acquired diseases of glomerular origin, eg, chronic pyelonephritis and chronic glomerulonephritis, present a mixed histologic picture of osteomalacia and hyperparathyroidism. Both osteomalacia and hyperparathyroidism are known to provoke abnormally high uptakes and 24-hour retentions of radiophosphate, but the relative contributions of these entities to the global uptake and retention is controversial. One group of investigators believes that the hyperparathyroid component is largely responsible, because they found a significant correlation of overall radiophosphate uptake with the immunoreactive parathormone, alkaline phosphatase blood levels, and the histologic findings of hyperparathyroidism. The correlations were maintained following treatment and subsidence of the signs of hyperparathyroidism. In contrast, correlations between skeletal

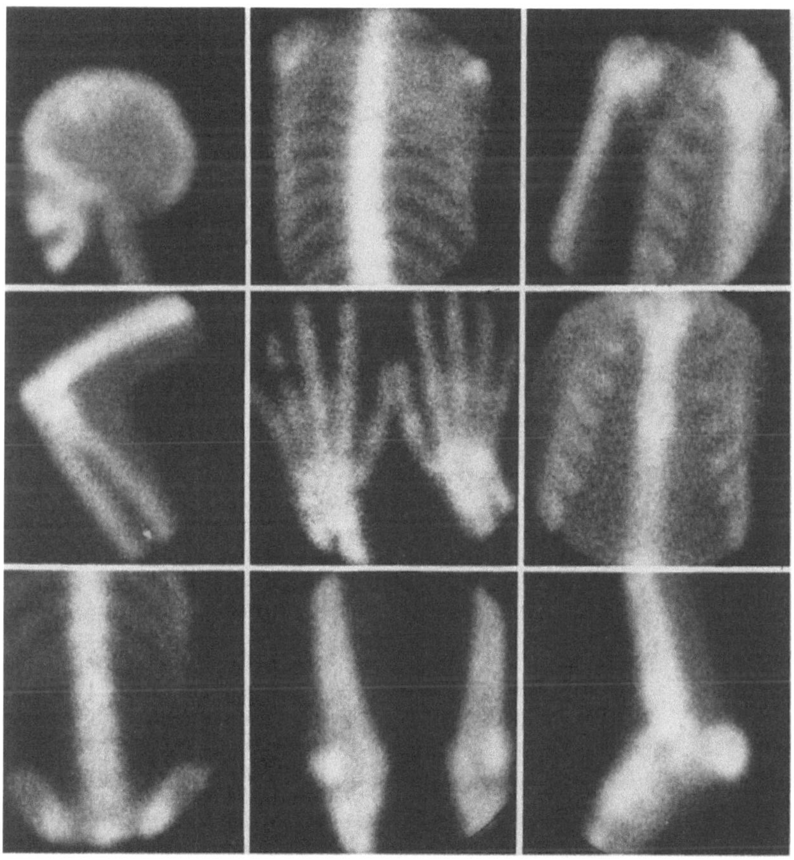

Fig. 3. Renal osteodystrophy in a patient with chronic renal failure. Tc-99m-MDP images show marked uptake universally and diffusely in the skeleton.

radioactivity and osteoid excess were either statistically of little or no significance (de Graaf et al, 1982; 1984).

In established renal osteodystrophy, the scan demonstrates markedly elevated concentrations of radiophosphate throughout the axial and appendicular skeleton (Fig. 3). Twenty-four hour total body retentions are high as might be expected when there is little or no renal excretion of radiophosphate. Mean values of 82-98% have been recorded. Bone/soft tissue ratios at 4 to 5 hours are also elevated in most of these patients (Lien et al, 1976). These ratios are not sensitive in the early stages of the disease because the high soft tissue background tends to decrease the quotient. It has been shown that the sensitivity of the ratios and the quality of the images are vastly improved by starting hemodialysis immediately after administration of radiophosphate and maintaining normal blood levels of the tracer (de Graaf et al, 1978).

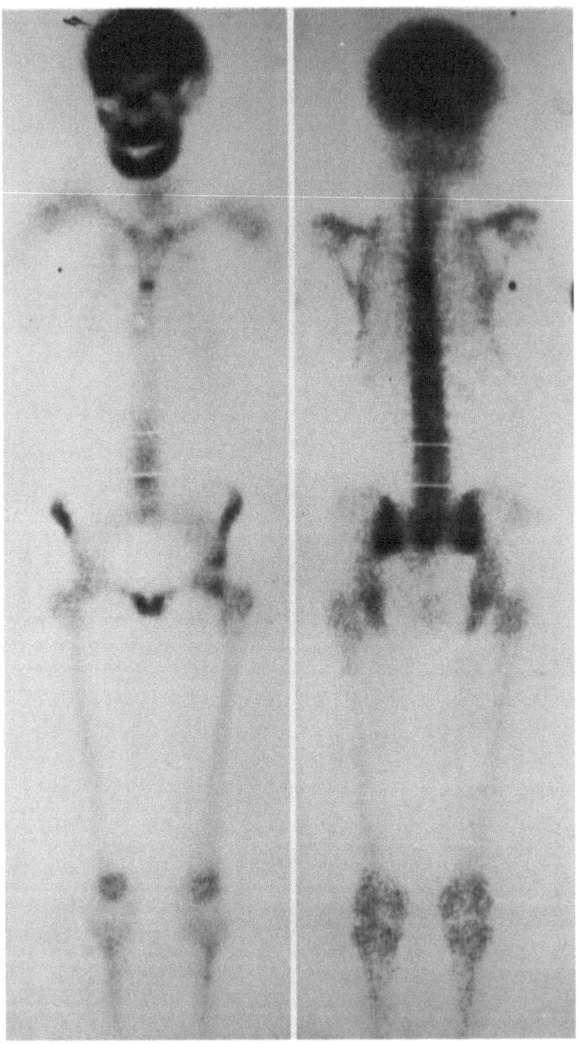

Fig. 4. Tertiary hyperparathyroidism in a 58-year old woman with a 20-year history of hypertension, progressive renal failure, bone pain and a loss of 2.4 inches in height over three years. Admitted in renal failure hypercalcemia and serum parathormone levels 20 x normal. At surgery two parathyroid glands weighing 7 g each were excised. The Tc-99m-MDP scan shows a diffusely increased skeletal concentration, most prominent in the calvarium, mandible and vertebral column.

Radiophosphate imaging appears to be more sensitive in disclosing the bone disorder than radiography. The sensitivity of radiophosphate is reported to range from 83 to 100% compared with a 46 to 58% range for routine radiographs (de Graaf et al, 1978; Fogelman and Carr, 1980).

Osteosclerosis is occasionally seen in radiographs of the spine in patients with renal osteodystrophy, and the bone scan shows linear areas of slightly increased radiophosphate uptake against a background of generalized high uptake in the spine (Fogelman and Citrin, 1981).

Sites of ectopic calcification may be recognized with bone imaging. At autopsy, the frequency of pulmonary calcification in patients with long standing uremia is 60 to 70% (Conger et al, 1975; Kuzela et al, 1977). In contrast, visible radiophosphate lung uptake is unusual, occurring when the degree of calcification is severe. This is due to the fact that uremic pulmonary calcifications are not of the apatite structure, but rather an amorphous or microcrystalline compound with a high magnesium and pyrophosphate content. The amorphous calcifications have one-quarter the affinity for radiophosphate than that of the apatite type. Nonvisceral calcification in uremia is of the apatite structure and one can rarely demonstrate radiophosphate uptake in the cutaneous and periarticular zones.

Tertiary Hyperparathyroidism

Tertiary hyperparathyroidism is a term referring to a situation in which the parathyroid escapes the regulatory effects of appropriate serum calcium levels in patients following prolonged stimulation. Some authorities do not recognize the existence of this condition. In the cases reported, the radiophosphate images demonstrated the usual generalized increased radiophosphate uptake characteristic of metabolic disorders (Fig. 4).

Pseudohypoparathyroidism

Pseudohypoparathyroidism is a rare hereditary disorder characterized by signs and symptoms of hypoparathyroidism and skeletal development defects, specifically short stature, and short metacarpi and metatarsi. The biochemical aberration is a deficient end organ response to endogenous parathormone. This leads to parathyroid hyperplasia and excessive elaboration of the hormone. Features of osteitis fibrosa have been seen radiographically and proven by biopsy in some of the reported cases. Radiophosphate images are nonspecific, and may demonstrate increased uptake in the periarticular regions of the hands, feet, or diffusely in the skeleton (Krishnamurthy et al, 1977).

Generalized Osteoporosis

Osteoporosis features a reduction in osteoid tissue formation and osteoblasts. A global loss of bone mass occurs with thinning of the cortex and trabeculae, and a decrease in the number of trabeculae. The degree of osteoporosis increases with age, but it occurs earlier and progresses more rapidly in women. It becomes evident soon after the menopause and results in the loss of 40 to 50% of bone tissue between the fifth and ninth decades of life. Other causes of this disorder are steroid therapy, alcoholism, nutritional deficiency, prolonged immobilization, weightlessness, and endocrinopathies such as thyrotoxicosis and Cushing's syndrome.

The bone scan outwardly appears normal in involutionary osteoporosis, unless it is complicated by fractures, in which case focal uptakes are observed. On careful analysis there seems to be a deterioration with increasing age in the quality of the scans and the sacrum/soft tissue ratios obtained between 2 and 5 hours (Buell et al, 1982; Wilson, 1981). In severe, end stage forms, the radiophosphate images may show poor uptake, which has been attributed to markedly reduced or absent osteoblastic activity (Levine et al, 1977). Total body 24-hour retention studies render a different insight into the process. An investigation comprising 250 normal persons demonstrated a fall between 20 and 35 years of age; after that time, the men showed a linear rise. Women's retentions parallel the men's until the menopause, and then show a steeper rise in retention. This implies increased osteoblastic activity; but since the bone mass is reduced, the osteoclastic activity must exceed osteoblastic activity (Fogelman and Bessant, 1982). The poorer bone scans obtained in the 2- to 5-hour interval may be due to the reduced rate of excretion of radiophosphate by the senile kidneys and consequent higher background levels. This is of lesser importance in a 24-hour span, where the background has more time to clear.

Hyperthyroidism may induce osteoporosis, particularly when chronic in postmenopausal women. Total body 24-hour retention measurements are reported to be significantly increased (Seto et al, 1982).

Excess steroid intake is known to cause osteoporosis either by suppressing bone formation and increasing bone resorption, or by suppressing bone formation alone. The effect on radiophosphate uptake is still unclear; some investigators report increases and others decreases (Caniggia et al, 1981; Seto et al, 1982; Steven et al, 1982). The question is not yet resolved.

Radiophosphate imaging has been used to monitor sodium fluoride treatment in postmenopausal women. Sodium fluoride stimulates bone formation rate and the increased osteoblastic activity is reflected in increased radiophosphate deposition. The enhanced metabolic activity antedates radiographic and densitometric manifestations of increased bone mass (Schultz et al, 1984).

Paget's Disease

Paget's disease has been considered to be an inborn error of connective tissue metabolism, disorder of hormone secretion, an acquired disorder or autoimmune state, and a hormone-sensitive benign tumor of bone. Current thinking favors a viral-induced disorder (Mills et al, 1980; Revel et al, 1980). It is postulated that virus-containing cells fuse with infected and noninfected cells to form large multinucleated osteoclasts, characteristic of Paget's disease (Frame and Marel, 1981).

The disease begins with intense osteoclastic resorption of normal bone by giant multinucleated cells. Moreover, there is reactive osteoblastic activity which causes an exuberant production of primitive bone, accompanied by increased vascularity and a substantial deposition of connective tissue that largely replaces the marrow space. These features are reflected in the radionuclide portrayal.

The radiographic appearance of the lesions can be purely lytic, mixed lytic and sclerotic, or predominantly sclerotic. In the histologically demonstrated purely lytic phase, the radiophosphate uptake will be low with a relatively higher concentration at the advancing front. Most of these radiographically lytic appearing lesions, however, will be intensely hyperactive throughout, an indication of diffuse osteoblastic activity but insufficient calcium deposition for roentgenographic detection. High accretions of radiophosphate occur in the mixed lytic and sclerotic, and predominantly sclerotic lesions as long as the disease is active. The radiophosphate uptake in pagetic bone can exceed normal bone by a factor of 15. When the disease becomes quiescent, uptake of radiophosphate reverts to normal.

Both qualititative and quantitative radiophosphate imagings have been used to monitor treatment, along with alkaline phosphatase and urinary hydroxyproline as biochemical measurements of bone turnover. Quantitative imaging can be in the form of a ratio of the counts over the afflicted bone to a normal reference bone 2 to 5 hours after delivery of radiophosphate, or a total body 24-hour retention. Perfusion and blood pool images of the pagetic lesions can be assessed visually or quantitated (Boudreau et al, 1983).

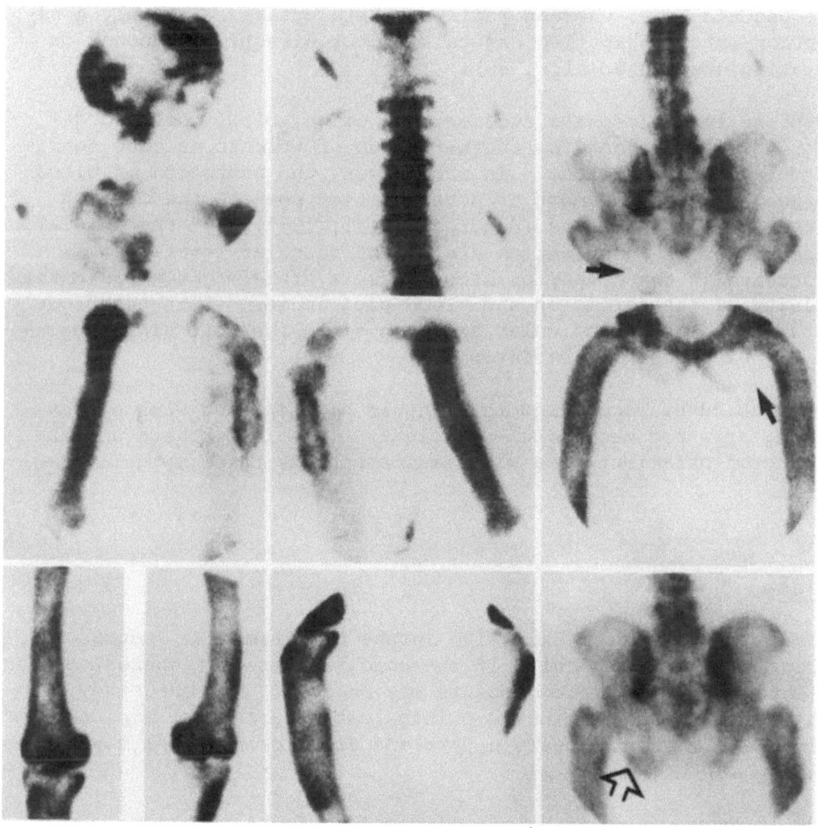

Fig. 5. Extensive Paget's disease involving calvarium, vertebral column, some ribs, sternum, pelvis, upper and lower extremities. Patient was on mithramycin and had a total body 24-hour retention of Tc-99m-MDP of 86% (normal 27%). Pretreatment retention was 98%. Solid arrow points to area of absent uptake, or photon-deficiency, in the left ischium which had been functioning but now undergoing destruction by malignant fibrous histiocytoma.

The radiophosphate method and biochemical measurements complement each other. In one report, reactivation of disease was detected by increased radiophosphate uptake in one-third of the patients before a rise in biochemical measurements; and in another third the biochemical measurements antedated the increased radiophosphate uptake (Pauwels et al, 1982). The radiophosphate manifestations of recurrence in order of frequency are diffuse and homogenous increased accretion in the affected part, focal and spotty increased uptake in the diseased area, and a progression of a lesion beyond its original boundaries into previously uninvolved bone. In polyostotic disease, deterioration can occur at one site while others remain static or improve. This variation from bone to bone is not necessarily reflected in the urinary hydroxyproline and alkaline phosphatase values, because they are global measurements of osteal metabolism like the total body 24-hour retention of radiophosphate. These variations in lesion activity can be seen with radiophosphate imaging. One group of workers advocates gallium-67-citrate as an imaging agent to monitor treatment because it seems to parallel the biochemical measurements more closely than radiophosphate. This alleged superiority of gallium-67 is attributed to its close association with the cellularity of pagetic bone, whereas radiophosphate uptake is largely a result of adsorption onto the apatite crystal and not directly dependent on the cell population (Waxman et al, 1980).

Serial triple-phase radiophosphate studies (perfusion, blood pool and delayed images) have been proposed by another group of workers as more sensitive than the delayed images alone. In some cases, the perfusion of blood pool images precede the improvement or deterioration seen in the delayed views and biochemical measurements (Boudreau et al, 1983). If the initial changes in improvement or reactivation are at the vascular level, ie, a decrease or increase in the number of blood vessels, this might explain the better sensitivity of the perfusion and blood pool images. This technique is only applicable to the appendicular skeleton since the soft tissue background is too high in the axial skeleton.

Malignant degeneration can occur and this should be suspected when a previously functioning area becomes photon-deficient. This is further substantiated if the photon-deficient area with radiophosphate takes up gallium-67 (Fig. 5).

Miscellaneous

Hypervitaminosis D results from excessive intake of vitamin D. Osteosclerosis may develop in the growing child if the condition is left untreated, and in the adult soft tissue calcific deposits may be found. In one study, three patients with alleged hypervitaminosis D intoxication presented a picture of generalized increased radiophosphate uptake and faint or no renal visualization (Fogelman et al, 1977a).

Hypersecretion of growth hormone by the acidophils of the anterior lobe of the pituitary causes *acromegaly*. Radiographically, there is subperiosteal appositional bone development in the skull and small bones of the hands and feet. The radiophosphate portrayal is more extensive, showing features of metabolic bone disease, ie, increased axial skeleton and long-bone uptake, prominent calvarium and mandible, increased periarticular and costochondral junction uptake, prominent sternum and faint kidney visualization (Fogelman et al, 1980b).

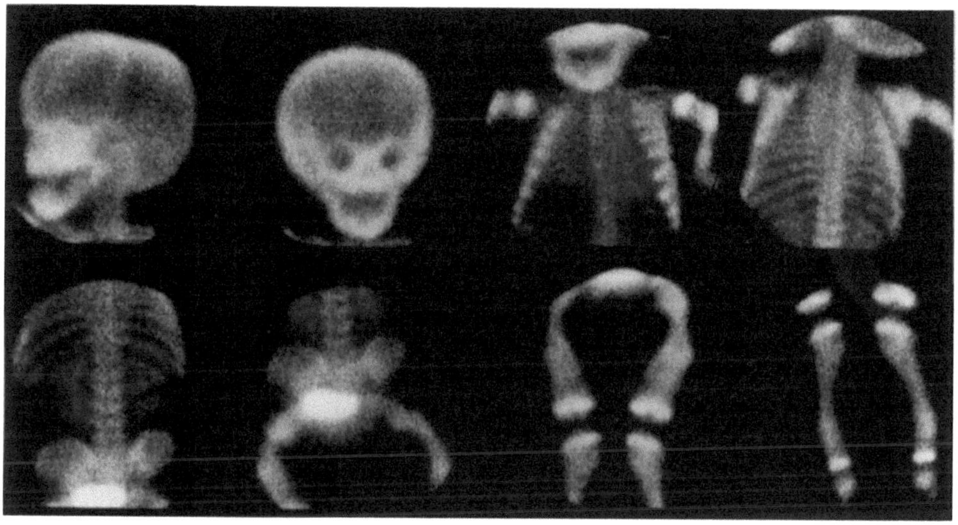

Fig. 6. Osteopetrosis in a child. Generalized increased accretion throughout the skeleton with lack of modeling in the distal extremities, most pronounced in the femurs.

The radiophosphate manifestations of *hypervitaminosis A* precede the radiographic indications. Two case reports of children showed increased radiophosphate deposition in the diaphyses of the ulnae, femora, tibiae, fibulae and metatarsi, and along the sutures of the calvarium. A normal bone scan was obtained four months after withdrawal of vitamin A intake in one of the patients who had a follow-up study (James et al, 1982; Miller and Hayon, 1985).

Osteopetrosis is a rare hereditary disorder of bone sclerosis and modeling which is believed to result from osteoclast dysfunction. It is caused by a failure of cartilage and bone matrix resorption and a consequent persistence of excess calcified matrix. This is seen as a universal and symmetrical sclerosis on the radiograph, with loss of distinction between medulla and cortex. The clinical manifestation varies from benign to a malignant course in which the infant fails to thrive (Fig. 6). In the malignant type, the radiophosphate scan exhibits an enhanced uptake throughout the axial and appendicular skeleton. The benign forms show variable characteristics, ranging from normal to increased uptake of radiophosphate at the ends of splayed long bones and in the epiphyseal ends of short tubular bones, while the rest of the skeleton is outwardly normal. (Park and Lambertus, 1977).

There is sparse information in literature on the bone scan appearance in *osteogenesis imperfecta*. Increased concentration is seen at fracture sites, and deformities as a result of previous multiple fractures are observed, but the bone uptake, per se, is normal.

Diffuse increased skeletal uptake of radiophosphate is nonspecific. The various metabolic bone diseases can all have similar radiophosphate images at some stage of their development. Other diseases not ordinarily classified as metabolic bone disease have been reported anecdotally as showing generalized skeletal response. Invariably, the corresponding radiographs are normal. These include progressive systemic sclerosis, secondary lues and psoriatic skin disease without articular involvement (Namey and Rosenthall, 1976; 1977). Some tumors produce a parathyroid hormone-like peptide that induces a clinical syndrome resembling hyperparathyroidism, and there is a report of higher sacrum/soft tissue ratios in patients with malignant disease not involving the sacrum (Buell et al, 1982).

References

1. Boudreau, R.J., Lisbona, R., Hadjipavlou, A.: Observations on serial radionuclide flow studies in Paget's disease. J.Nucl.Med. 28, 880, 1983.
2. Buéll, V., Kleenhaus, E., Zorn-Bopp, E., et al: A comparison of bone imaging with Tc-99m-DPD and Tc-99m-MDP. J.Nucl.Med. 23, 214, 1982.
3. Caniggia, A., Nute, R., Lore, F., et al: Pathophysiology of the adverse effects of glucoactive corticosteroids on calcium metabolism on man. J.Steroid Biochem. 15, 153, 1981.
4. Charkes, N.D., Brooks, M., and Mackler, P.T.: Studies of skeletal tracer kinetics. Evaluation of a 5 compartment model of F-18 fluoride kinetics in rats. J.Nucl.Med. 20, 1150, 1979.
5. Charkes, N.D., Mackler, P.T., Philips, C.: Studies of skeletal tracer kinetics. Digital-computer solution of a five compartment model of F-18 fluoride kinetics in humans. J.Nucl.Med. 19, 1301, 1978.
6. Conger, J.D., Hummond, W.C., Alfrey, A.C., et al: Pulmonary calcifications in chronic dialysis patients. Clinical and pathological studies. Ann.Intern.Med. 83, 330, 1975.
7. Cooper, R.A., Riley, J.W., Middleton, W.R., et al: Transient metastatic calcification in primary hyperparathyroidism. Aust.NZ J.Med. 8, 225, 1978.
8. de Graaf, P., Pauwels, E.K.J., Vos, P.H., et al: Observations on computerized quantitative bone scintigraphy in renal osteodystrophy. Eur. J.Nucl.Med. 9, 419, 1984.
9. de Graaf, P., Schicht, I.M., Pauwels, E.K.J., et al: Bone scintigraphy in renal osteodystrophy. J.Nucl.Med. 19, 1289, 1978.
10. de Graaf, P., Schicht, I.M., te Velde, J., et al: Quantitative bone scintigraphy in evaluating treatment of renal osteodystrophy. Neth. J.Med. 26, 125, 1983.
11. de Graaf, P., te Velde, J., Pauwels, E.K.J., et al: Increased bone radiotracer uptake in renal osteodystrophy. Clinical evidence of hyperparathyroidism as the major cause. Eur.J.Nucl.Med. 7, 152, 1982.
12. Fogelman, I. and Bessent, R.: Age-related alterations in skeletal metabolism - 24 hour whole body retention in 250 normal subjects. J. Nucl.Med. 23, 296, 1982.
13. Fogelman, I. and Carr, D.: A comparison of bone scanning and radiology in the evaluation of patients with metabolic bone disease. Clin. Radiol. 31, 321, 1980.
14. Fogelman, I. and Citrin, D.L.: Bone scanning in metabolic bone disease: A review. Appl.Radiol. 10, 158, 1981.

15. Fogelman, I., Bessent, R.G., Turner, J.G., et al: The use of whole body retention of Tc-99m diphosphonate in the diagnosis of metabolic bone disease. J.Nucl.Med. 19, 330, 1978.

16. Fogelman, I., Bessent, R.G., and Beastall, G.B.: Estimation of skeletal involvement in primary hyperparathyroidism. Ann.Intern.Med. 92, 65, 1980a.

17. Fogelman, I., Hay, I.D., Citrin, D.L., et al: Semi-quantitative analysis of the bone scan in acromegaly: Correlation with human growth hormone values. Br.J.Radiol. 53, 874, 1980b.

18. Fogelman, I., McKillop, J.H., Cowden, E.A., et al: Bone scan findings in hypervitaminosis D. J.Nucl.Med. 18, 1205, 1977a.

19. Fogelman, I., McKillop, J.H., Grieg, W.R., et al: Pseudofractures of the ribs detected by bone scanning. J.Nucl.Med. 18, 1236, 1977b.

20. Frame, B. and Marel, G.M.: Paget's disease: A review of current knowledge. Radiol. 141, 21, 1981.

21. Francis, M.D., Tofe, A.J., Benedict, J.J., et al: Imaging in the skeletal system. In, Proc. 2nd Int. Symp. on Radiopharmaceuticals, Seattle Society of Nuclear Medicine, New York, 1980. pp 603 - 615.

22. Holmes, R.A.: Quantitation of skeletal Tc-99m-labeled phosphates to detect metabolic bone disease. J.Nucl.Med. 19, 330, 1978.

23. Itoh, K. and Furudate, M.: Diffuse lung uptake on bone imaging in primary hyperparathyroidism before and after excision of a parathyroid adenoma. Clin.Nucl.Med. 4, 382, 1979.

24. James, M.B., Leonard, J.C., Fraser, J.J., et al: Hypervitaminosis A. Pediatrics 69, 112, 1982.

25. Jones, A.G., Francis, M.D., and Davis, M.: Bone scanning: radionuclide reaction mechanisms. Semin. Nucl. Med. 6, 3, 1976.

26. Krishnamurthy, G.T., Brickman, A.S., and Blahd, W.H.: Technetium 99m-Sn-pyrophosphate pharmacokinetics and bone image changes in parathyroid disease. J.Nucl.Med. 18, 236, 1977.

27. Kuzela, D.C., Huffer, W.E., Conger, J.D., et al: Soft tissue calcification in chronic dialysis patients. Am.J.Pathol. 86, 403, 1977.

28. Levine, S.B., Haines, J.E., Larson, S.M., et al: Reduced skeletal localization of 99m-Tc-diphosphonate in two cases of severe osteoporosis. Clin.Nucl.Med. 2, 318, 1977.

29. Lien, J.W.K., Wiegmann, T., Rosenthall, L., et al: Abnormal Tc-99m pyrophosphate bone scans in chronic renal failure. Clin.Nephrol. 6. 509, 1976.

30. MacFarlane, J.D., Lutkin, J.E., and Burwood, R.J.: The demonstration by scintigraphy of fractures in osteomalacia. Br.J.Radiol. 50, 369, 1977.

31. Miller, J.H. and Hayon, I.I.: Bone scintigraphy in hypervitaminosis A. Am.J.Roentgenol. 144, 768, 1985.

32. Mills, B.G., Singer, F.R., Weiner, L.P., et al: Cell cultures from bone affected by Paget's disease. Arthrit. Rheum. 23, 1115, 1980.

33. Namey, T.C. and Rosenthall, L.: Periarticular uptake of Tc-99m-diphosphonate in psoriatics. Arhtrit.Rheum. 19, 607, 1976.

34. Namey, T.C. and Rosenthall, L.: Generalized periarticular uptake of Tc-99m-pyrophosphate in progressive systemic sclerosis. Clin.Nucl.Med. 2, 26, 1977.

35. Park, H.M. and Lambertus, J.: Skeletal and reticuloendothelial imaging in osteopetrosis: Case report. J.Nucl.Med. 18, 1091, 1977.

36. Pauwels, E.K.J., Vellenga, C.J., Frijlink, W.B., et al: Bone scintigraphy in Paget's disease treated with APD. J.Nucl.Med. 23, 77, 1982 (abstr.)

37. Rai, G.S., Webster, S.G.P., and Wraight, E.P.: Isotope scanning of bone in the diagnosis of osteomalacia. J.Am.Geriat.Soc. 29, 45, 1981.

38. Revel, A., Basle, M., Poupard, K., et al: Bone tissue in Paget's dis-
88 ease of bone. Arthrit.Rheum. 23, 1104, 1980.

39. Rosenthall, L. and Arzoumanian, A.: Total body retention measurements of Tc-99m using a simple detector. Clin.Nucl.Med. 8, 210, 1983.

40. Rosenthall, L. and Kaye, M.: Technetium-99m pyrophosphate kinetics and imaging in metabolic bone disease. J.Nucl.Med. 16, 33, 1975.

41. Rosenthall, L. and Kaye, M.: Observations on the mechanism of Tc-99m-labeled phosphate complex uptake in metabolic bone disease. Semin. Nucl.Med. 6, 59, 1976.

42. Schultz, E.E., Libanati, C.R., Farley, S.M., et al: Skeletal scintigraphic changes in osteoporosis treated with sodium fluoride. J.Nucl. Med. 25, 651, 1984.

43. Seto, H., Futatsuya, R., Kamei, T., et al: Measurement of 24 hour whole body retention of Tc-99m-MDP with a thyroid probe: Quantitative assessment of metabolic and metastatic bone disease. Proc. 3rd World Congress in Nuclear Medicine and Biology, Paris, France, September 1982.

44. Singh, B.N., Kesala, A., Mehta, S.P., et al: Osteomalacia on bone scan simulating skeletal metastases. Clin.Nucl.Med. 2, 181, 1977.

45. Steven, M.M., Sturrock, R.D., Fogelman, I., et al: Whole body retention of diphosphonate in rheumatoid arthritis. J.Rheumatol. 9, 873, 1982.

46. Waxman, A.D., McKee, D., Siemsen, J.E., et al: Gallium scanning in Paget's disease of bone: Effect of calcitonin. Am.J.Roentgenol. 134, 303, 1980.

47. Wiegmann, T., Rosenthall, L., and Kaye, M.: Technetium-99m pyrophosphate bone scan in hyperparathyroidism. J.Nucl.Med. 18, 231, 1977.

48. Wilson, M.A.: The effect of age on the quality of bone scans using technetium-99m-pyrophosphate. Radiol. 139, 703, 1981.

Quantitative Assessment of Bone: Radiologic Methods

T. N. HANGARTNER

Introduction

Atraumatic or noninvasive methods for assessing the status of bone can be divided into two major groups: radiologic and nonradiologic. The former use ionizing radiation, including radiation produced by X-ray tubes, radioactive isotopes, and accelerators, namely photons and neutrons. Nonradiologic methods, such as ultrasound (Jurist, 1970; Langeton et al, 1984) and measurement of skinfold thickness (Brincat et al, 1984), are still in a developmental stage for application to bone, and therefore will not be discussed further.

The radiologic methods comprise three major subgroups: qualitative, semiquantitative, and quantitative methods. Qualitative methods depend largely on the more or less subjective interpretation of radiographs. Semiquantitative analysis of radiographs uses a defined system for grading qualitative features -- eg, the Singh index of the proximal end of the femur (Singh et al, 1970) and the index of striation of the metacarpi (Meema and Schatz, 1970). By far, most methods are quantitative, the subject of this review.

Description of Methods

1. Geometric analysis of radiographs (radiogrammetry)

Geometric analyses of bone from radiographs are the simplest methods available to assess the status of the skeleton. As long as the radiographic images are obtained under standardized conditions, results are reproducible.

a) Vertebral compression

Thinning of the spinal trabeculae weakens the vertebral bodies and can result in fractures, observable on radiographs.

In an early attempt to quantify vertebral compression fractures, both the anterior and the central height of the third lumbar vertebra were measured (Barnett and Nordin, 1960) and a spine score was calculated (Fig. 1). Later, wedge angles were computed from anterior and posterior height measurements (Gallagher et al, 1973), and measurements for parallel compression were obtained by comparing the heights of adjacent vertebrae (Hurxthal, 1968). The usual practice now is to compare the spinal measurements with norms; scores

Current Concepts of Bone Fragility

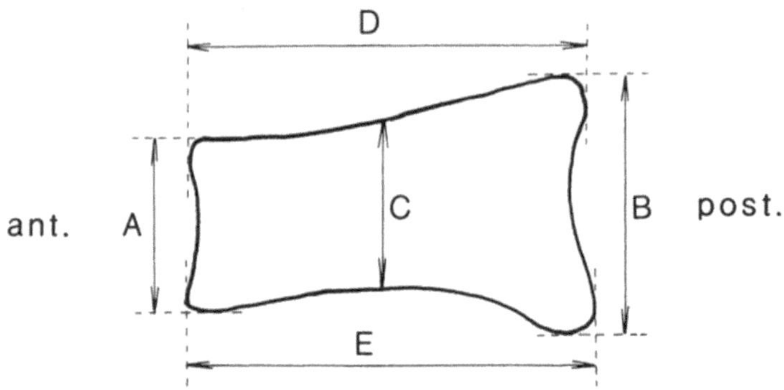

<u>Fig. 1</u>. Analysis of the spine by radiogrammetry: parameters for the quantitative evaluation of vertebral compressions.

Anterior compression	$B - A$	[mm]
Rel. anterior compression	$\frac{B - A}{B} 100$	[%]
Rel. central compression	$\frac{A + B - 2C}{A + B} 100$	[%]
Barnett-Nordin Score	$\frac{C}{A} 100$	[%]
Wedge Angle	$2 \sin^{-1} \frac{B - A}{D + E}$	[°]

---

of 0 to 3 are assigned for vertebrae that are normal, only wedged, or show central or parallel compression (Kleerekoper et al, 1984).

b) Cortical reduction

Reduction in cortical bone is always associated with osteopenia. The amount of cortical bone can be estimated from radiographs by measuring the width of the total bone and the marrow cavity (Fig. 2), and by calculating a cortical index; such measurements have been proposed for the femur (Barnett and Nordin, 1960; Virtama and Telka, 1962), second metacarpus (Barnett and Nordin, 1960; Garn, 1970), radius (Meema and Meema, 1963), humerus (Meema and Meema, 1963; Virtama and Telka, 1962), and the clavicle (Fujita et al, 1968). The combined cortical thickness represents an absolute width, whereas the relative cortical width is a value that is normalized for variations in bone size. Calculation of the amount of cross-sectional area covered by cortical bone is based on assumptions about the geometrical form of the cross section. The cylindrical geometry of a bone allows derivation of the mathematical expression for cortical area as in Figure 2 (Exton-Smith and Millard, 1969). The second metacarpus at midheight approximates a circular cross section fairly well (Dequeker and Roh, 1982); despite this, however, the cortical area of the metacarpus is systematically overestimated by measurements from radiographs (Dequeker and Roh, 1982; Horsman and Kirby, 1972).

c) Intracortical resorption

Rather than estimating osteopenia solely by measuring the thickness of cortical bone, the quantification of intracortical resorption provides an index

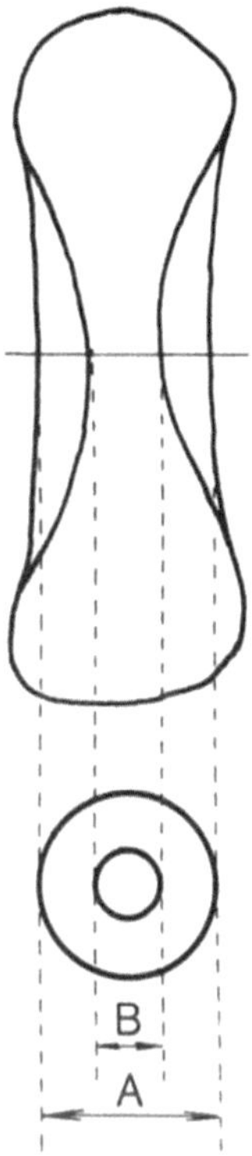

Fig. 2. Analysis of cortical bone by radiogrammetry: parameters for the quantitative evaluation of the cortical midshaft of long bones.

Combined cortical thickness	$A - B$	[cm]
Rel. cortical thickness	$\frac{A - B}{A} 100$	[%]
Cortical area	$\frac{\pi}{4} (A^2 - B^2)$	[mm²]
Rel. cortical area	$\frac{A^2 - B^2}{A^2}$	[%]

of the density of cortical bone. A section in the middle of the second metacarpus, 4 mm long, is viewed under magnification, and all resorptive tunnels lying entirely within the cortex are counted (Meema and Schatz, 1970). The index is the number of tunnels divided by the width of the cortex.

2. Analysis of radiographic density (photodensitometry)

Quantitative evaluation of the various grey levels in a radiograph constituted the first attempt to estimate the amount and density of tissue *in vivo*. As far back as 1901, a copper step wedge was being used for calibration (Price, 1901). Accuracy is enhanced by adding a compensating medium of soft tissue equivalent material above and below the body part to be measured, thus ensuring constancy of the length of the beam path over the area to be analyzed. One solution is the use of a water bath in which a subject submerses an arm, for example, so that it can be measured through the water (Jackson, 1951; Keane et al, 1959). Optical density readings thus obtained and referenced to a calibration wedge provide values (projection points) showing the amount of bone in the beam path. All projection points obtained along a line across the bone form a projection curve. The summation of all projection points (ie, the integral under the projection curve, as shown in Figure 3) represents the total amount of bone in the measured cross section. To give this calculated number a physical meaning requires standardization of the thickness of the slice, usually done by expressing the amount of bone in the cross section as if measured in a slice 1 cm thick. Thus, this parameter, Bone Mineral Content (BMC), is expressed as g/cm.

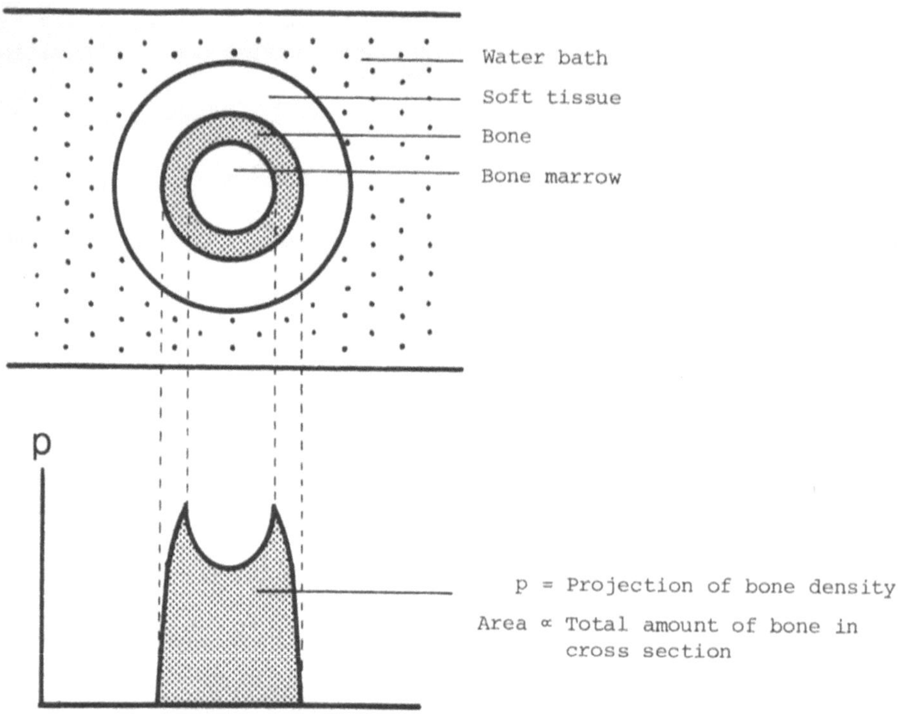

Fig. 3. Photodensitometric measurement of bone in a water bath. Water, soft tissue and marrow attenuate X-rays by about equal amounts; the projection profile, therefore, represents the bone tissue.

3) Absorptiometry

a) Single-photon absorptiometry

To avoid the problems associated with the film medium, direct measurement of a bone's projection curve can be made by counting the transmitted photons of a narrowly collimated photon beam (Fig. 4) while moving the source detector assembly across the bone (Cameron and Sorensen, 1963). This technique also requires a compensating water bath, and the index is essentially the same as with photodensitometry of radiographs (BMC).

b) Dual-photon absorptiometry

Certain bones, particularly in the spine, are not easily accessible for measurements with single-photon absorptiometry, but can be measured with the dual-photon system (Reed, 1966; Reed et al, 1970) in which the isotope emits photons at two distinct levels of energy. The isotope most widely used is ^{153}Gd (44 keV, 100 keV), but a combination of isotopes such as ^{125}I with ^{241}Am (29 keV, 60 keV) can also be employed. This method also measures the equivalent of BMC.

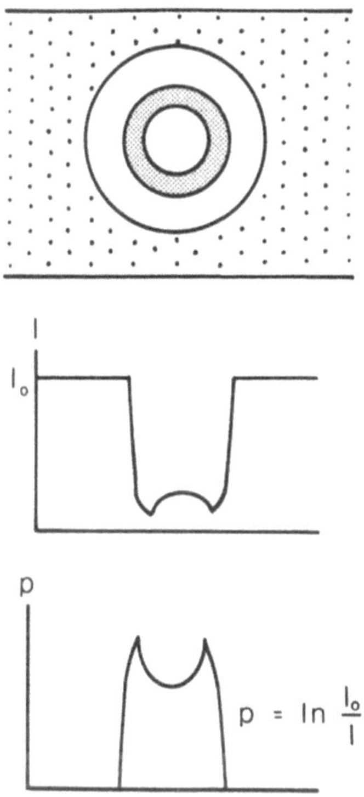

Fig. 4. Bone measurement by photon absorptiometry. A collimated photon beam is moved across the bone in the water bath, and the count rates I are recorded. Outside the bone, the count rate is I_0; the natural log of the ratio I_0/I gives the projection profile p.

4. Computed tomography (CT)

Computed tomography is the logical extension of absorptiometry. Instead of measuring only one profile across the bone, up to several hundreds are measured at various angles (Ruegsegger et al, 1974), and a two-dimensional map of the density of the cross section is computed. Each matrix element (pixel) represents the average linear attenuation coefficient of the material at that site in the cross section; this, in turn, is directly related to the physical density (expressed as g/cm^3). No water bath is necessary for this type of measurement, which can be applied to peripheral bones as well as vertebrae. Since a density matrix of the whole cross section is available, individual areas, particularly compact or trabecular bone, can be quantified separately.

The first commercially available CT scanner, a single-energy model, was dedicated to the measurement of cross sections of the head (Hounsfield, 1973).

a) Single energy CT

Although readings for bone density can be obtained from ordinary CT images, precision and accuracy are poor unless special precautions are taken. Two methods yield high-quality values. The first uses a special-purpose CT scanner with an ^{125}I source and photon-counting electronics. It is dedicated to the measurement of peripheral bones, particularly the radius (Ruegsegger et al, 1976). The second method, employing a commercial whole-body CT scanner, includes a calibration phantom that is measured concurrently with the patient (Cann and Genant, 1980).

b) Dual energy CT

As described before, each pixel of a CT image represents the average linear attenuation coefficient of the material at the particular location in the cross section. Assuming that a given pixel of trabecular bone contains only bone and marrow, both of known chemical composition, its linear attenuation coefficient will lie between that of bone and that of marrow. Based on this measured attenuation coefficient, we can calculate the relative amounts of bone and fat at that location. Since, however, the chemical composition of marrow is unknown -- because of variation in its fat content -- a second, independent measurement of the same cross section is needed. This is obtained with an X-ray beam of a different energy level (Genant and Boyd, 1977).

5. Compton scattering

This method of bone measurement relies on the physical effect of the interaction of photons of certain energies with atoms whereby the photons are scattered in various directions. When photons and electrons interact, the number of scattered photons is proportional to the number of electrons. For biologic materials, since the number of electrons in a volume element is proportional to physical density, Compton scattering provides an index of physical density (g/cm³). To define clearly the volume to be measured, source and detectors are collimated precisely and positioned at approximately a right angle to each other (Fig. 5). Two sources and detectors are usually

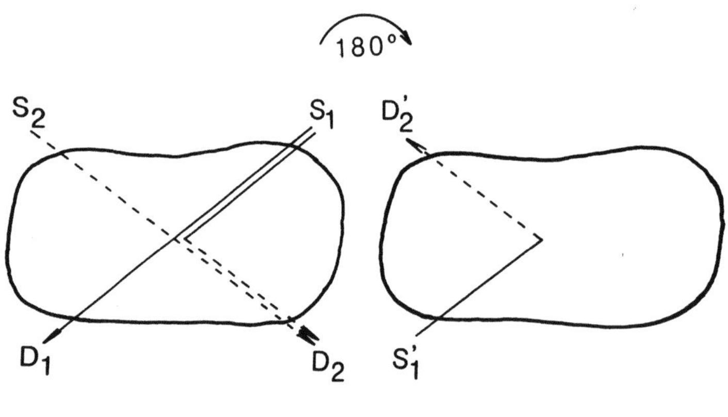

$$\rho \propto \sqrt{\frac{(S_1 \to D_2)(S_1' \to D_2')}{(S_1 \to D_1)(S_2 \to D_2)}}$$

Fig. 5. The Compton scattering method of bone measurement requires a photon source S_1 for the scattering measurement and à second source S_2 at the energy of the scattered radiation, for measuring attenuation. A total of 2 transmission and 2 scattering measurements are needed for the calculation of the bone density p.

needed to measure both scattered and transmitted radiation (Odeblad and Norhagen, 1956). The count rates recorded by the two detectors from the two sources are measured, the apparatus is turned 180°, and another set of readings is taken. These count rates allow computation of the physical density of the scattering volume. The bone most easily accessible *in vivo* is the calcaneus (Webber and Kennett, 1976). The distal end of the radius has also been measured (Hazan et al, 1977).

6. Neutron activation

Analysis of bone mass by neutron activation requires irradiation of parts or all of the body by neutrons. Sources of neutrons are accelerators or radioisotopes (eg, ^{238}Pu-Be, ^{241}Am-Be, ^{252}Cf). Irradiation converts a percentage of ^{48}Ca into ^{49}Ca, which emits photons at about 3.1 MeV; ordinary scintillation detectors can be used to count these photons. Since the amount of radioactive calcium produced is proportional to the total amount of calcium in the body volume irradiated, and because 99% of the calcium is concentrated in bone (Mitchell et al, 1945), the amount of activated calcium is a good measure of the amount of bone (mass, in g) in the irradiated volume.

Neutron activation has been used to measure bone mass in the hand (Catto et al, 1973), forearm (Smith and Tothill, 1979), lower part of the spine (Al-Hiti et al, 1976), trunk (McNeill et al, 1973), and in the entire body (Anderson et al, 1964).

Comparison of Methods

1. Measurement parameters

The quantitative methods yield a combination of a primary bone parameter and a geometrical one (Table I). The former is the descriptor of the amount of bone, and the latter indicates the number of geometrical dimensions measurable with the particular method. Secondary parameters, which are a combination of the primary bone parameters and geometric ones (eg, absorptiometry: Bone Mineral Index = BMC/Bone Width), have not been listed.

Radiogrammetry supplies only geometric information, whereas Compton scattering and neutron activation exclude geometric parameters.

Table I. Various parameters obtained by quantitative bone measurement methods

Method	Primary bone parameter	Dimension of geometrical parameter
Radiogrammetry	----	2
Photodensitometry	mass	1
Absorptiometry	mass	1
Computed tomography	density	3
Compton scattering	density	0
Neutron activation	mass	0

Photodensitometry and absorptiometry yield the same parameters, namely bone mass and one geometric dimension. When data are measured along adjacent pathways, a series of projection curves is obtained over a two-dimensional area. The anatomically-relevant parameter is the sum of all points of a projection curve, and one of the two geometric dimensions is lost by the summation process; the resulting values represent bone mass per unit length. These techniques permit examination of narrow bone cross sections, whereas neutron activation yields values of bone mass over a large volume.

Computed tomography provides a two-dimensional map of bone density over a bone cross section. A series of adjacent slices can then be put together to give a 3-dimensional representation of bone density. With this detailed information, any selected bone volume can be defined and evaluated separately, particularly trabecular bone or cortical bone. Three-dimensional mapping of bone density is theoretically possible also with the Compton scattering method but the practical limitations of measurement time and radiation dose restrict this method to the measurement of single, relatively large volumes of bone.

2. Precision and accuracy

The precision of most methods is between 2 and 5%. A noticeable exception is single photon absorptiometry of the distal end of the radius, with an error of 7.6% (Shimmins et al, 1972). The problem here is the rapid change of bone mass with axial position, but without a radiographic positioning device it is not possible to reduce this error.

Special-purpose CT of the distal end of the radius shows an error of only 0.5 to 0.9% (Hangartner and Overton, 1982; Ruegsegger et al, 1981; 1983). This is due to the high stability of the technique and the sensitivity of the parameter of axial position available from the cross-sectional area of the bone.

The major factor influencing accuracy is the unknown composition of some tissues in the volume to be measured. This is particularly true for bone marrow which may have a variable fat content. The only method capable of quantifying the amount of fat in marrow is dual-energy CT. Although dual-photon absorptiometry also uses two energy levels, these are needed to replace the water bath as a compensation medium and not to produce information about bone marrow composition.

3. Sensitivity

Trabecular bone and cortical bone behave differently, not only under the influence of disease but also in their way of normal remodeling (Frost, 1963). Clinical application determines which of the two bone types should be studied. Table II lists the methods and the type of bone accessible to them. It can be seen that CT is the only method capable of providing information separately about both types of bone.

Dual-photon absorptiometry is used both for the total body and for the spine. Since total bone only is accessible with this method, the spinal processes are included in the bone parameter measured. These processes increase the total amount of bone material and, therefore, decrease the sensitivity of the method to changes in trabecular bone in the vertebral body.

Table II. Bone type and skeletal site accessible by the various bone measurement methods

Method	Bone type			Skeletal site	
	trabecular	cortical	total	peripheral	axial
Vertebral compression index			X		X
Cortical index		X		X	
Intracortical resorption index		X		X	
Photodensitometry			X	X	
Single-photon absorptiometry			X	X	
Dual-photon absorptiometry			X	X	X
Computed tomography	X	X	X	X	X
Compton scattering	X			X	
Neutron activation			X	X	X

In the context of sensitivity, an important question is which bone in the skeleton is most representative for a particular disease or for the skeleton as a whole. In the past, the spine received most attention from radiologists. Several correlative studies have been published (Genant et al, 1984; Hangartner et al, 1983; Ott et al, 1984) in which various methods and sites of bone measurement are compared.

While many correlations among different sites are highly significant, the prime consideration is the standard error of the estimate. This is the error of prediction and exceeds 10% in most studies, with the result that bone density or bone mass measured at one site cannot be used to predict the density or mass at another site with an error of better than 10%. The precision of most methods, however, is considerably better than 5%. Thus, information about the axial skeleton has to be obtained from measurements of the axial skeleton and about the peripheral skeleton from measurements of the peripheral skeleton.

Clinical Use

The clinical use of a certain method for measuring bone is generally governed by its availability. Photogrammetry is most widely used since ordinary radiographic equipment is not only available in hospitals but also in private practice. For this reason, the number of vertebral compressions is the generally accepted criterion for deciding whether a patient has osteopenia.

Photodensitometry uses an automatic instrument to compare measured densities with those of the calibration wedge. While the films can be evaluated commercially, the considerable care required in the standardization of the radiographs limits this method to research.

Absorptiometry machines are commercially available, and single photon absorptiometry has been around long enough to be a reliable technique. Despite this, it is doubtful if single- as well as dual-photon absorptiometry will ever be used for single measurement screening purposes. The interindividual variation (2 SD) of the various bone measurements in a normal population of defined sex and age is about 20-30% (Genant et al, 1984; Mazess, 1984). A patient would have to be 30% below normal to be considered osteopenic, and a 30% density difference starts to show up on an ordinary radiograph. Allowing for the restrictions about the different behavior of cortical and trabecular bone, absorptiometry can be useful in following the effect of treatment.

Computed tomography for peripheral bone measurements requires special-purpose scanners if good precision and accuracy are desired. Such machines are, so far, only available at a few research centers. Axial CT measurements can be performed on most commercial whole-body scanners if the necessary quality control is implemented.

Obviously, many of the more sophisticated methods for bone measurement will never be widely used. However, research results produced with these machines may help to interpret more clearly the bone measurements obtained with less sophisticated methods and thus improve diagnosis and management.

Acknowledgement

The author is grateful to the Alberta Heritage Foundation for Medical Research for a scholarship and to Mrs. P.J. Cotterill for editorial assistance.

References

1. Al-Hiti, K., Thomas, B.J., Al-Tikrity, S.A., Ettinger, K.V., and Fremlin, J.H.: Spinal calcium: Its *in vivo* measurement in man. Int. J. Appl. Radiat. Isotopes 27, 97, 1976.

2. Anderson, J., Osborn, S.B., Tomlinson, R.W.S. Newton, D., Rundo, J., Salmon, L., and Smith, J.W.: Neutron-activation analysis in man *in vivo*. Lancet 2, 1201, 1964.

3. Barnett, E. and Nordin, B.E.C.: The radiological diagnosis of osteoporosis: a new approach. Clin. Radiol. 11, 166, 1960.

4. Brincat, M., Studd, J.W.W., Moniz, C.J., Parson, V., and Darby, A.J.: Skin thickness measurements. A simple screening method for determining patients at risk of developing postmenopausal osteoporosis. In, Osteoporosis 1. Eds: Christiansen, C., Arnaud, C.D., Nordin, B.E.C., Parfitt, A.M., Peck, W.A., Riggs, B.L. Glostrup Hospital, Copenhagen. 1984, pp 323-326.

5. Cameron, J.R. and Sorensen, J.: Measurement of bone mineral *in vivo:* an improved method. Science 142, 230, 1963.

6. Cann, C.E. and Genant, H.K.: Precise measurement of vertebral mineral content using computed tomography. J. Comput. Assist. Tomogr. 4, 493, 1980.

7. Catto, G.R.D., McIntosh, J.A.R., and MacLeod, M.: Partial body neutron activation analysis *in vivo*: A new approach to the investigation of metabolic bone disease. Phys. Med. Biol. 18, 508, 1973.

8. Dequeker, J. and Roh, Y.S.: Influence of morphometric properties of long bones on the radiogrammetric estimation of bone mass. In, Non-Invasive Bone Measurements: Methodological Problems. Eds: Dequeker, J. and Johnston, C.C., IRL Press, Oxford/Washington, D.C., 1982. pp 33-41.

9. Exton-Smith, A.N. and Millard, P.H.: Method for measuring quantity of bone. Lancet 2, 1153, 1969.

10. Frost, H.M.: Bone Remodelling Dynamics. Chas. C. Thomas, Springfield, Illinois, 1963, p. 72.

11. Fujita, T., Orimo, H., Ohata, M., and Yoshikawa, M.: Changes in the cortical thickness of the clavicle according to age. J. Am. Geriatr. Soc. 16, 458, 1968.

12. Gallagher, J.C., Aaron, J., Horsman, A., Marshall, D.H., Wilkinson, R., and Nordin, B.E.C.: The crush fracture syndrome in postmenopausal women. Clinics Endocrinol. Metab. 2, 293, 1973.

13. Garn, S.M.: The earlier gain and later loss of cortical bone in nutritional perspective. Springfield, IL, 1970.

14. Genant, H.K. and Boyd, D.: Quantitative bone mineral analysis using dual energy computed tomography. Invest. Radiol. 12, 545, 1977.

15. Genant, H.K., Cann, C.E., Ettinger, B., Gordan, G.S., Kolb, F.O., Reiser, U., and Arnaud, C.D.: Quantitative computed tomography for spinal mineral assessment. In, Osteoporosis 1. Eds: Christiansen, C., Arnaud, C.D., Nordin, B.E.C., Parfitt, A.M., Peck, W.A., Riggs, B.L. Glostrup Hospital, Copenhagen, 1984. pp 65-72.

16. Genant, H.K., Powell, M.R., Cann, C.E., Stebler, B., Rutt, B.K., Richardson, M.L., and Kolb, F.O.: Comparison of methods for *in vivo* spinal bone mineral measurement. In, Osteoporosis 1. Eds: Christiansen, C., Arnaud, C.D., Nordin, B.E.C., Parfitt, A.M., Peck, W.A., Riggs, B.L. Glostrup Hospital, Copenhagen, 1984. pp 97-102.

17. Hangartner, T.N. and Overton, T.R.: Quantitative measurement of bone density using gamma-ray computed tomography. J. Comput. Assist. Tomog. 6, 1156, 1982.

18. Hangartner, T.N., Overton, T.R., and Rigal, W.M.: Comparison of trabecular bone density at axial and peripheral sites using computed tomography. In, Clinical Disorders of Bone and Mineral Metabolism. Eds: Frame, B., Potts, J.T., Jr. Excerpta Medica, Amsterdam, 1983. pp 54-57.

19. Hazan, G., Leichter, I., Loewinger, E., and Weinreb, A.: The early detection of osteoporosis by Compton gamma ray spectroscopy. Phys. Med. Biol. 22, 1073, 1977.

20. Horsman, A. and Kirby, P.A.: Geometric properties of the second metacarpal. Calc. Tiss. Res. 10, 289, 1972.

21. Hounsfield, G.N.: Computerized transverse axial scanning (tomography): Part I. Description of system. Br. J. Radiol. 46, 1016, 1973.

22. Hurxthal, L.M.: Measurement of anterior vertebral compressions and biconcave vertebrae. Am. J. Roentgeno. 103, 635, 1968.

23. Jackson, H.: Problems in the measurement of bone density. Br. J. Radiol. 24, 613, 1951.

24. Jurist, J.M.: *In-vivo* determination of the elastic response of bone. I. Method of ulnar resonant frequency determination. Phys. Med. Biol. 15, 417, 1970.

25. Keane, B.E., Spiegler, G., and Davis, R.: Quantitative evaluation of bone mineral by radiographic method. Br. J. Radiol. 32, 162, 1959.

26. Kleerekoper, M., Parfitt, A.M., and Ellis, B.I.: Measurement of vertebral fracture rates in osteoporosis. In, Osteoporosis 1. Eds: Christiansen, C., Arnaud, C.D., Nordin, B.E.C., Parfitt, A.M., Peck, W.A., Riggs, B.L. Glostrup Hospital, Copenhagen, 1984, pp 103-109.

27. Langton, C., Palmer, S.B., and Porter, R.W.: The measurement of broadband ultrasonic attenuation in cancellous bone. In, Osteoporosis 1. Eds: Christiansen, C., Arnaud, C.D., Nordin, B.E.C., Parfitt, A.M., Peck, W.A., Riggs, B.L. Glostrup Hospital, Copenhagen, 1984, pp 223-225.

28. Mazess, R. B.: Advances in single- and dual-photon absorptiometry. In, Osteoporosis 1. Eds: Christiansen, C., Arnaud, C.D., Nordin, B.E.C., Parfitt, A.M., Peck, W.A., Riggs, B.L. Glostrup Hospital, Copenhagen, 1984. pp 57-63

29. McNeill, K.G., Thomas, B.J., Sturtridge, W.C., and Harrison, J.E.: *In vivo* neutron activation analysis for calcium in man. J. Nucl. Med. 14, 502, 1973.

30. Meema, H.E. and Meema, S.: Measurable roentgenologic changes in some peripheral bones in senile osteoporosis. J. Am. Geriatr. Soc. 11, 1170, 1963.

31. Meema, H.E. and Schatz, D.L.: Simple radiologic demonstration of cortical bone loss in thyrotoxicosis. Radiology 97, 9, 1970.

32. Mitchell, H.H., Hamilton, T.S., Steggerda, F.R., and Bean, H.W.: The chemical composition of the adult human body and its bearing on the biochemistry of growth. J. Biol. Chem. 158, 625, 1945.

33. Odeblad, E., and Norhagen, A.: Measurements of electron densities with the aid of the Compton scattering process. Acta Radiol. 45, 161, 1956.

34. Ott, S.M., Chesnut, C.H. III, Hanson, J.A., Kilcoyne, R.F., Murano, R., and Lewellen, T.K.: Comparison of bone mass measurements using different diagnostic techniques in patients with postmenopausal osteoporosis. In, Osteoporosis 1. Eds: Christiansen, C., Arnaud, C.D., Nordin, B.E.C., Parfitt, A.M., Peck, W.A., Riggs, B.L. Glostrup Hospital, Copenhagen, 1984, pp 93-96.

35. Price, W.A.: The science of dental radiography. Dental Cosmos 43, 483, 1901.

36. Reed, G.W.: The assessment of bone mineralization from the relative transmission of ^{241}Am and ^{137}Cs radiations. Phys. Med. Biol. 11, 174, 1966.

37. Reed, G.W., West, R.R., and Atkinson, P.J.: The measurement of bone mineralization *in vivo* using monoenergetic radiation. In, Symposium Ossium. Eds: Jelliffe, A.M., Strickland, B. E. & S. Livingstone, Edinburgh and London, 1970. pp 267-269.

38. Ruegsegger, P., Anliker, M., and Cambacher, M.: Quantification of trabecular bone with low dose computed tomography. J. Comput. Assist. Tomog. 5, 384, 1981.

39. Ruegsegger, P., Elsasser, U., Anliker, M., Gnehm, H., Kind, H., Prader, A.: Quantification of bone mineralization using computed tomography. Radiology 121, 93, 1976.

40. Ruegsegger, P., Medici, T.C., and Anliker, M.: Corticosteroid-induced bone loss. A longitudinal study of alternate day therapy in patients with bronchial asthma using quantitative computed tomography. Eur. J. Clin. Pharmacol. 25, 615, 1983.

41. Ruegsegger, P., Niederer, P., and Anliker, M.: An extension of classical bone mineral measurement. Ann. Biomed. Eng. 2, 194, 1974.

42. Shimmins, J., Smith, D.A., Aitken, M., Anderson, J.B., and Gillespie, F.C.: The accuracy and reproducibility of bone mineral measurements *in vivo*. (b) Methods using sealed isotope sources. Clin. Radiol. 23, 47, 1972.

43. Singh, M., Nagrath, A.R., and Maini, P.S.: Changes in trabecular pattern of the upper end of the femur as an index of osteoporosis. J. Bone Joint Surg. 52A, 457, 1970.

44. Smith, M.A. and Tothill, P.: Development of apparatus to measure calcium changes in the forearm and spine by neutron activation analysis using Californium-252. Phys. Med. Biol. 24, 319, 1979.

45. Virtama, P. and Telka, A.: Cortical thickness as an estimate of mineral content of human humerus and femur. Br. J. Radiol. 35, 632, 1962.

46. Webber, C.E. and Kennett, T.J.: Bone density measured by photon scattering. I. A system for clinical use. Phys. Med. Biol. 21, 760, 1976.

Bone Turnover Assessment Using Bone-Specific Biochemical Markers

K. G. MANN and B. L. RIGGS

Methodologic Problems in Assessing Bone Turnover

Simple, noninvasive methods for determining bone formation and bone resorption are urgently needed which are well-characterized, specific, and accurate. The lack of such methods severely contrains research of the pathophysiology of osteoporosis, other bone-losing metabolic disorders, and of the clinical evaluation of treatment. Radiocalcium kinetic studies combined with external calcium balance include a variable, nonresolvable long-term exchange component (which may represent as much as one-half of the computed bone turnover rate) (Riggs et al, 1971). Moreover, these methods, requiring the administration of radioactivity, are time-consuming and expensive. Bone histomorphometry, the other commonly employed technique measuring local rather than overall bone turnover, cannot quantify bone resorption rate accurately and requires an invasive procedure (Frost, 1973).

Biochemical markers for measuring bone turnover have the advantage of simplicity and convenience. However, serum alkaline phosphatase and urinary hydroxyproline measurements are nonspecific and relatively insensitive. Except in pregnant women, about 40% of total serum alkaline phosphatase is derived from the liver, about 40% from bone, and about 20% from the intestine (Farley et al, 1981). Attempts to separate the specific isoenzymes using heat inactivation or differences in electrophoretic mobility have been only moderately successful. Even when dietary hydroxyproline intake is controlled, urinary hydroxyproline is a nonspecific and insensitive measure of bone collagen breakdown. The skeleton contains only half of the body's stores of collagen. In addition, a rapid turnover component of the compliment system of proteins, Clq, contributes a large and variable amount to the urinary hydroxyproline excretion (Krane et al, 1977).

Bone-Specific Proteins

The recent discovery that bone contains specific proteins not found in other tissues has given rise to the hope that their measurement in the circulation will provide a quantitative estimate of bone turnover. The first such protein to be discovered, bone Gla-protein (BGP), also called osteocalcin, is a 5,800 dalton peptide which contains three-γ-carboxyglutamic acid (Gla) residues (Price, 1983). BGP comprises about 25% of the noncollagenous protein of bone matrix, is one of the most abundant proteins in the body, and is highly conserved in evolution. Its physiologic function is controversial. Studies in experimental animals, however, have suggested a role in

Current Concepts of Bone Fragility

preventing excessive mineralization of bone. In newborn rats maintained on warfarin therapy for eight months, complete fusion of the growth plates resulting in cessation of linear growth was observed (Price et al, 1982). Also, BGP-deficient bone particles were relatively resistant to resorption when implanted subcutaneously into normal rats (Lian et al, 1984), suggesting that BGP may facilitate bone resorption, perhaps by eliciting progenitor-cell recruitment and differentiation. BGP is synthesized by cultured rat osteosarcoma cells, and its production is increased by 1,25-dihydroxyvitamin D treatment (Price and Baukol, 1980). Recent studies have demonstrated that BGP is secreted by osteoblast-like cells from normal human bone (Beresford et al, 1984).

Termine et al (1981a) have identified three additional bone-specific proteins. One of them, osteonectin, is closely associated with calcified matrix and may bind hydroxyapatite to collagen (Termine et al, 1981b). Osteonectin has a molecular weight of 29,000 (Romberg et al, 1985; Termine et al, 1981a) It is an extremely potent inhibitor of hydroxyapaptite-seeded crystal growth, suggesting a regulatory function in bone mineralization (Romberg et al, 1985). Osteonectin, however, may not be completely bone-specific because it has been demonstrated that fibroblasts can synthesize small amounts of it (Wasi et al, 1984).

The other two components isolated from bone matrix by Termine et al (1981a) are a 62,000 dalton glycoprotein and a 24,000 dalton protein. Their function is not known. Other bone-specific noncollagenous proteins may also be present in matrix. Using two-dimensional electrophoresis, Delmas et al (1984) were able to identify 12 proteins, in addition to BGP and osteonectin, that are present in bovine bone extracts but not in blood (Fig. 1).

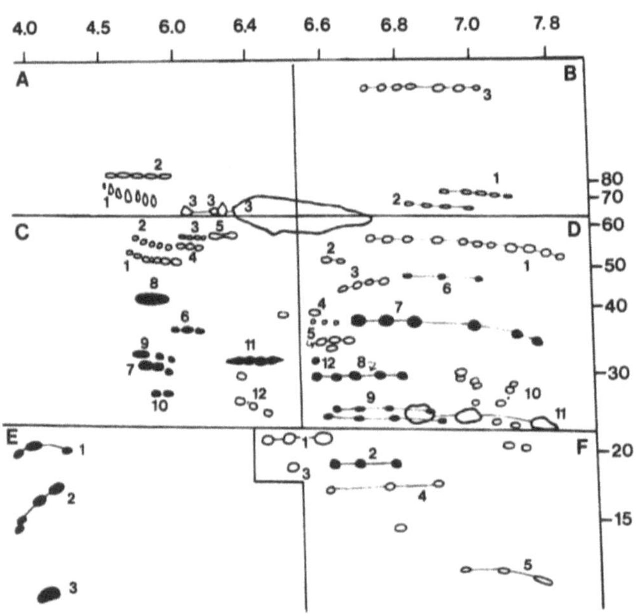

Fig. 1. Tracing of two-dimensional electrophoretic gel of bovine bone matrix extract. Spot E-3 represents bone Gla-protein and spot C-3 represents osteonectin.

Since osteoblasts are continually synthesizing new bone matrix and osteoclasts are resorbing bone (including old bone matrix), measurement of these bone-specific proteins or their fragments in blood and urine may allow the assessment of bone formation and bone resorption by biochemical measurements.

Radioimmunoassay of Serum Bone Gla-Protein

Of the various bone-specific proteins, thus far only BGP has been reliably measured in the circulation. Several groups have found that antiserum raised against bovine BGP cross-reacts with human BGP (Delmas et al, 1983a; Epstein et al, 1984; Gundberg et al, 1983; Price et al, 1980). Measurements of serum BGP using these radioimmunoassays have shown the normal range for young adults is about 4-12 ng/mL. One laboratory has recorded a circadian rhythm for serum BGP; levels fell during the morning, rose in the afternoon and early evening, and reached a peak nocturnally. Also, serum BGP increases with aging in both women and men, but the increase is greater in women (Delmas et al, 1983a; Epstein et al, 1984). The increase in serum BGP between young adulthood and extreme old age in women is almost twofold.

Measurement of serum BGP has proved to be a valuable biochemical marker for bone metabolism. Serum levels distinguish between high and low bone turnover in a variety of metabolic bone diseases characterized by high or low bone turnover (Deftos et al, 1982; Delmas et al, 1983b; Price et al, 1980) (Table I). Particularly impressive was the ability to detect low bone turnover in patients with hypoparathyroidism associated with normal levels of serum alkaline phosphatase (Delmas et al, 1983b; Price et al, 1980).

Table I. Relationships between serum BGP and serum alkaline phosphatase in human blood

	BGP ng/mL	AP IU/liter	r	P
Normal adults (n = 109)	6.78 (0.20)	26.7 (1.3)	0.10	NS
Men (n = 47)	7.89 (0.32)	28.1 (2.1)	0.40	<0.005
Women (n = 62)	4.85 (0.36)	25.2 (1.8)	-0.17	NS
Paget's disease (n = 13)	39.2 (16)*	587 (181)*	0.66	<0.025
Bone metastases (n = 5)†	15.8 (2.6)*	132 (26)*	0.93	<0.05
Hyperparathyroidism				
Primary (n = 11)	16.5 (1.7)*	64 (6.8)*	0.16	NS
Secondary (n = 38) §	47.3 (6.1)*	56 (8.5)*	0.64	<0.005
Hypoparathyroidism (n = 3)	2.40 (0.92)*	--	--	--
Liver disease (n = 11)	5.77 (1.0)	170 (41)*	0.10	NS
Osteopenia (n = 20)	9.05 (1.8)*	48 (4.6)*	0.64	<0.01

Except as indicated and in osteopenic group, all subjects are men. Results are mean ± SE.

* Significantly ($P < 0.05-0.005$) different from normal controls.

† Squamous cell carcinoma of the lung (2); adenocarcinoma of the colon (2), and of the breast (2).

§ Chronic renal disease on hemodialysis.

(Price et al, 1980).

Serum BGP determinations have also been shown to be useful in following the course of treatment of metabolic bone disease. Serum levels of BGP decreased in patients with Paget's disease following the acute and chronic administration of salmon calcitonin (Deftos et al, 1982). Following parathyroidectomy in patients with primary hyperparathyroidism, elevated levels of serum BGP decreased to within the normal range (Deftos et al, 1982). Treatment of postmenopausal women with estrogen also resulted in a significant decrease in serum BGP (Podenphant et al, 1984).

Controversy has arisen as to which component of bone turnover serum BGP measures. Although some BGP diffuses into the circulation after synthesis by osteoblasts, most is incorporated into bone matrix where it remains until removed by bone resorption (Price, 1983). Increasing evidence suggests, however, that serum levels of BGP reflect mainly, if not exclusively, bone formation. Price et al (1980) found, three hours after injecting rats with warfarin, an inhibitor of γ-carboxylation, and that BGP in serum was entirely decarboxylated whereas BGP in bone was fully γ-carboxylated. They concluded, therefore, that virtually all circulating BGP originated from recent cellular synthesis. Brown et al (1984), who compared serum levels with histomorphometric parameters in iliac crest biopsies in 26 patients with untreated postmenopausal osteoporosis, found highly significant correlations between levels of serum BGP and parameters relating to bone formation, but found no significant correlation with bone surfaces. Riggs et al (1984) infused synthetic PTH (1-34) for 24 hours to acutely increase bone resorption. They found that urinary hydroxyproline, an index of bone resorption, increased twofold whereas serum BGP showed a small but significant decrease. Collectively, these data suggest that serum BGP is a measure of bone formation but not of bone resorption. Presumably, during osteoclastic resorption BGP in bone matrix is degraded into fragments that either are not recognized by antisera raised against the native molecule or are rapidly cleared from the circulation.

Results in Postmenopausal Osteoporosis

Despite 40 years of investigation, it still is not clear whether the major cause of bone loss in women with postmenopausal osteoporosis is increased bone resorption or decreased bone formation. Experimental data supporting both mechanisms have been reported. Combined kinetic and calcium balance data strongly suggest that due to the menopause overall bone turnover increases but that resorption increases more than formation (Heaney et al, 1978). Most radiocalcium kinetic studies have reported normal accretion rates in postmenopausal osteoporosis despite a decrease in bone mass (Harris and Heaney, 1969). Jowsey (Jowsey et al, 1965) and Nordin et al (1981) found that patients with postmenopausal osteoporosis had significant increases in resorption surfaces in the iliac crest, and Wu et al (1967) reported an increase in the derived value for resorption rate in the rib. Studies with tetracycline double-labeling, however, have found that bone turnover in osteoporosis can be high, low, or normal in the iliac crest biopsy samples (Brown et al, 1984; Harris and Heaney, 1969; Heaney et al, 1978; Jowsey et al, 1965; Meunier et al, 1980; Nordin et al, 1981; Parfitt et al, 1980; Riggs et al, 1984; Whyte et al, 1982; Wu et al, 1967).

Because of this controversy, our group measured serum BGP (Delmas et al, 1983b) in 62 untreated patients with postmenopausal osteoporosis and vertebral compression fractures. Results were compared with those in 142 normal women. None of the normal or osteoporotic subjects was taking drugs or had any disease known to cause osteoporosis. All had normal values for serum calcium, phosphorus, protein electrophoresis, and 25-hydroxyvitamin D. Bone mineral density of the lumbar spine was assessed in all patients by dual photon absorptiometry. Differences between the osteoporotic and normal women were expressed as positive or negative standard deviation from the age-adjusted mean (Z-score).

Serum BGP was increased (+0.48 SD, P=0.002) in the osteoporotic patients as compared with the normal subjects. In the distribution of individual values given in Figure 2, 9.7% of the patients were >2 SD above but none was >2 SD below the normal mean. When the data from normal postmenopausal women (ages 51-75 years) and the osteoporotic patients were merged, there was a significant negative correlation ($r = -0.36$, $P < 0.001$) between serum BGP and bone density of the lumbar spine.

Thus, the data clearly show that basal levels of serum BGP were increased in osteoporotic patients and that the highest values were found in those with the greatest bone loss. Recently, this study was extended by measur-

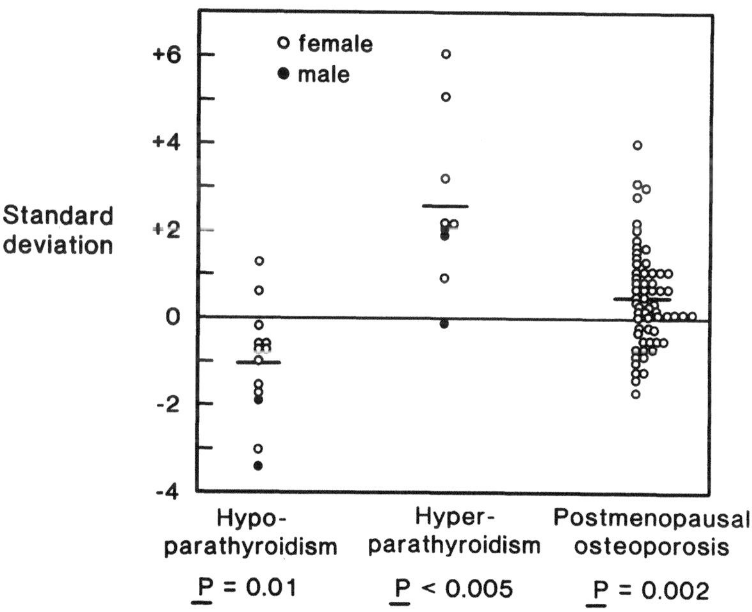

Fig. 2. Individual values for serum BGP in patients with postmenopausal osteoporosis. Units are standard deviations from predicted mean for normal subjects, obtained from sex-specific regression equations that predicted serum BGP as a function of age. Means are indicated by short horizontal lines. The mean for the osteoporotic patients is significantly increased; 9.5% of the patients are above but none below ±2 SD, about the age-adjusted normal mean. Values are also given for patients with hyperparathyroidism and hypoparathyroidism. These served as normal controls to demonstrate that the assay had a sufficiently dynamic range to measure elevated or depressed values in osteoporosis, if present.

ing stimulated levels of serum BGP following treatment with 1,25-dihydroxyvitamin D, a known secretogogue for serum BGP (Duda et al, 1985). Compared with an age- and sex-matched control group, stimulated levels of serum BGP were significantly greater in patients with postmenopausal osteoporosis.

The data, therefore, are consistent with the hypothesis that bone loss in patients with postmenopausal osteoporosis is mainly due to an increase in bone turnover. Possibly, the patients found to have low bone turnover in iliac crest biopsy samples have reached a burned-out stage for trabecular bone of the axial skeleton but still have normal or increased bone turnover in the remainder of the skeleton. Nonetheless, the issue of the level of bone turnover present in postmenopausal osteoporosis is complex and cannot be settled definitively by using a single method, albeit a highly specific one. Thus, as new biochemical markers for bone turnover are developed, they should be employed to attempt to settle this controversy more definitively.

References

1. Beresford, J.N., Gallagher, J.A., Poser, J.W., and Russell, R.G.G.: Production of osteocalcin by human bone cells *in vitro* effects of 1,25(OH)$_2$D$_3$, 24,25(OH)$_2$D$_3$, parathyroid hormone, and glucocorticoids. Metab. Bone Dis. Rel. Res. 5, 229, 1984.

2. Brown, J.P., Delmas, P.D., Malaval, L., Edouard, C., Chapuy, M.C., and Meunier, P.J.: Serum bone Gla-protein: a specific marker for bone formation in postmenopausal osteoporosis. Lancet i, 1091, 1984.

3. Deftos, L.J., Parthemore, J.G., and Price, P.A.: Changes in plasma bone Gla-protein during treatment of bone disease. Calcif. Tissue Int. 34, 121, 1982.

4. Delmas, P.D., Stenner, D., Wahner, H.W., Mann, K.G., and Riggs, B.L.: Increase in serum bone γ-carboxyglutamic acid protein with aging in women: implications for the mechanism of age-related bone loss. J. Clin.Invest. 71, 1316, 1983a.

5. Delmas, P.D., Wahner, H.W., Mann, K.G., and Riggs, B.L.: Assessment of bone turnover in postmenopausal osteoporosis by measurement of serum bone Gla-protein. J. Lab. Clin. Med. 102, 470, 1983b.

6. Delmas, P.D., Tracy, R.P., Riggs, B.L., and Mann, K.G.: Identification of the noncollagenous proteins of bovine bone by two-dimensional gel electrophoresis. Calcif. Tissue Int. 36, 308, 1984.

7. Duda, R.J., Jr., Mann, K.G., and Riggs, B.L.: Calcitriol stimulation test for osteoblast function: Results in postmenopausal osteoporosis. Proc. 7th Annual Scientific Meeting, American Society for Bone and Mineral Research, June 15-18, 1985. Abstract #129.

8. Epstein, S., Poser, J., McClintock, R., Johnston, C.C., Jr., Bryce, G., and Hui, S.: Differences in serum bone Gla-protein with age and sex. Lancet i, 307, 1984.

9. Farley, J.R., Chesnut, C.H., III, and Baylink, D.J.: Improved method for quantitative determination in serum of alkaline phosphatase of skeletal origin. Clin. Chem. 27, 2002, 1981.

10. Frost, H.M.: Bone remodeling and its relationship to metabolic bone diseases. In, Orthopedic Lecture Series, Charles C. Thomas, Springfield, Ill, Vol. 8, 1973.

11. Gundberg, C.M., Lian, J.B., and Gallop, P.M.: Measurements of γ-carboxyglutamate and circulating osteocalcin in normal children and adults. Clin. Chim. Acta 128, 1, 1983.

12. Harris, W.H., and Heaney, R.P.: Skeletal renewal and metabolic bone disease. N. Engl. J. Med. 280, 193, 1969.

13. Heaney, R.P., Recker, R.R., and Saville, P.D.: Menopausal changes in bone remodeling, J. Lab. Clin. Med. 92, 964, 1978.

14. Jowsey, J., Kelly, P.J., Riggs, B.L., Bianco, A.J., Scholz, D.A., and Gershon-Cohen, J.: Quantitative microradiographic studies of normal and osteoporotic bone. J. Bone Joint Surg. 47A, 785, 1965.

15. Krane, S.M., Kantrowitz, F.G., Byrne, M., Pinnell, S.R., and Singer, F.R.: Urinary excretion of hydroxylysine and its glycosides as an index of collagen degradation. J. Clin. Invest. 59, 819, 1977.

16. Lian, J.B., Tassinari, M., and Glowacki, J.: Resorption of implanted bone prepared from normal and warfarin-treated rats. J. Clin. Invest. 73, 1223, 1984.

17. Meunier, P.J., Sellami, S., Briançon, D., and Edouard, C.: Histological heterogeneity of apparently idiopathic osteoporosis. In, Osteoporosis: Recent Advances in Pathogenesis and Treatment. Eds: DeLuca, H.F., Frost, H.M., Jee, W.S.S., Johnston, C.C., Jr., Parfitt, A.M. University Park Press, Baltimore, 1980, p. 293.

18. Nordin, B.E.C., Aaron, J., Speed, R., and Crilly, R.G.: Bone formation and resorption as the determinants of trabecular bone volume in postmenopausal osteoporosis. Lancet ii, 277, 1981.

19. Parfitt, A.M., Mathews, C., Rao, D., Frame, B., Kleerekoper, M., and Villaneuva, A.R.: Impaired osteoblast function in metabolic bone disease. In, Osteoporosis: Recent Advances in Pathogenesis and Treatment. Eds: DeLuca, H.F., Frost, H.M., Jee, W.S.S., Johnston, C.C., Jr., Parfitt, A.M. University Park Press, Baltimore, 1980, p. 321.

20. Podenphant, J., Christiansen, C., Catherwood, B.D., and Deftos, L.J.: Serum bone Gla-protein variations during estrogen and calcium prophylaxis of postmenopausal women. Calcif. Tissue Int. 36, 536, 1984.

21. Price, P.: Osteocalcin. In, Bone and Mineral Research, Annual I. Ed: Peck, W.A., Excerpta Medica, Amsterdam, Oxford, Princeton, 1983, pp 157-190.

22. Price, P.A., and Baukol, S.A.: 1,25-dihydroxyvitamin D_3 increases synthesis of the vitamin D-dependent bone protein by osteosarcoma cells. J. Biol. Chem. 255, 11660, 1980.

23. Price, P.A., Parthemore, J.G., and Deftos, L.J.: New biochemical marker for bone metabolism: measurement by radioimmunoassay of bone Gla-protein in the plasma of normal subjects and patients with bone disease. J. Clin. Invest. 66, 878, 1980.

24. Price, P.A., Williamson, M.K., Haba, T., Dell, R.B., and Jee, W.S.S.: Excessive mineralization with growth plate closure in rats on chronic warfarin treatment. Proc. Ntl. Acad. Sci. USA 79, 7734, 1982.

25. Riggs, B.L., Marshall, J.H., Jowsey, J., Heaney, R.P., and Bassingthwaighte, J.B.: Quantitative ^{45}Ca autoradiography of human bone. J. Lab. Clin. Med. 78, 585, 1971.

26. Riggs, B.L., Tsai, K.-S., and Mann, K.G.: Evidence that serum bone Gla-protein is a measure of bone formation but not of bone resorption. Proc. 6th Annual Scientific Meeting, American Society for Bone and Mineral Research, June 26-29, 1984.

27. Romberg, R.W., Werness, P.G., Lollar, P., Riggs, B.L., and Mann, K.G.: Isolation and characterization of native adult osteonectin. J. Biol. Chem. 260, 2728, 1985.

28. Termine, J.D., Belcourt, A.B., Conn, K.M., and Kleinman, H.K.: Mineral and collagen-binding proteins of fetal calf bone. J. Biol. Chem. 256, 10403, 1981a.

29. Termine, J.D., Kleinman, H.K., Whitson, S.W., Conn, K.M., McGarvey, M. L., and Martin, G.R.: Osteonectin, a bone-specific protein linking mineral to collagen. Cell 26, 99, 1981b.

30. Wasi, S., Otsuka, K., Yao, K.-L., Tung, P.S., Aubin, J.E., and Sodek, J.: An osteonectin-like protein in porcine periodontal ligament and its synthesis by periodontal ligament fibroblasts. Can. J. Biochem. Cell Biol. 62, 470, 1984.

31. Whyte, M.P., Bergfeld, M.A., Murphy, W.A., Avioli, L.V., and Teitelbaum, S.L.: Postmenopausal osteoporosis: a heterogeneous disorder as assessed by histomorphometric analysis of iliac crest bone from untreated patients. Am. J. Med. 72, 193, 1982.

32. Wu, K., Jett, S., and Frost, H.M.: Bone resorption rates in rib in physiological, senile and postmenopausal osteoporosis. J. Lab. Clin. Med. 69, 810, 1967.

The Role of Bone Biopsy in Metabolic Bone Disease

C.-P. ADLER

In patients with bone fractures the question arises whether the traumatic event was severe enough to break the bone. In the absence of trauma, we call it a pathologic bone fracture.

In a 25 year old man who has a severe accident while skiing and breaks his leg, obviously the trauma was the only cause of that bone fracture. The roentgenogram will show a fracture within a normally-structured bone. The biopsy material taken from the fractured region four weeks later will show a fibrous and bony callus tissue formed by repair processes; no other pathologic tissue would be observed, nor would there be morphologic signs of increased bone fragility.

A bone fracture often occurs, on the other hand, without a trauma, or if the trauma was not strong enough to produce a bone fracture. In all these cases we are dealing with a bony weakness that may have several different causes. In some individuals, the underlying pathologic process may be local and concentrated in the fractured region; in other cases, the patient may have a generalized disease of the skeleton such as metabolic bone disease. Usually, the underlying structural alteration responsible for bone fragility can be definitely identified only by means of bone biopsy. In the roentgenogram of a fracture of the left proximal femur of a 56 year old woman, we identified a faint disturbance of the bony structures of the spongiosa. The bone biopsy from this field showed necrotic bone trabeculae without osteocytes and fibrotic areas in the bone marrow. Histologically, we could therefore diagnose aseptic bone necrosis as the cause of this pathologic bone fracture.

In another bone fracture which had occurred spontaneously in the left proximal humerus of a 10 year old child the roentgenogram showed the classical structures of a juvenile bone cyst. The lesion was curetted, and in the histologic slides fragments of the cyst wall could be identified within the fracture material.

Similarly, even a malignant bone tumor is sometimes diagnosed following a pathologic fracture. This was the case in a 22 year old man with an osteosarcoma of the left distal femur which was not discovered until a sudden fracture had occurred. In the roentgenogram, we could easily recognize the malignant tumor masses together with the fracture. In the biopsy material, the characteristic tissue pattern of an osteoblastic osteosarcoma was seen as the cause of this pathologic bone fracture.

Current Concepts of Bone Fragility

In the case of generalized bone diseases, it is assumed that the morphologic changes responsible for fractures in one location are widespread and are present at the site of biopsy performed in other locations. The most common site of such biopsy in these cases is the iliac crest. Numerous general skeletal diseases may show representative structural bone changes responsible for a pathologic bone fracture in this location (Vitalli, 1970).

Osteoporosis in elderly persons, for example, is a widepread skeletal disorder associated with a loss of bone mass. Many of these patients sustain a pathologic fracture mainly in a vertebral body or femoral neck. Radiologically, osteoporosis can first be identified when more than 30% of the bone mineral has been lost (Babiantz, 1947). We then observe a loosening of the spongiosa and thinning of the cortex mixed with some pronounced bone trabeculae. It is impossible, on the other hand to identify an osteoporosis of lesser degree and in an early stage of development.

To clarify the cause of fracture in such a case, a bone biopsy has to be performed. The spongy substance of an osteoporotic vertebral body appears wide-meshed, macroscopically, with slender bone trabeculae reduced in size and number. Histologically, wide-meshed spongiosa with reduced spongy trabeculae is obvious. The remaining trabeculae are very small and contain small osteocytes. They have smooth outlines and no osteoclasts are attached. The marrow space is widened and filled with fatty tissue. In a bone biopsy the histologist has to estimate the quantitative relationship between marrow space and spongy bone volume to diagnose osteoporosis. The same structural alteration can be seen in the osteoporotic iliac crest macroscopically as well as microscopically. The wide-meshed spongiosa is the characteristic structure of this disease. In the histologic slides we can see only the atrophic spongiosa with slightly slender bone trabeculae and wide marrow space without any bone-resorbing cells such as osteoclasts. It is understandable that this bone loss is the cause of the pathologic fracture in question, but we cannot determine histologically the pathogenetic factor of this kind of osteoporosis. Primary osteoporosis of this kind may occur in elderly patients as postmenopausal osteoporosis or as a consequence of immobilization. In all cases, bone mineralization is normal.

While primary osteoporosis develops mainly in the axial skeleton, most secondary osteoporoses can be found in the whole skeleton (Kruse et al, 1976). In case of a pathologic bone fracture, a transiliac biopsy may detect the underlying structural alteration in both. A metabolic or endocrinologic bone disease can, in most cases, be identified by an iliac bone biopsy.

In primary hyperparathyroidism, the bone is osteoporotic. In the roentgenogram, flaking of the cortical bone with cortical cysts due to bone resorption may indicate the underlying disease. Especially in the vertebral bodies one can see a so-called "horizontal triple layering" of the spongiosa. As well as osteopenia, increased production of new bone takes place in an irregular manner. In macerated preparations of the vertebral body, the spongiosa in hyperparathyroidism is much more close-meshed than in normal bone.

In completely developed osseous manifestations of primary hyperparathyroidism, described by von Recklinghausen in 1891 as "osteodystrophia fibrosa cystica", the histologic changes of the bone are characteristic and pathognomonic of the disease. It is not necessary to prepare undecalcified bone biopsies from the iliac crest to recognize these structures. In a

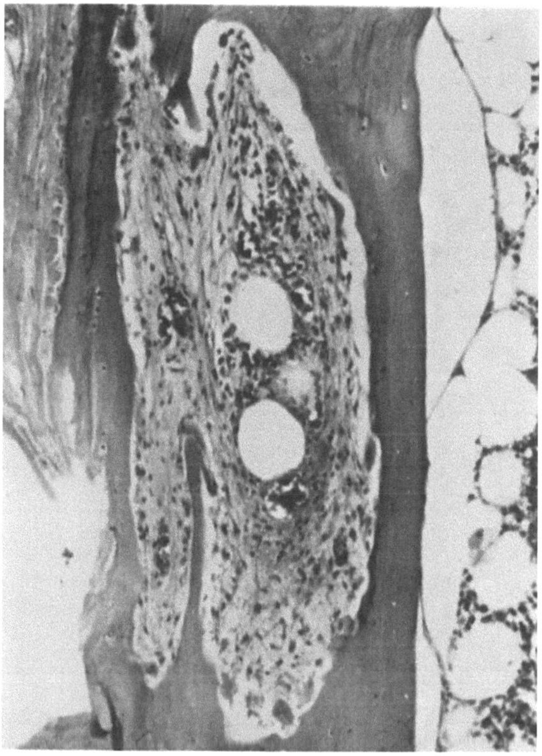

Fig. 1. Decalcified transiliac biopsy with osteodystrophia fibrosa in primary hyperparathyroidism showing characteristic fibroosteoclasia. (H and E stain, x 60

decalcified bone biopsy the most significant structure is the so-called dissecting fibroosteoclasia in which fibrous granulation tissue has invaded the bone trabeculae together with numerous osteoclasts and activated osteoblasts (Fig. 1). The fatty tissue in the marrow space is more or less replaced by fibrous tissue. In less severe cases, only discrete endosteal fibrosis with increased osteoclasts can be found (Byers and Smith, 1971; Delling, 1984; Olah, 1973). The same histologic picture can been seen in undecalcified bone sections: the structures of dissecting fibroosteoclasia are obvious and some broader osteoid seams are noticable as a consequence of osteoblastic activity which should not be interpreted as osteomalacia.

About 35% of patients with an adenoma of the parathyroid gland show no specific bone changes (Delling, 1984). In the transiliac biopsy, we see only an osteoporosis that does not indicate hyperparathyroidism. In other cases, discrete endosteal fibrosis and some widened osteoid seams may point to hyperparathyroidism which has to be determined by estimating blood parathyrin levels. On the other hand, in advanced stages of hyperthyroidism, so-called brown tumors may develop that are in reality resorptive giant cell granulomas resulting in microfractures in the osteodystrophic bone. In the roentgenogram, one or more cystic bone lesions can be seen indicating a malignant bone tumor. The biopsy from this type of lesion reveals cell-rich granulation tissue with irregular distribution of many osteoclasts. From the histologic standpoint several other osteoclastic bone lesions have to be considered for a differential diagnosis, such as true giant cell tumor, giant cell granuloma of short tubular bones, reparative giant cell granuloma of jaws, or even aneurysmal bone cyst.

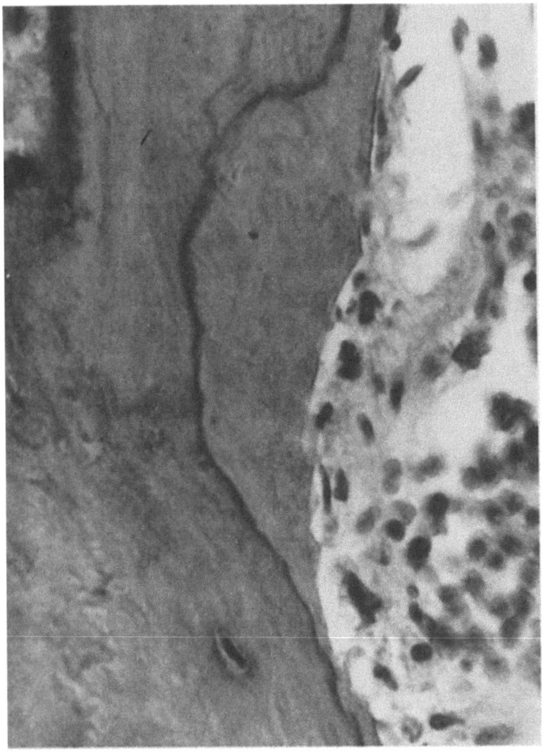

Fig. 2. Decalcified transiliac biopsy with osteomalacia with clearly visible, broadened osteoid seams. (H and E stain, x 120)

A bone fracture can also occur in patients with osteomalacia. This is a skeletal disorder of calcification due to deficiency of vitamin D or calcium resulting in a reduction of the density of the skeleton with blurred outline of the spongiosa in the roentgenograms (Ellegast, 1961). Osteomalacia may involve all bones of the skeleton and may lead to bony deformations. True fractures seldom occur; but stress fractures, mainly in the so-called Looser's zones, are prone to develop. These lesions tend to be chronic and are rarely detected in the stage of acute infraction (Murray and Jacobson, 1977). Bone repair occurs by forming an osteoid callus only. Absence of mineralization means that a pseudarthrosis remains.

In such cases, a transiliac biopsy enables one to identifiy definitely the underlying disease. Histologically, osteomalacia is characterized by broad osteoid seams lining bone trabeculae (Fig. 2). Whereas some authors maintain that osteoid cannot be identified in decalcified bone material (Schulz and Delling, 1985), we always see this structure in decalcified as well as in undecalcified bone sections. The original bone trabeculae are often narrowed and some osteoblasts may be attached to the osteoid seams. This so-called osteoidosis is either a consequence of delayed mineralization of normal bone apposition or an expression of increased bone apposition with equal mineralization. When we diagnose osteomalacia from a transiliac bone biopsy, we have to consider several metabolic diseases for differential diagnoses. In children it may be rickets. In adults, it may be alimentary insufficiency, malabsorption, maldigestion, disturbance of vitamin D metabolism, or liver or renal diseases. In all these metabolic disorders, we find similar bone changes indicating osteomalacia (Drueke and Cournot-Witmer, 1982).

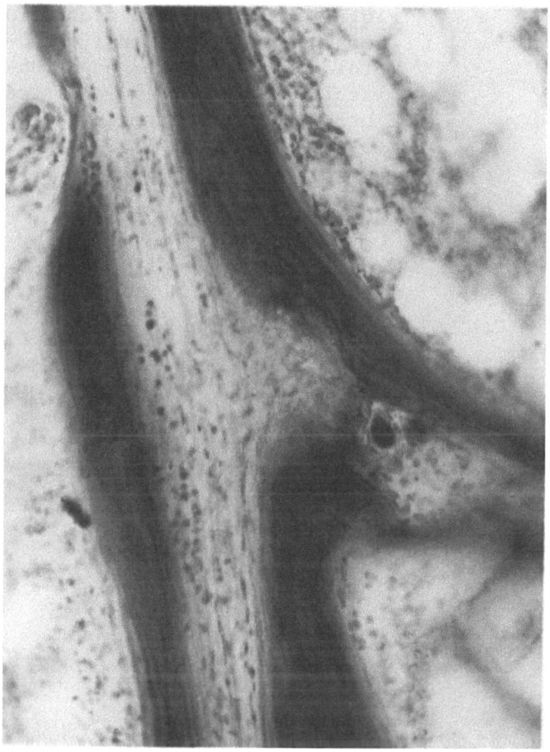

Fig. 3. Decalcified transiliac biopsy with renal osteopathia showing all three structural components of the disease. (H and E strain, x 60)

The real underlying disease has to be found by medical examinations. From the biopsy material we can easily differentiate between simple osteoporosis without osteoid seams and osteomalacia with broad osteoid seams.

In case of renal insufficiency, a more complicated multifactorial spectrum of bone changes occurs, called "renal osteopathia". As a result of endogenic factors, such as secondary hyperparathyroidism, disturbance of vitamin D metabolism or parathyrin-resistance, or exogenic factors such as phosphate restriction or insufficient supply of vitamin D, the bone structures change into osteodystrophia fibrosa, osteomalacia and osteoporosis (Adler, 1983; Freudenberg et al, 1975). This means a weakening of bone and that bone fractures may occur without serious trauma.

In the roentgenogram, moderate to severe osteoporosis with signs of osteomalacia and a so-called milkman fracture may be seen. These radiologic changes require a transiliac biopsy in cases of fracture to reveal the underlying disease. In a decalcified bone section we can already notice all three components of renal osteopathia (Fig. 3). These include osteoporotically-reduced bone trabeculae, broad osteoid seams as in osteomalacia, and structural changes of osteodystrophia, such as dissecting fibroosteoclasia and marrow sclerosis.

To estimate the extent of renal osteopathia, Delling (1972; 1975; 1984) has introduced a morphologic classification that is generally in use in Germany, including three types of renal osteopathias. Type I renal osteopathia is characterized by increased osteoclastic bone resorption as a consequence of

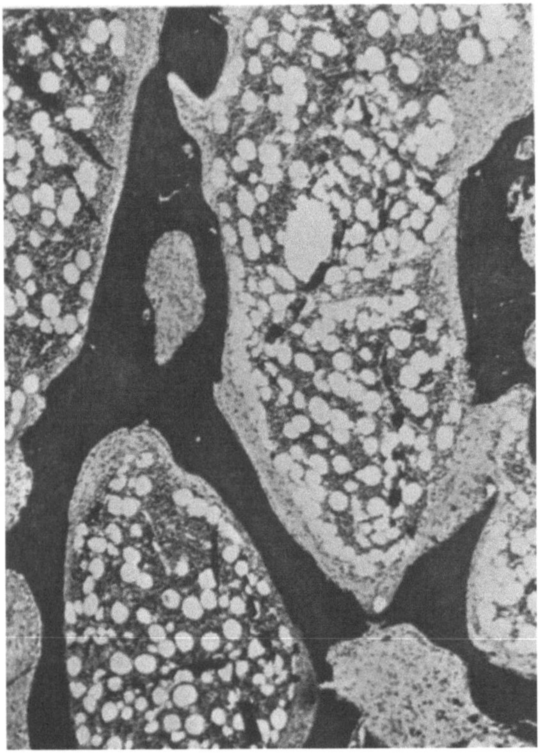

Fig. 4. Undecalcified transiliac biopsy with Type I renal osteopathia showing increased osteoclastic resorption and endosteal fibrosis but no osteoidosis. (Goldner stain, x 25)

secondary hyperparathyroidism and low bone apposition. Bone mineralization is not disturbed. In the histologic section, we see most signs of fibroosteoclasia (Fig. 4). The trabeculae have normal osteoid surfaces as well as normal osteoid volume, and increased osteoclastic resorption can be seen. Remarkable is endosteal fibrosis. This bone pattern is seen in 5% of all patients with renal insufficiency and also in patients with rapidly progressing renal diseases such as glomerulonephritis and acute renal failure (Delling, 1984).

Type II (a and b) renal osteopathia is characterized by osteomalacia alone without fibroosteoclasia. Histologically, in Type IIa renal osteopathia we see small osteoid seams without osteoblasts or endosteal fibrosis. The total bony mass is reduced. No osteoclastic bone resorption can be found. In Type IIb renal osteopathia bone mineralization is completely stopped, resulting in broad osteoid seams (Fig. 5). Due to the reduced calcified bone mass, the risk of spontaneous fractures increases. After labeling with tetracycline, the absence of mineralization can be confirmed through ultraviolet microscopy. This kind of bone change can be found in 20% of patients with chronic renal insufficiency without hemodialysis, and in 30% of these patients on chronic hemodialysis (Delling, 1984).

Approximately 70% of patients with chronic renal failure have Type III renal osteopathia. In these patients, a transiliac biopsy reveals osteoidosis and fibroosteoclasia. This indicates the influence of secondary hyperparathyroidism and a disorder of vitamin D metabolism. In Type IIIa renal osteopathia, we see slight fibroosteoclasia and clear osteoidosis with broad

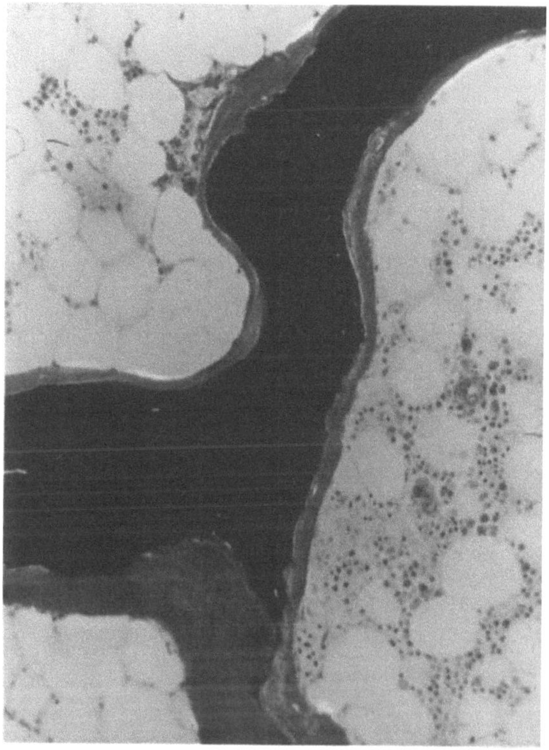

Fig. 5. Undecalficied transiliac biopsy with Type II renal osteopathia showing broad osteoid seams as in osteomalacia but no fibroosteoclasia. (Goldner stain, x 48

osteoid seams. The remodeling of spongiosa is reduced. Type IIIb renal osteopathia is characterized by a disturbance of bone mineralization, apparent through broad osteoid seams; in addition, there is secondary hyperparathyroidism with increased osteoclastic resorption (Fig. 6). Perforating resorption channels can be seen in the center of trabecular bone. In addition, the number of osteoblasts with cytoplasmic vacuoles is increased. Severe endosteal fibrosis is obvious. Remodeling of spongiosa is normal or slightly reduced. Type IIIc renal osteopathia shows an advanced stage of trabecular remodeling with renewal of woven bone. Fibroosteoclasia is excessive and osteoidosis fairly moderate. These bony changes are a clear indication for revision of the parathyroid glands.

Under the influence of different therapies, some changes may occur in the bone pattern. For example, in a patient with chronic pyelonephritis the first transiliac biopsy showed a moderate renal osteopathia Type II. After three years of vitamin D administration, a marked increase in osteoclastic bone resorption and small increase of osteoid could be observed. A patient with severe renal osteopathia Type IIIa was treated with 1,25-dihydroxycholecalciferol, resulting in progressive mineralization and reduction of osteoid. Under the influence of aluminum hydroxide or during long-term uptake of aluminum in hemodialyzed patients, this element is deposited in the mineralization front of the osteoid seams, in the cement lines as well as in the osteoid itself (Delling et al, 1983). This leads to a nearly total cessation of mineralization, resulting in severe osteoidosis (Ellis et al, 1979). Therefore, patients with chronic renal diseases may sustain bone fractures

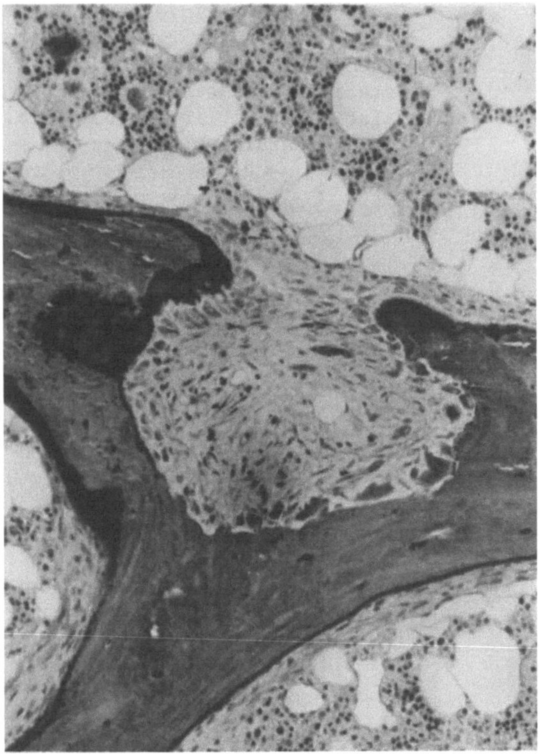

Fig. 6. Undecalcified transiliac biopsy with Type III renal osteopathia showing broad osteoid seams, fibroosteoclasia and endosteal fibrosis. (Goldner stain, x 48

under the influence of hemodialysis. Here, the transiliac biopsy may show deposits of aluminum in the bone as a cause of fracture (Walker et al, 1982).

Renal transplantation reduces the bony changes of renal osteopathia within a few months. On the other hand, long-term steroid therapy induces osteopenia with the risk of bone fractures. This steroid-induced osteoporosis is characterized by a reduction of bone apposition together with increased bone resorption (de Valderrama and Munuera, 1966; Eisenberg and Gordan, 1961; Nordin, 1964; Sissons, 1956). The bone trabeculae are thinned and show many resorption lacunae. No osteoid seams can be seen. Fracture in steroid-induced osteoporosis usually is associated with a characteristic hyperplastic callus formation that may suggest the underlying skeletal alteration.

Using tetracycline labeling, bone formation dynamics can be measured microscopically and directly in bony tissue (Boyde and Reid, 1983; Frost, 1969; Milch et al, 1957). Rates can be obtained by measuring change between two successive moments in time, a principle which allows both formation and resorption rates (Frost, 1969). Tetracycline -- administered orally or by injection -- will be deposited at sites of bone mineralization and subsequently can be made visible under fluorescent light in undecalcified sections from a bone biopsy (Eger et al, 1964; Frost, 1968). Contrary to all the other histologic investigations of metabolic bone diseases which can be performed on decalcified and undecalcified sections, for tetracycline labeling only undecalcified sections must be prepared.

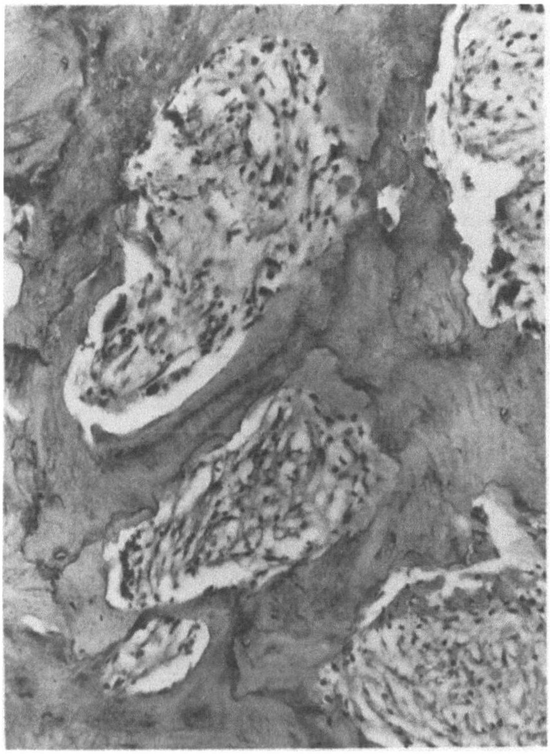

Fig. 7. Decalcified transiliac biopsy with Paget's disease showing advanced remodeling of bone trabeculae lined by activated osteoclasts and osteoblasts and with many mosaic-like reversal lines. (H and E stain, x 30)

Using tetracycline labeling in normal bone from the iliac crest, the mineralization border is marked by an intense yellow seam showing normal amounts of mineralizing osteoid. In a tetracycline double-labeled bone biopsy in primary hyperparathyroidism, labeled three weeks before exstirpation of a parathyroid adenoma and 14 days after the operation, a broad, diffuse fluorescence is visible in the mineralization borders; postoperative reduction indicates improved mineralization. In experimental hypoparathyroidism, performed by Delling (1975), tetracycline labelings showed severe disturbances of mineralization. The periosteal apposition contained large mineralization defects with fuchsin-permeable zones and a diffuse tetracycline fluorescence. After three months' calcitonin treatment, normal mineralization with sharply defined tetracycline labels was visible. The interval between two tetracycline labels was one week.

Investigation of bone biopsies on undecalcified sections combined with tetracycline labeling can be expanded with morphometric measurements (Burkhardt et al, 1981; Delling, 1975; Frost, 1969), biochemical estimations of substances such as calcium or hydroxyproline (Kuhlencordt, 1979; Laitinen, 1976), microradiographic analysis (Heuck, 1965; 1979; Jowsey, 1977) and other techniques. All these methods are complicated and costly, and should be restricted to special cases or to scientific investigations. In most patients with pathologic fractures, it is sufficient to analyze a transiliac bone biopsy microscopically by using decalcified sections to determine the underlying skeletal alterations. In Paget's disease, for instance, in which a pathologic fracture probably occurs, a normal biopsy from the involved bone shows the full histologic pattern of the disease with advanced remodeling of bone trabeculae lined by many activated osteoclasts and osteoblasts and a fibrous marrow tissue rich in blood vessels (Adler, 1983)(Fig. 7).

Adult patients with osteopetrosis tend to suffer from many bone fractures during their life. The bone biopsy reveals a heavily mineralized cartilaginous matrix containing no osteoclasts, or insufficiently active osteoclasts which do not remodel the bone in a proper manner. This underlying disease can be diagnosed radiologically and histologically in cases of pathologic fractures. Most spontaneous fractures occur in patients with carcinoma, and often the primary tumor is unknown. A biopsy from the fractured region then reveals the underlying alteration as bone metastasis. Occasionally we see patients with advanced skeletal carcinosis, and a transiliac biopsy may help to find the primary tumor. In one such patient, for example, we observed signet-ring cells in the marrow space, from which we presumed that the patient had gastric cancer.

A transiliac bone biopsy may detect the underlying structural alteration responsible for bone fragility. In most patients, the histologic analysis of decalcified sections with routine methods is sufficient. In special cases of metabolic bone diseases, however, we must prepare undecalcified sections to find the exact diagnosis and to estimate bone remodeling.

References

1. Adler, C.P.: Knochenkrankheiten. Diagnostik makroscopischer, histologischer und radiologischer Strukturveränderungen des Skeletts. Thiieme, Stuttgart, New York, 1983.
2. Babiantz, L.: Les ostéoporoses. Radiol. Clin. (Basel) 16, 291, 1947.
3. Boyde, A., and Reid, S.A.: Tetracycline cathodoluminescence in bone, dentine and enamel. Histochemistry 77, 525, 1983.
4. Burkhardt, R., Bartl, R., Demmler, K., and Kettner, G.: Zwölf histobioptische Thesen zur Pathogenese der primären und sekundären Osteoporose. Klin. Wschr. 59, 5, 1981.
5. Byers, P.D., and Smith, R.: Quantitative histology of bone in hyperparathyroidism. Its relation to clinical features, x-ray, and biochemistry. Quart. J. Med. 40, 471, 1971.
6. Delling, G.: Quantitative Auswertung von Skelettveränderungen bei chronischer Hämodialyse. Verh. Dtsch. Ges. Path. 56, 436, 1972.
7. Delling, G.: Endokrine Osteopathien (Endocrine Bone Diseases). G. Fisher , Stuttgart, 1975.
8. Delling, G.: Skelettsystem. In, Pathologie, Bd. 3, Ed: Remmele, W.: Springer-Verlag, Berlin-Heidelberg-New York-Tokyo, 1984, pp 639-740.
9. Delling, G., Schäfer, H.-J., Krumme, H., and Schulz, W.: Renale Osteopathie und Aluminium-Pathomorphologie. Nieren- u. Hochdruckerkrgn. 12, 207, 1983.
10. Delling, G., Schulz, A., and Schulz, W.: Morphologische Klassifikation der renalen Osteopathie. Mels. Med. Mitt. 49, 133, 1975.

11. de Valderrrama, J.A.F., and Munuera, L.M.: The effect of cortisone and anabolic agents on bone. Proc. 3rd Europ. Symp. Calc. Tissue, 1965. Eds: Fleisch, H., Blackwood, H.J.J. and Owen, M., Springer-Verlag, Berlin -Heidelberg-New York, 1966, p. 245.

12. Drueke, T., and Cournot-Witmer, G.: Die Dialyse Osteomalazie. Dtsch. med. Wschr. 107, 1259, 1982.

13. Eger, W., Goetz, F., and Kaemmerer, H.: Herstellung von Dünnschliffen aus Knochen und Weichgewebe nach Markierung mit Tetracyclinen. Langenbeck's Arch. klin. Chir. 306, 205, 1964.

14. Eisenberg, E., and Gordan, G.S.: Skeletal dynamics in man by non-radioactive strontium. J. Clin. Invest. 40, 1809, 1961.

15. Ellegast, H.: Zur Röntgensymptomatologie der Osteomalazie. Radiologica Austriaca 11, 85, 1961.

16. Ellis, H.A., McCarthy, J.H., and Herrington, J.: Bone aluminum in hemodialyzed patients and rats injected with aluminum chloride. J. Clin. Path. 32, 832, 1979.

17. Freudenberg, N., Adler, C.P., Halbfaß, H., and Kröpelin, T.: Renale Osteopathie. Med. Welt (Stuttgart) 26, 1061, 1975.

18. Frost, H.M.: Tetracycline bone labeling in anatomy. Am. J. Phys. Antrop. 29, 183, 1968.

19. Frost, H.M.: Tetracycline-based histological analysis of bone remodeling. Calc. Tissue Res. 3, 211, 1969.

20. Heuck, F.: Die Messung des Kalksalzgehaltes im Knochen bei Osteopathien. Med. Klin. 60, 954, 1965.

21. Heuck, F.: Qualitative und quantitative radiologische Analyse des Knochens. In, Lehrbuch der Röntgendiagnostick. Eds: Schinz, H.R., Baensch, W.E., Frommhold, W., Glauner, R., Uehlinger, E., and Wallauer, J., Bd. II, Teil 1, Thieme, Stuttgart, 1979 pp 145-212.

22. Jowsey, J.: Metabolic Diseases of Bone. Saunders Co., Philadelphia-London-Toronto, 1977.

23. Kruse, H.-P., Kuhlencordt, F., and Ringe, J.-D.: Correlation of clinical densitometric and histomorphometric data in osteoporosis. In, Calcified Tissue. Eds: Nielsen, S.P., and Hjørting-Hansen, E. Fadl, Copenhagen, 1976, pp 457-461.

24. Kuhlencordt, F.: Osteoporose. Verh. Dtsch. Ges. Inn. Med. 85, 269, 1979.

25. Laitinen, O.: Relation to osteoporosis of age- and hormone-induced changes in the metabolism of collagen and bone. Israel J. Med. Sci. 12, 593, 1976.

26. Milch, R.A., Rall, D.P., and Tobie, J.E.: Bone localization of the tetracyclines. J. Nat. Cancer Inst. 19, 87, 1957.

27. Murray, R.O., and Jacobson, H.G.: The Radiology of Skeletal Disorders. Vol. 1, 2nd Ed. Churchill Livingstone, Edinburgh-London-New York, 1977, p. 653.

28. Nordin, B.E.C.: The application of basic science to osteoporosis. In, Bone Biodynamics. Ed: Frost, H.M. Little Brown, Boston, 1964, pp 521-542.

29. Olah, A.J.: Quantitative relations between osteoblasts and osteoid in primary hyperthyroidism, intestinal malabsorption and renal osteodystrophy. Virch. Arch. Abt. A. Path. Anat. 358, 301, 1973.

30. Schulz, W., and Delling, G.: Knochenstoffwechselstörungen bei Dauerdialysepatienten. In, Blutreinigungsverfahren, Technik und Klinik. Ed: Franz, H.E., Thieme, Stuttgart-New York, 1985.

31. Sissons, H.A.: The osteoporosis of Cushing's syndrome. J. Bone Joint Surg. 38B, 418, 1956.

32. Vitalli, H.P.: Knochenerkrankungen. Histologie und Klinik. Sandoz Mon., Basel (Schweiz), 1970.

33. Walker, G.S., Aaron, J.E., Peacock, M., Robinson, P.J.A., and Davidson, A.M.: Dialysate aluminum concentration and renal bone disease. Kidney Int. 21, 411, 1982.

Bone Microdamage: Factors That Impair Its Repair

H. M. Frost

Introduction

Discussions of bone microdamage (MDx) by other investigators have addressed the mechanical nature and causes of some of its fragilizing effects on intact bone but not the role of its repair in accumulating MDx and resulting clinical problems (Carter, 1984). Table I lists some clinical problems in which MDx physiology should play a significant role, in fibrous tissues as well as bone.

Companion articles discuss early forms of MDx in bone and how to demonstrate them (Frost, 1985b), some pathogenetic mechanisms of osteoporoses and some roles of MDx in the skeletal mechanical incompetence (MIn) that forms part of the pathophysiologic osteoporotic triad (Frost, 1985a). However, MIn

Table I. Some clinical problems that involve microdamage physiology

Bone endoprostheses: design and service life
Internal fixation: design and service life
Dental endoprostheses: design and service life
Bone pain in metabolic bone disease and athletics
Bone fragilization in metabolic bone disease
Sports medicine: shin splints, tendonitis, arthralgias
Spontaneous fractures; pathologic fractures; radiation damage
Stress fractures; spontaneous tendon ruptures
Adult acquired osteoporoses and osteomalacias
Children's acquired osteoporoses and osteomalacias
Osteogenesis imperfecta (all types) and osteopetrosis (all types)
Spontaneous fascial and ligament ruptures; hernia; aneurysm
Osteoarthritis (some forms); traumatic arthritis
Arthrokatadesis; collapsed tibial plateaus; osteochondritis dissecans
Idiopathic aseptic necrosis of the femoral head and humeral head

Current Concepts of Bone Fragility

and the MDx that usually underlies it can occur in other conditions besides osteoporosis (OPs) (Table I).

Review of Pertinent Physiology

Basic MDx relation

Increasing accumulations of MDx occur when, for whatever reason, its production exceeds its repair. It describes a balance between certain mechanical phenomena and the biologic ones that repair MDx. That state of balance can occur when MDx production increases or its repair decreases, or if both occur, or if both decrease but the latter the most, or if both increase but the former the most. Each possibility occurs in life. Examples are listed in Table II. Thus, whenever MDx production minus MDx repair is a positive quantity, MDx burdens accumulate, and that situation must lead in time to a complete fatigue fracture of the bone (or rupture of the tendon, fascia or ligament) in which it occurs. Thus:

If:

new MDx - repair = 0, the system is stable

new MDx - repair = <0, the structure is healing

new MDx - repair = >0, fracture will occur in time

The less studied matter of MDx and MIn in fibrous tissues has some parallels with the bone problem. Thus, some of the latter's properties should apply to tendon, fascia and ligament (Frost, in press, a; b). Also, the biodynamic mechanisms that can lead to a complete fatigue fracture of bone differ in kind from the subsequent processes that heal complete fractures and that have been called the macrorepair process (Frost, in press, a). The latter

Table II. Particular clinical examples of pathologically increased MDx burdens

New MDx	Repair	Sign of Repair - MDx	Clinical example
N	N	0	The mechanically competent skeleton
N, I	D	-	Osteomalacias
I	N	-	Strenuous sports; draftees in boot camp
I	D	-	Osteoporoses
II	I	-	Thyrotoxicosis
D	DD	-	Osteopetrosis
D	I	+	Healing MDx burden, as in casted stress fracture

N = produced at normal rate; I = increased; D = decreased;
II = markedly increased; DD = markedly decreased

organ-level phenomenon can be normal or abnormal independently of the former IO-domain matter, and vice versa.

The microscopic MDx repair system should have the following general properties:

First, when repeated strains create an MDx locus somewhere in bone and advance it to a frank microcrack (Frost, 1985a; Frost et al, 1961), it creates a signal that activates a new remodeling BMU (basic multicellular unit). (The osteocytes may play a role in that detection-signaling process (Frost, in press, a)).

Second, that remodeling BMU begins with resorption at a cutting cone which, as Jaworski et al have shown, normally advances through bone at ~.05 mm/day (Jaworski and Lok, 1972; Jaworski et al, 1981). The cutting cone should pursue or follow the advancing MDx locus through the bone.

Third, if the MDx locus advances more slowly than the pursuing BMU, the latter would eradicate the locus. If the MDx advances faster than the BMU, however, the locus will enlarge with time and add to any other fragilizing MDx in the bone. If the locus does not evoke a repairing BMU, it will progress completely unrepaired with further mechanical usage.

Accordingly, suppressing BMU activation could cause MDx accumulation (Frost, in press, a); furthermore, retarding the progression through bone already ongoing BMU could do likewise, and both effects could combine.

Biologically and operationally, activating new BMU (and the speed of progress of already ongoing ones have different bone effects) depends in part on different cellular mechanisms and responds to different controlling agents (Frost, 1985a; in press, a). In principle then, in some situations the former might be abnormal but not the latter, or vice versa, or both could be abnormal. To evaluate such possibilities requires measuring those two activities.

Measuring the repair

Investigators (Recker, 1983; Shenck and Olah, 1980) have devised ways to measure those activities by dynamic histomorphometry and double fluorochrome bone labeling *in vivo* (Frost, 1969; 1973a; Recker, 1983).

The measure of the initiation of new BMU is the activation frequency. Greek lower case mu, μ, usually signifies it and typical adult human values would equal ~1.0 new BMU/mm^3 of compacta/yr, or ~2/mm^2 of bone surface/yr (Frost, 1969). In spongiosa its index is the bone formation rate (Frost, 1973a; Malluche et al, 1982; Melsen et al, 1983). How quickly an already activated BMU proceeds is usually expressed as an inverse function named its sigma value, expressed as the total time the typical BMU takes to evolve from A to the end of its F (Frost, 1969). Typical normal values for adult humans: ~3-4 months (Frost, 1966a; 1969; Vedi et al, 1984).

The time the typical BMU takes to evolve is found by multiplying the sigma value for its formation phase, σ_f, by the factor S_r/S_f, and then adding the result to Sigma$_f$. S_r is the fractional resorption surface in the bone, and S_f is the fractional formation or osteoid surface, as measured in the bone and including both active and inactive fractions of each kind of surface. The simple histomorphometric algebra follows (Frost, 1969)(Table III):

$$\sigma_f = mwt/M_f \qquad \text{Equation 1}$$

$$\sigma_r = \sigma_f \cdot S_r/S_f \qquad \text{Equation 2}$$

$$\sigma = \sigma_r + \sigma_f \qquad \text{Equation 3}$$

Table III. Histomorphometric parameters involved in measuring MDx repair efficency

mwt	Mean wall thickness of completed new bone packets
M	The appositional rate: the mean thickness of new bone deposited at bone forming centers that are in the "On" state.
M_f	The radial closure rate: the mean thickness of new bone deposited daily at the typical new bone forming center, averaged over the whole time period taken to complete the packet by including "Off" as well as "On" states (see below).
σ_r	Sigma$_r$, the resorption period: the time taken to complete the resorption phase of the typical BMU.
σ_f	Sigma$_f$, the formation period: the time taken to complete the formation phase of the typical BMU.
σ	Sigma: $\sigma_r + \sigma_f = \sigma$. The time taken to complete the whole BMU, from cutting cone to the end of its formation phase.
S_f	The fractional formation surface, or surface covered by osteoid, both active and inactive.
S_r	The fractional resorption surface, or surface scalloped by Howship's lacunae, whether active or inactive.
μ	The activation frequency: number of new BMU created per unit volume or surface of bone, in unit time.

Confusion over the value of sigma for bone remodeling in spongiosa stems from the fact that in the aged and in many diseases (including most osteoporoses and all true osteomalacias) a given bone forming site spends part of its time in the "On" state and part in the "Off". During the latter state no new osteoid matrix deposition or mineralization of existing osteoid occurs, but an obvious resting osteoid seam or border persists (Frost, 1969; 1973a; Hori et al, 1983). No double fluorochrome labels deposit during "Off" states; they deposit only during "On" states, which vary from ~95% of the lifetime of the seam in healthy people to <10% of that lifetime in some OPs and osteomalacias.

Accordingly, the mineral appositional rate (M) can be measured only in osteoid foci in the "On state", and typical values range from 120% to 50% of normal. That value used in Equation 1 to compute a sigma$_f$ value provides an active-only sigma that is rarely 2x longer than normal and can actually be subnormal if mwt is subnormal, as it is in some OPs (range: 30-70 days). Meunier's group has reported such values (Arlot et al, 1983; Boivin et al, 1984; Briançon and Meunier, 1979; Meunier et al, 1979).

But when corrected for "Off" states to obtain the radial closure rate, M_f (by multiplying M by S_{lab}/S_f, where S_{lab} is the fractional instantaneously active or labeled bone forming surface) (Epker et al, 1964; Frost, 1969; Melsen et al, 1983), the true total $sigma_f$ period is obtained, and it can prolong to many years in OPs and most osteomalacias (range: 2->10 years). It is the generally agreed correct way to define sigma, as per Equation 3 (Courpron, 1981; Danylchuk, 1978; Duncan, 1972; Epker et al, 1964; Flora et al, 1981; High et al, 1980; Jaworski et al, 1980; Keshawarz and Recker, 1984; Kimmel et al, 1981; Malluche et al, 1982; Melsen et al, 1983; Norrdin and Shih, 1983; Parfitt, 1984a; Takahashi et al, 1980; Teitelbaum et al, 1981; Vedi et al, 1984; Wronski et al, 1981). The shorter 40-50 day values reported by Meunier's group assume that a doubly labeled osteoid region is continuously "On" from the beginning of its formation to the end.

Some histomorphometrists have misunderstood one meaning of the sigma value provided by Equation 3. In compacta it is usually measured on cross sections, yet the length of the evolving BMU usually exceeds its diameter by ~30x (Jaworski and Lok, 1972). Some investigators thought that cross-sectional value did not reveal how long a new BMU takes to progress longitudinally from one end to the other. However, as calculated above, sigma does equal the time between the location of the cutting cone's front and the final formation that follows it at that same location. Since the cutting cone advances ~.05 mm/day and sigma ~100 days, the total length of a typical BMU approximates ~.05 mm X 100 days or ~5 mm, and it takes one sigma period to advance that 5 mm through the bone. However, that sigma value does not reveal the total length of the completed BSU (basic structural unit of lamellar bone) made by the BMU; as the diagram below shows, that could vary from ~5 mm to >20 mm. Therefore, the above sigma value indicates reliably how quickly BMU move through bone, and its inverse ($^1/\sigma$) is a rate in units of the fraction of the length of the typical active BMU completed in unit time.

As illustrated in the following diagram, a BMU proceeds to the right through compacta, signified by FRA (rather than ARF). Its completed part on the left is signified by periods, the virgin bone ahead of and behind it by x's. then, at five successive times, the following situations could exist, where the BMU's activation (A) begins at t_0, and has finished at t_4:

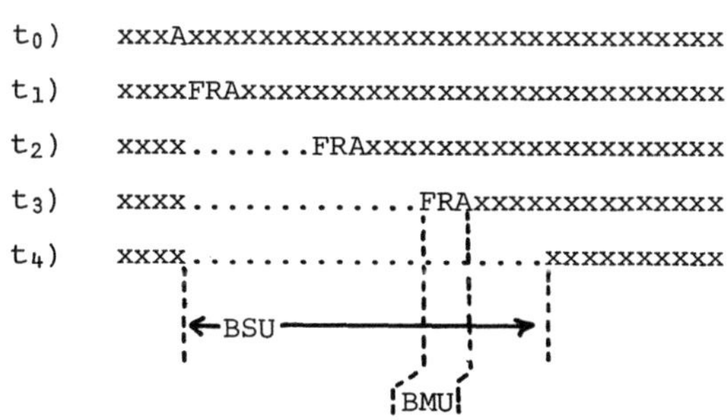

The distance FRA corresponds to both the sigma period and the length of the histologically active BMU itself. The distance BSU is the length of the completed BSU created by the FRA activities when the BMU has finished its work; it also corresponds to the total time taken to create it. That BSU length could vary from half or less of that at t_4 to over twice that without changing sigma for the FRA sequences that made it, or the actual length of the FRA in the bone. Accordingly, the measured sigma indicates how quickly a BMU would chase any bone microcrack propagating ahead of it; measuring it would therefore permit comparing normal to abnormal subjects. Since the basic measuring techniques have been applied by many investigators to human and laboratory animal affections, considerable published data have accumulated. These data have shown both the existence and nature of any dynamic abnormalities in MDx repair (Frost, 1985a).

The Histomorphometric Evidence

For human compact bone turnover dynamics, the most comprehensive data remain that obtained for the 6th, 10th and 11th ribs (Frost, 1969). These data came from more than 600 normal and diseased individuals. Other investigators have published comparable data for compacta in man and laboratory animals and for human spongiosa, including Anderson (Anderson and Danylchuk, 1979), Danylchuk (1978), High (High et al, 1980), Jaworski (Jaworski and Lok, 1972; Jaworski et al, 1980; 1981), Malluche (Malluche et al, 1976; 1982), Melsen (1978; Melsen and Moskilde, 1977; 1978a; 1978b; 1981; Melsen and Nielsen, 1977; Melsen et al, 1983), Meunier (Meunier et al, 1972; 1973; 1979), Mosekilde (Mosekilde and Melsen, 1978a; 1978b; 1979; 1980), Norrdin (Norrdin and Shih, 1983; Norrdin et al, 1977), Parfitt (1983a; 1983b; 1984a; 1984b), Recker (1983), and Takahashi (Takahashi et al, 1966; 1980).

In the following discussion, prolonged sigma values imply "lazy" BMU that repair individual MDx loci more slowly than normal. In compacta, the BMU activation frequency can be calculated from direct measurements (Frost, 1969), but in spongiosa the bone formation rate provides an index (Frost, 1983a), albeit a reliable one in steady states (Frost, 1985a).

Sigma and BMU activation are age-dependent (but not appreciably sex-dependent) so they were normalized for age in Table IV, which abstracts some of the above data.

The BMU activation-MIn association

Table IV shows that when MIn exists, activation usually has declined, but moderately. Typical reductions range from 30-80% of normal.

One example is idiopathic aseptic necrosis of the femoral head in young adults. Since approximately 1955 it has conventionally been attributed to an initial infarction which caused a bony collapse by unspecified means. However, it has been shown that infarcts, when they occurred, resulted from bony collapse rather than causing it; that accumulating MDx burdens led to that collapse; and that depressed BMU activation caused the accumulations. While presented in 1961 (McFarland and Frost, 1961) and on several other occasions up to and including 1985, that idea was rejected by others even though numerous attempts to reproduce the phenomenon in animals by infarcting their femoral heads failed. No direct evidence identifies ischemia as the primary cause of the above affection, yet as late as 1979 Glimcher reiterated that dogma (Glimcher and Kenzora, 1979). However, other studies now confirm the early viability of such femoral heads (Boutelier et al, 1983) and the depressed remodeling parameters (Arlot et al, 1983; Charon et al, 1982; Melsen and Nielson, 1977) inferred from pathologic and histomorphometric evidence, noting that certain other kinds of aseptic necrosis begin with an infarct (post hip dislocation, post femoral neck fracture).

Table IV. Summary of histomorphometric findings in human bone affections

Affection	Bone type	OPn	MIn	μ	σ	Citations
Normal aged	C	C	O	N	N	Frost, 1969
	S	O	O	N	N	Malluche et al, 1982 Melsen et al, 1983 Vedi et al, 1984
Normal aged**	C	+	O	N	N	Frost, 1969
	S	+	O	N	N	Malluche et al, 1982 Melsen et al, 1983 Vedi et al, 1984
Senile OPs	C	+	+	D,V	II*	Jett et al, 1967 Villaneuva et al, 1966a Wu et al, 1967
	S	+	+	D,V	II*	Giroux et al, 1975 Melsen et al, 1983
Postmenopausal OPs	C	+	+	D,V	II*	Jett et al, 1967 Villaneuva et al, 1966a Wu et al, 1967
	S	+	+	D,V	II*	Courpron, 1981 Melsen et al, 1983
Adrenocorticosteroid OPs	C	+	+	DD	II*	Jett et al, 1970 Klein et al, 1965
	S	+	+	D	II*	Bressot et al, 1976; 1979
Osteogenesis imperfecta	C	+	+	I	I	Jett et al, 1966 Villanueva and Frost, 1970
	S	+	+	D	I	Meunier

Table IV (continued)

Affection	Bone type	OPn	MIn	μ	σ	Citations
Osteopetrosis	C	O	O	DD	I*	Frost et al, 1961; Frost†
Acromegaly, early	C	O	O	I*	N	Ramser et al, 1966b
Acromegaly, late	C	+	+V	D	I	
Primary hyperparathyroidism	C	O,V	O,V	I,V	I*	Villanueva et al, 1970 Wilde et al, 1972
	S	+,V	O,V	D,V	II*	Bressot et al, 1976 High et al, 1980
Osteomalacia, malabsorption	C	O,V	+	D,V	II*	Leite et al, 1966 Ramser et al, 1966a
	S	O,V	+	D,V	II*	Melsen et al, 1983
Renal osteodystrophy	C	+,V	V	V	II*	Hitt et al, 1970 Norrdin and Shih, 1983 Norrdin et al, 1977 Sarnsethsiri et al, 1969
	S	V	V	V	II	de Vernejoul et al, 1981 Frost et al, 1981 Kimmel et al, 1981 Malluche et al, 1976
Familial vitamin D resistant rickets	C	O	O	D*	II*	Marie and Glorieux, 1982; 1984 Villaneuva et al, 1966b
Etidronate intoxication	C	O	+*	DD*	II*	Alexandre et al, 1981 Flora et al, 1981

† Unpublished observations and data

Table IV (continued)

Affection	Bone type	OPn	MIn	μ	σ	Citations
Radiation necrosis	C	O	+	DD*	?	Frost†; Jee
Idiopathic aseptic necrosis	S	V	+	D	I	Arlot et al, 1983 Charon et al, 1982 Frost† McFarland and Frost, 1961
Pathologic fractures	C	+	+	NC(?)	N(?)	Frost†
Stress fractures, healthy adults	C	O	+	N	N	Frost†
Spontaneous fractures, adults	C	O	+	D	?	Frost†
Thyrotoxicosis	C	+	O*	II*	D	Frost†; High et al, 1980
	S	+	O*	I	D	Jastrup et al, 1982 Melsen and Mosekilde, 1977 Meuner et al, 1972 Mosekilde and Melsen, 1978b
Postparalysis, acute	C	+	O*	I-D	I	Jaworski et al, 1980 Uhthoff and Jaworski, 1978
	S	+	O*	I-D	I	Minaire, 1973
Postparalysis, chronic	C	+	O*	D	I	Frost†
	S	+	O*	O	I	Frost† Jaworski et al, 1980 Uhthoff and Jaworski, 1978

† Unpublished observations and data

Table IV (concluded)

Affection	Bone Type	OPn	MIn	μ	σ	Citations
Estrogen effect	C	O	O*	DD*	?	Frost, 1964; in press, a
	S	O	O	D	N	Anderson
Naturally reversible OPn	C	+	O	II	N	Jaworski et al, 1980
Fluoride treatment, low dose	S	O	O	I	I	Bolvin et al, 1984 Briançon and Meunier, 1979 Kragstrop et al, 1984
Fluoride treatment, high dose	S	O	O	D	I	Jastrup; Olah
Disuse, acute	C	O	O	I	I	Frost† Jaworski et al, 1980 Uhthoff and Jaworski, 1978
	S	O	O	I	I	Frost†; Parfitt Jaworski et al, 1980 Uhthoff and Jaworski, 1978
Disuse, chronic	C	+	O	D	I	Frost†; Minaire, 1973
	S	+	O	D	I	Frost†; Minaire, 1973
Zero gravity, acute	C	O	O	I	I	Minaire; Parfitt; Wronski
	S	O	O	I	I	Minaire; Parfitt; Wronski
Regional acceleratory phenomenon (RAP)	C	+	V	I	?	Duncan; Frame; Frost
	S	+	+	I	?	Duncan; Frame; Frost

O = does not exist; + = exists; I = increased; II = markedly increased; D = decreased; DD = markedly decreased; V = variable; ? = unknown; N = normal. μ = mu, the BMU activation frequency; σ = sigma, the time taken to complete already enabled BMU. S = in spongiosa; C = in compacta. * = occurs in >95% of cases; ** = an OPn occurs with normal remodeling parameters and no MIn in large numbers of individuals.

Some exceptions to the activation-MIn association occur, as in compacta in osteogenesis imperfecta where activation is increased ~3x yet MIn occurs too (Jett et al, 1966; Villanueva and Frost, 1970; Villaneuva et al, 1966a; 1966c). Also, about 1/6 of postmenopausal and senile osteoporotic women show increased BMU activation (Frost, 1964; Jett et al, 1967; Teitelbaum et al, 1981; Wu and Frost, 1969; Wu et al, 1967). It is not known if such patients maintain continuously high activation and turnover, or if they alternate between high and low rates, which can, however, be determined by biopsy timing. Activation also increases in most thyrotoxic and many hyperparathyroid patients (Melsen and Mosekilde, 1977; 1978a; 1981; Meunier et al, 1972; Mosekilde and Melsen, 1978a; 1978b), but few such patients show much evidence of MIn; when they do, their disease is usually severe and prolonged, and their sigma values (see below) tend to be prolonged too. Activation is also increased in migratory osteoporosis (Arnstein, 1972).

Nevertheless, a general association between depressed BMU activation and MIn occurs although moderately and not consistent. However, in some postmenopausal (Villanueva et al, 1966a) and many corticosteroid osteoporotic patients (Bressot et al, 1979; Duncan, 1972) as well as in some cases of osteomalacia (Frost et al, 1981), virtually no active bone turnover could be detected in biopsy and autopsy studies (de Vernejoul et al, 1981; Duncan, 1972; Frame et al, 1965; Frost et al, 1981; Giroux et al, 1975; Hitt et al, 1970; Klein et al, 1965; Leite et al, 1966; Malluche et al, 1976; Meunier et al, 1973; 1979; Ramser et al, 1966a; Takahashi et al, 1980; Villanueva et al, 1966a-c; Wu and Frost, 1967). Furthermore, the clinical indications of MIn in such patients were usually severe, implying a virtually complete lack of BMU activation (and thus of bone turnover) could have been the major biodynamic cause of their MDx accumulations and MIn.

As an anecdotal observation, while markedly depressed activation usually means MIn, it did not in most nonosteoporotic and nonosteomalacic patients show such depressions. This observation is difficult to interpret because most such patients were already selected from the general population by the medical care complex. However, biopsies of 357 medically normal subjects, 5-95 years of age, showed little or no detectable bone turnover at the time of sampling in ~5% of the adults. That may reflect at least in part a normal annual variation in bone turnover between a maximum and a minimum, and the above people were sampled during a minimum. Such alternations could be regional as well as global in the bony skeleton.

The Sigma-MIn association

Table IV shows that when MIn exists, sigma prolongs too, and nearly invariably in most diseases but variably in a few. The prolongations are consistently large in some diseases and moderate in others. However, the major exceptions to the increased sigma association are stress fractures, thyrotoxicosis, and the so far unstudied radiation necrosis.

In most stress fractures (but not all) the person's usually high physical activity level implies the increased MDx production exceeded the capacity of remodeling to repair it.

The temporal properties of remodeling create an obligatory time lag between the beginning of the repair of an MDx locus by a BMU, and its histologic completion. That histologic time lag, the aforesaid sigma period, normally equals 3-4 months (Frost, 1969; Melsen and Mosekilde, 1978b; 1981; Vedi et al, 1984), but a special mechanical time lag follows. This is the time, the stiffness lag (Frost, in press, a), that a newly formed bone moiety or BSU (which is usually compliant mechanically*) needs to mineralize sufficiently to become stiff enough to carry its share of the local bone unit loads. That stiffness lag can last from ~3 months after the end of the histologic sigma period in healthy people, to >2 years in certain diseases (including some OPs and most osteomalacias) or under the influence of some drugs. Because of the stiffness lag, the older bone around a still compliant new BSU must carry the latter's share of the bone loads as well as its own. That increases its unit loading and stresses, and makes it more likely to develop its own MDx (see also OPn-MIn association, below). The biologic sigma value does not reveal the duration of the subsequent mechanical stiffness lag, which has not been studied systemically. The biologic plus mechanical time lags can allow a sudden escalation in mechanical usage to cause large enough accumulations of new MDx to result in complete stress fractures in healthy subjects.

Given those exceptions, nevertheless, the data summarized in Table IV indicate that: a prolonged sigma and the retarded MDx repair it implies are a major factor in most skeletal MIn. As examples, sigma has proven greatly increased (ranging from 4x - >10x normal) in nearly all cases (~98%) of postmenopausal, senile and corticosteroid-induced osteoporoses and osteomalacias (de Vernejoul et al, 1981; Duncan, 1972; Frame et al, 1965; Frost et al, 1981; Giroux et al, 1975; Hitt et al, 1970; Klein et al, 1965; Leite et al, 1966; Malluche et al, 1976; Meunier et al, 1973; 1979; Ramser et al, 1966a; Takahashi et al, 1980; Villanueva et al, 1966a-c; Wu and Frost, 1967). It is moderately increased (~1.3x normal) in osteogenesis imperfecta (Villanueva and Frost, 1970), pycnodysostosis (Canalis et al, 1980), and aseptic necrosis (Arlot et al, 1983). So far, it has been found actually decreased (~.7x normal) only in thyrotoxicosis (Melsen et al, 1983; Meunier et al, 1972; Mosekilde and Melson, 1978b).

The OPn-MIn association

When MIn exists, an OPn also usually exists (Table IV).

Exceptions include the stress and march fractures commented on above, osteopetrosis (Frost et al, 1969), and pycnodysostosis (Canalis et al, 1980; Sarnsethsiri et al, 1971). Also, in radiation necrosis, no OPn exists, but BMU activation markedly decreases in bone damaged by that means, probably due to radiation damage to the precursor cell populations on which remodeling depends. Accordingly, MDx burdens accumulate in such bones. That precursor cell damage also impairs the macrorepair process that heals complete fractures. No such impairment of macrorepair occurs in most cases of osteoporoses but it does in most cases of osteomalacias (an exception -- familial vitamin D-resistant rickets, where it has been shown that histomorphometrically severe osteomalacia seldom accompanies problems in healing gross fractures or surgical osteotomies (Frost, 1963; 1966b; 1973b).

Exceptions to the OPn-MIn association also occur in some osteomalacias, where MIn occurs but the ABV is either only moderately reduced or actually

* Compliant means flexible, rubber-like, the opposite of stiff.

supranormal (Frost et al, 1981). However, in such patients another special biomechanical phenomenon occurs which might be called a virtual osteopenia.

Briefly, a big fraction of osteomalacic bone is incompletely mineralized and thus mechanically hypercompliant, but it intermingles at the microscopic level with older and stiffer fractions. The effect is as though a thick stick of blackboard chalk had numerous holes drilled through it longitudinally which were filled with a sludge of powdered chalk mixed with gelatin. The sludge would be far more flexible than the stiff, intact chalk around it. The sludge would represent incompletely mineralized osteons or other BSU, and the intact chalk would represent the older and stiffer osteons and interstitial lamellae. The total volume of a column or trabeculum made of such materials might be normal or even supranormal, but its loads would be carried mainly by the stiff fraction, which would therefore be overloaded. Since stiff materials fatigue more than compliant ones under equal strains, and since in an intact, internally nonhomogeneous bone the stiff and compliant fractions strain almost equally during mechanical usage, the stiffer fractions of osteomalacic bone (or of any other mechanically nonhomogeneous bone) will carry more than their share of the total bone loads and will supply more than their share of the internal stresses that support those loads. That represents a "virtual" OPn, in which the stiffer moieties are more prone to MDx, as are planes where stiff and compliant moieties join, as at cement lines. The virtual osteopenia and the MDx caused in the stiffer bone fractions, plus the prolonged sigma values that retard MDx repair in osteomalacias, probably explain why pseudofractures occur in osteomalacia. The impaired mineralization of new fracture callus in most osteomalacias probably explains why those fractures fail to heal properly (Avioli, 1982; Bogumill and Schwamm, 1984; Krane, 1981; Kumar and Riggs, 1980). Exactly that failure distinguishes pseudofractures from stress fractures. A virtual OPn also exists when much micropetrosis occurs in compacta, for micropetrotic bone is dead, fully mineralized, and quite stiff (Frost, 1960). It can also occur in high turnover states, as in Paget's disease of bone, and after some forms of internal fixation of fractures where new stress fractures can occur after apparently satisfactory healing of the original fracture. That stiffness lag and a local virtual OPn which it can cause, plus the greatly increased local remodeling caused by the surgical trauma and its attendant RAP, probably underlie some service-life problems of bone and joint endoprostheses (Frost, in press, a).

The MIn-OPn association

When an OPn exists, MIn also often exists, but now with more exceptions (Table IV).

Less important exceptions include thyrotoxicosis where BMU activation typically increases and sigma decreases (Melsen et al, 1983; Meunier et al, 1972). That implies unusually effective repair of new MDx. Osteomalacias and the renal osteodystrophies can show an interesting schism, for occasionally their trabecular bone volumes can be normal or increased but their compacta thinned. That usually accompanies a virtual OPn, which is biomechanically important and also relatively frequent.

Postparalytic situations can also show an OPn without MIn, but the paralysis markedly reduces the usual bone loads in the paralyzed regions and, thus, the usual strains; MDx production therefore should also reduce markedly. Yet, BMU activation usually increases after acute paralysis or disuse, as shown in man by Minaire (1973), and in dogs by Jaworski and Uhthoff (Jaworski et al, 1980; Uhthoff and Jaworski, 1978), although 6-36 months later it usually declines to normal or subnormal values (Minaire, 1973). Therefore, if the osteopenic bones of chronically paralyzed limbs are mechanically weak compared with normal limbs, they are nevertheless well suited mechanically to their profoundly reduced typical mechanical usage (Frost, in press, a).

Naturally reversible osteoporoses are not really osteoporoses in the sense defined here, because MIn does not usually occur too (although it can in migratory osteoporosis (Arnstein, 1972; Duncan et al, 1967; Lengloh et al, 1973) which Europeans know as algodystrophy). The usually greatly increased activation and the relatively normal sigma values found in such states, for example in RAP (Frost, 1983b), probably explain much of that.

The most important and frequent exception to the OPn-MIn association (the second entry in Table IV, marked by double asterisks) occurs in apparently healthy older persons with no known medical cause of an osteoporosis or clinical evidence of MIn, but whose ABV is one or more standard deviations below normal for their age. Histomorphometric analyses of these persons reveal normal dynamic bone remodeling variables (Frost, 1969; Malluche et al, 1982; Melsen and Mosekilde, 1978b; 1981; Melsen et al, 1983; Vedi et al, 1984). Since they comprise ~15% of all clinically healthy individuals over 60 years of age in the U.S.A. (15% approximately equals the lower side of one standard deviation from the ABV mean), they outnumber all kinds of osteoporotic patients combined, and by ~5x (since only about 2% of all adults over age 60 have some evidence of spinal MIn, either active or past). They prove the OPn alone cannot be the sufficient pathology, or the sole pathogenesis of the MIn, in OPs.

Suggested conclusions

a) Retarded evolution of ongoing BMU (revealed by prolonged sigma values) will usually cause MIn, whether an OPn exists or not. It alone can cause MIn, although it is usually associated with other causes. Consequently, its study deserves more attention.

b) Increased MDx production can alone cause MIn, as in march and stress fractures. However, more often it is associated with an OPn in the presence of normal mechanical usage.

c) Greatly depressed BMU activation can alone cause MIn, although more often its depression is accompanied by other factors such as prolonged sigma and a true and/or virtual OPn, and therefore requires further investigation.

d) An OPn alone seldom causes MIn, although in health and disease the two often associate.

e) Most pathologic bone fragility arises from pathologically large MDx burdens. It seldom arises solely from structural weakening due to an OPn of otherwise normal bone. An obvious exception is: some pathologic fractures associated with great bone destruction, as in bone cysts, primary tumors and destructive metastases.

f) Pathologic fragility occurs in a variety of osseous and fibrous tissue affections (Table I). It is not unique to the OPs or to OPn.

g) MIn is a separate pathologic feature. It is distinct from and not necessarily associated with an OPn alone, and its causes are multifactorial. An OPn is also a separate pathologic feature, distinct from and not necessarily associated with MIn. Its causes are multifactorial and several kinds exist. MDx is a separate and real pathologic feature too, with its own multifactorial causes and variants.

Comment

New concepts

The above terms and concepts will be new to many who work with metabolic bone disease and bone fragility. The terms include MIn, MDx, ABV, BMU, mu and sigma, the stiffness lag, virtual OPn, compliance, strain, mechanical usage, modeling, remodeling; companion articles have also used the terms ΔB.BMU, "L"-gated (or site specific) biologic control, the RAP and the MES (Frost, 1985a; 1985b).

Others may modify this terminology and much remains to be learned about the features it stands for. Still, the basic ideas should endure as useful tools and seeds.

The new perspective

Abundant evidence now reveals meaningful associations between mechanical incompetence and osteopenia on the one hand, and MDx and remodeling disorders that retard MDx repair. The sigma-MIn association is the strongest of all. Those associations are too numerous to be coincidental. They are real pathogenetic mechanisms of bone fragility and MIn.

Table V. Pathogenetic mechanisms of accumulating MDx burdens in clinical affections

Condition	Tissue affected	New MDx	Mu	Sigma	ABV
Stress fractures	Bone	II	N	N	N
Pathologic fracture	Bone	II	N	N	DD
Postmenopausal OPs	Bone	I	D	II	D
Spontaneous fracture	Bone	N	DD	?	N
Idiopathic aseptic necrosis	Bone	N	DD	?	D
Spontaneous Achilles tendon rupture	Tendon	N	DD	?	N
Rheumatoid tendon rupture	Tendon	D	DD	II	N
Osteochondritis dissecans	Bone	I	DD	?	N

I = increased; II = greatly increased; D = decreased; DD = markedly decreased; N = normal; ? = unknown; ABV = total amount of tissue in the structure

That conclusion challenges prevalent ideas of the pathogenesis of the osteoporoses (Aergerter and Kirkpátrick, 1975; Avioli, 1982; Bogumill and Schwamm, 1984; Cruess, 1982; Emmertgen et al, 1982; Krane, 1981; Kumar and Riggs, 1980). The more recent understanding of the MIn and MDx elements of OPs means we must learn what depresses BMU activation and prolongs the sigma values in disease, and then, separately, how to restore them to normal to improve MDx repair and reduce MIn of already existing bone. Table V summarizes some pertinent examples.

The above material also means that at least two basically different routes could cure the mechanical disability of osteoporosis (Frost, 1963; 1966b; 1973b). One would correct the osteopenia, and investigators and clinicians have tried that route almost exclusively since the 1930's. A second and so far unexplored route would correct the remodeling abnormalities that contribute to the MDx accumulations that underlie most MIn. A recent study by Gallagher and Recker (in which 1,25-dihydroxy vitamin D apparently improved MIn without affecting the ABV of patients with OPs) suggests that is a viable approach.

Signals for MDx repair, MU and bone remodeling

Remodeling usually responds to mechanical use (Frost, 1985a). However, those responses can have little to do with how remodeling responds to MDx. As one example of that dissociation, the profound disuse caused by an acute paraplegia virtually eliminates major bone strains and therefore any new MDx in the paralyzed limbs. Nevertheless, bone remodeling increases in them promptly, regularly and considerably (Jaworski et al, 1980; Minaire, 1973; Uhthoff and Jaworski et al, 1978), so MDx is not the sole mechanical factor that can enable remodeling.

BMU-based bone remodeling provides a kind of "final common pathway" for bone responses to both mechanical usage (MU) and to MDx, but the signals each generates to control remodeling must differ somehow (Frost, 1984). If the MU responses followed the general route of: load (L) → bone (B) → strain (E) → primary signals (S_1) → first receptor (R_1) → secondary signal (S_2) → observed remodeling response by the second receptor (R_2), then the separate MDx signal (S_3) could route differently, at least in part, perhaps as in one of these relations (Frost, 1984).

$$\begin{array}{l} L \rightarrow B \rightarrow E \rightarrow S_1 \rightarrow R_1 \rightarrow S_2 \rightarrow R_2 \\ \qquad\qquad\qquad\quad \uparrow \\ \qquad\qquad MDx \rightarrow S_3 \end{array}$$

or:

$$\begin{array}{l} L \rightarrow B \rightarrow E \rightarrow S_1 \rightarrow R_1 \rightarrow S_2 \rightarrow R_2 \\ \qquad\qquad MDx \rightarrow S_3 \longrightarrow\uparrow \end{array}$$

or:

$$\begin{array}{l} L \rightarrow B \rightarrow E \rightarrow S_1 \rightarrow R_1 \rightarrow S_2 \rightarrow R_2 \\ \qquad\quad MDx \rightarrow R_3 \rightarrow S_3 \longrightarrow\uparrow \end{array}$$

or:

$$\begin{array}{l} \text{Endocrine/humoral agents} \longrightarrow | \\ MU \longrightarrow R_1 \longrightarrow | \text{---} R_3 \\ MDx \longrightarrow R_2 \longrightarrow | \end{array}$$

Those examples of "serial-parallel gating" of physiologic control (Frost, in press, a) encode the fact that remodeling provides a final pathway for expressing the different and independent but often concurrent needs of the endocrine milieu, homeostasis, growth, mechanical usage and microdamage repair (Frost, in press, a).

The above cell signal-response mechanisms (ie, S → R) might all occur within the same kind of cell or, possibly within a series of different kinds of cells. Other possibilities exist too, but the above synthesis suggests some factors that existing clinical evidence already strongly supports. For example, it suggests a disease could occur in which the normal inhibition of remodeling by MU is impaired; remodeling increases, but the MDx signal is also impaired; burdens of MDx increase and bone fragilizes in spite of the increased remodeling. Exactly that happens in compacta in osteogenesis imperfecta (Frost, 1985a; in press, a; 1984), as well as in spongiosa in two rarer congenital bone disorders.

The above situation, plus other evidence not presented here, in effect prove the signal-receptor mechanisms, that relate remodeling to MU and to MDx, differ in some respects; thus, some drugs and diseases can affect one but not the other, or can affect each but in different ways.

References

1. Aegerter, E., and Kirkpatrick, J.A.: Orthopaedic Diseases, 4th ed. W.B. Saunders Co., Philadelphia, 1975.

2. Alexandre, C., Meunier, P.J., Edouard, C., Khair, R.A., and Johnston, C.C. Jr.: Effects of ethane-1 hydroxy-1, 1-diphosphonate (5 mg/kg/day dose) on quantitative bone histology in Paget's disease of bone. J. Metab. Bone Dis. Rel. Res. 4, 309, 1981.

3. Anderson, C., and Danylchuk, E.D.: Age-related variations in cortical bone remodeling measurements in male beagles 10 to 26 months of age. Am. J. Vet. Res. 40, 869, 1979.

4. Arlot, M.E., Bonjean, M., Chavassieux, P.M., and Meunier, P.J.: Bone histology in adults with aseptic necrosis. J. Bone Joint Surg. 65A, 1319, 1983.

5. Arnstein, A.R.: Regional osteoporosis. Orthop. Clin. North Am. 3, 585, 1972.

6. Avioli, L.: Bone diseases. In, Cecil's Textbook of Medicine, 16th ed. Eds: Wyngaarden, J.B. and Smith, L.H., Jr., W.B. Saunders Co., Philadelphia, 1982, pp 1318-1553.

7. Bogumill, G.P., and Schwamm, H.A.: Orthopaedic Pathology, W.B. Saunders Co., Philadelphia, 1984

8. Bolvin, G., Edouard, C., Chapuy, M.C., and Meunier, P.J.: Iliac bone histomorphometry in skeletal fluorosis. Presented at Fourth International Workshop on Bone Histomorphometry, Aarhus, Denmark, 1984.

9. Boutelier, G., Arlet, J., Blasco, A., Vigoni, F., and Ekfterion, A.: Is osteonecrosis of the femoral head avascular? Bone blood flow measurements after long term treatment with corticosteroids. J. Metab. Bone Dis. Rel. Res. 4, 313, 1983.

10. Bressot, C., Courpron, P., Edouard, C., and Meunier, P.J.: Histomorphométrie des Ostéopathies Endocriniennes. Univ. Claude Bernard, Lyon, 1976.

11. Bressot, C., Meunier, P.J., Chapuy, M.D., Lejeune, E., Edouard, C., and Darby, A.J.: Histomorphometric profile, pathophysiology and reversibility of corticosteroid induced osteoporosis. J. Metab. Bone Dis. Rel. Res. 1, 303, 1979.

12. Briançon, D., and Meunier, P.J.: Le Traitement de l'Ostéoporose par l'Association Fluorure de Sodium, Calcium, Vitamine D. Univ. Claude Bernard, Lyon, 1979.

13. Canalis, E.M., Reardon, G.E., Baron, R., and Raisz, L.G.: Dynamic bone morphometry and studies on the effects of serum on bone metabolism *in vitro* in a case of pyconodysostosis. J. Metab. Bone Dis. Rel. Res. 2, 99, 1980.

14. Carter, D.R.: Mechanical loading histories and cortical bone remodeling. Calcif. Tissue Int. 36, S19, 1984.

15. Charon, S., Bavery, E., Malik, M.E., Touraine, J.L., Edouard, C., Arlof, M., Traeger, J., and Meunier, P.J.: Osteonécrose de la transplantation rénale. Lyon Medicale 247, 339, 1982.

16. Courpron, P.: Bone tissue mechanisms underlying osteoporoses. Orthop. Clin. North Am. 12, 513, 1981.

17. Cruess, R.L.: Physiology of bone formation and resorption. In, The Musculoskeletal System: Embryology, Biochemistry and Physiology. Ed: Cruess, R.L. Churchill-Livingstone, New York, 1982, pp 219-252.

18. Danylchuk, K.D.: The effects of environmental pollutants on bone remodeling. Thesis, Univ. Western Ontario, 1978.

19. de Vernejoul, M.C., Kuntz, D., Miravet, L., Gueris, J., Bielakoff, J., and Ryckewaert, A.: Bone histomorphometry in dialysed patients. J. Metab. Bone Dis. Rel. Res. 3, 175, 1981.

20. Duncan, H.: Osteoporoses in rheumatoid arthritis and corticosteroid induced osteoporosis. Orthop. Clin. North Am. 3, 571, 1972.

21. Duncan, H., Frame, B., Frost, H.M., and Arnstein, A.R.: Migratory osteolysis of the lower extremities. Ann. Int. Med. 66, 1165, 1967.

22. Emmertgen, F., Melsen, F., Mosekilde, L., Lund, Bi, Lund, Bj, Sørensen, O.H., Neilson, H.E., Sølling, H., and Hansen, H.H.: Altered vitamin D metabolism and bone remodeling in patients with medullary thyroid carcinoma and hypercalcitonemia. J. Metab. Bone Dis. Rel. Res. 4, 17, 1982.

23. Epker, B.N., Hattner, R., and Frost, H.M.: Radial rate of osteon closure: Its application to the study of bone formation in metabolic bone disease. J. Lab. Clin. Med. 64, 643, 1964.

24. Evans, R.A., Hughes, W.G., Dunstan, C.R., Lennon, W.P., Kohan, L., Hills, E., and Wong, S.Y.P.: Adult osteosclerosis. J. Metab. Bone Dis. Rel. Res. 5, 111, 1984.

25. Flora, L., Hassing, G.S., Parfitt, A.M., and Villanueva, A.R.: Comparative skeletal effects of two diphosphonate drugs. In, Osteoporosis. Eds: DeLuca, H.F., Frost, H.M., Jee, W.S.S., Johnston, C.C., Jr., and Parfitt, A.M. University Park Press, Baltimore, 1981, pp 389-407.

26. Frame, B., Arnstein, A.R., Frost, H.M., and Smith, R.W., Jr.: Resistant osteomalacia. Studies with tetracycline bone labeling and metabolic balance. Am. J. Med. 38, 134, 1965.

27. Frost, H.M.: Micropetrosis. J. Bone Joint Surg. 42A, 144, 1960.

28. Frost, H.M.: Bone Remodeling Dynamics. Charles C. Thomas, 1963.

29. Frost, H.M.: Dynamics of bone remodeling. In, Bone Biodynamics. Ed: Frost, H.M. Little, Brown and Co., Boston, 1964, pp 315-333.

30. Frost, H.M.: Bone dynamics in metabolic bone diseases. J. Bone Joint Surg. 48A, 1192, 1966a.

31. Frost, H.M.: Bone Dynamics in Osteoporosis and Osteomalacia. Charles C. Thomas, 1966b.

32. Frost, H.M.: Tetracycline based histological analyses of bone remodeling. Calcif. Tissue Res. 3, 211, 1969.

33. Frost, H.M.: A method of analysis of trabecular bone dynamics. In, Bone Histomorphometry. Ed: Meunier, P.J. Armour-Montagu, Paris, 1973a, pp 445-475.

34. Frost, H.M.: Bone Remodeling and Its Relation to Metabolic Bone Disease. Charles C. Thomas, 1973b.

35. Frost, H.M.: Bone histomorphometry: Analysis of trabecular bone dynamics. In, Bone Histomorphometry: Techniques and Interpretation. Ed: Recker, R.R. C.R.C. Press, Boca Raton, 1983a, pp 109-132.

36. Frost, H.M.: The regional acceleratory phemonemon: A review. Henry Ford Hosp. Med. J. 31, 3, 1983b.

37. Frost, H.M.: Series of manuscripts circulated to the sigma bone group, 1984.

38. Frost, H.M.: Pathogenetic mechanisms of the osteoporoses. In, Basic Concepts of Bone Fragility in Orthopaedics and Medicine. Eds: Uhthoff, H.-K., and Stahl, E. Springer-Verlag, Berlin-Heidelberg-New York, 1985.

39. Frost, H.M.: Early forms of bone microdamage: Types and techniques to demonstrate them. In, Basic Concepts of Bone Fragility in Orthopaedics and Medicine. Eds: Uhthoff, H-K. and Stahl, E. Springer-Verlag, Berlin-Heidelberg-New York, 1985.

40. Frost, H.M.: The Skeletal Intermediary Organization. C.R.C. Press, Boca Raton, in press (a).

41. Frost, H.M.: Mechanical determinants of skeletal architecture: Fibrous tissue modeling. In, Basic Science of Orthopaedis, Vol. II. Eds: Albright, J.A., and Brand, R.A. Appleton-Century Crofts, New York, in press (b).

42. Frost, H.M., Griffith, D.L., Jee, W.S.S., Kimmel, D.B., McCandlis, R.P., and Teitelbaum, S.L.: Histomorphometric changes in trabecular bone of renal failure patients treated with calciferol. J. Metab. Bone Dis. Rel. Res. 2, 285, 1981.

43. Frost, H.M., Roth, H., and Villanueva, A.R.: Physical characteristics of bone. IV: Microscopic failure and prefailure patterns. Henry Ford Hosp. Med. Bull. 9, 163, 1961.

44. Frost, H.M.: Villanueva, A.R., Jett, S., and Eyring, E.: Tetracycline-based analysis of bone remodeling in steopetrosis. Clin. Orthop. 65, 203, 1969.

45. Giroux, J.M., Courpron, P., and Meunier, P.J.: Histomorphométrie de l'Ostéopenie Physiologique Sénile. Univ. Claude Bernard, Lyon, 1975.

46. Glimcher, M.J., and Kenzora, J.E.: The biology of osteonecrosis of the human femoral head and its clinical implications. III. Discussion of the etiology and genesis of the pathological sequellae; Comments on treatment. Clin. Orthop. Rel. Res. 140, 273, 1979.

47. High, W.B., Capen, C.C., and Black, H.E.: Histomorphometric evaluation of the effects of 1,25 dihydroxycholecalciferol, parathormone and thyroxine on trabecular bone remodeling in adult dogs. Thesis. Dept. Veterinary Pathology, Ohio State University, 1980.

48. Hitt, O.K., Jaworski, Z.F.G., Shimizu, A.O., and Frost, H.M.: Tissue level bone formation rates in chronic renal failure, measured by means of tetracycline bone labeling. Canad. J. Physiol. Pharmacol. 48, 824, 1970.

49. Hori, M., Takahashi, H., Konnot, T., and Haba, T.: A classification of double labels in iliac trabecular bone in beagles. In, Handbook of Bone Morphometry. Ed: Takahashi, H. Nipponia, Tokyo, 1983, pp 147-153.

50. Jastrup, B., Mosekilde, L., Melsen, F., Lund, B.J., and Sørensen, O.H.: Serum levels of vitamin D metabolites and bone remodeling in hyperthyroidism. Metabolism 31, 126, 1982.

51. Jaworski, Z.F.G., and Lok, E.: The rate of osteoclastic bone erosion in haversian remodeling sites of adult dog rib. Calcif. Tissue Res. 10, 103, 1972.

52. Jaworski, Z.F.G., Duck, B., and Sekaly, G.: Kinetics of osteoclasts and their nuclei in evolving secondary osteons. J. Anat. 133, 397, 1981.

53. Jaworski, Z.F.G., Liskova-Kiar, M., and Uhthoff, H.: Effect of long term immobilization on the pattern of bone loss in older dogs. J. Bone Joint Surg. 62B, 104, 1980.

54. Jett, S., Ramser, J.E., Frost, H.M., and Villanueva, A.R.: Bone turnover and osteogenesis imperfecta. Arch. Path. 81, 112, 1966.

55. Jett, S., Wu, K., and Frost, H.M.: Tetracycline-based histological measurement of cortical endosteal bone formation in normal and osteoporotic rib. Henry Ford Hosp. Med. J. 15, 325, 1967.

56. Jett, S., Duncan, H., and Frost, H.M.: Adrenalcorticoid and salicylate actions on human and canine haversian bone remodeling. Clin. Orthop. 68, 301, 1970.

57. Keshawarz, N.M., and Recker, R.R.: Expansion of the medullary cavity at the expense of cortex in postmenopausal osteoporosis. J. Metab. Bone Dis. Rel. Res. 5, 223, 1984.

58. Kimmel, D., Ritz, E., Krempien, B., Mehls, O.: Bone cell kinetics and function during experimental uremia. J. Metab. Bone Dis. Rel. Res. 3, 191, 1981.

59. Klein, M., Villanueva, A.R., and Frost, H.M.: A quantitative histological study of rib from 18 patients treated with adrenal cortical steroids. Acta Orthop. Scand. 35, 171, 1965.

60. Kragstrop, J., Richards, A., Fejerskor, O.: Experimental osteofluorosis in the domestic pig. A stereologic study of vertebral trabecular bone. Presented at the Fourth International Workshop on Bone Histomorphometry. Aarhus, Denmark, 1984.

61. Krane, S.M.: Connective tissue. In, Pathophysiology. The Biological Principles of Disease. Eds: Smith, L.H., Jr., and Thier, S.O. W.B. Saunders Co., Philadelphia, 1981, pp 755-798.

62. Kumar, R., and Riggs, B.L.: Pathologic bone physiology. In, Fundamental and Clinical Bone Physiology. Ed. Urist, M.R. J.B. Lippincott Co., Philadelphia, 1980, pp 394-406.

63. Lengloh, N.D., Hunder, G.G., Riggs, B.L., and Kelley, P.J.: Transient painful osteoporoses of the lower extremities. J. Bone Joint Surg. 55A, 1188, 1973.

64. Leite, C.A., Frame, B., Frost, H.M., and Arnstein, A.R.: Osteomalacia following ureterosigmoidostomy. Clin. Orthop. 49, 103, 1966.

65. Malluche, H.H., Meyer, W., Sherman, D., and Massry, S.G.: Quantitative bone histology in 84 normal American subjects. Calcif. Tissue Int. 34, 449, 1982.

66. Malluche, H.H., Ritz, E., Lange, H.P., Kutshera, J., Hodgson, M., Sieffert, U., and Schoeppe, W.: Bone histology in incipient and advanced renal failure. Kidney Int. 9, 355, 1976.

67. Marie, P.J., and Glorieux, F.H.: Bone histomorphometry in asymptomatic adults with hereditary hypophosphatemic vitamin D resistant osteomalacia. J. Metab. Bone Dis. Rel. Res. 4, 249, 1982.

68. Marie, P.J., and Glorieux, F.H.: Stimulation of cortical bone mineralization and remodeling by phosphate and 1,25-dihydroxyvitamin D in vitamin D-resistant rickets. J. Metab. Bone Dis. Rel. Res. 3, 159, 1984.

69. McFarland, P.H., and Frost, H.M.: A possible new cause for aseptic necrosis of the femoral head. Henry Ford Hosp. Med. Bull. 9, 115, 1961.

70. Melsen, F.: Histomorphometric analysis of iliac bone in normal and pathological conditions. Aarhus Amtssygehus, Aarhus, 1, 1978.

71. Melsen, F., and Mosekilde, L.: Morphometric and dynamic bone changes in hyperthyroidism. Acta Path. Microbiol. Scand. 85, 141, 1977.

72. Melsen, F., and Mosekilde, L.: Dynamic studies of trabecular bone formation and osteoid maturation in normal and certain pathological conditions. J. Metab. Bone Dis. Rel. Res. 1, 45, 1978a.

73. Melsen, F., and Mosekilde, L.: Tetracycline double labelling of iliac trabecular bone in 41 normal subjects. Calcif. Tissue Res. 26, 99, 1978b.

74. Melsen, F., and Mosekilde, L.: The role of bone biopsy in the diagnosis of metabolic bone disease. Orthop. Clin. North Am. 12, 571, 1981.

75. Melsen, F., and Nielson, H.E.: Osteonecrosis following renal allotransplantation. Acta Path. Microbiol. Scand., Sect. A 85, 99, 1977.

76. Melsen, F., Mosekilde, L., and Kragstrup, J.: Metabolic bone diseases as evaluated by bone histomorphometry. In, Bone Histomorphometry. Techniques and Interpretation. Ed: Recker, R.R. C.R.C. Press, Boca Raton, 1983, pp 265-284.

77. Meunier, P.J., Bianchi, G.G.S., Edouard, C.M., Bernard, J.C., Courpron, P., and Vignon, G.E.: Bony manifestations of thyrotoxicosis. Orthop. Clin. North Am. 3, 745, 1972.

78. Meunier, P.J., Courpron, P., Edouard, C.M., Bernard, J., Bringuier, J., and Vignon, G.: Physiological senile involution and pathological rarefaction of bone. Quantitative and comparative histological data. Clin. Endocrinol. Metab. 2, 239, 1973.

79. Meunier, P.J., Courpron, P., Edouard, C.M., Alexandre, C., Bressot, C., Lips, P., and Boyce, B.F.: Bone histomorphometry in osteoporotic states. In, Osteoporosis II. Ed: Barzel, U.S. Grune and Stratton, New York, 1979, pp 27-47.

80. Minaire, P.: L'Ostéoporose d'Immobilisation. Données Biologiques et Histologiques Quantitatives. Ediprim, Lyon, 1973.

81. Mosekilde, L., and Melsen, F.: Morphometric and dynamic studies of bone changes in hypothyroidism. Acta Path. Microbiol. Scand. 86, 56, 1978a.

82. Mosekilde, L., and Melsen, F.: A tetracycline based histomorphometric evaluation of bone resorption and bone turnover in hyperthyroidism and hyperparathyroidism. Acta Med. Scand. 204, 97, 1978b.

83. Mosekilde, L., and Melsen, F.: A tetracycline based histomorphometric evaluation of the maturation period of osteoid in normal and certain pathological conditions. Calcif. Tissue Int. 27, 117, 1979 (abstract)

84. Mosekilde, L., and Melsen, F.: Dynamic differences in trabecular bone remodeling between patients after jejuno-ileal bypass for obesity and epileptic patients receiving anticonvulsant therapy. J. Metab. Bone Dis. Rel. Res. 2, 77, 1980.

85. Norrdin, R.W., and Shih, M.S.: Profiles of cortical remodeling sites in longitudinal rib sections of beagles with renal failure and parathyroid hyperplasia. J. Metab. Bone Dis. Rel. Res. 5, 353, 1983.

86. Norrdin, R.W., Villafane, F.A., and Lopresti, C.A.: Haversian remodeling activity in various bones of beagles and the effect of chronic renal failure. In, Bone Histomorphometry-1976. Ed: Meunier, P.J. Armour-Montagu, Paris, 1977, pp 171 - 178.

87. Parfitt, A.M.: Steriologic basis of bone histomorphometry: Theory of quantitative microscopy and reconstruction of the third dimension. In, Bone Histormophometry: Techniques and Interpretation. C.R.C. Press, Boca Raton, 1983a, pp 53-88.

88. Parfitt, A.M.: The physiologic and clinical significance of bone histomorphometric data. In, Bone Histomorphometry: Techniques and Interpretation. C.R.C. Press, Boca Raton, 1983b, pp 143-224.

89. Parfitt, A.M.: The cellular basis of bone remodeling: The quantum concept reexamined in the light of recent advances in the cell biology of bone. Calcif. Tissue Int. 36, 537, 1984a.

90. Parfitt, A.M.: Age-related structural changes in trabecular and cortical bone: Cellular mechanisms and biomechanical consequences. Calcif. Tissue Int. 36, S123, 1984b.

91. Ramser, J.E., Frost, H.M., Arnstein, A.R., Frame, B., and Smith, R.W.: Tetracycline based studies of bone dynamics in rib of 6 cases of osteomalacia. Clin. Orthop. 46, 219, 1966a.

92. Ramser, J.E., Frost, H.M., and Smith, R.W.: Tetracycline-based measurements of the tissue and cell dynamics in rib of a 25 year old man with active acromegaly. Clin. Orthop. 49, 169, 1966b.

93. Recker, R.R.: Bone Histomorphometry. Techniques and Interpretation. C.R.C. Press, Boca Raton, 1983.

94. Sarnsethsiri, P., Jaworski, Z.F.G., Shimizu, A.G., and Frost, H.M.: New bone formation and osteoid seam thickness: Appositional rate in patients undergoing renal dialysis. Arch. Path. 88, 49, 1969.

95. Sarnsethsiri, P., Hitt, O.K., Eyring, E.J., and Frost, H.M.: A tetracycline-based study of bone dynamics in pycnodysostosis. Clin. Orthop. 74, 301, 1971.

96. Shenck, R.K., and Olah, A.J.: Histomorphometrie. In, Klinische Osteologie, 6th Ed. Eds: Kuhlencordt, F., and Bartelheimer, H. Springer-Verlag, Heidelberg, 1980, pp 437-494.

97. Takahashi, H., Frost, H.M., and Kuhn, T.: Bone tissue and cell dynamics determined by tetracycline labelling in a case of pseudohypoparathyroidism (and the patient's mother). Clin. Orthop. 43, 163, 1966.

98. Takahashi, H., Norimatsu, H., Watanabe, G., Konno, T., Inoue, J., and Fukuda, M.: The remodeling period (sigma) in canine and human cortical bone. In, Calcium Endocrinology. Eds: Yoshitoshi, Y. and Fujita, T. Chugai, Igaku, Tokyo, 1980, pp 13-31.

99. Teitelbaum, S.L., Bergfield, M.A., Avioli, L., and Whyte, M.P.: Failure of routine biochemical studies to predict histological heterogeneity of untreated postmenopausal osteoporosis. In, Osteoporosis. Eds: DeLuca, H.D., Frost, H.M., Jee, W.S.S., Johnston, C.C., Jr., and Parfitt, A.M. University Park Press, Baltimore, 1981, pp 303-309.

100. Uhthoff, H., and Jaworski, Z.F.G.: Bone loss in response to long term immobilization. J. Bone Joint Surg. 60B, 420, 1978.

101. Vedi, S., Compston, J.E., Webb, A., and Tighe, J.E.: Histomorphometric analysis of dynamic parameters of trabecular bone formation in the iliac crest of normal British subjects. J. Metab. Bone Dis. Rel. Res. 5, 69, 1984.

102. Villanueva, A.R., and Frost, H.M.: Bone formation in osteogenesis imperfecta measured by tetracycline bone labeling. Acta Orthop. Scand. 41, 531, 1970.

103. Villanueva, A.R., Frost, H.M., Ilnicki, L., Frame, B., Smith, R.W., and Arnstein, A.R.: Cortical bone dynamics in 21 cases of osteoporosis measured by means of tetracycline bone labelling. J. Lab. Clin. Med. 68, 599, 1966a.

104. Villanueva, A.R., Ilnicki, L., Frost, H.M., and Arnstein, A.R.: Measurement of the bone formation rate in a case of familial hypophosphatemic vitamin D resistant rickets. J. Lab. Clin. Med. 67, 973, 1966b.

105. Villanueva, A.R., Ilnicki, L., Duncan, H., and Frost, H.M.: Bone and cell dynamics in the osteoporoses: A review of measurements by tetracycline bone labelling. Clin. Orthop. 49, 163, 1966c.

106. Villanueva, A.R., Jaworski, Z.F.G., Hitt, O.K., Sarnsethsiri, P., and Frost, H.M.: Cellular level bone resorption in chronic renal failure and primary hyperparathyroidism. Calcif. Tissue Res. 5, 289, 1970.

107. Wilde, C.D., Jaworski, Z.F.G., Villanueva, A.R., and Frost, H.M.: Quantitative histological measurements of bone turnover in primary hyperparathyroidism. Calcif. Tissue Res. 12, 137, 1972.

108. Wronski, T.J., Smith, J.M., and Jee, W.S.S.: Variation in mineral apposition rate of trabecular bone within the beagle skeleton. Calcif. Tissue Int. 33, 1981.

109. Wu, K., and Frost, H.M.: Bone formation in osteoporosis: Appositional rate measured by tetracycline labeling. Arch. Path. 88, 508, 1969.

110. Wu, K., Jett, S., and Frost, H.M.: Bone resorption rates in physiological, senile and postmenopausal osteoporoses. J. Lab. Clin. Med. 69, 810, 1967.

Loads versus Bone Strength

Impaired Bone Strength and Fracture Patterns at Different Skeletal Sites

L. J. MELTON III and B. L. RIGGS

Introduction

Disease patterns are not only clinically useful for identification of high-risk patients, but are often of greater value as clues to important etiologic factors. The epidemiologic patterns of disease are of most interest here, raising the question of fracture patterns at different skeletal sites. Furthermore, what hypotheses can one establish as to the causes of age-related fractures?

Fracture Patterns

It has long been recognized (Buhr and Cooke, 1959) that some fractures are of the so-called "L" type, eg, distal humerus and skull. Such fractures are more common among the young, are more prevalent in men than in women, and are usually caused by obviously severe trauma (Nelson et al, 1984; Rose et al, 1982); the question of impaired bone strength rarely arises. Other fractures, such as Colles' fractures of the distal forearm, comprise the composite type and occur among adolescents as well as the elderly (Buhr and Cook, 1959). Parfitt covers the implications of fracture patterns in these younger subjects elsewhere in this symposium (Parfitt, 1985). Our emphasis will be on the "J" type fractures (Fig. 1), including proximal femur (Melton et al, 1982), proximal humerus (Rose et al, 1982), pelvic fractures (Melton et al, 1981), and Colles' fractures among adults (Owen et al, 1982). All these fractures show the same general pattern: increasing incidence with age and higher incidence rates among elderly women than elderly men (Melton and Riggs, 1983). Preliminary data from our studies in Rochester, Minnesota show, as expected, that vertebral fractures among women have the same pattern (L.J. Melton, unpublished data). Moreover, the fractures of this type usually result from only moderate trauma, in the case of the limb fractures most often a simple fall to the floor (Melton and Riggs, 1985).

A number of hypotheses have been proposed to account for this pattern of fracture:

1. *Increased risk of falling.* The frequency of falls increases with age (Campbell et al, 1981; Gryfe et al, 1977) and may be greater among women than men (Gryfe et al, 1977; Prudham and Evans, 1981). However, the incidence of falls does not appear to increase 30-fold (Gryfe et al, 1977), as does the incidence of hip fractures between the ages of 50 and 80 years;

Current Concepts of Bone Fragility

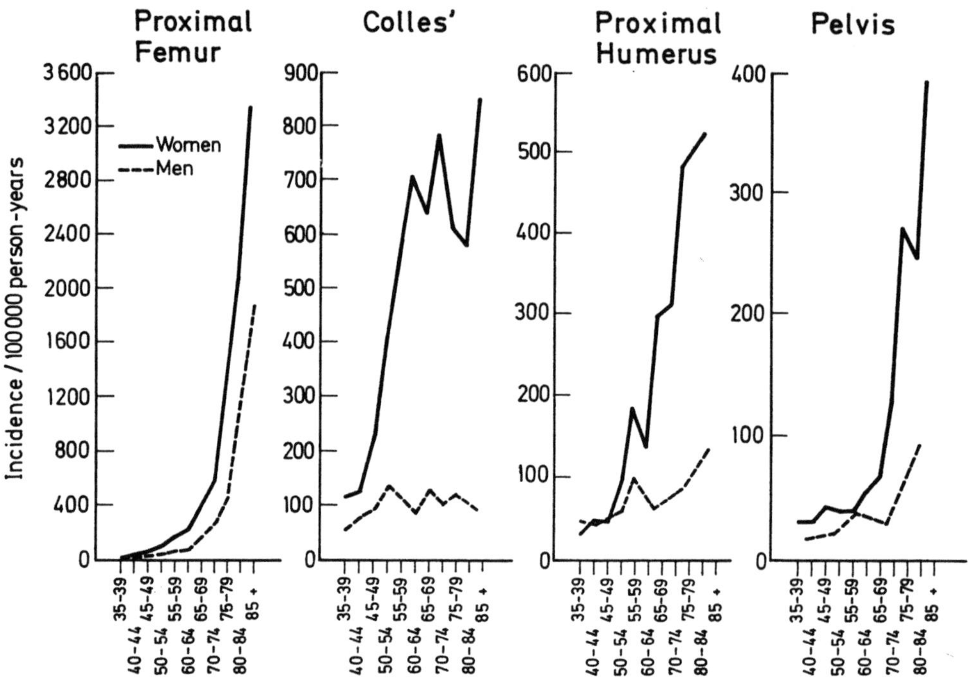

Fig. 1. Age- and sex-specific incidence per 100,000 person-years for four age-related fracture sites among Rochester, Minnesota residents. (Reprinted from Melton, L.J., and Riggs, B.L.: Epidemiology of age-related fractures. In, The Osteoporotic Syndrome, Avioli, L.V. (Ed.) Grune and Stratton, New York, 1983). Reproduced with permission of the publisher and authors.

and vertebral fractures are not at all closely associated with falls. Moreover, most falls do not result in a fracture even among the elderly (Ashley et al, 1977; Baker and Harvey, 1985; Rodstein, 1964).

2. *Increased traumatic energy.* Most age-related fractures occur as a result of simple falls, without evidence that the height of these falls increases with age (Melton and Riggs, 1985) or that the landing surface gets harder (Waller, 1978). It is generally believed, however, that coordination is impaired and reflexes are slowed in the elderly (Isaacs, 1978), perhaps resulting in decreased ability to break the impact of a fall (Muckle et al, 1978). Fracture incidence rates, however, begin to rise many years before the ages at which one might expect the capability for protective responses to be lost. Impaired reflexes may also interfere with energy dissipation through muscle action (Muckle et al, 1978; Parfitt, 1979; Stelmach, 1985), and reduced muscle strength in the elderly (Wolfson et al, 1985) might also contribute to this problem. Reduced muscle mass along with the reduction in adipose tissue, often seen in the aged, could also impair the effectiveness of energy absorption by soft tissue (Curry, 1968).

3. *Reduced bone strength.* It has been suggested that an age-related reduction in microfractures repair (Frost, 1981) might lead to vertebral col-

lapse (Vernon-Roberts and Pirie, 1973), but a role for this mechanism in the pathogenesis of femoral neck fractures has been questioned (Wicks et al, 1982). Osteomalacia is relatively common among patients with femoral fractures in Britain (Aaron et al, 1974; Jenkins et al, 1973), although others have not observed this (Wootton et al, 1979). Osteomalacia does not seem to be a major risk factor for age-related fractures in the United States generally, although impaired vitamin D metabolism may induce secondary hyperparathyroidism and osteoporosis (Riggs, 1984). Some investigators report that changes in the physical properties of bone are associated with the age-related increase in fracture risk (Chatterji et al, 1981; Dickenson et al, 1981; Kent et al, 1983; Mongiori et al, 1983). Evaluation of such factors is complicated, however, by compensatory structural changes, such as increased diameter of long bones (Mazess, 1982) or load-shifting from trabecular to cortical bone in the vertebrae (Rockoff et al, 1969). There is some evidence for and against each hypothesis, however, and they consequently remain controversial.

Osteoporosis and Fracture Risk

Some investigators believe that the changes in structure associated with age-related bone loss are sufficient to account for the effects observed above (Bell et al, 1967; Carter and Hayes, 1976; Vernon-Roberts and Pirie, 1973), and most believe osteoporosis to be the primary explanation for the bone fragility that underlies the "J" type pattern of fracture incidence (Consensus Conference 1984; Newton-John and Morgan, 1970; Nordin, 1971). Overall, bone mass appears to account for about 80% of the variance in the compressive strength of trabecular bone and 90% in cortical bone (Mazess, 1982); and the *in vivo* measurements, as bone mineral content or bone mineral density (BMD), are highly correlated with resistance to compressive forces in the femoral neck (Dalén et al, 1976; Leichter et al, 1982) and in the vertebra (Bell et al, 1967; Hansson et al, 1980).

BMD declines with age and reaches lower levels among women than men (Riggs et al, 1982). Moreover, fractures are common only when BMD has fallen considerably from its peak values in the young (Fig. 2). There is no clear bimodality in the distribution of bone mineral in the population, however, and values overlap widely for age- and sex-matched individuals with and without various fractures (Riggs et al, 1982). Consequently, investigators have been unable to distinguish reliably a pathologic degree of bone loss from physiologic osteopenia, and this has even led some to doubt an etiologic relationship between osteoporosis and age-related fractures (Aitken, 1984; Cummings, 1985; Evans et al, 1981; Wicks et al, 1982). We suggest that fracture risk is associated with the absolute level of BMD (Melton and Riggs, 1983), not the level relative to age- and sex-matched peers. Consequently, we have taken an entirely different approach in evaluating the relevance of bone fragility to fracture risk.

To obtain more detailed data about the relationship between BMD and fractures, we measured spinal (L_1-L_4) BMD with dual photon absorptiometry (Riggs et al, 1982) in an age-stratified random sample of Rochester, Minnesota women, ≥35 years old, to estimate the distribution of spinal BMD in the population of adult women. We also assessed BMD among women in the sample who had had one or more vertebral fractures, to estimate both the total number of women with vertebral fractures in the population and the distribution of spinal BMD among such women.

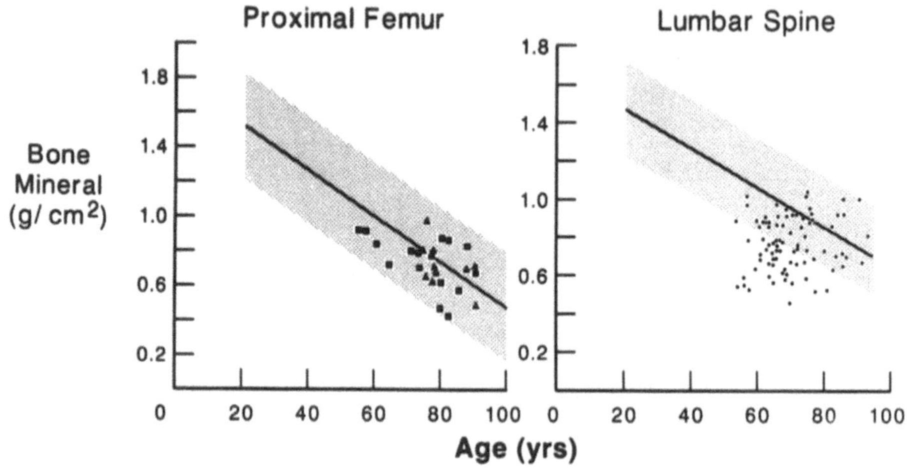

Fig. 2. Individual values of bone mineral density (BMD) for cervical region of proximal femur in 28 women with hip fractures (■ = femoral neck and ▲ = intertrochanteric fractures) and values of lumbar spine BMD in 84 women with one or more nontraumatic vertebral fractures. Lines denote age regressions for normal women, and shaded areas represent 90% confidence limits (Reprinted from Riggs, B.L., et al, J. Clin. Invest. 70, 716, 1982). Reproduced with permission of the publisher and authors.

These population-based estimates were then used to calculate the prevalence rate of vertebral fracture at various levels of spinal BMD. As expected, the prevalence of vertebral fractures was negligible among Rochester women 35 years old and over who had bone density levels ≥1.0 g/cm². Fracture rates were much higher among women with BMD below 1.0 g/cm², however, and a gradient of increasing fracture risk with decreasing BMD levels was observed.

We also estimated the numerators and denominators necessary to calculate hip fracture incidence rates for specific femoral BMD levels. The denominators were obtained by measuring BMD at the cervical and intertrochanteric regions of the proximal femur in each subject included in the random sample described above. BMD at each site was related to age through a multiple regression model weighted for the age-stratified sampling fractions, and the appropriate multiple regression model for each femoral site was used to estimate the distribution of BMD values in each age group. These distributions were then weighted by multiplication with the number of Rochester women in each age stratum; and the resulting numbers were then summed across the age strata to obtain the total number of Rochester women who would be expected to lie in each BMD interval. The numerators were obtained by multiplying the expected number of cervical and intertrochanteric proximal femur fractures for the Rochester population by the distributions of cervical and intertrochanteric BMD among Rochester women with cervical or intertrochanteric hip fractures.

These numerators and denominators were then used to estimate the incidence of cervical and intertrochanteric proximal femur fractures at each level of cervical and intertrochanteric BMD, respectively. The incidence of hip fractures, at either the cervical or intertrochanteric sites, was low among women with BMD levels ≧1.0 g/cm² (measured at the same two sites in the femur). As with vertebral fractures, however, incidence rates for hip fracture increased as BMD declined below this level, although even in the lowest category of femoral BMD used, <0.6 g/cm², less than 2% of women experienced hip fractures each year.

Since fracture risk is a function of boney resistance to fracture as well as the force that is applied (Melton and Riggs, 1983), it was anticipated that the frequency of fractures would increase as BMD declined. Many individuals were still free of fractures, however, even within the subgroups at greatest risk. This is not particularly surprising in view of a number of possible explanations. Vertebral bone density, for example, might be spuriously increased by subtle compression of whole segments of the spine or inclusion in the scanning site of nonskeletal areas of calcification. This would tend to shift the distribution of bone density values upward (Cann et al, 1985) and, to the extent that patients with vertebral fractures were affected more than others, might cause us to underestimate vertebral fracture prevalence at the lowest levels of spinal bone mineral. Such a scenario would not explain the hip fracture findings, however, In the case of the hip data, presumably reduced BMD in specific smaller areas, such as supporting trabeculae in the proximal femur (Singh et al, 1970) or Ward's triangle (Vose and Mack, 1963), is even more closely associated with fracture risk. If that is the case, we might be underestimating the risk somewhat by evaluating the sites as we did. Moreover, BMD is not the only indicator of bone loss and alternative variables might be of value (Hayes and Gerhart, 1985).

Conclusion

The current study demonstrates that vertebral fracture prevalence and hip fracture incidence both vary with the level of BMD. The rise in fracture rates as BMD declines indicates that fracture risk depends on the absolute level of BMD. These findings, associated with other observations (Cann et al, 1985; Iskrant and Smith, 1969; Jensen et al, 1983; Krølner and Nielsen, 1982; Newton-John and Morgan, 1970; Odvina et al, 1984; Smith et al, 1975), suggest that it is reasonable to consider reduced BMD as a necessary cause of age-related fractures, although low bone mass alone may not be a sufficient cause (Melton and Riggs, 1985). With further refinement, the current model may serve as an index permitting prediction of fracture risks from bone mineral measurements and thus provide the basis for a definition of osteoporosis.

Acknowledgements

The authors would like to thank Miss Mary Ramaker for her help in preparing the manuscript.

This work was supported in part by research grants AM-27065 and AM-30582 from the National Institutes of Health.

References

1. Aaron, J.E., Gallagher, J.C., Anderson, J., Stasiak, L., Longton, E.B., Nordin, B.E.C., and Nicholson, M.: Frequency of osteomalacia and osteoporosis in fractures of the proximal femur. Lancet 1, 229, 1974.

2. Aitken, J.M.: Relevance of osteoporosis in women with fractures of the femoral neck. Br. Med. J. 288, 597, 1984.

3. Ashley, M.J., Gryfe, C.I., and Amies, A.: A longitudinal study of falls in the elderly population. II. Some circumstances of falling. Age Ageing 6, 211, 1977.

4. Baker, S.P. and Harvey, A.H.: Fall injuries in the elderly. Symposium on Falls in the Elderly: Biological and Behavioral Aspects. Clin. Geriatr.Med. 1, 501, 1985.

5. Bell, G.H., Dunbar, O. and Beck, J.S.: Variations in strength of vertebrae with age and their relation to osteoporosis. Calcif.Tiss.Res. 1, 75, 1967.

6. Buhr, A.J. and Cooke, A.M.: Fracture patterns. Lancet 1, 531, 1959.

7. Campbell, A.J., Reinken, J., Allan, B.C., and Martinez, G.S.: Falls in old age: A study of frequency and related clinical factors. Age Ageing 10, 264, 1981.

8. Cann, C.E., Genant, H.K., Kolb, F.O., and Ettinger, B.: Quantitative computed tomography for prediction of vertebral fracture risk. Bone 6, 1, 1985.

9. Carter, D.R., and Hayes, W.C.: Bone compressive strength: The influence of density and strain rate. Science 194, 1174, 1976.

10. Chatterji, S., Wall, J.C., and Jeffery, J.W.: Age-related changes in the orientation and particle size of the mineral phase in human femoral cortical bone. Calcif.Tiss.Int. 33, 567, 1981.

11. Consensus Conference - Osteoporosis. JAMA 252, 799, 1984.

12. Cummings, S.R.: Are patients with hip fractures more osteoporotic? Review of the evidence. Am.J.Med. 78, 487, 1985.

13. Currey, J.D.: The effect of protection on the impact strength of rabbits' bones. Acta Anat. 71, 87, 1968.

14. Dalén, N., Hellström, L.G., and Jacobson, B.: Bone mineral content and mechanical strength of the femoral neck. Acta Orthop.Scand. 47, 503, 1976.

15. Dickenson, R.P., Hutton, W.C., and Stott, J.R.R.: The mechanical properties of bone in osteoporosis. J. Bone Joint Surg. 63B, 233, 1981.

16. Evans, R.A., Ashwell, J.R., and Dunstan, C.R.: Lack of metabolic bone disease in patients with fracture of the femoral neck. Aust.N.Z.J. Med. 11, 158, 1981.

17. Frost, H.M.: Mechanical microdamage, bone remodeling, and osteoporosis: A review. In, Osteoporosis: Recent Advances in Pathogenesis and Treatment. Eds: DeLuca, H.F., Frost, H.M., Jee, W.S.S., Johnston, C.C. Jr., Parfitt, A.M., University Park Press, Baltimore 1981, pp 185-190.

18. Gryfe, C.I., Amies, A., and Ashley, M.J.: A longitudinal study of falls in an elderly population: I. Incidence and morbidity. Age Ageing 6, 201, 1977.

19. Hansson, T., Roos, B., and Nachemson, A.: The bone mineral content and ultimate compressive strength of lumbar vertebrae. Spine 5, 46, 1980.

20. Hayes, W.C., and Gerhart, T.N.: Biomechanics of bone: Applications for assessment of bone strength. In, Bone and Mineral Research/3. Ed: Peck, W.A.; Elsevier Science Publishing Co., Inc., New York, pp 259-294. 1985

21. Isaacs, B.: Are falls a manifestation of brain failure: Age Ageing 7 (Suppl.), 97, 1978.

22. Iskrant, A.P., and Smith, R.W., Jr.: Osteoporosis in women 45 years and over related to subsequent fractures. Publ. Health Rep. 84, 33, 1969.

23. Jenkins, D.H.R., Roberts, J.G., Webster, D., and Williams, E.O.: Osteomalacia in elderly patients with fracture of the femoral neck: A clinico-pathological study. J.Bone Joint Surg. 55B, 575, 1973.

24. Jensen, G.F., Christiansen, C., Boesen, J., Hegedüs, V., and Transbøl, I.: Relationship between bone mineral content and frequency of postmenopausal fractures. Acta Med.Scand. 213, 61, 1983.

25. Kent, G.N., Dodds, R.A., Klenerman, L., Watts, R.W.E., Bitensky, L., and Chayen, J.: Changes in crystal size and orientation of acidic glycosaminoglycans at the fracture site in fractured necks of femur. J.Bone Joint Surg. 65B, 189, 1983.

26. Krølner, B., and Nielsen, S.P.: Bone mineral content of the lumbar spine in normal and osteoporotic women: Cross-sectional and longitudinal studies. Clin.Sci. 62, 329, 1982.

27. Leichter, I., Margulies, J.Y., Weinreb, A., Mizrahi, J., Deutsch, D., Robin, G.C., Makin, M., and Conforti, B.: Mechanical strength of the femoral-neck in relation to density and mineral-content of bone. In, Osteoporosis. Eds: Menczel, J., Robin, G.C., Makin, M., and Steinberg, R. John Wiley and Sons, Ltd., Chichester, 1982. pp 166-173.

28. Mazess, R.B.: On aging bone loss. Clin.Orthop. 165, 239, 1982.

29. Melton, L.J. and Riggs, B.L.: Epidemiology of age-related fractures. In, The Osteoporotic Syndrome. Ed: Avioli, L.V. Grune and Stratton, Inc., New York, 1983. pp 45-72.

30. Melton, L.J., and Riggs, B.L.: Risk factors for injury after a fall. Symposium on Falls in the Elderly: Biological and Behavioral Aspects. Clin.Geriatr.Med. 1, 525, 1985.

31. Melton, L.J., Ilstrup, D.M., Riggs, B.L., and Beckenbaugh, R.D.: Fifty-year trend in hip fracture incidence. Clin.Orthop. 162, 144, 1982.

32. Melton, L.J., Sampson, J.M., Morrey, B.F., and Ilstrup, D.M.: Epidemiologic features of pelvic fractures. Clin.Orthop. 155, 43, 1981.

33. Melton, L.J., Wahner, H.W., Richelson, L.S., O'Fallon, W.M., and Riggs, B.L.: Osteoporosis and the risk of hip fractures. In press.

34. Mongiorgi, R., Romagnoli, R., Olmi, R., and Moroni, A.: Mineral alterations in senile osteoporosis. Biomaterials 4, 192, 1983.

35. Muckle, D.S., Bentley, G., Deane, G., and Kemp, F.H.: Basic sciences of the hip. In, Femoral Neck Fractures and Hip Joint Injuries. Ed.: Muckle, D.S., John Wiley and Sons, New York, 1978.

36. Nelson, E.L., Melton, L.J., Annegers, J.F., Laws, E.R., and Offord, K.P.: Incidence of skull fractures in Olmsted County, Minnesota. Neurosurg. 15, 318, 1984.

37. Newton-John, H.F., and Morgan, D.B.: The loss of bone with age, osteoporosis, and fractures. Clin.Orthop. 71, 229, 1970.

38. Nordin, B.E.C.: Clinical significance and pathogenesis of osteoporosis. Br.Med.J. 1, 571, 1971.

39. Odvina, C.V., Wergedal, J.E., Libanati, C., Schulz, E.E., and Baylink, D.J.: Relationship between quantitative computerized tomography scan values and vertebral fractures in osteoporotics. In, 1984 Program and Abstracts of the Sixth Annual Scientific Meeting of the American Society for Bone and Mineral Research, Harford, Connecticut, June 26-29, 1984. A47.

40. Owen, R.A., Melton, L.J., Johnson, K.A., Ilstrup, D.M. and Riggs, B.L.: Incidence of Colles' fracture in a North American community. Am.J.Publ. Hlth. 72, 605, 1982.

41. Parfitt, A.M.: What causes osteoporotic fractures? In, International Symposium on Osteoporosis, St. John, U.S. Virgin Islands, October 25-27, 1978. Biomedical Information Corporation, New York, 1979.

42. Parfitt, A.M.: Cortical porosity in the pathogenesis of wrist fractures: Similarities between adolescence and postmenopause. Proc. Current Concepts of Bone Fragility In Orthopaedics and Medicine, Ottawa, May 16-18, 1985. Springer-Verlag.

43. Prudham, D., and Evans, J.G.: Factors associated with falls in the elderly: A community study. Age Ageing 10, 141, 1981.

44. Riggs, B.L.: Vitamin D and involutional osteoporosis. In, Vitamin D: Basic and Clinical Aspects. Ed: Kumar, R. Martinus Nijhoff Publishing, Boston, 1984, pp 559-577.

45. Riggs, B.L., Wahner, H.W., Seeman, E., Offord, K.P., Dunn, W.L., Mazess, R.B., Johnson, K.A., and Melton, L.J.: Changes in bone mineral density of the proximal femur and spine with aging: Differences between the postmenopausal and senile osteoporosis syndromes. J.Clin.Invest. 70, 716, 1982.

46. Rockoff, S.D., Sweet, E., and Bleustein, J.: The relative contribution of trabecular and cortical bone to the strength of human lumbar vertebrae. Calcif.Tiss.Res. 3, 163, 1969.

47. Rodstein, M.: Accidents among the aged: Incidence, causes and prevention. J.Chronic Dis. 17, 515, 1964.

48. Rose, S.H., Melton, L.J., Morrey, B.F., Ilstrup, D.M., and Riggs, B.L.: Epidemiologic features of humeral fractures. Clin.Orthop. 168, 24, 1982.

49. Singh, M., Nagrath, A.R., Maini, P.S., and Haryana, R.: Changes in trabecular pattern of the upper end of the femur as an index of osteoporosis. J.Bone Joint Surg. 52A, 457, 1970.

50. Smith, D.M., Khairi, M.R.A., and Johnston, C.C. Jr.: The loss of bone mineral with aging and its relationship to risk of fracture. J.Clin. Invest. 56, 311, 1975.

51. Stelmach, G.: Motor control deficits related to falling. Symposium on Falls in the Elderly: Biological and Behavioral Aspects. Clin.Geriatr. Med. 1, 679, 1985.

52. Vernon-Roberts, B., and Pirie, C.J.: Healing trabecular microfractures in the bodies of lumbar vertebrae. Ann.Rheum.Dis. 32, 406, 1973.

53. Vose, G.P., and Mack, P.B.: Roentgenologic assessment of femoral neck density as related to fracturing. Am.J.Roentgenol. 89, 1296, 1963.

54. Waller, J.A.: Falls among the elderly - Human and environmental factors. Accid.Anal.Prev. 10, 21, 1978.

55. Wicks, M., Garrett, R., Vernon-Roberts, B., and Fazzalari, N.: Absence of metabolic bone disease in the proximal femur in patients with fracture of the femoral neck. J.Bone Joint Surg. 64B, 319, 1982.

56. Wolfson, L.I., Whipple, R., Amerman, P., Kaplan, J., and Kleinberg, A.: Gait and balance in the elderly: Two functional capacities which link sensory and motor ability to falls. Symposium on Falls in the Elderly: Biological and Behavioral Aspects. Clin.Geriatr.Med. 1, 649, 1985.

57. Wootton, R., Brereton, P.J., Clark, M.B., Hesp, R., Hodkinson, H.M., Klenerman, L., Reeve, J., Slavin, G., and Tellez-Yudilevich, M.: Fractured neck of femur in the elderly: An attempt to identify patients at risk. Clin.Sci. 57, 93, 1979.

Fracture Patterns in Children

J. J. WILEY and W. M. McINTYRE

Introduction

Fractures respect no age group. The patterns of fractures in respective age groups, however, are somewhat unique, mainly in their dissimilarities (Melton and Riggs, 1983). Likewise, certain groups of individuals, such as the young, are more prone to fractures associated with environmental hazards, whereas in others, such as the older population, endogenous causes are more frequent (Alframm and Bauer, 1962). Few studies report fracture patterns in the pediatric population (Landin, 1983; Reed, 1977), primarily because such injuries defy current methods of recording and retrieval in most hospitals, and because of the difficulties of capturing the pediatric population at risk.

This study is a retrospective review of fracture patterns encountered during the course of one year, 1984, in the emergency room of the Children's Hospital of Eastern Ontario (CHEO), Ottawa. It should be stressed that this is a descriptive review of the patient sample, the referral patterns in our community leading to a relatively higher incidence of more complicated fractures. Consequently, there is an obvious disproportion in the number of primary, secondary, and tertiary type patients, inseparable in such a retrospective study. Nonetheless, many of the observations were surprisingly similar to those obtained in Landin's survey in 1983 of the pediatric population in Malmo, Sweden.

Clinical Material

We examined 2,640 consecutive fractures in our hospital emergency room and referred to the Division of Orthopaedic Surgery during 1984. Of these injuries, 1,881 (72.1%) involved the upper extremities, whereas 739 (27.9%) involved the lower extremities. Twenty cases involved the spine. Fractures of the skull, facial bones and thorax were excluded. Twenty patients with pathologic fractures were also excluded, most of whom had osteogenesis imperfecta or fractures going through a unicameral bone cyst.

Of interest was the infrequent occurrence of joint dislocations in this pediatric group (63 patients).

Although the upper age limit for admission to this pediatric hospital is 18 years of age, patients over 16 years of age were excluded from this re-

Current Concepts of Bone Fragility

view, surmising that many beyond 16 years of age seek treatment at adult hospitals in preference to a pediatric institution.

As well as overall incidence, certain aspects were investigated in this study -- ie, age, sex, seasonal variations, and certain environmental problems. Other aspects not evaluated were bone morphometry in children, the characteristics of pathologic fractures, pediatric versus adult fracture patterns, sprains and strains, mechanisms of injury, school-related injuries, repeated injuries, and treatment modalities. No attempt was made to differentiate between major and minor fractures or severity of injury.

Age and Sex Incidence

With the exception of infants under 1 year of age, when fractures are less common, age alone as a risk factor reflects a progressive increase in fracture incidence, peaking in early adolescence followed by a rapid decline (Fig. 1). In both upper and lower extremity fractures, approximately 55%

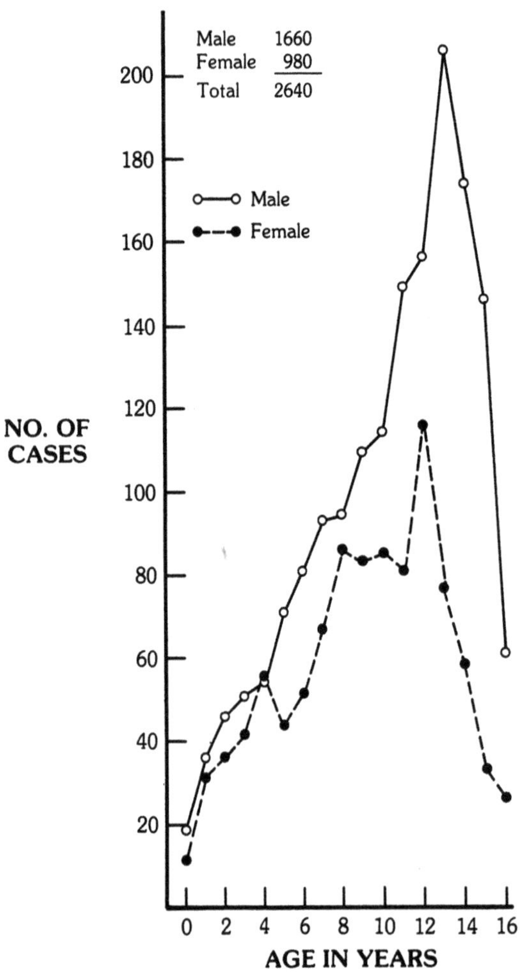

Fig. 1. Total number of extremity fractures and sex ratio admitted to the emergency room of the Children's Hospital of Eastern Ontario (CHEO) in 1984.

of fractures (upper 59.2%; lower 53.9%) occurred in the group 10-15 years of age.

The incidence of fractures in boys predominates in all age groups. Overall, 63% (1,660 fractures) occurred in boys, and 37% (980 fractures) in girls. In Landin's (1983) controlled study, 62% of the fractures occurred in boys. From early childhood onward, the age group incidence rises sharply, the boys' distribution curve paralleling that of girls. Interestingly, an abrupt decrease occurs starting after age 12 in girls and age 13 in boys, corresponding to early phasing of skeletal maturation with puberty.

Considering the rather small number of dislocations, the incidence rises in adolescence, perhaps heralding joint capsule vulnerability versus the augmented bony strengthening from physeal plate closure and metaphyseal remodeling (Fig. 2).

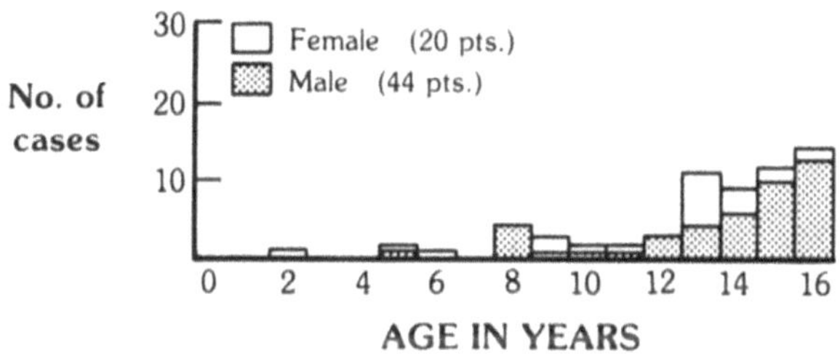

Fig. 2. Occurrence of dislocation, sex ratio (CHEO, 1984)

A unique fracture pattern was noted about the elbow region. Unlike other age-related patterns in the upper extremity, the supracondylar fracture is most common in the younger child, in fact more common than all other elbow fractures combined (121 of 220 elbow injuries). Other elbow injuries reveal no specific pattern except diminishing incidence with epiphyseal plate closure.

Environmental Fractures

Certain environmental factors in this particular geographic area reflect fracture patterns. The popularity of skating and skiing is noted by an increase in distal forearm and tibial fractures respectively during the winter months (Fig. 3). As the seasons change, another sudden increase in fracture incidence occurs with the onset of spring weather and daylight saving time, beckoning long evenings of outdoor play and the attendant risks. The onset of summer marks the exodus of large numbers of children to summer camps, resulting in a decrease in fracture incidence. Landin (1983) made the same observation in his study. The incoming pediatric summer tourist , well behaved in the presence of supervising parents, does not really replace the former locals who carry their personal risk factors to whichever camp or cottage they may go. As school reconvenes, the fracture incidence rises again, only to diminish in the autumn as daylight saving time comes to an end, and cooler weather and evening school study preclude outdoor activities.

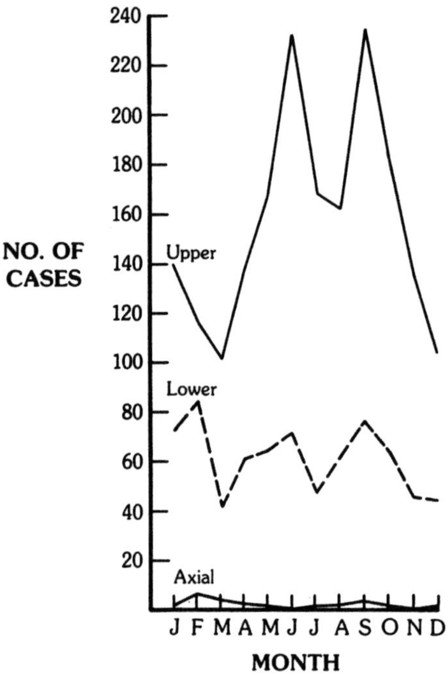

Fig. 3. Fracture incidence related to seasonal variation (CHEO, 1984)

Fracture Sites (Fig. 4A and 4B)

Some investigators have reported that pediatric diaphyseal fractures are more common than those involving the distal ends of bone (Reed, 1977; Tredwell et al, 1984), exceptions being distal radial epiphyseal fractures. This study, however, revealed that diaphyseal fractures were more common than metaphyseal fractures in the lower extremities only, the reverse being true in the upper extremity (Fig. 5).

Fractures about the distal end of the radius are exceedingly common in the young and old alike, this anatomic region being the most common site for confrontation with a breaking load (Alffram and Bauer, 1962; Beekman and Sullivan, 1941; Giberson and Ivins, 1952).

With some exceptions, epiphyseal fractures rarely occur in infancy, begin to rise in incidence after the age of 8 or 9 years, and rapidly decrease with skeletal maturation and epiphyseal plate closure (Buhr and Cooke, 1959; Hanlon and Estes, 1954; Tredwell, 1984). In the upper extremity, the epiphyses about the elbow region are somewhat unique in that lateral condylar and radial head/neck fractures are not age-specific and have well known diagnostic problems because of this.

Epiphyseal fractures of the proximal and distal tibia tend to parallel the incidence of shaft fractures in the toddler group (age 1-2 years) and the comparable decrease after 14 years of age in both the epiphyseal and shaft fractures. Incidentally, tibial shaft fractures were noted to be the commonest fracture in the lower extremity (328 of 739 total -- 44.4%), and the third most common site of all fractures.

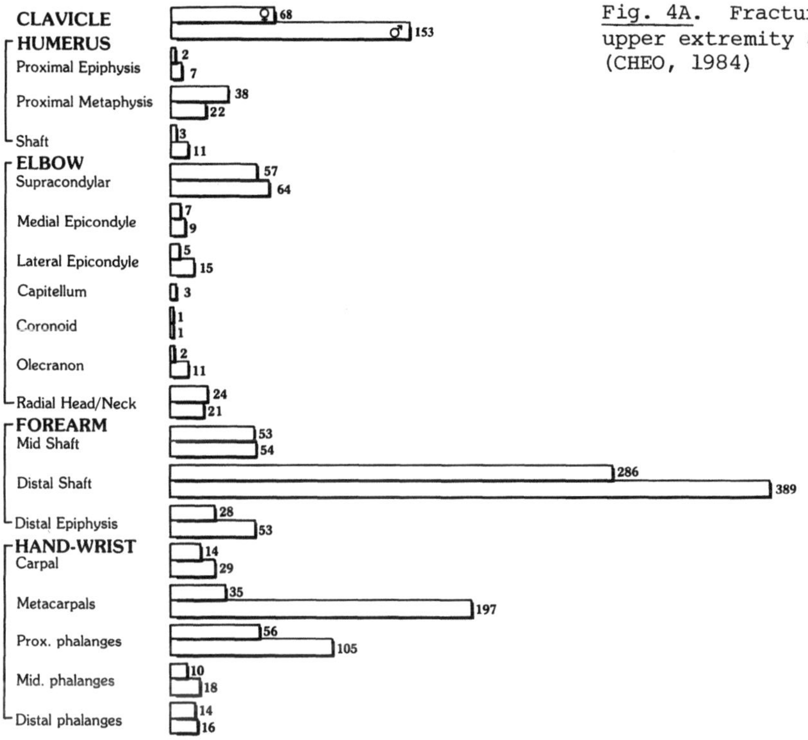

Fig. 4A. Fractures involving upper extremity and sex ratio. (CHEO, 1984)

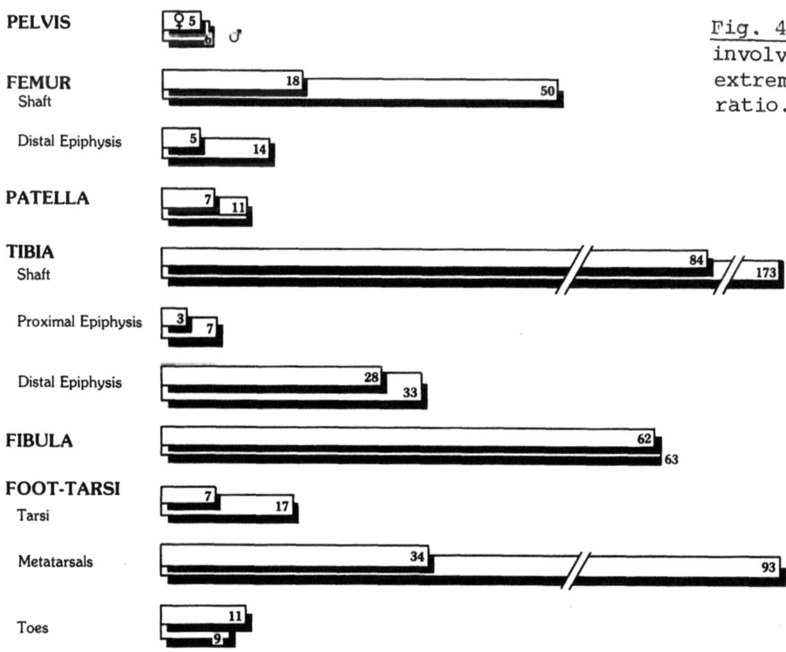

Fig. 4B. Fractures involving lower extremity and sex ratio. (CHEO, 1984)

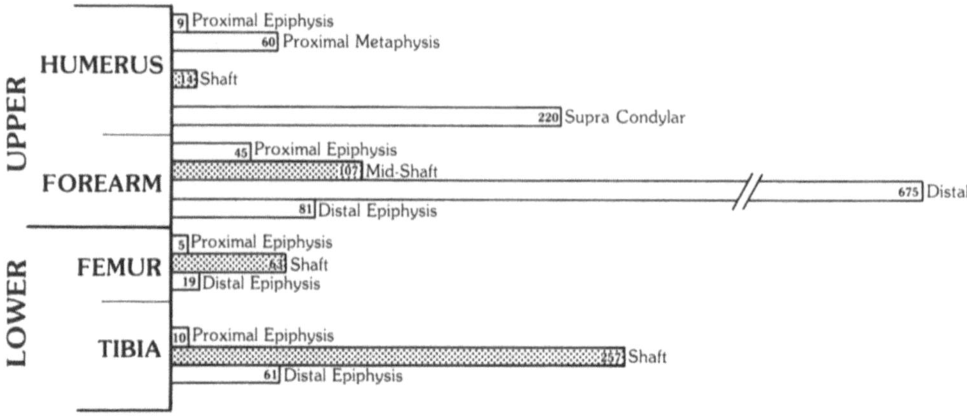

Fig. 5. Incidence of diaphyseal fractures compared to metaphyseal fractures in upper and lower extremities (CHEO, 1984)

Although the number of fractures involving the carpal and tarsal bones seems inordinately high, many were described as chip fractures of minor significance, although correctly reported as true fractures.

Conclusion

From this study of consecutive fractures encountered during the course of one year, 1984, in one pediatric institution, we believe that the data support the facts that the risk in the pediatric population is a combination of age, sex, behavior, and skeletal maturation. Inherent bone weakness is not a problem. Certain anatomic locations are more specific for the childhood injury, including the clavicle, tibia, and supracondylar region of the humerus. Certain anatomic areas in the child are conspicuous in their relative freedom from fracturing compared with adults -- the hips, pelvis, and surgical neck of the humerus. The single exception is the curiously high incidence of fractures of the distal forearm in both the young and the aged. Experimental evidence has demonstrated a lesser elastic modulus in the young bone, increasing progressively with age until attaining that of the skeletally-mature adolescent (Currey and Butler, 1975; Hirsch, 1965). Diminished bone density is not the problem of the young, and consequently leaves little common ground for a comparative study.

However, one has to note the curious morbidity associated with children's fractures. Fractures bring little or no loss in the quality of life in this young age group. Rehabilitation is not a major problem in managing these injuries. Relatively few require in-patient care. Unlike fractures in the aged, mortality is not associated with the pediatric musculoskeletal injury.

The study of fracture patterns offers much to stimulate fracture awareness, fractury injury prevention, search for better treatment modalities, and, finally, substantiating many aspects of prognosis.

References

1. Alffram, P.A., and Bauer, G.C.: Epidemiology of fractures of the forearm. A biochemical investigation of bone strength. J. Bone Joint Surg. 44A, 105, 1962.
2. Beekman, F., and Sullivan, J.E.: Bone observation on fractures of long bone in children. Am. J. Surg. 51, 722, 1941.
3. Buhr, A.J., and Cooke, A.M.: Fracture patterns. Lancet 1, 531, 1959.
4. Currey, J.D., and Butler, G.: The mechanical properties of bone tissue in children. J. Bone Joint Surg. 57A, 810, 1975.
5. Giberson, R.G., and Ivins, J.C.: Fractures of the distal part of the forearm in children. Minn. Med., 744, August 1952.
6. Hanlon, C.R., and Estes, W.L.: Fractures in childhood - a statistical analysis. Am. J. Surg. 87, 312, 1954.
7. Hirsch, C., and Evans, F.G.: Studies on some physical properties of infant compact bone. Acta Orthop. Scand. 35, 300, 1965.
8. Landin, L.A.: Fracture patterns in children. Acta Orthop. Scand. (Suppl. 202), 54, 49, 1983.
9. Melton, L.J., and Riggs, B.L.: Epidemiology of Age-Related Fractures. The Osteoporotic Syndrome. Ed: Alvioli, L.V.; Grune and Stratton, New York, 1983, pp 45-72.
10. Reed, M.H.: Fractures and dislocations of the extremities in children. J. Trauma 17, 351, 1977.
11. Tredwell, S.J., van Peteghem, K., and Clough, M.: Pattern of forearm fractures in children. J. Pediat. Orthop. 4, 604, 1984.

Cortical Porosity in Postmenopausal and Adolescent Wrist Fractures

A. M. Parfitt

Fractures of the lower forearm, known as wrist or Colles fractures, are frequently classified with fractures of the vertebral body and upper femur as manifestations of age-related bone loss (Melton, III and Riggs, 1983; Parfitt, 1982). At all three sites, the incidence of fracture increases with age and is higher in women than in men; for wrist fractures the cumulative prevalence by age 70 is estimated to be 15-20% in women and 3-4% in men (Melton, III and Riggs, 1983). For all three fracture types, the mean value for bone mass at the fracture site is less than in persons of the same age without fracture (Cann et al, 1985; Horsman et al, 1981; Jensen et al, 1982; Nilsson and Westlin, 1977; Riggs et al, 1981, 1982), and the occurrence of one type of osteoporotic fracture increases the likelihood of another (Crilly et al, 1979; Jensen et al, 1982; Horsman et al, 1981; Melton III and Riggs, 1983). A further common feature is that estrogen replacement therapy prevented most vertebral deformations in a prospective controlled trial (Lindsay et al, 1980) and significantly reduced the risk of both wrist and hip fractures in retrospective case control studies (Hutchinson et al, 1979; Weiss et al, 1980). The seasonal fluctuation in incidence, unique to wrist fractures, can be explained by their relationship to falls outdoors rather than indoors as for hip fractures (Melton, III and Riggs, 1983).

The distinction made by Albright between two forms of age-related osteoporoses -- postmenopausal and senile -- has recently been refined and extended, with the former renamed Type I, since a similar syndrome can occur in men, and the latter renamed Type II, since senility in its usual sense is often absent (Riggs and Melton, III, 1983; Riggs et al, 1983). In Type I osteoporosis, a greater loss of trabecular bone is observed relative to cortical bone and an increased risk of vertebral compression fractures, while in Type II osteoporosis a similar relative loss of trabecular and cortical bone is observed and increased risk of hip fractures. The frequency of both types is increased by unopposed estrogen-dependent bone loss. Wrist fractures resemble vertebral fractures more than hip fractures as to their early age of onset (Crilly et al, 1979; Melton, III and Riggs, 1983), large sex difference (Horsman et al, 1981; Melton, III and Riggs, 1983), degree of overlap and predictive value (Crilly et al, 1979; Owen et al, 1982a), lack of geographic variation (Matkovic et al, 1980), lack of relationship to lifelong calcium intake (Matkovic et al, 1979), and occurrence at sites where the ratio of trabecular to cortical bone is higher than for the skeleton as a whole (Riggs and Melton, III, 1983; Riggs et al, 1983). On this basis, wrist fractures are currently regarded as a manifestation of Type I rather than of Type II osteoporosis (Riggs and Melton, III, 1983; Riggs et al, 1983), unless they occur after 70 years of age (Owen et al, 1982a).

Current Concepts of Bone Fragility

That wrist fractures are an expression of the skeletal response to menopausal estrogen deficiency seems well established, but the epidemiologic facts cannot be explained solely by accelerated loss of trabecular bone from the distal radius. First, at this site trabecular bone has a much lower rate of turnover than trabecular bone in the axial skeleton, most likely because of the absence of hematopoietic marrow (Parfitt et al, in press). Second, there is no evidence of disproportionate loss of trabecular bone at sites other than the spine (Mazess, 1982). Third, the difference in local bone mass between demographically similar persons with and without wrist fracture is smaller and less consistent than for vertebral fracture (Nilsson and Westlin, 1977; Riggs et al, 1981), resembling more closely the situation for hip fractures (Cummings, 1985). Indeed, when proper allowance is made for the effects of handedness and of bone loss resulting from fracture, there may be no difference in distal radius bone mineral even though spinal bone mineral is significantly lower in patients with wrist fracture than in control subjects (Krølner et al, 1982). Together with the absence of such a difference in upper femoral bone mineral (Lamke et al, 1978) these data confirm the value of a wrist fracture as a marker for Type I osteoporosis (Parfitt, 1982; Riggs and Melton, III, 1983) but leave the reason for this relationship unexplained.

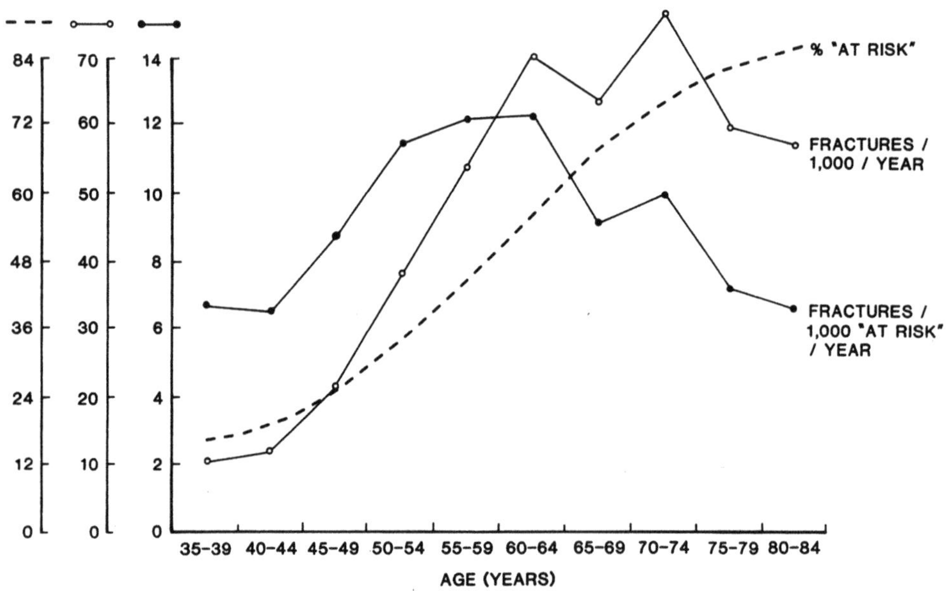

Fig. 1. Application of Newton-John and Morgan model of wrist fractures and bone loss (Newton-John and Morgan, 1970) to data from Rochester, Minnesota. Subjects at risk (interrupted line) defined as those whose distal radial bone mineral determined by single energy photon absorptiometry is more than 1 SD below the mean peak adult value (Riggs et al, 1981). Observed fracture rates (solid line, open circles) based on all occurrences in a defined population during the period 1945-1974 (Owen et al, 1982b). Fracture rates in those at risk as defined (solid line, closed circles) calculated for each successive 5-year period. Note that this rate approximately doubles between the ages of 45 and 60 years and does not fall to the young adult level until after age 75.

Most important, the incidence of wrist fractures has already increased significantly in the age group 45-50 years (Alffram and Bauer, 1962; Owen et al, 1982b), before the median age of menopause -- currently 51.4 years in the United States (McKinlay et al, 1985) -- and at a time when bone loss from the distal radius is still trivial. According to the Newton-John and Morgan hypothesis, the change in wrist fracture rate with age corresponds to the change in the proportion of women whose bone mass falls more than one standard deviation below the mean peak adult value (Newton-John and Morgan, 1970). When applied to the data from Rochester, Minnesota, however, with both fracture rates (Alffram and Bauer, 1962) and distal radial bone mass (Riggs et al, 1981) determined in the same population, this calculation fails to account for the early increase in wrist fracture rates; rather the data suggest the existence of one or more additional factors that increase wrist fracture risk between 45 and 60 years of age (Fig. 1). A more complex model that treats fracture risk as a continuous rather than a divided variable predicts a much larger increase in wrist fracture rates for men than is observed (Horsman et al, 1985).

Middle-aged women do not suddenly become more liable to fall on the outstretched hand, so that the missing piece of the puzzle must still be sought in bone. During the perimenopausal period, does the distal radius undergo a qualitative change that would make it more susceptible to fracture? In the spine, focal disruption of architecture due to trabecular plate perforation increases the vertebral fracture risk (Kleerekoper et al, in press), but it is highly unlikely that a similar change would occur 5 to 10 years earlier at a site where bone turnover is lower. A clue is provided by an examination of wrist fracture epidemiology throughout life, not just in middle and old age. In both sexes, lower forearm fracture rates increase substantially during the adolescent growth spurt, subsequently falling to the low levels characteristic of young adults as growth slows down (Alffram and Bauer, 1962; Buhr and Cooke, 1959; Wiley and McIntyre, 1985). In young in total bone mineral would suggest. Cortical porosity is high throughout childhood (Frost, 1969; Handelsman, 1983; Wilson and Genant, 1979), suggesting that the type and extent of physical activity is an additional factor contributing to the adolescent peak in fracture rates (Wiley and McIntyre, 1985). Nevertheless, increased porosity of the thin cortex of the distal radius appears a reasonable explanation for the early peri- and postmenopausal increase in lower forearm fracture rates.

References

1. Alffram, P.-A., and Bauer, G.C.H.: Epidemiology of fractures of the forearm. A biomechanical investigation of bone strength. J. Bone Joint Surg. 44A, 105, 1962.

2. Buhr, A.J., and Cooke, A.M.: Fracture patterns. Lancet i, 531, 1959.

3. Cann, C.E., Genant, H.K., Kolb, F.O., and Ettinger, B.: Quantitative computed tomography for prediction of vertebral fracture risk. Metab. Bone Dis. Rel. Res. 6, 1, 1985.

4. Crilly, R., Horsman, A., Marshall, D.H., and Nordin, B.E.C.: Prevalence, pathogenesis and treatment of post-menopausal osteoporosis. Aust. NZ J. Med. 9, 24, 1979.

5. Cummings, S.R.: Are patients with hip fractures more osteoporotic? Review of the evidence. Am. J. Med. 78, 487, 1985.

6. Frost, H.M.: Tetracycline-based histological analysis of bone remodeling. Calc. Tissue Res. 3, 211, 1969.

7. Genant, H.K., Cann, C.E., Ettinger, B., and Gordan, G.S.: Quantitative computed tomography of vertebral spongiosa: A sensitive method for detecting early bone loss after oophorectomy. Ann. Int. Med. 97, 699, 1982.

8. Handelsman, J.E.: Management of fractures in children. Surg. Clin. North Am. 63, 629, 1983.

9. Heaney, R.P., Recker, R.R., and Saville, P.D.: Menopausal changes in bone remodeling. J. Lab. Clin. Med. 92, 964, 1978.

10. Horsman, A., Marshall, D.H., and Peacock, M.: A stochastic model of age-related bone loss and fractures. Clin. Orthop. 195, 207, 1985.

11. Horsman, A., Nordin, B.E.C., Aaron, J., and Marshall, D H.: Cortical and trabecular osteoporosis and their relation to fractures in the elderly. In, Osteoporosis: Recent Advances in Pathogenesis and Treatment. Eds: DeLuca, H.F., Frost, H., Jee, W., Johnston, C., and Parfitt, A.M. University Park Press, Baltimore, 1981, pp 175-184.

12. Hutchinson, T.A., Polansky, S.M., and Feinstein, A.R.: Post-menopausal oestrogens protect against fractures of hip and distal radius. A case-control study. Lancet ii, 705, 1979.

13. Jaworski, Z.F.G.: Parameters and indices of bone resorption, In, Bone Histomorphometry, 2nd Int. Workshop, Lyon. Ed: Meunier, P.J. Armour Montague, 1976.

14. Jensen, G.F., Christiansen, C., Boesen, J., Hegadüs, V., and Transbøl, I.: Epidemiology of postmenopausal spinal and long bone fractures. Clin. Orthop. 166, 75, 1982.

15. Kleerekoper, M., Villanueva, A.R., Stanciu, J., Rao, D.S., and Parfitt, A.M.: The role of three dimensional trabecular microstructure in the pathogenesis of vertebral compression fractures. Calc. Tissue Int. (in press).

16. Krølner, B., Tøndevold, E., Toft, B., Berthelsen, B., and Nielsen, S.P.: Bone mass of the axial and the appendicular skeleton in women with Colles' fracture: Its relation to physical activity. Clin. Physiol. 2, 147, 1982.

17. Lamke, B., Sjöberg, H.-E., and Sylven, M.: Bone mineral content in women with Colles' fracture: Effect of calcium supplementation. Acta Orthop. Scand. 49, 143, 1978.

18. Lindsay, R., Hart, D.M., Forrest, C., and Baird, C.: Prevention of spinal osteoporosis in oophorectomised women. Lancet ii, 1151, 1980.

19. Matkovic, V., Ciganovic, M., Tominac, C., and Kostial, K.: Osteoporosis and epidemiology of fractures in Croatia. Henry Ford Hosp. Med. J. 28, 116, 1980.

20. Matkovic, V., Kostial, K., Simonovic, I., et al: Bone status and fracture rates in two regions of Yugoslavia. Am. J. Clin. Nutr. 32, 540, 1979.

21. Mazess, R.B.: On aging bone loss. Clin. Orthop. 165, 239, 1982.

22. McKinlay, S.M., Bifano, N.L., and McKinlay, J.B.: Smoking and age at menopause in women. Ann. Int. Med. 103, 350, 1985.

23. Meema, H.E.: Recognition of cortical bone resorption in metabolic bone disease *in vivo*. Skel. Radiol. 2, 11, 1977.

24. Melton, L.J., III, and Riggs, B.L.: Epidemiology of age-related fractures. In, The Osteoporotic Syndrome. Ed: Avioli, L.V. Grune & Stratton, 1983. pp 45-72.

25. Newton-John, H.F., and Morgan, D.B.: The loss of bone with age, osteoporosis and fractures. Clin. Orthop. 71, 229, 1970.

26. Nilsson, B.E., and Westlin, N.E.: Bone mineral content and fragility fractures. Clin. Orthop. 125, 196, 1977

27. Owen, R.A., Melton, L.J., Ilstrup, D.M., Johnson, K.A., and Riggs, B.L.: Colles' fracture and subsequent hip fracture risk. Clin. Orthop. 171, 37, 1982a.

28. Owen, R.A., Melton, L.J., III, Johnson, K.A., Ilstrup, D.M., and Riggs, B.L.: Incidence of Colles' fracture in a North American community. Am. J. Public Health 72, 605, 1982b.

29. Parfitt, A.M.: The morphologic basis of bone mineral measurements. Transient and stead state effects of treatment in osteoporosis. Min. Electrolyte Metab. 4, 273, 1980.

30. Parfitt, A.M.: Lower forearm fracture in the midle-aged woman. A neglected opportunity for preventing osteoporosis. I. Age-related bone loss and fractures. Continuing Education for the Family Physician, April 1982, 46-49.

31. Parfitt, A.M.: The physiologic and clinical significance of bone histomorphometric data. In, Bone Histomorphometry. Techniques and Interpretations. Ed: Recker, R. CRC Press, Boca Raton, 1983, pp 143-223.

32. Parfitt, A.M., Rao, D.S., Stanciu, J., Villanueva, A.R., Kleerekoper, M., and Frame, B.: Irreversible bone loss in osteomalacia: Comparison of radial photon absorptiometry with iliac bone histomorphometry. J. Clin. Invest. (in press).

33. Riggs, B.L., and Melton, L.J., III.: Evidence for two distinct syndromes of involutional osteoporosis. Am. J. Med. 75, 899, 1983.

34. Riggs, B.L., Melton, L.J., III, and Wahner, H.W.: Heterogeneity of involutional osteoporosis: Evidence for two distinct osteoporosis syndromes. In, Clinical Disorders of Bone and Mineral Metabolim. Eds: Frame, B. and Potts, J.R. Jr. Excerpta Medica, Amsterdam. 1983. pp 337-342.

35. Riggs, B.L., Wahner, H.W., Dunn, W.L., Mazess, R.B., Offord, K.P., and Melton, L.J., III.: Differential changes in bone mineral density of the appendicular and axial skeleton with aging. Relationship to spinal osteoporosis. J. Clin. Invest. 67, 328, 1981.

36. Riggs, B.L., Wahner, H.W., Seeman, E., Offord, K.P., Dunn, W.L., Mazess, R.B., Johnson, K.A., and Melton, L.J. III: Changes in bone mineral density of the proximal femur and spine with aging. Differences between the postmenopausal and senile osteoporosis syndromes. J. Clin. Invest. 70, 716, 1982.

37. Schiele, F., Henny, J., Hitz, J., Petitclerc, C., Gueguen, R., and Siest, G.: Total bone and liver alkaline phosphatases in plasma: Biological variations and reference limits. Clin. Chem. 29, 634, 1983.

38. Stepan, J.J., Pospichal, J., Presl, J., and Pacovsky, V.: Plasma tartrate resistant acid phosphatase, bone isoenzyme of serum alkaline phosphatase and urinary hydroxyproline for early identification of the patients at risk for developing osteoporosis. In, Osteoporosis. Proc. Copenhagen Int. Symp. on Osteoporosis. Aalborg Stiftsbogtrykkeri. Eds: Christiansen, C., Arnaud, C.D., Nordin, B.E.C., Parfitt, A.M., Peck, W.A., and Riggs, B.L. 1984. pp 139-143.

39. Weiss, N.S., Ure, C.L., Ballard, J.H., Williams, A.R., and Daling, J.R.: Decreased risk of fractures of the hip and lower forearm with postmenopausal use of estrogen. N. Engl. J. Med. 303, 1195, 1980.

40. Wiley, J.J., and McIntyre, W.M.: Fracture patterns in pediatric patients. In, Current Concepts of Bone Fragility in Orthopaedics and Medicine. Eds: Uhthoff, H.-K., and Stahl, E. Springer-Verlag, 1985.

41. Wilson, J.S., and Genant, H.K.: *In vivo* assessment of bone metabolism using the cortical striation index. Invest. Radiol. 14, 131, 1979.

Pathologic Fractures and Stress Fractures: A Review of Pathogenesis and Assessment

M. Finnegan

Pathologic Fractures

Pathologic fractures are classically defined as fractures resulting from physiologic forces applied to abnormal bone (Biewener et al, 1983). This definition, however, is too all-embracing considering the wide variation in both physiologic forces and abnormal bone. The most common pathologic fractures are those seen in osteoporosis regardless of origin. The Singh

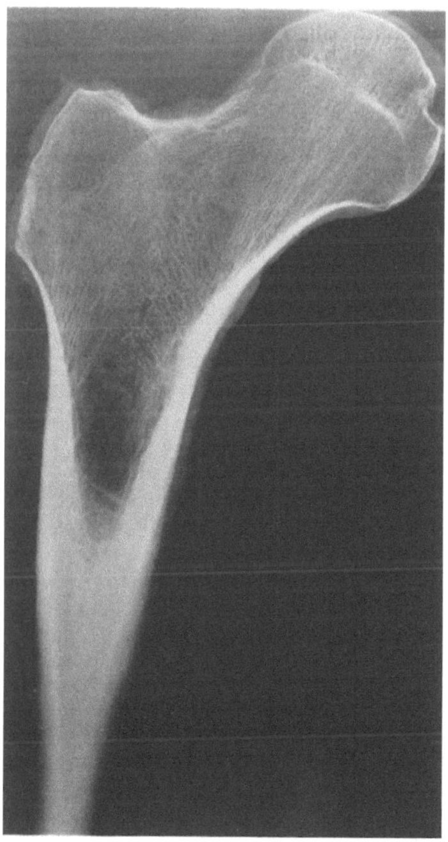

Fig. 1. Cross section of proximal femur.

Current Concepts of Bone Fragility

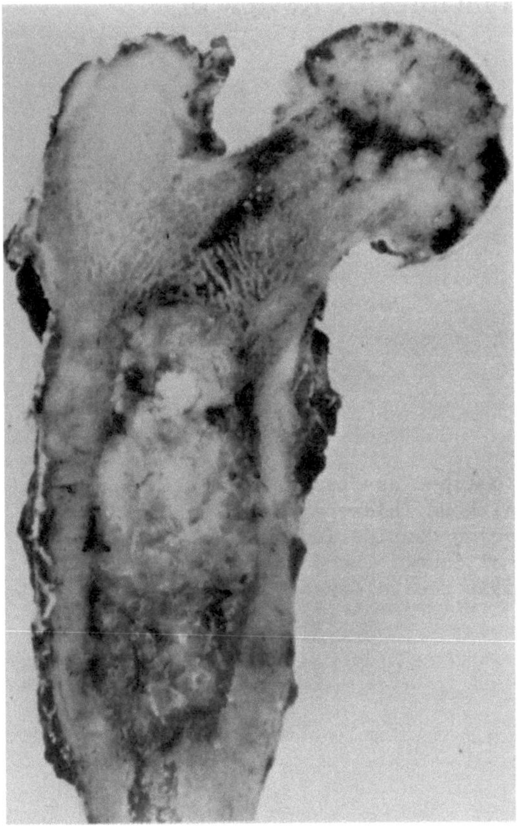

Fig. 2. Chondrosarcoma. (Courtesy of H.A. Sissons: Bones. In, Systemic Pathology. Vol. 5, p. 2466. Ed: W. St.C. Symmers)

index was an early attempt to predict impending fractures of the proximal femur in both postmenopausal and senile osteoporosis (Singh et al, 1970). Normal distribution of forces across the hip joint leads to a standard pattern of trabecular bone (Fig. 1). A significant alteration in these forces, either in time or in load, will result in a reproducible pattern of bone loss in the proximal femur. Singh attempted to determine at what point fracture was inevitable. Predicting similar fragility points in other anatomic sites has been even less successful, and is a continued clinical problem particularly when dealing with disuse osteoporosis. Early reports (McBroom and Hayes; Ruegsegger et al, 1984) suggest that quantitative computerized tomography may help solve some of this dilemma.

Osteoporosis is a state of decreased bone mass therefore imposing increasing stresses on bone. Analogies are not possible with other pathologic states where the material is altered or replaced, or where the total volume of material being stressed may even increase (Fig. 2). Case histories have shown that frequently in these patients larger forces are needed to produce pathologic fractures and significant displacement is a lesser problem. This observation leads to the postulate that the biologic constituents of the pathologic tissue contribute to the strength of the bone rather than the prevalent postulate that a hole in bone weakens it. Perhaps the most common, least understood, example is a unicameral bone cyst (Fig. 3). This

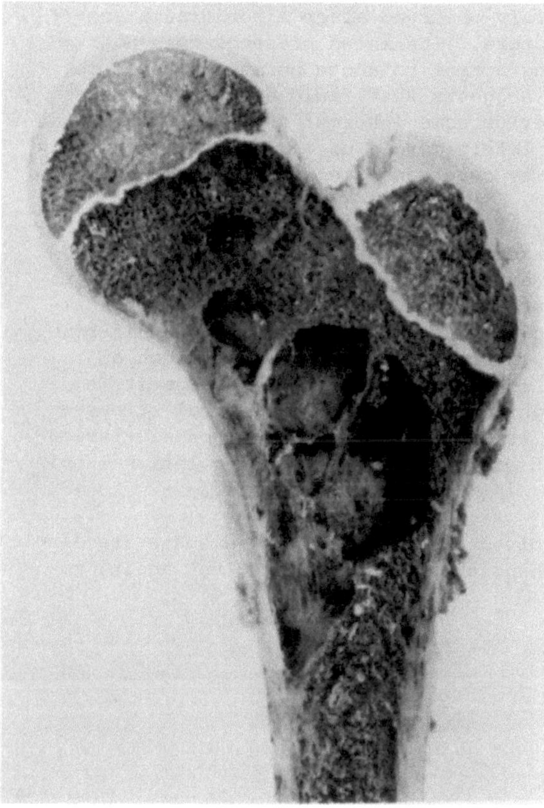

Fig. 3. Unicameral bone cyst. (Courtesy of H.A. Sissons: Bones. In, Systemic Pathology, Vol. 5, p. 2450. Ed: W. St.C. Symmers)

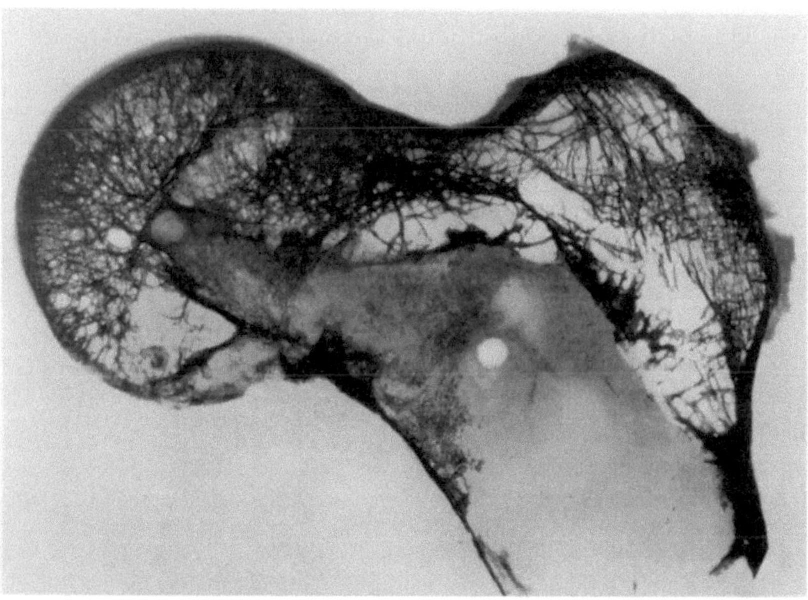

Fig. 4. Fibrous dysplasia. (Courtesy of H.A.Sissons: Bones. In, Systemic Pathology, Vol. 5, p. 2445. Ed: W. St.C. Symmers)

potentially large lytic lesion is rarely observed after minor trauma and rarely, if ever, displaces after fracture. Its known presence does not deter healthy youngsters from applying normal to above normal stresses on the lesion. This uncontrolled study suggests that fluid and the bony ridged architecture of the lesion provide some inherent mechanical strength. In contrast, a hole of this size completely devoid of tissue would certainly fracture under these loads, as shown by curetted osteomyelitic lesions.

Another puzzling entity is fibrous dysplasia. As seen in Figure 4, the normal trabecular pattern of the proximal femur has been replaced by pathologic tissue. The flowing of the material into the remaining bone suggests that it is an integral part of the material structure and therefore contributes to the inherent strength, although this strength is less than if trabecular bone were in the same site. In contrast, some lesions, such as osteoid osteomas, increase bone mass in certain areas and decrease it in others. In this circumstance one might question whether abnormal stresses are occurring at the junction of the sclerotic bone with the normal trabecular bone. The role of the subsequent microfractures producing lesional pain will need further investigation.

The mechanical responses of bone involved in metabolic bone disease are also ill-defined. Paget's disease is perhaps the best described; but again, me-

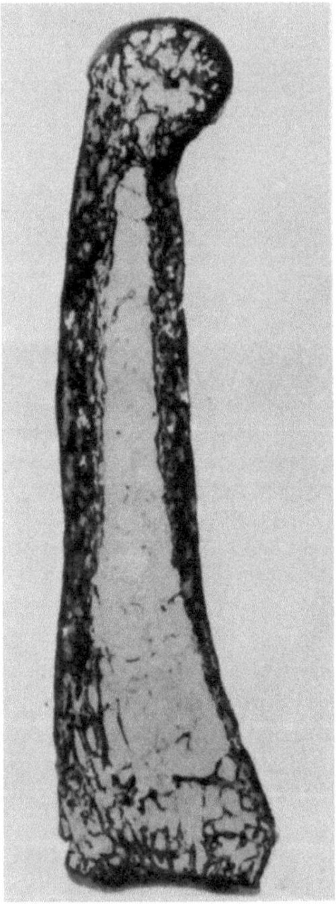

Fig. 5. Renal osteodystrophy. (Courtesy of H.A. Sissons: Bones. In, Systemic Pathology, Vol. 5. p. 2437. Ed: W. St.C. Symmers)

chanical weakness has been related mainly to bone resorption, although the contribution of woven bone has been discussed. Certainly, no mechanical or theoretical studies have yet been undertaken to delineate which factor contributes most to fracturing. Another metabolic disease presenting many problems is renal osteodystrophy. The mechanical response of this lattice work of bone and fibrous tissue (Fig. 5) to various loading conditions has never been studied.

One of the most urgent clinical problems at the present time is the metastatic lesion in bone. The orthopedic and oncologic literature is replete with debates as to the determination of impending fracture and the best treatment of various lesions (Harrington et al, 1976; Nicolson et al, 1983; Reddy et al, 1983; Tong et al, 1982; Wallace, 1984). No studies have been carried out, however, to investigate the mechanical strength of various lesions or the clinical correlation between size of lesion at the time of fracture and tissue diagnosis. Currently, some early work has been reported (McBroom and Hayes) on the creation of diaphyseal lesions with intramedullary reaming devices followed by mechanical testing. This testing technique does not take into consideration the contribution from the tumor mass which may be a significant factor as demonstrated in Figure 2 by a chondrosarcoma of the proximal femur.

To date, all pathologic fractures have been lumped together in terms of definitions and strength. All predictions of mechanical bone strength have been based on the size of the lesion within the bone, equating lesion size with bone and thus material loss. A review of pathologic specimens and typical clinical presentations suggests that the tissue replacing bone contributes to the material strength, making diagnosis of impending fracture difficult, if not impossible. Further experimental and clinical review work is necessary before we have a clearer understanding of the response of pathologic bone to stress.

Stress Fractures

In recent years, stress fractures have become increasingly more common due to a significant rise in sports participation. Current reports describe these lesions as resulting from microcracks secondary to cyclic overloading. Review of clinical cases frequently shows no radiologic change initially, followed later by callus formation (Fig. 6). Bone scans are now taken in the early stages; here the activity is often seen as an oval area rather than the linear increase characteristic of fractures. Interest in these lesions was aroused on reviewing the histologic specimens of remobilized dogs in a disuse osteoporosis study carried out at the Bone and Joint Research Laboratory at the University of Ottawa (Jaworski et al, 1980; Uhthoff et al, 1983).

Stress fractures were noted in several metacarpi (Uhthoff et al, 1985). A complete radiologic and histologic review of the metacarpi was then carried out. Eighteen beagles had the right forelimb immobilized in a shoulder spica and were divided into three groups. The animals in group I were immobilized for six weeks and remobilized for ten weeks before they were killed. Those in group II were immobilized for 12 weeks and remobilized for four, 12 or 28 weeks before being killed. The animals in group III were immobilized for 32 weeks and remobilized for 28 weeks. The metacarpi of the immobilized and of the free limbs were then radiographed in two planes using Kodak M fine grain film. The third metacarpus was prepared

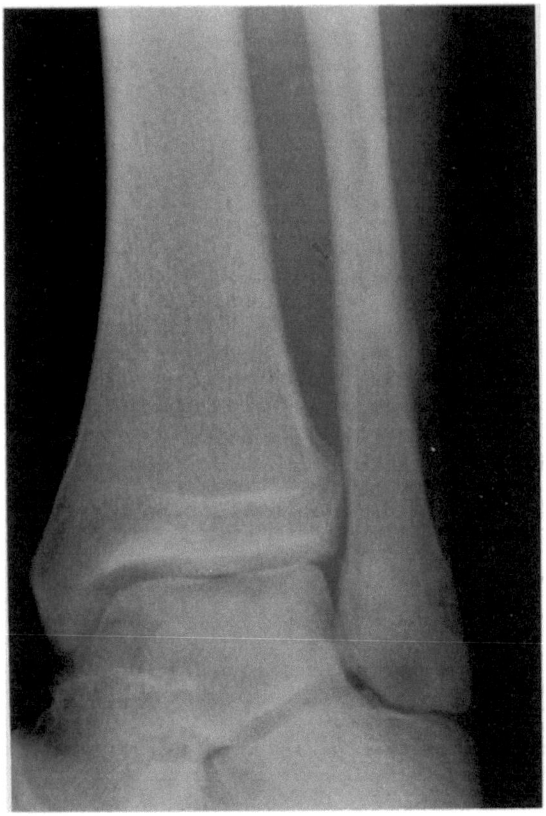

Fig. 6. Stress fracture distal fibula in 25-year old. (Courtesy of H.K. Uhthoff and Z.F.G. Jaworski. Clin. Orthop. Rel. Res. 199:284, 1985)

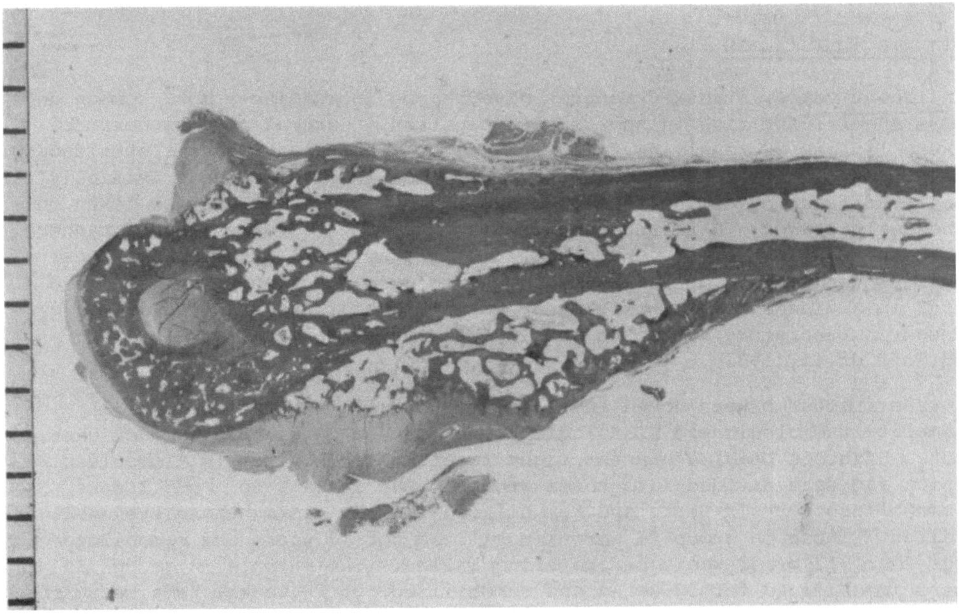

Fig. 7. Histologic specimen, periosteal stress reaction in the second metacarpus of a dog.

in an undecalcified state for histomorphometric studies. The remaining metacarpi were decalcified in EDTA, cut longitudinally in an anterior posterior plane, and stained with Goldner's trichrome.

Periosteal reactions were found in eight dogs. Radiographs of these lesions showed periosteal callus consistently found on the palmar aspect of the neck of the metacarpus (Fig. 7). Minimal callus was found laterally and almost none on the dorsal aspect. Careful histologic review of the slides failed to reveal any signs of fracture. The callus was composed of both woven and lamellar bone. The histomorphometric results of the disuse osteoporosis study were then reviewed in light of these findings. The periosteal envelope of the third metacarpus in young beagles showed a precipitous drop at 12 weeks, bottoming at 32 weeks. In contrast, the older dogs showed a gradual decrease in the periosteal envelope from the twelfth to the sixtieth week. The results of this review showed that none of the animals in Group I developed a periosteal reaction. Three animals in Group II showed a periosteal reaction, of which all were young dogs. All animals in group III had periosteal reactions (Uhthoff and Jaworski, 1985).

On reviewing the cause of a classic stress fracture in humans, one finds that a periosteal reaction develops and remodels without any fracture line seen during this time (Fig. 8). Frost (1973) has described the current theory of bone reaction to stress. In this outline (Fig. 9), normal bone may sustain microdamage following a certain mechanical force. This microdamage stimulates an osteocyte response and the bone modeling unit then repairs the microdamage. The results of our review suggest that microfractures may not be the only response of bone to stress. Further support for this observation is the work of Lanyon and coworkers (Biewener et al, 1983; Goodship et al, 1979), who placed *in vivo* strain gauges on the metacarpi of horses. The animals were then moved at various speeds (walk, trot, and canter). At all speeds, the highest strain was recorded on the palmar aspect of the metacarpus. With increasing speed, the palmar strain increased. As the animals moved slowly on the involved limb, it is possible that the

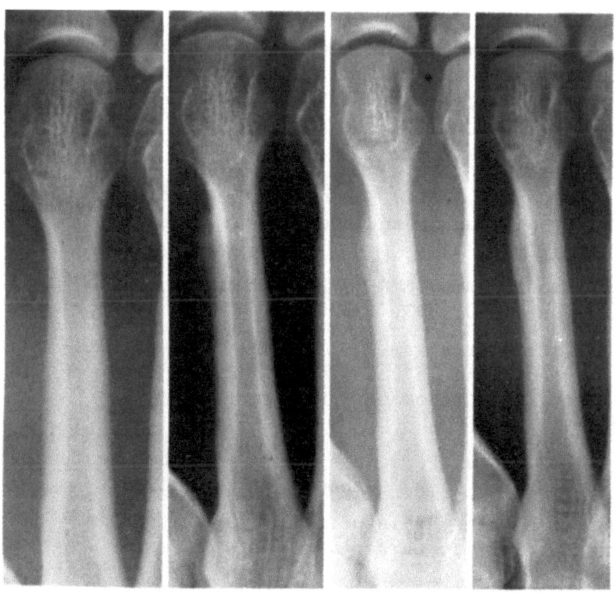

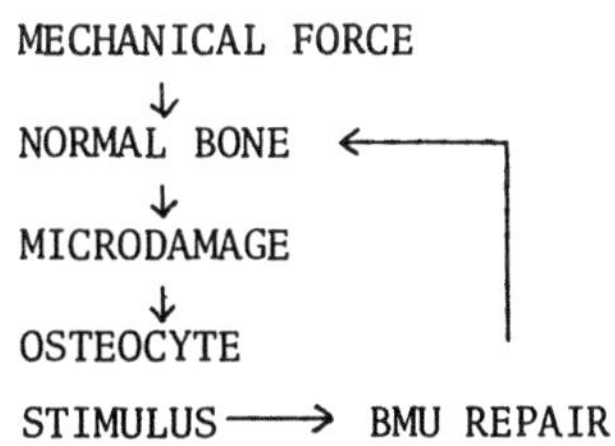

Fig. 9. Frost's outline of bone remodelling (Frost, 1973).

Fig. 8. Stress fracture in a 45-year old woman followed over 3 months.

bone was subjected to increasing increments of stress rather than acute overloading.

We therefore propose that there may be, in fact, more than one response of bone to stress. With forces of low magnitude, the periosteum may respond directly to the stress whereas with forces of high magnitude a microcrack may occur, provoking the bone remodeling unit response. This bone reaction to stress may be either a periosteal stress reaction or a stress fracture.

References

1. Biewener, A.A., Thompson, J., Goodship, A., and Lanyon, L.E.: Bone stress in the horse forelimb during locomotion at different gaits: A comparison of two experimental methods. J. Biomech. 16, 565, 1983.
2. Frost, H.M.: In, Orthopaedic Lectures, Volumes I-IV. Charles C. Thomas, 1973.
3. Goodship, A.E., Lanyon, L.E., and McFie, H.: Functional adaptation of bone in increased stress. J. Bone Joint Surg. 61A, 539, 1979.
4. Harrington, K., Sims, F., Enis, J., Johnston, J., Dick, H., and Gristina, A.: Methylmethacrylate as an adjunct in internal fixation of pathological fractures. J. Bone Joint Surg. 58A, 1047, 1976.
5. Jaworski, Z.F.G., Liskova-Kiar, M., and Uhthoff, H. K.: Effect of long term immobilization on the pattern of bone loss in older dogs. J. Bone Joint Surg. 62B, 104, 1980.
6. McBroom, R., and Hayes, W.T.: Personal communication.
7. Nicolson, G., and Poste, G.: Tumor cell diversity and host responses in cancer metastasis. Current Problems in Cancer. Vol. VII (6) and (7), 1983.
8. Reddy, S., Hendrickson, F.R., Hoeksema, J., and Gelber, R.: Role of radiation therapy in the palliation of metastatic genitourinary carcinoma. Cancer 52, 25, 1983.
9. Ruegsegger, P., Dambacker, M.A., Ruegsegger, E., Fisher, J.A., and Anliker, M.: Bone loss in premenopausal and postmenopausal women. A cross sectional and longitudinal study using quantitative computerized tomography. J. Bone Joint Surg. 66A, 1015, 1984.
10. Sissons, H.A.: Bones. In, Systemic Pathology, Vol. 5. Ed: Symmers, W. St.C. Churchill Livingstone, 1979.
11. Singh, M., Magrath, A.R., and Maini, P.S.: Changes in trabecular pattern of the upper end of the femur as an index of osteoporosis. J. Bone Joint Surg. 52A, 457, 1970.
12 Tong, P., Gillick, L., and Hendrickson, F.R.: Palliation of symptomatic osseous metastasis. Cancer 50, 893, 1982.
13. Uhthoff, H.K., Sekaly, G., and Jaworski, Z.F.G.: The effect of immobilization on compact and spongy bone in young adult and old beagle dogs. Trans. 29th Ann. Meetings, Orthopaedic Research Society. Anaheim, CA, 1983. p. 142.
14. Uhthoff, H.K., and Jaworski, Z.F.G.: Periosteal stress-induced reactions resembling stress fractures. Clin. Orthop. 199, 284, 1985.
15. Wallace, S.: Percutaneous transcatheter infusion and infarction in the treatment of human cancer. Part I. Current Problems in Cancer. VIII:1, 1984.

Disuse Osteoporosis: Current Status and Problems

Z. F. G. JAWORSKI and H. K. UHTHOFF

Introduction

Disuse osteoporosis clearly demonstrates the effect of mechanical factors on bone structure. Sudden withdrawal of mechanical loading, ie, of weight bearing and physical exertion against gravity, initiates a rapid bone loss (Whedon, 1960; Whedon et al, 1948) that will abate, however, even during continued immobilization (Minaire et al, 1974; Uhthoff and Jaworski, 1978; Whedon, 1960). This phenomenon suggests an adjustment of bone mass to reduced mechanical demands.

While most studies indicate that the initial rapid bone loss due to immobilization tends to slow down with time (Jowsey and Gordon, 1971; Minaire et al, 1974; Uhthoff and Jaworski, 1978), not all bones or types of bone show the same pattern of loss (Uhthoff et al, 1985).

The potential for recovery of bone deficit after remobilization has been denied by some investigators (Lindgren and Mattsson, 1977; Nilson, 1966; Rose, 1970), while others have observed recovery (Donaldson et al, 1970; Geiser and Truetta, 1958; Hattner and McMillan, 1968; Krolner and Toft, 1983; Sevastic and Lindgren, 1984). The diversity of opinions may stem from several factors, such as study of different species; age; bone type; method of immobilization; study method; and, most important, the duration of immoblization and remobilization (Uhthoff and Jaworski, 1978).

Always of concern to the orthopedic surgeon, disuse osteoporosis has acquired renewed importance since similar bone loss due to weightlessness has been observed during space flights (Mack and LaChance, 1967; Pace, 1971; Whedon et al, 1976). Thus, the unresolved problems of disuse osteoporosis on earth appear to apply to osteoporosis of weightlessness.

We propose to review the current status of disuse osteoporosis, based mainly on our experience with disuse osteoporosis in the dog whose bone structure and bone metabolism are similar to those of man.

As shown in Figure 1, the foreleg of young adult and old beagle dogs was placed in a spica cast for up to 60 weeks. In some, the cast was removed after 12 or 32 weeks of immobilization and the recovery of bone loss was observed for 28 weeks thereafter (Jaworski et al, 1980; Uhthoff and Jaworski, 1978; Uhthoff et al, 1985).

Current Concepts of Bone Fragility

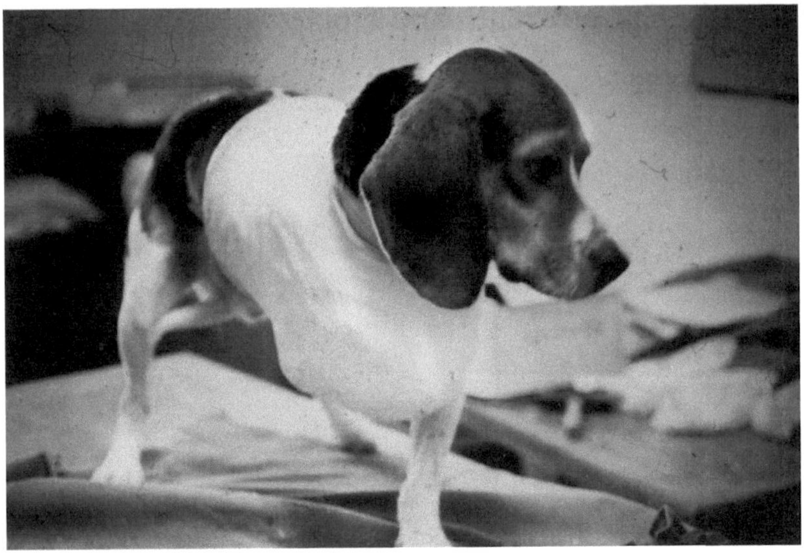

Fig. 1. Beagle dog immobilized in shoulder spica.

Bone Envelopes

Distinction between bone envelopes and their specific behavior is crucial to understand the pathogenesis of disuse osteoporosis and its eventual reversal on reloading because the cellular mechanisms mediating bone loss or gain operate on bone surfaces.

The spongy parts of the skeleton, ie, short bones as well as the epiphyses and metaphyses of long bones, are encased between the periosteal envelope (with the muscle and tendon insertions) on the outside, and the endosteal envelope (cortical and trabecular) in contact with the bone marrow, on the inside. In the large, long-living animals, such as dogs, the network of the haversian and Volkmann's canals communicating with the periosteal and endosteal envelopes constitute an additional envelope (Fig. 2).

The envelopes are the site of bone turnover. In microscopic loci osteoclasts first create a cavity through resorption that osteoblasts subsequently refill with new bone, as shown in Figure 2. In the diaphyseal compacta, the haversian systems represent the outcome of such local turnover.

The expansion or contraction on a given envelope is due to the cumulative balances within the individual sites of bone turnover, ie, mainly between the mean depth of erosion (MDE) and the thickness of lamellar bone deposited, also called the wall thickness (MWT) (Jaworski, 1984a; 1984b).

One of the important features of MWT is that because of the mode of osteoblasts' recruitment and operation, it cannot exceed a potential maximum (Jaworski and Wieczorek, 1985).

Characteristically, the turnover sites on the endosteal envelope and in paramedullary haversian systems are in negative balance, ie, MDE exceeds MWT,

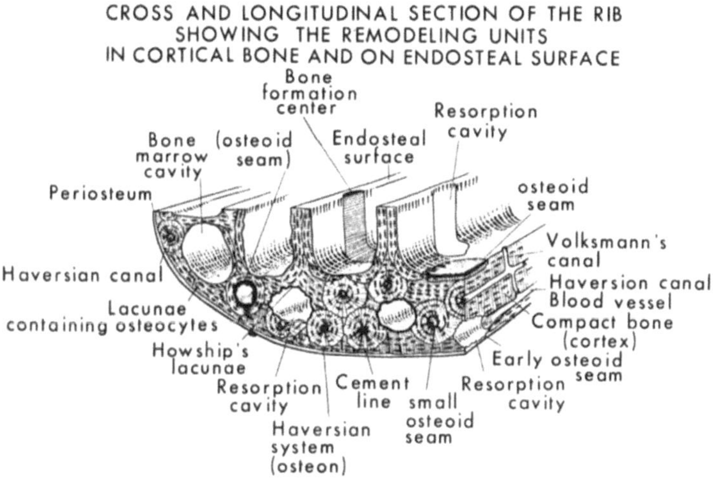

Fig. 2. Three-dimensional representation of a section of rib showing cortical compacta and some trabeculae. Cement (reversal) lines subdivide bone tissue into BSUs, both in the compacta (haversian systems) and on the endosteal, cortical, and trabecular surfaces. BSUs are the outcome of local bone turnover sites in which formation follows the resorption of a cavity. The radius of resorption cavity, in cross section, is referred to as mean depth of erosion or MDE while the thickness of lamellar bone deposited as MWT. In the compacta such bone turnover units or BMWs are represented by the evolving haversian systems; although morphologically and dimensionally different, BMWs operate also on endosteal and periosteal bone surfaces (Jaworski, 1972).

while slightly positive on the periosteal envelope, where presumably the MDE is less than MWT. The balance is neutral in the haversian systems of the external two-thirds of diaphyseal compacta (Frost, 1973).

The negative bone balance on paramedullary and endosteal envelopes accounts for the continuous erosion and trabeculation of the cortex from within, and the thinning and loss of the trabeculae in the center of the medullary cavity (Arnold, 1970) which thus continuously expands throughout life (Garn, 1975).

It is important to note that the rate of generation of new turnover sites, ie, their activation frequency (Frost, 1973), will affect the envelope balance, basically determined by the MDE and MWT relationship. It will, therefore, amplify the bone loss on the paramedullary and endosteal envelopes (Jaworski, 1984b).

The whole bone volume is, therefore, at any given time a product of balance of individual envelopes. Since the expansion of bone marrow cavity in the adult is greater than the expansion of the periosteal envelope:

$$\text{P env. exp.} < \text{E env. exp.}$$

the endosteal envelope balance basically determines the changes in the whole bone volume.

Stages of Disuse Osteoporosis

If followed for an adequate period of time (40-60 weeks) the three stages of disuse osteoporosis can be discerned (Fig. 3).

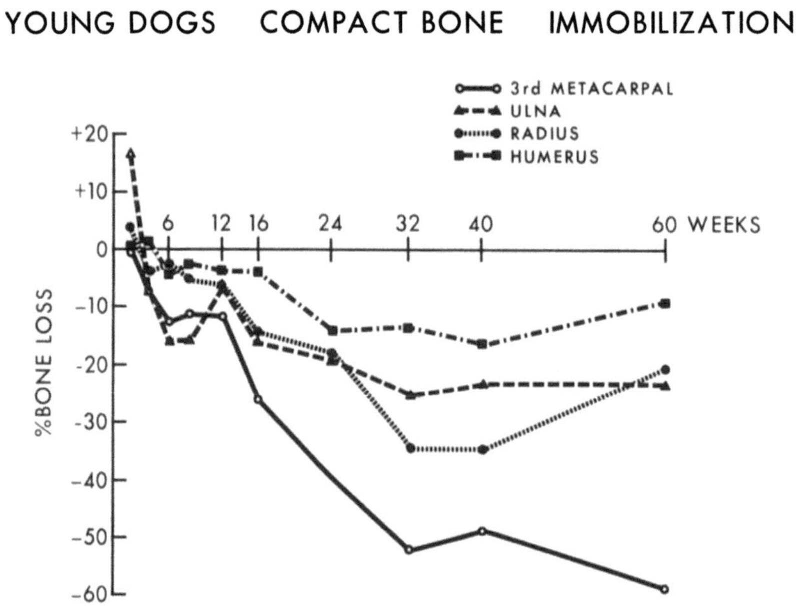

Fig. 3. A graph relating the pattern of total bone loss in the third metacarpus, radius, ulna and humerus to the duration of immobilization, expressed as percentage of the control. The first stage of reaction to immobilization (from 0 to 12 weeks approx.) shows its triphasic course: rapid bone loss followed by recovery. After the 12th week, there is a more protracted bone loss (second stage) leveling off between 12 to 32 weeks or more according to type of bone, heralding the third stage of bone volume stabilized at 20-50% of the original volume.

The first biphasic stage immediately follows immobilization. It is characterized by a burst of resorption cavities on all three envelopes (Fig. 4) which, a few weeks later, revert to bone forming sites, with bone volume tending to return to normal even while immobilization continues (Uhthoff et al, 1985). This first stage may represent a nonspecific response to any trauma, such as putting the foreleg in the cast as in our experiments. This reaction is referred to as regional acceleratory phenomenon or RAP (Frost, 1981). In other words, neurocirculatory and hormonal factors may play a more important role here than the immobilization or disuse (Semb, 1971).

The second stage begins with the protracted bone loss lasting approximately 40 weeks. In the spongy parts of the skeleton it is limited to the endos-

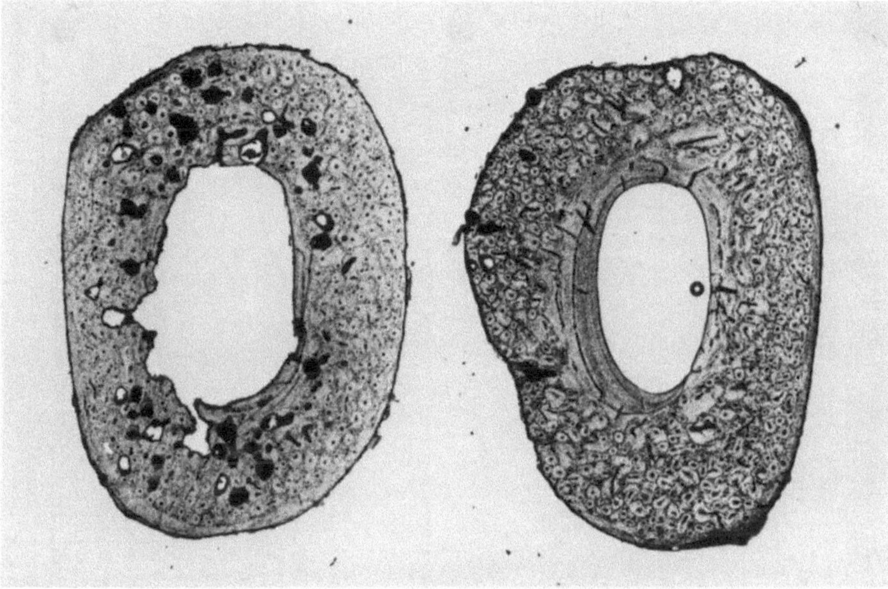

Fig. 4. Cross section of the third metacarpus at 12 weeks of immobilization, showing transient increase in cortical porosity (Uhthoff and Jaworski, 1978. Reproduced with permission of the Journal of Bone and Joint Surgery, British Edition).

teal envelope in both young adult and old dogs -- in diaphyses to the periosteal envelope in young adult dogs and to the endosteal in older dogs (Jaworski et al, 1980; Uhthoff and Jaworski, 1978). This specific loss in disuse osteoporosis may result in a bone volume reduction of 50-60% before bone loss levels off, 40-60 weeks after immobilization depending on the location of the bone (Fig. 5).

The third stage, beginning with the levelling off of bone loss, represents established or inactive disuse osteoporosis (Fig. 3 and 5).

Reversibility

Remobilization after 12 or 32 weeks of immobilization showed considerable recovery of the original bone loss (Fig. 5). Thus, 28 weeks after removal of the cast after 32 weeks of immobilization, the following changes were observed: in the third metacarpal diaphysis of younger dogs a 54% loss (mostly from the periosteal envelope) decreased to 16% (a 70% recovery); in the old dogs a 38% loss (mostly from the endosteal envelope) decreased to 23% (a 40% recovery). In metaphyseal spongiosa in young adult dogs, a 50% loss decreased to 17% (a 66% recovery), while in the older dogs a 47% loss decreased to 19% (a 60% recovery).

The amount of recovery, however, depended on the duration of immobilization, ie, the relative amount of bone loss, the bone envelope, type of bone involved, and age. Thus, as net bone losses increase with the duration of

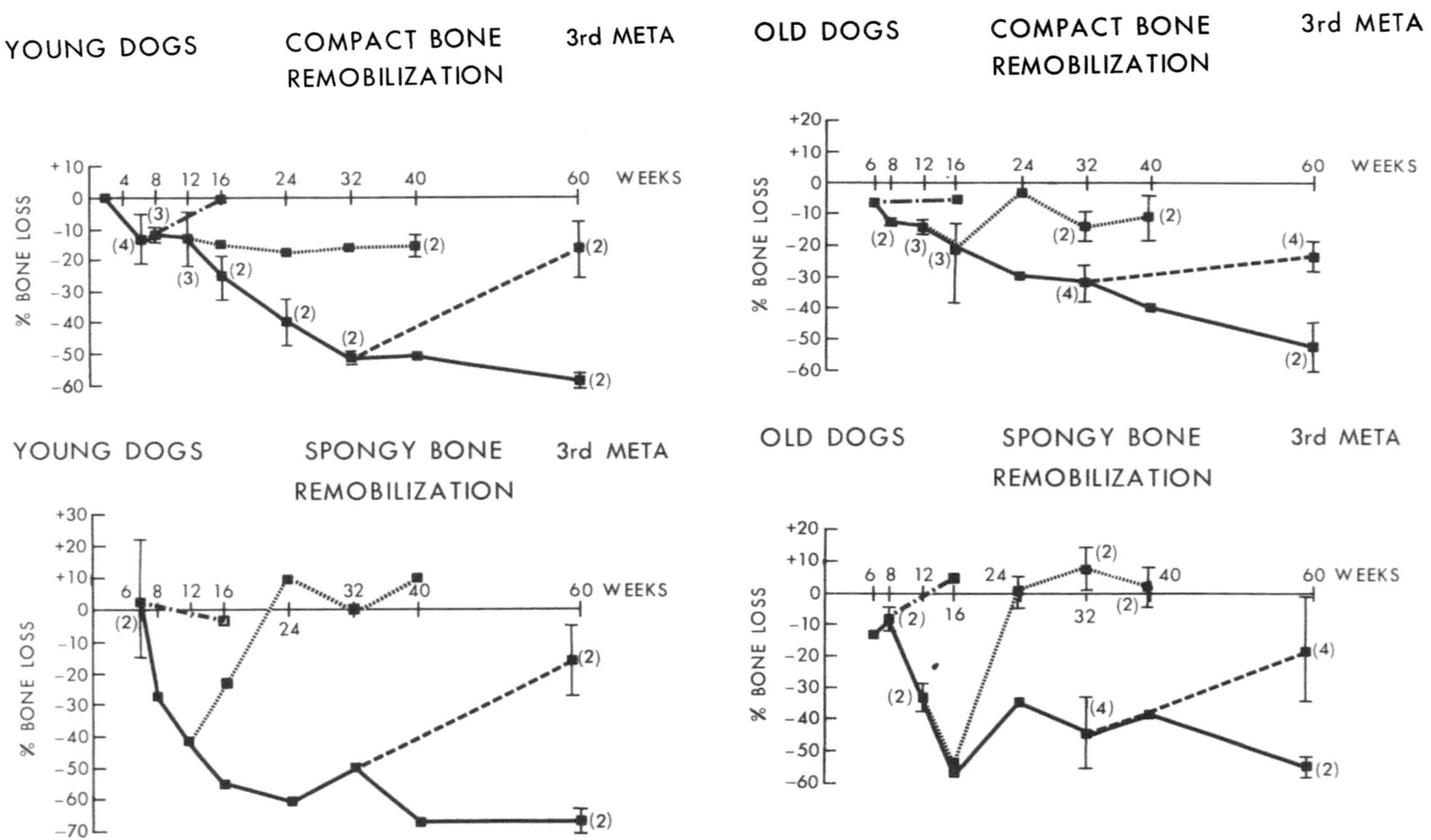

Fig. 5. Bone volume changes in response to remobilization at two stages of disuse osteoporosis in the third metacarpus. Compact (diaphyses) bone: upper row; spongy bone: below; young adult dogs on the left, old dogs on the right side. The continuous line at the bottom in each panel represents the pattern and magnitude of bone loss during immobilization against which (interrupted lines) the recovery following the remobilization is assessed. In the diaphyses, changes in bone volume correspond to the sum total of the contributions of individual envelopes: periosteal, haversian and endosteal. In the young adult dogs, the response to immobilization and recovery at remobilization occurred mainly on the periosteal envelope while in the old dogs on the endosteal envelope. In the spongiosa, total bone changes are due only to changes on the endosteal envelope.

immobilization (remobilization at 12 versus 32 weeks), so, on the whole, do the residual deficits on all surfaces of all bones in both age groups (Fig. 5).

Generally, the metaphyseal spongiosa, which sustained greater losses than the diaphyses, also showed a greater recovery potential, especially during remobilization after 12 weeks of immobilization.

It is important to note that the third metacarpus, a small, peripheral weight bearing bone, showed the greatest global losses of all bones in both age groups, but it also showed greater recovery than the larger and more proximal bones in almost all situations.

As previously noted in man (Minaire et al, 1974), the bone volume of the older dogs at the onset of these experiments was reduced by 10% compared with younger dogs. This, obviously, indicates an age-related bone loss. Older dogs also showed smaller relative losses than the young dogs and less recovery both in the diaphysis and in metaphyseal spongiosa.

Cellular Mechanisms Underlying Disuse Osteoporosis and Its Reversal

The first stage, that of RAP, is characterized by the appearance of numerous resorption cavities, ie, local osteoclasts which in due course are replaced by osteoblasts refilling the cavities, as in normal remodeling. In the diaphyseal compacta, however, the cavities appear to be larger than normal and more numerous (Fig. 4), suggesting not only a sudden increase in the number of activated sites but also an increase in local recruitment of osteoclasts accounting for the increased MDE.

The second, more specific stage of reaction to immobilization, a protracted bone loss, is characterized microscopically by a marked extension of the resorption surface (Fig. 6) on the predominantly affected envelope. It is due both to the increased number of active resorption sites covered by osteoclasts and the extension of the so-called transitional zone (Baron et al, 1981), ie, empty Howships lacunae. The extension of the transitional zone (inactive resorption surface) occurs when the recruitment of osteoblasts from the dividing, committed progenitors is delayed. Besides increased resorption, therefore, it is likely, as suggested by several investigators (Chai Benfu et al, 1980; Chartraine, 1979; Minaire et al, 1974; Obrant, 1984; Wronski and Morey, 1983), that throughout the immobilization period deficient bone formation due to impaired recruitment or function of osteoblasts may contribute to the observed negative bone balance. In fact, areas of bone formation during the active second stage of disuse osteoporosis are so few that it is difficult to measure the rate of bone apposition. Although the appositional rate is usually taken as a measure of the osteoblast function or efficiency (Frost, 1969), recent studies suggest that the decreased rate of osteoblast recruitment will affect independently both the MWT and the appositional rate as measured by double tetracycline marking (Jaworski and Wieczorek, 1985; Marotti, 1976).

The leveling off of bone loss between 40-60 weeks, despite continued immobilization, was shown histologically by the contraction of the resorption surface and reappearance of osteoblasts, bone-forming surfaces approximating the control values (Fig. 6). Thus, the bone turnover rate and bone balance resumed at the preimmobilization level with a permanently reduced

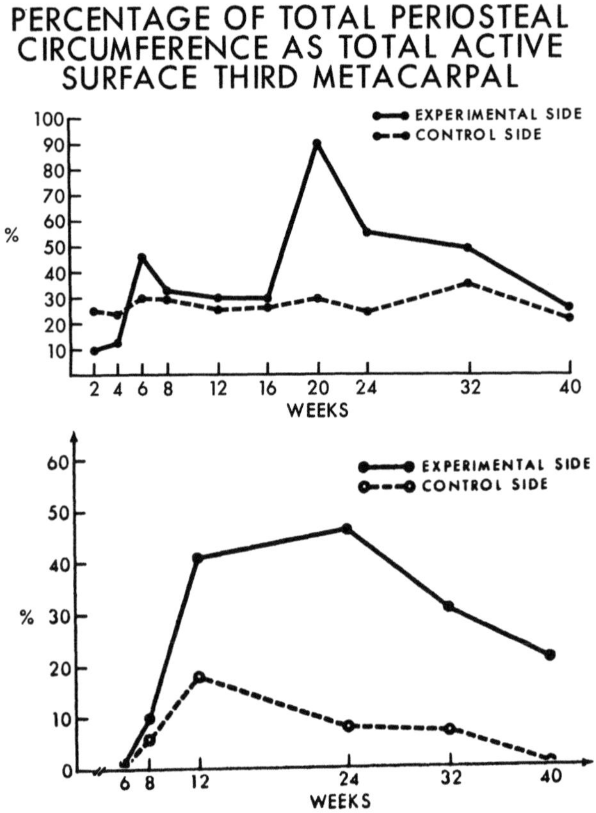

a)

b)

Fig. 6. The total active surface (resorption and formation) as a percentage of the total periosteal circumference of the third metacarpus (a), and of the total endosteal circumference in the old dogs (b). (Jaworski et al, 1980; Uhthoff and Jaworski, 1978) (Reproduced with the permission of the Journal of Bone and Joint Surgery, British Edition.)

bone volume. As to the ultimate cause of this leveling off with continued immobilization, we presume that the bone mass and new reduced mechanical demands eventually equilibrate. Furthermore, the reduction in bone mass permitted mechanical strains to reappear which begin to control again the cellular mechanisms which escaped from such control during the preceding stage. To account for a significant recovery of bone on remobilization during the active phase of disuse (second stage), a different sequence of events has to be postulated than that stabilizing bone volume while immobilization continued. Thus, not only the generation of new resorption sites, ie, of osteoclasts, must have declined but also the bone formation which follows it must have substantially improved. This is most likely achieved by the increased rate of osteoblast recruitment allowing the MWTs to reach their maximum at all sites where the resorption surfaces were converted to bone-forming ones.

Residual Deficit

As noted in Figure 5, the recovery after remobilization at 32 weeks is not complete and is less in old than in young dogs, suggesting an irreversible component to bone loss. This may be due, as already mentioned, to the honeycomb structure of spongy bone and of perimedullary compacta where the increase in the rate of bone resorption will result in the perforation of

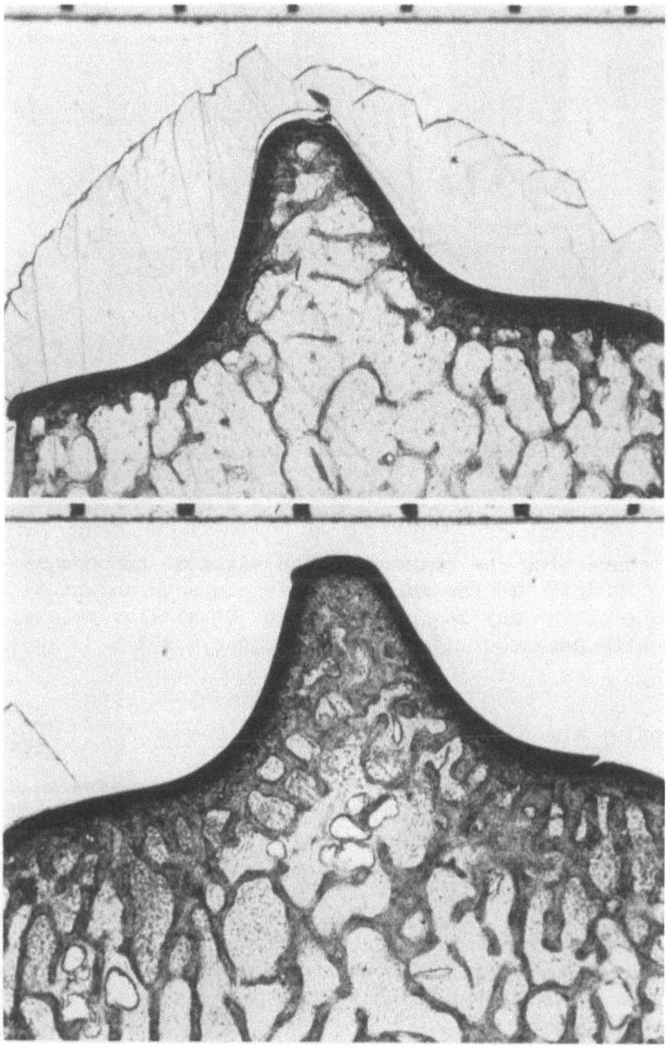

Fig. 7. Eighty micron thick cross section of a distal metacarpal diaphysis of the immobilized side (a) and the opposite side 60 weeks after immobilization (b). Note the reduction in the size and number of trabeculae. Besides thinning of trabeculae, their apparent loss is noted; the latter is due to a defect in the plates. (Uhthoff et al, 1985. Reproduced with permission of Clinical Orthopaedics and Related Research)

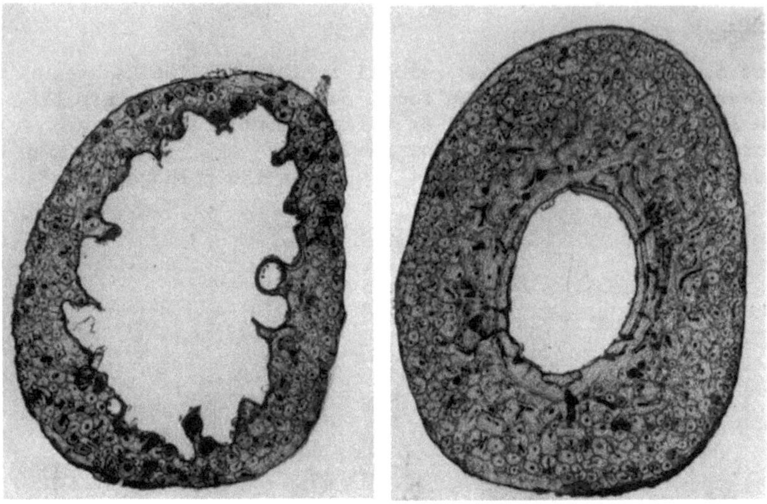

a) b)

Fig. 8. Cross section of the third metacarpus at 40 weeks of immobilization in old dogs, the experimental side (a) and the control side (b). Note a marked expansion (sloughing of the perimedullary area) of bone marrow cavity. (Jaworski et al, 1980. Reproduced with permission of Journal of Bone and Joint Surgery, British Edition)

thinner plates (Fig. 7) connecting the transverse and vertical trabeculae (Arnold, 1970; Jaworski, 1984b). In the perimedullary compacta an actual sloughing of the innermost cortex may be observed (Fig. 8) similar to that seen in rabbits treated with adrenocorticosteroids (Duncan, 1967).

Implications Concerning the Disuse of Weightlessness

Studies in humans on earth suggest that disuse osteoporosis is self-limiting, ie, bone loss not continuing indefinitely (Minaire et al, 1974; Uhthoff et al, 1985; Whedon, 1960). To date, astronauts have not remained in space long enough (up to 24 weeks) to reveal whether the bone loss due to weightlessness is self-limiting. If the experience of disuse osteoporosis on earth can be extrapolated to disuse in weightlessness, the astronauts probably are still actively losing bone when returning to earth. Consequently, they may be regaining much of the loss incurred in space, especially younger individuals. This may not be true, however, after longer periods in space.

Since a complete recovery of bone loss may not be possible after remobilization during the active phase of disuse, and since treatment of established osteoporosis presents a new set of problems, prevention of bone loss becomes the only practical avenue available.

Theoretically, the first stage of reaction to immobilization or RAP could be prevented by suppression of activation of new turnover sites, ie, the appearance of osteoclasts recruited from their dividing committed progenitors. The only agents known so far to have this potential are calcitonin

(Muhlbauer et al, 1971) and diphosphonate analogues (Fleisch, 1983). Furthermore, these agents should be applied before immobilization or weightlessness is initiated.

Although there are a few reports that diphosphonates may decrease the degree of bone loss specific for disuse (Minaire et al, 1981), there are no reports that its prior administration may prevent RAP or subsequent stages commonly observed in disuse bone loss.

Physical activity in a weightless environment does not, on the other hand, produce within bones mechanical strains sufficient to affect bone turnover or reduce bone loss. Consequently, conditions have to be created in space flights which would impose muscle and tendon pull on bone surfaces and weight bearing effects comparable to those which result on earth from gravity (Abramson and Delagi, 1961; Pace, 1977).

On the other hand, once the inactive phase of disuse osteoporosis supervenes, ie, the bone turnover rate and balance return to normal with bone volume considerably reduced, as observed in the affected limb in our dogs after 60 weeks of continuous immobilization, the conditions may be less favorable for the recovery of bone deficit. The situation then resembles the established or residual osteoporosis of any etiology encountered in clinical medicine.

Summary and Conclusions

Bone loss following a sudden immobilization has practical and theoretical implications. Disuse osteoporosis appears clearly related to biomechanical factors, such as weight bearing and muscular activity against gravity.

It appears that mechanical usage mitigates the excess of endosteal and paramedullary envelope expansion over the periosteal one, accounting for the universal age-related bone loss, while unloading accelerates it until the bone volume matches the new reduced mechanical demands.

Whether the cellular mechanisms mediating these adaptations respond to intensity of strains, related to the degree of weight bearing and physical exertion or some circulatory changes related to muscle use, is not yet entirely clear.

The reimposition of customary loads can reverse bone loss incurred during the active phase of disuse. This appears to be accomplished not only by inhibiting bone resorption induced by immobilization, but also by enhancing bone formation on resorption surfaces, ie, the recruitment and function of osteoblasts.

It remains uncertain whether disuse osteoporosis can be prevented by other than biomechanical means, for example, by drugs or hormones blocking the initial burst of resorption activity and its continuation.

Once the rate of bone loss subsides and bone turnover rate and associated balance return to predisuse levels, the situation is changed. The problem then is to increase bone volume, as it were, *de novo*, as in any type of established osteoporosis of any etiology in clinical medicine.

Acknowledgements

The authors wish to thank Christiane Menard for the preparation of the manuscript. This paper was in part based upon work supported by the Medical Research Council of Canada.

References

1. Abramson, A.S., and Delagi, E.F.: Influence of weight bearing and muscle contraction on disuse osteoporosis. Arch. Phys. Med. 42, 147, 1961.
2. Arnold, J.S.: Focal excessive endosteal resorption in aging and in senile osteoporosis. In, Osteoporosis. Ed: Barzel, U.S. Grune and Stratton, New York, 1970, pp 80-100.
3. Baron, R., Vignery, A., and Lane, R.: Reversal phase and osteopenia: Defective coupling of resorption to formation in the pathogenesis of osteoporosis. In, Osteoporosis: Recent Advances in Pathogenesis and Treatment. Eds: DeLuca, H.F., Frost, H.M., Jee, W.S.S., Johnston, C.C. Jr., Parfitt, A.M. University Park Press, Baltimore, 1981, pp 311-320.
4. Chai Benfu, Zhu Xiulin, Yang Lianfang: Effect of cast immobilization on bone turnover, a tetracycline double labelling investigation. Chin. Med. J. 93, 316, 1980.
5. Chantraine, A.: L'Ostéoporose et les Para-Ostéo-Arthropathies au Cours de la Paraplegie. Editions Arsica SA, Bruxelles, 1979.
6. Donaldson, C.L., Hulley, S.B., Vogel, J.M., Hattner, R.S., Bayers, J.H., and McMillan, D.E.: Effect of prolonged bed rest on bone mineral. Metabolism 19, 1071, 1970.
7. Duncan, H.: Bone dynamics in rheumatoid arthritis treated with adrenal corticosteroids. Arthrit. Rheum. 10, 716, 1967.
8. Fleisch, H.: Biphosphonates: Mechanics of action and clinical applications. In, Bone Mineral Research (Chapter 8). Ed: Peck, W.A. Excerpta Medica, Amsterdam, 1983, pp 319-357.
9. Frost, H.M.: Tetracycline-based histologic analysis of bone remodeling. Calcif. Tissue Res. 3, 211, 1969.
10. Frost, H.M.: Bone Remodeling and Its Relationship to Metabolic Bone Disease. Charles C. Thomas, Springfield, Ill., 1973.
11. Frost, H.M.: The regional acceleratory phenomenon. Orthop. Clin. North Am. 12, 725, 1981.
12. Garn, S.M.: Bone Loss and Aging: Physiology and Pathology of Aging. Academic Press, New York, 1975, pp 39-57.
13. Geiser, M., and Truetta, J.: Muscle action, bone rarefaction and bone formation. J. Bone Joint Surg. 40B, 282, 1958.
14. Hattner, R.S., and McMillan, D.E.: Influence of weightlessness upon the skeleton. Aerospace Med. 39, 849, 1968.
15. Jaworski, Z.F.G.: Pathophysiology, diagnosis and treatment of osteomalacia. Orthop. Clin. North Am. 3, 623, 1972.

16. Jaworski, Z.F.G.: Lamellar bone turnover system and its effector organ. Calcif. Tissue Int. 36, S46, 1984a.

17. Jaworski, Z.F.G.: Coupling bone formation to bone resorption: A broader view (Editorial). Calcif. Tissue Int. 36, 531, 1984b.

18. Jaworski, Z.F.G., and Wieczorek, E.: Constants in lamellar bone formation determined by osteoblast kinetics. Bone 6, 361, 1985.

19. Jaworski, Z.F.G., Liskova-Kiar, M., and Uhthoff, H.K.: Effect of long-term immobilization on the pattern of bone loss in older dogs. J. Bone Joint Surg. 62B, 104, 1980.

20. Jowsey, J., and Gordon, G.: Bone turnover and osteoporosis. In, The Biochemistry and Physiology of Bone, Ed. 2, Vol. 3. Ed: Bourne, E.H. New York Academic Press, 1971, pp 201-238.

21. Krolner, B., and Toft, B.: Vertebral bone loss: An unheeded side effect of therapeutic bed rest. Clin. Sc. 64, 537, 1983.

22. Lindgren, U., and Mattson, S.: The reversibility of disuse osteoporosis. Calcif. Tissue Res. 23, 179, 1977.

23. Mack, P.B., and LaChance, P.L.: Effects of recumbency and space flight on bone density. Am. J. Clin. Nutr. 20, 1194, 1967.

24. Marotti, G.: Decrement in volume of osteoblasts during osteon formation and its effect on the size of the corresponding osteocytes. In, Bone Histomorphometry. 2nd International Workshop. Ed: Meunier, P.J. Armour Montagu, Paris, 1976, pp 385-397.

25. Minaire, P., Berard, E., Meunier, P.J., Edouard, C., Goebert, G. and Pilonchery, G.: Effects of disodium dichloromethylene diphosphonate on bone loss in paraplegic patients. J. Clin. Invest. 68, 1086, 1981.

26. Minaire, P., Meunier, P., Edouard, C., Bernard, J., Courpron, P., and Bourret, J.: Quantitative histologic data on disuse osteoporosis: Comparison with biological data. Calcif. Tissue Res. 17, 57, 1974.

27. Mühlbauer, R.C., Russel, R.G.G., Williams, D.A., and Fleisch, H. The effects of diphosphonates, polyphosphates and calcitonin on "immobilization osteoporosis" in rats. Eur. J. Clin. Invest. 1, 336, 1971.

28. Nilsson, B.E.R.: Post-traumatic osteopenia: A quantitative study of the bone mineral mass in the femur following fracture of the tibia in man, using Americium-241 as a photon source. Acta Orthop. Scand. 37 (Suppl) 91, 1, 1966.

29. Obrant, K.J.: The Morphology of Post-Traumatic Osteopenia. Lidbergs Blanchett AB, Skurup, Sweden, 1984.

30. Pace, N.: Weightlessness: A matter of gravity. New Engl. J. Med. 297, 32, 1977.

31. Rose, G.A.: Irreversibility of osteoporosis. In, Osteoporosis. Ed: Barzel, U.S. Grune and Stratton, New York, 1970, pp 123-132.

32. Semb, H.: Experimental limb disuse and bone blood flow. Acta Orthop. Scand. 40, 552, 1971.

33. Sevastic, J.A., and Lindgren, J.V.: Osteoporosis. Experimental and clinical studies. Clin. Orthop. Rel. Res. 191, 35, 1984.

34. Uhthoff, H.K., and Jaworski, Z.F.G.: Bone loss in response to long-term immobilization. J. Bone Joint Surg. 60B, 420, 1978.

35. Uhthoff, H.K., Sekaly, G., and Jaworski, Z.F.G.: Effect of long-term non-traumatic immobilization on metaphyseal spongiosa in young adult and old beagle dogs. Clin. Orthop. 192, 278, 1985.

36. Whedon, G.D.: Disuse osteoporosis. In, Bone as a Tissue. Eds: Rodahl, K., Nicholson, J.T., and Brown, E.M. McGraw-Hill, New York, 1960, pp 67-69.

37. Whedon, G.D., Deitrick, J.E., and Shorr, E.: Modification of the effects of immobilization upon metabolic and physiologic functions of normal men by the use of an oscillating bed. Am. J. Med. 6, 684, 1948.

38. Whedon, G.D., Lutwak, L., Rambault, A., Whittle, M., Leach, C., Reid, J., and Smith, M.: Mineral and nitrogen balance study observations: The second manned Skylab mission. Aviat. Space Environ. Med. 47, 391, 1976.

39. Wronski, T.J., and Morey, E.R.: Inhibition of cortical and trabecular bone formation in the long bones of immobilized monkeys. Clin. Orthop. Rel. Res. 181, 269, 1983.

Osteoporosis: Limitations of Strain-Related Bone Remodeling in Its Prevention

L. E. LANYON

The structural competence of the skeleton is determined by the mass, material properties, and architecture of the bones within it. These features are in turn the product over time of the balance and intensity of the remodeling process at each location. Under normal circumstances, assuming that all requirements are met (ie, sufficient calcium, phosphate, vitamin D) the principal extrinsic influences on this remodeling process are those derived from mechanical loading and circulating hormones. In the past, the predominant interest in bone remodeling was directed towards its hormonal control. Recently, however, the effects of mechanically-related variables have received more attention. It is now generally accepted that the question of the etiology of osteoporosis be rephrased from 'what dietary or hormonal imbalances give rise to the condition' to 'why does the mechanism which appropriately matches structure to function during the first four decades of life subsequently fail to do so?' Of course, the answer to this question is as yet beyond our understanding. Some known features of the way in which mechanical events influence remodeling, however, enable us to make a tentative hypothesis.

Let us assume that the principal functional determinant of an individual's bone mass is the strength of an 'osteogenic' stimulus derived from the mechanical strains which physical load bearing engenders in bone tissue. For each skeletal location, evolution has determined a level of functional strain which is appropriate in terms of tissue bulk, tissue damage, and the probability of fracture. Provided all requirements are fulfilled, any deviation from this appropriate level will stimulate the remodeling necessary to eliminate it. Since natural selection only influences populations with breeding potential, the appropriate strain at each location will be that relevant to the fracture risks and activity patterns in young and young adult age groups.

In our accompanying paper in this volume we have referred to at least two aspects of bone's mechanical strain environment which have been shown to influence bone remodeling, namely the strain change waveform and the strain distribution.

Strain Distribution

The level of bone mass which natural selection has determined to be appropriate at each location is likely to be related to the cumulative strain related stimulus derived from a number of separate loading situations. One

Current Concepts of Bone Fragility

of the characteristics distinguishing young and old individuals is the difference in their diverse activities. Even if the strength of the stimulus derived from each separate loading situation persisted with age, the total mechanically-related stimulus would decline as the range of loading situations decreased. The result of a diminished strain-related osteogenic stimulus would therefore be a decline in bone mass and an increase in functional strain. This strain increase, while intensifying the osteogenic stimulus produced by the existing loading situations, does not compensate for the loading activities which are absent. Bone loss thus continues with a progressive reduction in the margin of safety to fracture and an increase in the level of fatigue damage. In a certain proportion of individuals the situation is serious enough to cause fracture and osteoporosis.

Strain Change Waveform

In one series of experiments we have been able to demonstrate a dose:response relationship between peak strain magnitude and the strength of the osteogenic stimulus which a dynamic strain situation produces. In another experiment we have demonstrated that an even more important determinant of osteogenic potential may be the maximum strain rate. Thus, it is quite possible, by reducing the rate at which the strain changes, to produce increasingly high strains without engendering a compensating osteogenic stimulus.

Another feature of changing activity patterns with age is their decreased vigor, which is presumably associated with a decreased strain rate. Thus, with regard to strain rate, as with strain distribution, we can provide explanations for an activity-related decline in strain-related osteogenic stimulus which would permit increased functional strain to coexist with decreased bone mass. To approach the clinical situation of osteoporosis, we must add to this scenario the probable age-related decrease in effectiveness of the cellular response to any particular level of strain-related stimulus, and an increased requirement for resorptive remodeling associated with dietary insufficiencies and/or malabsorption. These features would naturally exacerbate the situation.

All the factors so far mentioned are potentially common to both men and women, whereas the obvious difference between the pattern of bone remodeling between the sexes is the rapid decline in bone mass which follows the menopause. This loss is clearly related to withdrawal of estrogen which in some way appears to increase the bone's sensitivity to reabsorptive effects of parathormone. Thus, in women after the menopause the strain-related (primarily osteogenic) stimulus is in equilibrium with a hormonally-derived (primarily net osteolytic) stimulus which has become stronger. This may have the effect of increasing the appropriate strain threshold at each location by setting the strain 'thermostat' at a newer and higher level. The rapid postmenopausal loss of bone following withdrawal of estrogen may represent the decline in bone mass necessary to restore the balance between local and systemic stimuli at this higher strain level.

The question regarding exercise and postmenopausal osteoporosis is therefore: 'to what extent can an exercise regimen be formulated which, by maximizing the osteogenic stimulus, successfully modulates or prevents postmenopausal loss, and yet avoid the potentially damaging effect of physical loadbearing?'. The answer to this question is, of course, as yet unknown but the topic is amenable to study if suitable investigations are undertaken in normal and potentially osteoporotic human populations.

Disorganized Bone Structure

Congenital Osteopetrosis

J. D'ASTOUS and J. CORKAL

Introduction

Osteopetrosis is a rare disorder, characterized mainly by radiographically evident excessive density of the bony skeleton. The pathogenesis of osteopetrosis is thought to be due to a decreased resorption of endochondral cartilage in bone in the presence of a normal rate of bone formation (Shapiro et al, 1980).

The causes of decreased bone resorption can be listed as follows:

1) decreased number of osteoclasts;

2) decreased production of lysosomal enzymes;

3) partial or total absence of the ruffled border in osteoclasts;

4) decrease in the stem cell population for osteoclasts;

5) a compromised ability of the skeletal microenvironment to support the proliferation, differentiation and function of osteoclast precursors.

Histologically, most studies have concentrated on the juvenile recessive form of osteopetrosis and have shown that rickets, with its wide osteoid seams, is common (Marks, 1984). The morphology and number of osteoblasts appear to be normal (Reeves et al, 1981; Sieff et al, 1983; Teitelbaum et al, 1976). The osteoclasts may be increased in juvenile osteopetrosis, and increased, decreased or normal in adult osteopetrosis (Marks, 1984). The ruffled borders on the osteoclasts are absent in most cases of human osteopetrosis (Shapiro, 1982).

Most of the dynamic bone metabolic studies have shown a decrease in bone resorption (Marks, 1984). With respect to laboratory data, the serum calcium is usually normal while the parathyroid hormone levels may be increased, decreased or normal (Marks, 1984). Another observation is an increase in the stem cells and immature cells in the circulation (Milgram and Jasty, 1982; Shapiro et al, 1980).

Marks, in 1984, proposed the following classification of human osteopetrosis:

Type I: A recessive, lethal, infantile form, which may be in itself heterogenous.

Current Concepts of Bone Fragility

Type II. A later onset "juvenile" recessive form.

Type III. Recessive osteopetrosis with mild clinical manifestations.

Type IV. Recessive osteopetrosis with renal tubular acidosis and cerebral calcification "carbonic and hydrase II deficiency".

Type V. Benign adult-dominant osteopetrosis.

In the infantile lethal recessive form of osteopetrosis, the diagnosis is usually made at birth. The child has severe anemia and thrombocytopenia, and clinically one can note severe hepatosplenomegaly. This is secondary to the fact that all the potential marrow spaces are taken over by sclerotic bone. These patients have frequent fractures, fail to thrive, and often have optic atrophy, secondary to compression of the optic nerve. They also present with osteomyelitis, delayed tooth eruption, caries, hydrocephalus and bony encroachment of cranial fossa and nerve foramina. Death usually occurs in early childhood from overwhelming infection.

The adult dominant benign type of osteopetrosis is generally asymptomatic, but the patients may present with pathologic fractures, coxa vara and a limp, bone pain or osteomyelitis.

As to treatment, experiments have shown that bone marrow transplantation or temporary parabiotic union can reverse the changes of osteopetrosis in certain strains of osteopetrotic mice (Walker, 1973). In human osteopetrosis, bone marrow transplant has been used for the lethal infantile recessive form and, although the numbers are small, a 55% cure rate has been reported (Ballet et al, 1977; Marks, 1984). Because of the diverse pathogenetic mechanism implicated in human osteopetrosis, failure of bone marrow transplantation in some children is not surprising and further research is required to develop other modes of therapy.

Coxa Vara: A Feature of Osteopetrosis

Coxa vara was found in five members of the same family who had osteopetrosis. The development of a typical coxa vara deformity arising from an anatomically normal proximal femur is illustrated by Case I. The abnormal hip findings in the other family members are also described.

Case I

This 2-1/2 year old boy was seen in 1977 for a one-week history of pain in the knee, fever and tenderness on the medial aspect of the proximal tibia. Roentgenographs of the hips and knees (Fig. 1) revealed no abnormalities except osteopetrosis. He returned three years later with a one-week history of knee pain. Roentgenographs at that time revealed a peculiar linear lucency extending distally from the epiphyseal plate on the medial side of the tibia, simulating a Type II epiphyseal fracture of the proximal tibial epiphysis (Fig. 2). At 6-1/2 years of age, radiographs of his asymptomatic left hip revealed the presence of what appears to be a Type II epiphyseal fracture of the proximal femoral capital epiphysis (Fig. 3). No treatment was initiated or planned, a decision directed largely by the benign natural history of the coxa vara deformities, secondary to osteopetrosis in other members of his family.

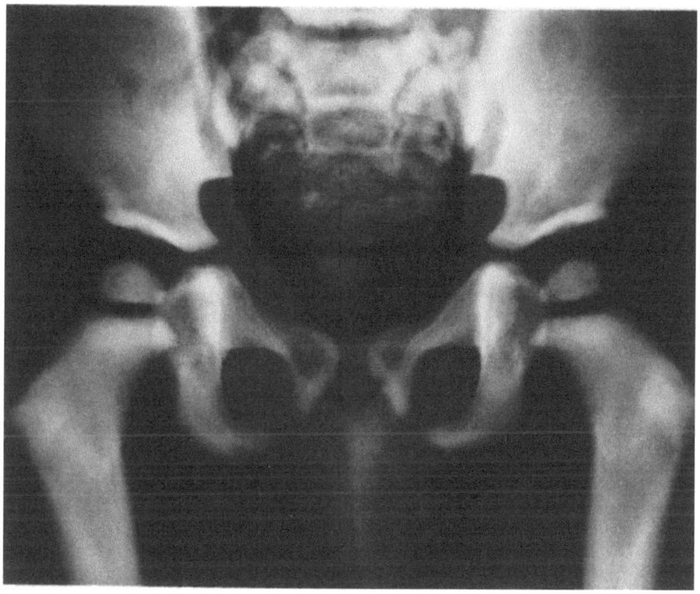

Fig. 1. Case I. Normal hips with features of osteopetrosis.

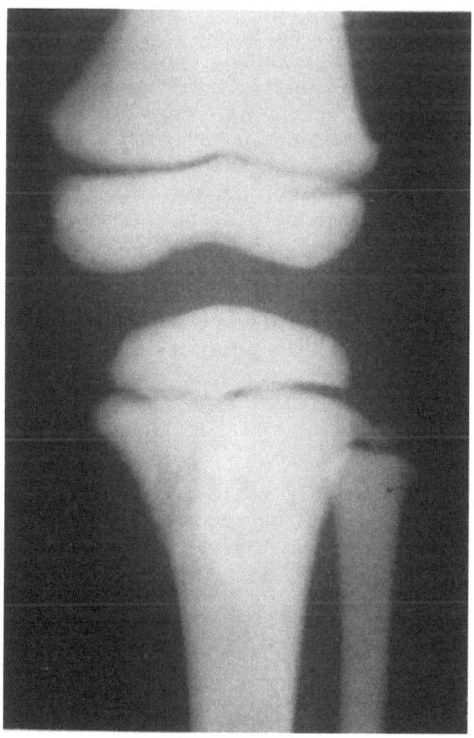

Fig. 2. Case I: Lucent line on medial tibial metaphysis simulating a Type II epiphyseal fracture.

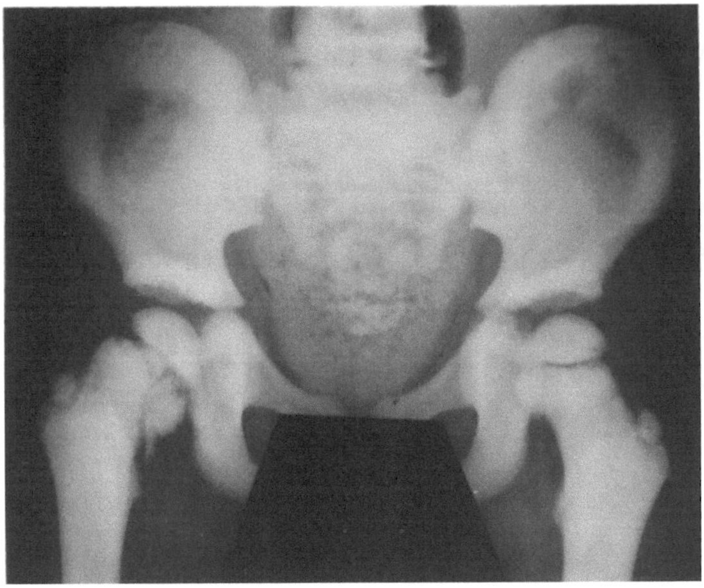

Fig. 3. Case I: Appearance of a Type II epiphyseal fracture in the proximal femur of his asymptomatic left hip.

Case II

A 9 year 1 month old girl, first cousin of Case I, suffered from a painful limp after a trivial fall while figure skating. Roentgenographs revealed a previously undiagnosed osteopetrosis as well as an undisplaced Type II epiphyseal fracture of the proximal femoral capital epiphysis (Fig. 4). Bone scan revealed a generalized increased uptake of technetium 99 with a roughly equal uptake in both hips. Roentgenographs of the right hip taken one month later revealed a further displacement and at that time she was seen by a surgeon at another hospital who performed an emergency pinning for her so-called "displaced Type II fracture . There were no technical problems associated with the pinning, but she developed avascular necrosis of the right femoral head, for which sepsis and chondrolysis were considered as causes, although blood cultures and hip aspiration did not confirm the presence of sepsis. Roentgenographs taken two years after her hip pinning show essentially a destroyed hip joint. Clinically, her hip remained extremely stiff.

Case III

The 35 year old mother of Case II had pain in the hip following a fall as a teenager. Currently, she is active in sports and is asymptomatic except for a minor limp after exercise. Roentgenographs revealed a coxa vara on the left.

Case IV

The 37 year old father of Case I was initially seen at 12 years of age with the classical features of the infantile type of coxa vara and osteopetrosis.

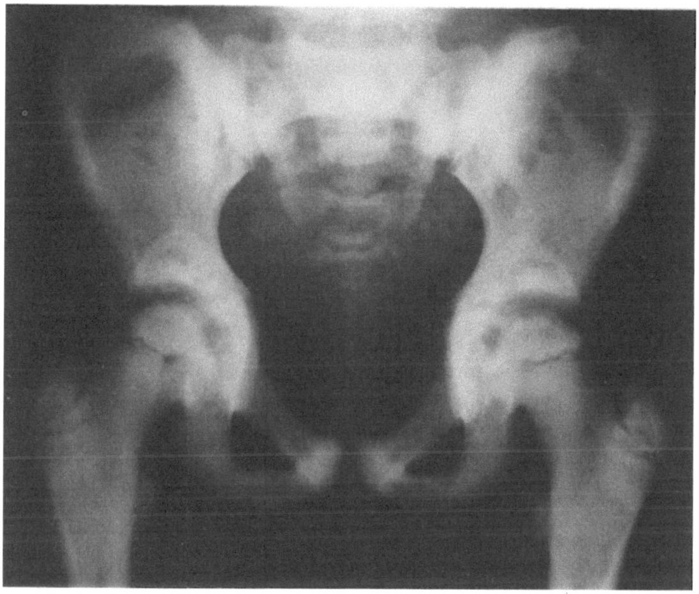

Fig. 4. Case II: Undisplaced Type II epiphyseal fracture of proximal femur in a young girl with osteopetrosis.

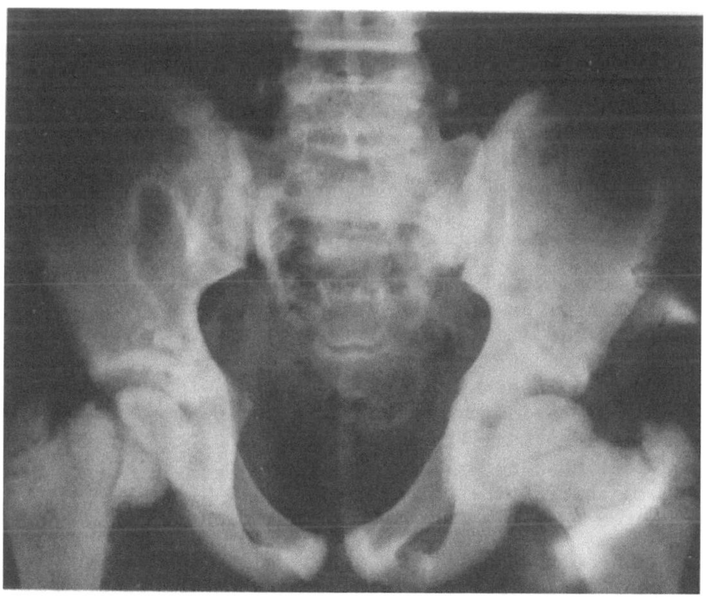

Fig. 5. Case V: Unilateral coxa vara right hip, age 12.

He remembers a limp and some discomfort as a child but he never underwent treatment other than a few chiropractic manipulations. At 37 years of age, he remains physically active and asymptomatic except for a minor limp. Roentgenographs show a typical coxa vara with evidence of the lucent lines of the inverted V sign of a metaphyseal defect.

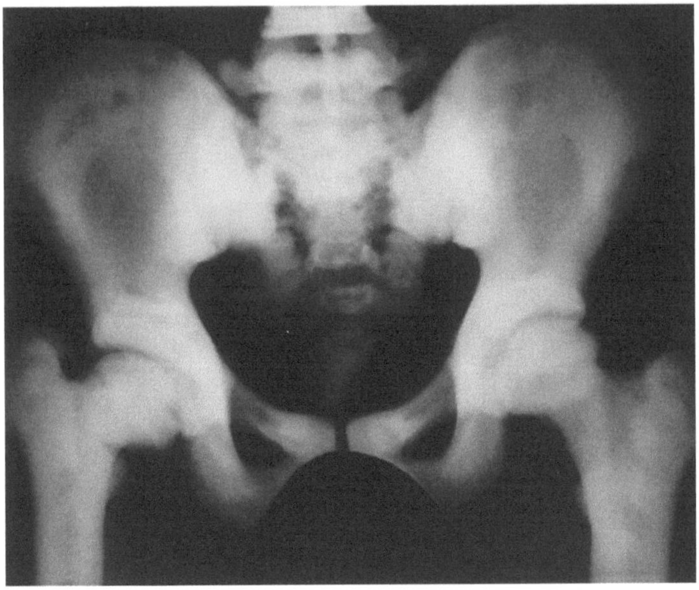

Fig. 6. Case V: Unilateral coxa vara right hip, age 23 with no treatment.

Case V

A 23 year old uncle of patients I and II, and brother of Cases III and IV, is asymptomatic except for a mild limp. He has a unilateral coxa vara as seen in his films taken at age 12 (Fig. 5) and at age 23 (Fig. 6).

Discussion

One question we have asked ourselves is, what does this radiolucent line in the metaphysis represent? A similar defect has also been seen in congenital coxa vara and has been called a clear zone, a zone of rarefaction, an insufficiency fracture, or a zone of aberrant cartilage. Other than the evidence of a shearing strain across the pathologic tissue of the femoral neck, no explanation can be given for the rather high incidence of this phenomenon. Having seen the identical linear defect in the proximal tibial metaphysis of Case I, we feel that this linear defect in coxa vara of osteopetrosis is probably due to aberrant cartilage which the osteoclasts have failed to resorb, although we have no histologic proof of this.

Hasenhuttl, in 1962, documented the radiologic progression of coxa vara in osteopetrosis over a 24-year period but does not comment on the functional status of the hip. Of passing interest is that the follow-up of one of our patients (Case IV) is 25 years. The patient has minimal disability although his roentgenographs show marked coxa vara (Robichon et al, 1968). Review of the literature for the results of surgical treatment for coxa vara in osteopetrosis reveals only one case by King and Lovejoy (1973). The patient did well with a valgus-subtrochanteric osteotomy performed at 9 years of age. Observations during surgery in osteopetrotic patients have shown that bones are hard and brittle, and extreme care must be taken to avoid fractures.

The literature is replete with surgical cases in osteopetrosis fraught with complications such as fractures and breaking of the implant (Beck et al, 1957; King and Lovejoy, 1973).

Conclusions

We have presented five patients with coxa vara and osteopetrosis. In one, pinning in situ was unsuccessful; another patient is doing well without surgery but is still under observation; and three patients are well without surgical intervention.

In conclusion, coxa vara is definitely observed in some cases of osteopetrosis. It is not necessarily associated with any specific incident or event, and is often an incidental radiographic finding. Few reports in the literature refer to the pathogenesis or treatment of this hip deformity, other than detailing the difficulty encountered with various techniques of internal fixation. It is likely that a healed coxa vara is the least of the major bony problems associated with osteopetrosis and that one should exercise great care before embarking on the surgical treatment of coxa vara in osteopetrosis.

References

1. Ballet, J.J., Griscelli, C., Courtris, C., Michaud, G., and Maroteaux, P.: Bone marrow transplantation in osteopetrosis. Lancet ii, 1137, 1977.
2. Beck, L., Cornell, R.C., and Emmett, J.E.: Intramedullary fixation of fractures of the femur in a case of osteopetrosis. J. Bone Joint Surg. 39A, 1389, 1957.
3. Hasenhuttl, L.K.: Osteopetrosis. Review of the literature and comparative studies on a case with a twenty-four year follow-up. J. Bone Joint Surg. 44A, 359, 1962.
4. King, R., and Lovejoy, J.F.: Familial osteopetrosis with coxa vara. J. Bone Joint Surg. 55A, 381, 1973.
5. Marks, S.: Congenital osteopetrotic mutations as probes of the origin, structure, and function of osteoclasts. Clin. Orthop. 189, 239, 1984.
6. Milgram, J., and Jasty, M.: Osteopetrosis - A morphological study of twenty-one cases. J. Bone Joint Surg. 64A, 912, 1982.
7. Reeves, J., Arnaud, S., Gordon, S., Subryan, B., Block, M., Huffer, W., Arnaud, C., Mundy, G., and Haussler, M.: The pathogenesis of infantile malignant osteopetrosis: Bone mineral metabolism and complications in five infants. Metab. Bone Dis. Rel. Res. 3, 135, 1981.
8. Robichon, J., Wiley, J.J., and Germain, J.P.: Osteopetrosis. Can. J. Surg. 2, 424, 1968.
9. Shapiro, F.: Ultrastructural abnormalities of osteoclasts in malignant-recessive osteopetrosis. Arch. Path. Lab. Med. 106, 425, 1982.
10. Shapiro, F., Glimcher, M.J., Holtrop, M.E., Tashjian, A.H., Brickley-Parsons, D., and Kenzora, J.E.: Human osteopetrosis - A histological, ultrastructural, and biochemical study. J. Bone Joint Surg. 62A, 384, 1980.

11. Sieff, C.A., Levinsky, R.J., Rogers, D.W., Muller, K., Chessells, J.M., Pritchard, J., Casey, A., and Hazil, C.M.: Allogeneic bone-marrow transplantation in infantile malignant osteopetrosis. Lancet i, 437, 1983.

12. Teitelbaum, S.L., Coccia, P.F., Brown, D.M., and Kahn, A.J.: Malignant osteopetrosis: A disease of abnormal osteoclast proliferation. Metab. Bone Dis. Rel. Res. 3, 99, 1981.

13. Walker, D.: Experimental osteopetrosis. Clin. Orthop. 97, 158, 1973.

Osteogenesis Imperfecta: Current Concepts

J. R. Shapiro and D. W. Rowe

Introduction

Exceptional progress in the understanding of osteogenesis imperfecta (OI) during the past decade is due to improved methods for the characterization of procollagens and collagen alpha chains, and the remarkable progress achieved in the molecular biology of collagen genes (Prockop and Vivirikko, 1984). These found ready application in the study of OI and other heritable disorders of connective itssue.

OI was clinically characterized by Ekman in 1788. Definition of the full clinical spectrum took approximately another 125 years. The evolution of this story has been told by U.H. Weil (1981). It was observed that in addition to fragile bones, the OI syndrome includes blue sclerae, adult onset hearing loss, and dentinogenesis imperfecta (DI). Only recently have clinicians also noted the frequency with which hyperextensible joints, scoliosis, and short stature occur in the OI patient. The various OI phenotypes present clinically and biochemically heterogenous syndromes encompassing a generalized disorder of connective tissue. Understanding the molecular basis of this disorder promises to clarify not only the other heritable disorders of connective tissue, but disorders not usually grouped with them, such as the adult osteoporoses and the pediatric osteochondrodysplasias.

Clinical Classification of OI

A crisp clinical classification of OI has been impeded by the genetic heterogeneity and variable expressivity inherent in this disorder. The traditional nosology "congenita" and "tarda" forms of the disease should be discarded since they are inaccurate. Approximately 10% of mild cases of OI present with fractures at birth, but these may be absent in the severe forms of the disease. Terms such as mild, without long bone deformity, and severe OI with long bone deformity are useful but estimation of the degree of deformity is subject to individual bias (Bauze et al, 1975). Sillence has proposed that four major types be recognized (Table I) (Sillence et al, 1979). This classification is insufficient, however, because of uncertainty regarding the mode of inheritance in sporadic cases, difficulty in judging scleral color, and the fact that approximately 10% of patients cannot be adequately categorized. Nevertheless, it represents a categorization which is clinically useful.

Current Concepts of Bone Fragility

Table I. Classification of OI syndromes by increasing severity

Mild OI, Bauze et al Type I, Sillence	
Absent to mild skeletal deformity, blue sclerae, 25% DI, may have presenile hearing loss	Autosomal dominant
Moderate OI, Bauze et al Type IV, Sillence	
Skeletal fragility is moderate, also obvious skeletal deformity that may require bracing or cane. Sclerae blue in some; many families have white sclerae. 25% DI; presenile hearing loss	Sporadic; Autosomal dominant
Severe OI, Bauze et al Type III, Sillence	
Prenatal fractures, cranial and skeletal deformities, scoliosis, growth retardation severe. Sclerae usually white; DI common.	Autosomal dominant or recessive
Lethal OI, Buaze et al Type II, Sillence	
Perinatal death. Severe defect in mineralization, cranial and long bone deformities; deep blue sclerae. Pulmonary insufficiency	Autosomal dominant or recessive

Modified from Bauze et al, 1975, and Sillence, 1979.
DI = dentinogenesis imperfecta

Clinical Maxims

There are several principles which serve to identify and evaluate the OI patient as distinct from other childhood and adult osteopenias. Considerable uncertainty still remains regarding diagnosis and management of this syndrome, a fact disturbing to patients and their families. Failure to identify a significant history of fractures and of blue sclerae in siblings or parents, or dentinogenesis imperfecta or wormian occipital bones in infants with fractures has led to failed diagnosis and, at times, a mistaken charge of child abuse.

First, in terms of transmission of the disorder, OI tends to breed true -- eg, the severity is fairly uniform within a family. While variations in fracture rate or extent of deformity occur secondary to the level of activity, age or site of fracture, only rarely does one encounter a severely affected member in a family whose previously affected members exhibit a mild form of the disease.

Second, OI is a systemic disorder of type I collagen, the body's major structural protein. OI patients are shorter than their peers, the short stature being related to the severity of the disease (Wynne-Davies and Gormely, 1981). Most patients are in the lower 5-11th percentile for height; severely affected subjects may not be taller than 3 or 4 feet. The issue of limited growth is of great concern to most OI parents.

Third, in each of the nonlethal types of OI, the fracture rate falls precipitously following puberty (Smars, 1961). However, as discussed by Wiley in this Symposium, a decrease in the incidence of wrist fractures has been observed in normal children. The reason for change in bone strength following puberty is unknown, but a changed hormonal milieu influencing protein synthesis or enzyme activity is possible.

At an early age, most fractures involve the lower extremities. Older children may fracture digits or their upper extremities. Although joint dislocations are relatively uncommon in OI, joint laxity occurs in most patients, more commonly in the more severely affected. We have observed joint laxity in relatives who have not had any fractures. The biochemical basis for this is not known.

Echocardiographic analysis of a large number of patients suggests that mitral valve prolapse occurs in approximately 5% of patients (Hortop et al, 1985; White et al, 1983). Dilatation of the aortic valve occurs in a few patients, but when present affects individual families suggesting a specific gene mutation affecting type I collagen synthesis in the aorta. However, a tissue specific posttranslation modification of the gene product could be at fault.

No consistent biochemical abnormality in serum or urine chemistries is found in OI. Alkaline phosphatase values may be increased in the presence of a fracture. Aminoaciduria has been reported in some individuals. Urinary hydroxyproline excretion is usually normal. Serum acid phosphatase levels are normal. Thyroid homeostasis is normal in OI, as revealed by serum thyroid levels and a normal response to testing with TRH (Shapiro et al, 1985). Growth hormone levels are normal. Certain children with short stature have low somatomedin C serum levels, but the significance of this finding is uncertain.

Lastly, fractures in the OI patient heal in expected time. Hyperplastic callus, an acute inflammatory lesion which complicates healing of a fracture, occurs in less than 1% of OI fractures (Roberts, 1976). It is puzzling why deformity complicates fracture healing in the more severe conditions while mildly-affected patients experience multiple fractures without residual deformity. This serves to focus on the role normal collagen synthesis plays in cell differentiation and orientation. The specific molecular gene defect influences tissue healing, and as it is now recognized, collagen influences the spatial organization of skeletal tissue in the embryo.

Clinical Phenotypes in OI (Table I)(Smith et al, 1983)

Type I - Mild

The majority, approximately 60%, of OI patients have a mild disease. Subjects with this degree of the disorder have fewer fractures than other phenotypes, and may escape detection until their later years. They have a short stature, triangular faces, minimal scoliosis, and in spite of several fractures, their long bones heal without deformities. This category includes patients with blue sclerae. Approximately 25% have dentinogenesis imperfecta, and are categorized as type IB. A similar proportion develop hearing loss during the second or third decade. Many will exhibit mild skin and joint laxity, particularly in the smaller distal joints. The disorder is transmitted as an autosomal dominant trait so that 50% of offspring may be affected.

Mild OI may go undetected in many subjects until an older age when, for example, fractures recur in postmenopausal women or blue sclerae are noted for the first time. However, both sexes have been found to be osteopenic throughout their lives.

Type II - Lethal, or perinatal lethal

An infant of this phenotype, approximately 15% of patients, is incapable of living beyond the first few weeks. As the result of a severe defect in the synthesis of type I collagen, these infants suffer multiple intrauterine fractures which produce a characteristic radiologic picture at birth. A soft, poorly ossified skull, short crumpled extremities with fractures (concertina deformity), and a characteristic beading (callus) of previously broken ribs are seen at birth. Extremities may be either broad and rectangular or narrow with a widened metaphysis. Sclerae are deep blue. Because of the severe connective tissue lesion, dismemberment may occur at birth. Death occurs due to respiratory failure during the first several weeks. The disorder may be the result of a dominant mutation, or may be transmitted as a recessive trait. The parents are clinically normal. Multiple pregnancies with OI deformities have been observed in individual families.

Type III - Severe or progressively deforming

These children, approximately 20% of OI patients, are born with multiple fractures involving the extremities, pelvis and chest. The skull appears large, with frontal bossing, and the soft skull is flattened in the AP diameter. Wormian occipital bones are common. Settling of the soft skull ultimately gives rise to the "Tam-O-Shanter" occipital overhang. With time, settling of the skull on the spine can produce basilar impression with neurologic complications. The "sunset" appearance of the face is a result of a relatively large skull, small face, and frontal bossing. The extremities are twisted or angulated at birth, the result of fractures or unequal muscle pull on softened bones. Sclerae are typically white. A small percentage, perhaps 20%, are affected with dentinogenesis imperfecta. Scoliosis tends to be marked and pectus deformities of the sternum and chest wall are frequently observed. Later, these deformities reduce chest volume and lead to pulmonary insufficiency. Joint laxity tends to be more prominent in type III patients. Growth retardation is severe; most patients do not grow taller than three feet. Osteopenia is severe; fractures occur with minimal trauma and heal with increased deformity, but as indicated above, fracture rate declines after puberty. Hearing loss is more common in this group during adulthood.

Type IV - Moderate

This category is both genetically and clinically disparate. Clinically, the disease is intermediate between types I and III, and overlaps with each.

Included are patients with moderately severe disease as to incidence of fractures and extent of deformities. Typically, they have white sclerae, although some patients who fit the disease may have blue sclerae. Osteopenia is usually severe. Dentinogenesis imperfecta and hearing loss are relatively common in this group. Scoliosis may be progressive during adolescence. There is moderate growth retardation. Many patients in this group have obvious deformities, particularly of their lower extremities, and require either a cane or brace for walking. Type IV disease may appear sporadically, or be transmitted as an autosomal dominant trait.

The Pathophysiology of OI

Studies of collagen synthesis by dermal fibroblasts in culture from patients with various types of OI show mutations in the synthesis of normal type I collagen in this connective tissue lesion (Shapiro and Rowe, 1983). Since only a limited number of such studies have been performed, the data do not yet permit assignment of a specific mutation to one or another phenotype. It is likely that, as in the thalassemic disorders of hemoglobin synthesis, a limited number of mutations will underlie various phenotypes. Responsible for the variation in expression are tissue specific modifications of the primary gene product. These modifications have been summarized by Byers and Bonadio (1985).

Type I OI: Diminished production of type I collagen, increased III/I ratio, normal ratio of a-1(I)/a-2(I) chains.

Decreased type I content in skin
Decreased synthesis of a-1(I) with normal gene copy number, and no apparent defect in gene structure.
Decrease mRNA for type I a-1 chains.

Limited availability of Pro-A-1(I) chains (51% of normal) is balanced by intracellular degradation of the excess a-2(I) so that secreted extracellular procollagen alpha chain ratio is normal.

Type II OI: As outlined by Byers, there are four mutations which, thus far, have been recognized in this phenotype (Byers and Bonadio, 1985)

1) deletions from the triple helical region of Pro-A-1(I);
2) deletions from the triple helical region of Pro-A-2(I);
3) deletions from the triple helical region of Pro-A-2(I) associated with a nonfunctional allele of Pro-A-2(I);
4) amino acid substitution (cysteine for glycine) in the triple helical region of Pro-A-1(I) which interferes with alpha chain assembly and secondarily leads to overmodification (eg, excess lysyl hydroxylation).

It is important to note that several strains have been studied in which no deletions, insertions, or structural modifications have been identified.

Type III OI: Synthesis of type I trimer, Pro-A-1(I)3 due to failure to incorporate Pro-A-2(I) into the triple helix associated with a deletion near the carboxy terminus of Pro-A-2(I):

excessive oligosaccharide in carboxy-terminal propeptide extension, probably due to slowed procollagen processing.

Type IV OI: Mutations in the helical portion of Pro-A-2(I), and restriction length fragment polymorphism analysis of type IV families with an a-2(I) probe suggest linkage for the type-2 alpha chain. The synthesis of both normal and abnormal Pro-A-2(I) chains has been demonstrated in these cell lines.

Other deletions which involved the Pro-A-2(I) chain leading to intermediate phenotypes have been described, including one in a type IV patient with blue sclerae.

The histopathologic expression of these mutations in collagen fiber synthesis involves diminished trabecular bone volume, defective cortical bone formation, and in those with reduced diameter of long bone, defective periosteal remodeling (Bullough et al, 1981). Woven bone, which is immature trabecular or cortical bone, is found in the severe grade of the disease. Hyperosteocytosis is found in all OI phenotypes. Osteoclasts and resorption spaces may be increased in certain specimens. Bone turnover may be increased; however, excessive osteoid deposition is not commonly associated with OI. Electron microscopy may reveal collagen fibers smaller than normal in diameter but with normal periodicity.

Collagen fibers may show fraying, breakage or appear unravelled. Type II OI may demonstrate a lack of type I collagen fibers in the extracellular matrix due to failure of the cell to secrete abnormal or excessively modified (excess lysine hydroxylation or mannosylation) procollagen molecules.

Therapy of OI

The use of a variety of rods or pins to straighten deformed or weakened limbs is an important tool which improves ambulation in many patients, and functional status in the wheelchair bound patient (Root, 1984). Cosmetic improvement in a school-age child with deformed bones cannot be overestimated for its positive effect on performance and social adaptation.

The medical therapy of OI has involved a series of nutritional and medicinal trials, none of which has proved successful (Albright, 1981). The list includes calcium, magnesium, and sodium fluoride supplements, vitamin D, ascorbic acid, salmon calcitonin, and several hormones including estrogens and anabolic (androgenic) steroids. Estrogen replacement is indicated for the postmenopausal woman with OI as it is in the unaffected postmenopausal woman.

At this time, no medicinal therapy of OI is effective; however, an adequate calcium intake appears reasonable for growing children and postmenopausal women, or men over 61 years of age.

In collaboration with Dr. Lynn Gerber (Clinical Center, NIH) and Dr. Helga Binder (Children's National Medical Center, Washington, DC), we have promoted the use of orthotic therapy as soon as the child begins to walk, using light weight circumferential or bivalved polypropylene braces as first suggested by Dr. Eugene Bleck (Bleck, 1981; Binder et al, 1984). In these braces, which include ischial support, children are encouraged to stand erect and walk. Thus far, success is limited to children with high motivation; recurrent fracture, while in the brace, has not been a problem as long as the brace comes high enough to support the upper femur.

Finally, those having any therapeutic role with OI children and OI families must be sensitive to their special needs. Parents are understandably terrified by the prospect of causing a fracture through carelessness. Having a child at prolonged rest in a spica cast places the family and siblings under a particular strain. The developmental and educational needs of children and adults with OI must be taken into consideration. Each patient lives with the knowledge that a minor fall or accident can turn into an expensive and painful disaster. Physical medicine and rehabilitative care are essential to maintaining good muscle tone and minimizing the effects of immobility on growing bones. Swimming in heated pools under supervision is a particularly effective method for strengthening both bone and muscle in the OI child.

References

1. Albright, J.A.: Systemic treatment of osteogenesis imperfecta. Clin. Orthop. Rel. Res. 159, 88, 1981.
2. Bauze, R.J., Smith, R., and Francis, M.J.O.: A new look at osteogenesis imperfecta. J. Bone Joint Surg. 57B, 2, 1975.
3. Binder, H., Hawks, L., Graybill, G., Gerber, N.L., and Weintraub, J.C.: Osteogenesis imperfecta: Rehabilitation approach with infants and young children. Arch. Phys. Med. Rehabil. 65, 537, 1984.
4. Bleck, E.E.: Nonoperative treatment of osteogenesis imperfecta: Orthotic and mobility management. Clin. Orthop. Rel. Res. 159, 111, 1981.
5. Bullough, P.G., Davidson, D.D., and Lorenzo, J.C.: The morbid anatomy of the skeleton in osteogenesis imperfecta. Clin. Orthop. Rel. Res. 159, 42, 1981.
6. Byers, P.H. and Bonadio, J.F.: The molecular basis of clinical heterogeneity in osteogenesis imperfecta: Mutations in Type I collagen genes have different effects on collagen production. In press, 1985.
7. Hortop, J., Tsipouras, P., Maron, B., and Shapiro, J.R.: Echocardiographic findings in osteogenesis imperfecta. In press, 1985.
8. Prokop, D.J. and Kivirikko, K.I.: Heritable diseases of collagen. New Engl. J. Med. 311, 376, 1984.
9. Roberts, J.: Bilateral hyperplastic callus formation in osteogenesis imperfecta. J. Bone Joint Surg. 58A, 1164, 1976.
10. Root, L.: The treatment of osteogenesis imperfecta. Orthop. Clin. North Am. 15, 775, 1984.
11. Shapiro, J.R. and Rowe, D.W.: Collagen genes and brittle bones. Ann. Int. Med. 99, 711, 1983.
12. Shapiro, J.R., Bercu, B., and Levine, J.: Thyroid function in osteogenesis imperfecta. In press, 1985.
13. Sillence, D.O., Senn, A.S., and Danks, D.M.: Genetic heterogeneity in osteogenesis imperfecta. J. Med. Genetics 16, 111, 1979.
14. Smars, G.: Osteogenesis Imperfecta in Sweden. Svenska Bokforlaget, Stockholm, 1961. p. 69.
15. Smith, R., Francis, M.J.O., and Houghton, G.R.: The Brittle Bone Syndrome: Osteogenesis Imperfecta. Butterworths, London, 1983.

16. Weil, U.H.: Osteogenesis imperfecta: Historical background. Clin. Orthop. Rel. Res. 159, 6, 1981.

17. White, N.J., Wineris, C.B., and Smith, R.: Cardiovascular abnormalities in osteogenesis imperfecta. Am. Heart J. 116, 1416, 1983.

18. Wynne-Davies, R. and Gormely, J.: Clinical and genetic patterns in osteogenesis imperfecta. Clin. Orthop. Rel. Res. 159, 26, 1981.

Setpoint Proposal for Osteogenesis Imperfecta

H. M. Frost

Introduction

This article summarizes the details of a possible pathogenetic mechanism in osteogenesis imperfecta (OGIM). It concerns the minimum effective strain (MES) described in a companion article in this volume (Frost, 1985a), specifically the strains involved in the control, by the mechanical usage of the skeleton, of its bone modeling, remodeling, and microdamage repair. The MES phenomenon was described by the author, based on clinical evidence, in 1963 (Frost, 1963). It has been supported by *in vivo* strain gauge studies of bone carried out in laboratory animals by a number of investigators since 1975 (Frost, in press).

The MES is a threshold range that separates strains too small to affect living bone's biologic systems from larger strains that consistently affect them (Frost, 1985a). The location of that range on the horizontal axis of the MES-biologic response graph (Frost, 1985a, Fig. 12) would represent its setpoint, biochemically trivial or ineffective stains lying to its left, and nontrivial ones to the right. Available evidence suggests that bone modeling, remodeling and microdamage repair activities may each have their own physical kinds and magnitude of MES (Frost, 1985a), and that predictable architectural and dynamic abnormalities can occur if their setpoints become too low or too high. Certain clinicopathologic features of OGIM might appear in a typical patient between 5 and 12 years of age.

The Elevated Setpoint Predictions

Clinical pathology in osteogenesis imperfecta

Table I lists 19 major features of OGIM in 5-12 year old patients (Sillence, 1981). Some of the features listed usually change at or after the time of skeletal maturation around 18 years of age.

Setpoint predictions

a) Modeling

Strains caused by mechanical usage enable bone modeling which then, and beyond the effects of mechanically unmodified growth alone, normally increases outside diaphyseal bone diameter and tends to retard diaphyseal marrow cav-

Current Concepts of Bone Fragility

Table I. Clinical pathology of osteogenesis imperfecta*

Subnormal outside diaphyseal bone diameter
Relatively large diaphyseal marrow cavity diameter
Reduced cortical cross section area
Osteopenic primary and secondary spongiosa
Bone fragility and increased fractures
Postfracture malunions correct slowly and incompletely
A global osteopenia of the growth-modeling type is present
Compact bone BMU-based remodeling is supranormal (Frost, in press)
The younger the disease becomes apparent, the more severe it is
No diagnostic changes in serum, urine, hepatic, renal, hematologic, GI, pulmonary, endocrine or neuromotor variables
Blue sclerae, thin tendon, ligament, fascia, dermis
Dentinogenesis imperfecta, otosclerosis
Complete fractures usually heal normally

* The setpoint proposal correctly predicts all the above reatures except otosclerosis

ity expansion (Frost, 1985a; Frost, in press). A congenitally-elevated MES setpoint for modeling should therefore retard growth in outside diameter and cause slender bones, plus a relative increase in the marrow cavity, resulting in a decreased cortical cross section area.

Since the modeling function specifically corrects postfracture malunions of long bones in normal children (Frost, 1985; Frost, in press), an elevated modeling setpoint would cause such corrections to occur both more slowly than normal and incompletely, the deformities of multiple fractures thus tending to accumulate.

b) Remodeling

Since increasing mechanical usage inhibits BMU-based remodeling, and thus turnover of compacta and primary and secondary spongiosa, and since the ΔB.BMU that controls the bone balance affects remodeling < 0 on trabecular and cortical-endosteal surfaces (Frost, 1985; Frost, in press), an increased remodeling setpoint should allow increased remodeling. This, in turn, would accelerate net losses of spongiosa and cause an OPn of spongiosa, plus enlargement of the marrow cavity and thus thinning as well.

c) MDx repair

Since mechanical microdamage usually initiates its own repair by remodeling (Frost 1985b), an increased setpoint for that initiation should retard repair and let microdamage pile up, which would cause the clinical phenomena of increased bone fragility and increased numbers of fractures. Since subsequent fracture healing is a pathologic and quite different activity from physiologic modeling and remodeling, there is no apparent reason why it should also be impaired.

d) The age-severity relation

Since the mechanical strains caused by normal mechanical usage are typically larger in infants than in adolescents, which in turn exceed those in adults, small setpoint increases have no obvious effects until later during growth when the control of modeling and remodeling by mechanical usage usually depends on smaller strains. However, large setpoint increases have obvious effects in infancy or even *in utero* (Frost, 1985a; Frost, in press). Accordingly, the greater the setpoint increases the more severe the disease and the sooner it becomes apparent.

e) Global bone mass (ABV)

ABV normally peaks between age 20 and 30 years and much of its increase is determined by partly predictable mechanical usage effects on the growing skeleton (Frost, 1985a; Frost, in press). From *a* and *b* above, a congenitally increased MES setpoint for modeling and remodeling would cause that ABV to increase more slowly than normal, to peak at a lower value, and probably also peak at a later age than normal. Because of that OPn, the production of new MDx during normal mechanical usage increases (Frost 1985a) which would also tend to increase bone fragility.

f) Other structures

The setpoint proposal can also apply to growing dentin and fibrous tissues, including sclera, dermis, tendon, fascia and ligament. The predicted effects on those tissues of an elevated modeling MES setpoint are described elsewhere (Frost, 1985a; Frost, in press). Without exception they match the observed pathologic findings.

g) Those increased MES setpoints do not seem to require or cause any known serum, urine, hematologic, pulmonary, renal, cardiovascular, GI, GU, or CNS abnormalities (Frost, in press)

Discussion

Comparison of theory to fact

The setpoint proposal described briefly above correctly predicts all but one of the entries (otosclerosis) listed in Table I which may serve to enhance the understanding of bone physiology and the theory behind it.

The common denominator(s)

The pathology listed in Table I represents the direct results of behavioral malfunctions of eight histologically and clinically distinct organized multicellular IO mechanisms. These are BMU-based remodeling of growth plates, primary spongiosa, secondary spongiosa and compacta, modeling of compact bone, fibrous tissue and dentin, and MDx physiology (Frost, in press). The diversity of those activities, mechanisms, and tissues suggests they may not all use the same physical means to generate controlling signals from their mechanically-induced strains, thus lacking a common denominator.

However, the biologic part of their MES mechanisms (to the right of the vertical dashed lines below) should involve an intermediary signal detector cell-secondary signal generator coupled (Frost, 1985a) as schematically shown below:

load → bone → strain → primary signal ⇸ detector cell → secondary signal

→ responding I) unit (remodeling, modeling)

That cellularly based detector-secondary signal couple or mechanism should be a common denominator in the modeling, remodeling and microdamage repair responses of each of the above tissues. It could be the only one or one of the mechanisms specifically defective in OGIM. While the idea is frankly speculative, the precision with which it predicts the real pathology lends it credibility, and I believe it will prove to be another among the many truths that could ultimately explain the pathologic and pathogenetic spectra of OGIM. It should be understood that the present proposals do not imply that no other pathologic or pathogenetic mechanisms occur in OGIM. Whatever they are, however, these proposals probably are additional. If, to explain each entry in Table I, the setpoint proposal had an equal probability of being correct or wrong, then the likelihood of being correct by chance alone in 19 of 20 consecutive matters would be $p \ll .0001$.

Genetic roots

While abnormalities in Type I collagen chemistry have been found in most of the OGIM variants studied to date (Brown, 1981), it is not apparent to me how they might cause the cell behavioral abnormalities described above, which do occur. The hypothesis presented here does not concern those behavioral abnormalities, for they are, in my opinion, unquestionably the real and direct causes of the pathologic process. In this regard it seems possible that the known abnormalities in collagen chemistry need not and may not directly cause the above cell behavioral abnormalities of OGIM nor the postulated increase in the MES setpoint. While that suggests more than one basic genetic defect in this group of diseases, the clinical variants described by Sillence (1981) among others already indicate that more than one such defect must exist. The idea is therefore not unreasonable at this time. Space limitations prevent discussing some further pertinent phenomena of OGIM in the fetus and neonate, and in adults. I would state, however, that the setpoint proposal, analytically speaking, seems to offer reasonable explanations for many of those problems too.

References

1. Brown, D.M.: Biochemical abnormalities in osteogenesis imperfecta. Clin. Orthop. Rel. Res. 159, 75, 1981.
2. Frost, H.M.: An Introduction to Biomechanics, Charles C. Thomas, Springfield, 1963.
3. Frost, H.M.: Pathogenic mechanisms of the osteoporosis. In, Current Concepts of Bone Fragility in Orthopaedics and Medicine. Eds: H.-K. Uhthoff and E. Stahl, Springer-Verlag, 1985a.
4. Frost, H.M.: Osteogenesis imperfecta: The setpoint proposal. Clin. Orthop. Rel. Res. In press

5. Frost, H.M.: Bone microdamage: Factors that impair its repair. In, Current Concepts of Bone Fragility in Orthopaedics and Medicine. Eds: H.-K. Uhthoff and E. Stahl, Springer-Verlag, 1985b.

6. Sillence, D.: Osteogenesis imperfecta. An expanding panorama of variants. Clin. Orthop. Rel. Res. 159, 11, 1981.

Osteogenesis Imperfecta: Orthopedic Aspects

J. G. Birch

Introduction

Osteogenesis imperfecta (OI) is a hereditary disorder characterized primarily by excessive bone fragility. Associated abnormalities can include blue sclera, generalized ligamentous laxity, dentinogenesis imperfecta and pre-senile hearing loss. The presence and severity of the various manifestations of the disorder vary markedly. Furthermore, the exact biochemical abnormality is as yet unidentified.

Sillence (Sillence and Danks, 1978) has presented a useful classification identifying four major groups of patients based on genetic and morphologic features. Clinical severity can markedly vary within each group, limiting the usefulness of the system in the orthopedic evaluation of individual patients. The modification of Looser's classification (Looser, 1906) presented by Falvo and associates (1974), consisting of osteogenesis imperfecta congenita, tarda I (with bowing), and tarda II (without bowing), remains a clinically useful classification to determine the prognosis for ambulation and the need for orthopedic intervention.

Conservative Orthopedic Care

The degree of bone fragility varies between patients who have thin cortices and sparse trabeculae with only a few fractures throughout life, and the severely involved patients with "popcorn" epiphyses, undetectable physes, and significant bony deformity due to repeated fractures. The presence or absence of birth fractures does not appear to be a significant prognostic factor for either progressive bony deformity or ambulation potential. Severe osteopenia and repeated fractures with resultant deformity of the long bones of the lower extremity are more significant.

Fractures in osteogenesis imperfecta are generally treated by routine conservative methods. Since disuse osteoporosis will aggravate any tendency to fracture, the extent and duration of immobilization should be kept to a minimum; early weight bearing and rapid mobilization are recommended. Frequently, patients will complain of pain and local tenderness suggestive of a fracture but without radiographic confirmation. In this circumstance, they should be immobilized until symptoms resolve. Further investigation by tomography or bone scan to document the presence of a fracture is usually unnecessary. Most fractures in OI heal fairly rapidly. However, malunion is frequent and can lead to progressive deformity.

Current Concepts of Bone Fragility

Nonunion of fractures is uncommon. In a review of 53 patients treated at Texas Scottish Rite Hospital for Crippled Children over the past 15 years, only three patients (all with OI congenita) were identified as having pseudarthroses. One case each of pseudarthrosis of the humerus and of the radius and ulna were encountered, both resulting from repeated fractures and associated with severe bowing of the affected long bone. Both patients were asymptomatic, and the pseudarthroses were left untreated. One patient had pseudarthroses of both femora, requiring corrective osteotomy and intramedullary fixation to alleviate excessive tenderness and instability.

Recognized physeal injury in OI is likewise uncommon. Three patients in our series suffered Salter-Harris Type II injuries, one of the proximal humerus and two of the distal tibia. Subsequent growth disturbance did not occur.

Intra-articular fractures are also rare. In our series, one patient suffered an acetabular fracture associated with a traumatic posterior dislocation of the hip in a water-skiing accident; this fracture was managed nonsurgically without sequelae. Two patients suffered three displaced intra-articular fractures of the olecranon which were treated by open reduction and internal fixation, using an AO tension band wiring technique. This is our preferred method of treatment, with careful consideration given to the increased bone fragility intraoperatively. Early removal of internal fixation is recommended to prevent subsequent growth disturbance of the olecranon apophysis. All three fractures healed uneventfully following this procedure.

Four patients in this series suffered transcervical fractures of the femoral neck. Three were minimally displaced and healed uneventfully with pin fixation and spica immobilization. One patient, however, had significant displacement and union failed after two attempts at closed reduction and pin fixation. The fracture healed after valgus osteotomy and compression screw fixation but avascular necrosis of the femoral head ensued. Despite obvious irregularity of the femoral head on radiographs, he remains asymptomatic four years after the fracture.

Bracing of the lower extremities may be very helpful in managing repeated fractures which might otherwise interfere with mobility in the absence of significant bony deformity. Because of the reduced stature of these patients and their generally poor muscular strength, braces should be as lightweight as possible. Plastic braces with lightweight metals are generally preferable; significant swelling with continued fractures, however, may be better managed with conventional braces which allow greater tolerance of acute swelling while permitting weight bearing. Long leg braces in the presence of proximal femoral deformity can lead to a stress-riser effect and fracture at the upper end of a brace; for this reason, the addition of a brace with an external articulation at the level of the hip and a pelvic band are often required.

Despite generalized ligamentous laxity, symptomatic subluxations and dislocations were infrequent in our series. One patient suffered a traumatic dislocation of the hip. Another patient had an unreduced dislocation of the radial head associated with a Monteggia fracture; the radial head was eventually excised for local symptoms. Ligamentous laxity was associated with marked planovalgus feet in many of our patients. Orthotic management, such as UCBL* inserts, were occasionally required to improve shoe wear. Most

---

* University of California Biomechanics Laboratory

patients in our series did not develop more severe symptoms relative to their feet.

Excessive bone fragility leads to repeated vertebral fractures causing codfish vertebrae, and contributes to progressive scoliosis and kyphosis. Significantly displaced spinal fractures, however, are unusual. One patient in this series suffered a hangman type fracture of the second cervical vertebra which was treated successfully with immobilization in a soft collar.

Management of Long Bone Deformity

Sofield (Sofield and Millar, 1959) presented a ten-year evaluation of fragmentation, realignment, and intramedullary rod fixation of the long bones in children with deformity, most of whom had OI. Sofield's technique consists of subperiosteal exposure of the entire shaft of the affected long bone. The shaft is removed from its bed and divided into a sufficient number of fragments to allow realignment. The fragments are reamed and then threaded on a rod. Sofield recommended Rush rods or bent Steinman pins. In a series of 117 patients, he reported two serious infections, no nonunions, and no major vascular embarrassment in any patient.

Bailey and Dubow (1963) introduced the concept of the extensible intramedullary rod. This has the theoretic and clinically-substantiated benefit of reducing the frequency of rod replacement. When solid rods (such as a Rush rod) are used in skeletally immature patients, the bone can angulate or fracture at the end of the rod. With the Bailey-Dubow rods fixed in the epiphysis, these problems are avoided. The insertion of an extensible rod is a more extensive procedure, and some authors had the impression of a higher rate of infection occurring than when fixed length rods were used. The surgical procedure is usually combined with Sofield fragmentation. The rods themselves have two components: an outer hollow rod with a removable, threaded T-end, and an inner solid rod with a fixed T-end. The threaded T-end may disconnect and be found to lie free in the tissues when it is not embedded in the bone (such as in the proximal femur). Bailey (1981) subsequently recommended using a fixed T-end for the outer hollow rod as well. We have continued to use the removable variety since intra-articular insertion of a fixed T-rod requires significant articular exposure, particularly in the ankle.

The Sofield procedure is most often indicated in the lower extremities where fractures are more frequent and where deformity often interferes with ambulation. We generally use the solid inner rod, distally in the femur and proximally in the tibia, to avoid the possibility of the removable T-end coming free in the knee joint. Bailey recommended that the T-end not be embedded in the articular cartilage in the knee; we normally embed it in the bone to prevent migration. The T-end must be embedded through the articular cartilage into the epiphyseal bone in the proximal humerus, distal humerus, and the distal tibia, to avoid interference with joint function.

Repeated fracture and significant long bone deformity in ambulatory patients are considered the primary indications for Sofield osteotomies and intramedullary fixation. We have also found the procedure helpful in nonambulatory patients who have problems with repeated fractures.

Fifteen of our 53 patients underwent 42 procedures of Sofield fragmentation and Bailey-Dubow rodding. They showed satisfactory results overall in what were otherwise difficult clinical situations. Even in nonambulatory patients, significant reduction in fracture frequency occurred and long bone integrity was maintained. This occurred even when the radiographic appearance was less than satisfactory from the point of view of inadequate rod lengthening, separation of the T-end, or protrusion of a portion of the rod beyond the cortex. Significant complications included one infection which resolved with debridement and removal of the implant; one nonunion in a preexisting humeral pseudarthrosis; and six implant failures. These implant failures included three cases of cutout requiring removal; two cases of articular encroachment requiring removal; and one case of bending of a femoral rod requiring replacement. Eight other patients had undergone fragmentation with intramedullary fixation using Rush rod or Steinman pin fixation two or more years before skeletal maturity. Each of these patients required revision for rod migration, deformity beyond the end of the rod, or fracture beyond the end of the rod.

Spinal Deformity in Osteogenesis Imperfecta

A particularly challenging task in patients with OI has been adequate management of progressive scoliosis. Lordo- and kyphoscoliosis secondary to ligamentous laxity and repeated microfractures can be progressive and quite severe. Brace treatment is generally believed to be ineffective, and has been demonstrated to produce potentially harmful secondary rib deformity (Benson et al, 1978). *In situ* posterior spinal fusion is hampered by difficult postoperative immobilization. Routine Harrington instrumentation is frequently difficult due to laminar fracture at hook sites (Cristofaro et al, 1979; Yong-Hing and MacEwen, 1982). Polymethylmethacrylate augmentation of the Harrington hook site can reduce the incidence of hook site failure.

Five patients have been treated at Texas Scottish Rite Hospital with posterior spinal fusion combined with Luque-type segmental spinal instrumentation with satisfactory results. Despite sometimes severe bone fragility, sufficient stability has been achieved to maintain curve correction and avoid immobilization in most patients.

Only minimal curve correction was obtained (averaging 17% in these patients) so that early surgery was indicated once a curve had been documented to progress beyond 40°. Intraoperative blood loss exceeded standard cases, averaging 70% of estimated blood volume in these patients. Furthermore, since the iliac crests are not adequate sources of autogenous bone, allograft bone must be available for grafting purposes. In this series, no failure of internal fixation occurred, and no progression of a fused curve after follow-ups averaging one year.

Anesthetic Considerations

Several specific problems are associated with OI that the anesthesiologist must consider (Libman, 1981). First, the patient is obviously quite fragile, and even the application of a blood pressure cuff may cause fracture. Bone and tooth fragility as well as narrow airways may lead to difficult intubation. The most significant anesthetic consideration in OI is the presence of a hypermetabolic state which can lead to rising intraoperative body temperature similar to malignant hyperthermia. The exact etiology is unclear, possibly related to a disturbance of calcium metabolism. On this basis, the elevation in body temperature can be blocked by preoperative administration of dantrolene. Life-threatening arrhythmias generally associated with true malignant hyperthermia do not usually occur. Preoperative agitation or fever, however, should lead to cancellation of scheduled surgery. Finally, capillary fragility, cortical fragility, and demanding technical details during most orthopedic procedures combine to create greater than average blood loss which should be anticipated.

Summary

The broad spectrum of clinical severity of bone fragility in patients with OI can be a difficult and challenging problem for the orthopedic surgeon. Fractures should be managed in a routine fashion, with heavy emphasis on conservative treatment, minimal degree of immobilization, early weight bearing, and rapid mobilization where possible. Protective bracing may be effective in controlling repeated fractures. Sofield fragmentation with Bailey-Dubow intramedullary fixation in skeletally immature patients has been very satisfactory in our hands. Progressive scoliosis can be a significant problem in these patients; brace management is ineffective and probably detrimental. Segmental spinal instrumentation has been extremely helpful in alleviating technical difficulties in the surgical management and the postoperative immobilization of patients with progressive scoliosis.

References

1. Bailey, R.W., and Dubow, H.I.: Studies of longitudinal bone growth resulting in an extensible nail. Surgical Forum, Am. Coll. Surg. XIV, 1963.

2. Bailey, R.W.: Further clinical experiences with the extensible nail. Clin. Orthop. Rel. Res. 159, 171, 1981.

3. Benson, D.R., Donaldson, D.H., and Millar, E.A.: The spine and osteogenesis imperfecta. J. Bone Joint Surg. 60A, 925, 1978.

4. Cristofaro, R.L., Hoek, K.J., Bonnett, C.A., and Brown, J.C.: Operative treatment of spine deformity in osteogenesis imperfecta. Clin. Orthop. Rel. Res. 139, 40, 1979.

5. Falvo, K.A., Root, L., and Bullough, P.G.: Osteogenesis imperfecta: Clinical evaluation and management. J. Bone Joint Surg. 56A, 783, 1974.

6. Libman, R.H.: Anesthetic considerations for the patient with osteogenesis imperfecta. Clin. Orthop. Rel. Res. 159, 123, 1981.

7. Looser, E.: Für Kenntnis de Osteogenesis Imperfecta Congenita et Tarda. Mitt Grenzgeb. Med. u. Chir. 15, 161, 1906.

8. Sillence, D.O., and Danks, D.M.: The differentiation of genetically distinct varieties of osteogenesis imperfecta in the newborn period. Clin. Res. 26, 178A, 1978.

9. Sofield, H.A., and Millar, E.A.: Fragmentation, realignment and intramedullary rod fixation of deformities of the long bones in children. J. Bone Joint Surg. 41A, 1371, 1959.

10. Yong-Hing, K., and MacEwen, G.D.: Scoliosis associated with osteogenesis imperfecta: Results of treatment. J. Bone Joint Surg. 64B, 36, 1982.

Paget's Disease of Bone (Osteitis deformans)

J. R. SHAPIRO

Introduction

Sir James Paget presented five cases illustrating a chronic, slowly progressive and disabling bone disorder to the Medical and Chirurgical Society of London on November 14, 1876 (Handy, 1981). A century later, we are able to apply medical therapy which slows the progress of the disease in many patients but cures none. The etiology of Paget's disease remains obscure, although recent evidence suggests (but does not prove), that its cause is a putative viral infection of skeletal osteoclasts.

Paget's disease is notable for a large number of subjects who remain mostly asymptomatic. On the other hand, significant morbidity occurs in a relatively small group of patients, probably due to concomitant osteoarthritis or erosive arthritis associated with the primary disorder. Complications of Paget's disease -- fractures, spinal or cranial nerve compression, deafness, heart failure, osteosarcoma -- are, with the exception of fractures, relatively uncommon. Pain, skeletal deformity and limited mobility are common but highly variable, even in one individual. Certain patients are frequently resistant to both medical and surgical therapy.

The epidemiology of Paget's disease is interesting. It affects approximately 3% of the population over age 41 in the Western hemisphere, Australia and New Zealand, but is extremely uncommon in Asia, the Middle East and Africa. In Great Britain, its prevalence varies from 8.3% of hospitalized patients over 51 years of age in the town of Lancaster, to 2.3% for a comparable group in the town of Aberdeen (Barker et al, 1981). It is slightly more common in men than women, but occurs equally in blacks and whites in North America.

Physicians dealing with the clinical problems of Paget's disease must confront several issues and questions:

- How strong is the evidence for a viral etiology? Will curing Paget's disease require eliminating the putative virus?

- What is the meaning of familial clustering: is osteitis deformans a heritable disorder?

- What is the explanation for the spontaneous flares and remissions which occur in Paget's disease?

Current Concepts of Bone Fragility

- Which are the best measurements for evaluating the activity of the disease, before or during therapy?
- Which patients should be treated?
- Which symptoms will respond to therapy, and which will not?

Evidence for a Viral Etiology of Osteitis deformans

Microtubular filamentous inclusion bodies in osteoclast nuclei and cytoplasm of Paget's disease have been described by Gherardi et al (1981), Mills and Singer (1976), and Revel et al (1975). They are not present in other metabolic bone diseases (Mills and Singer, 1976; Revel et al, 1975). They consist of paracrystalline arrangements of microfilaments which at times are seen to surround a granular core similar to dense chromatin. Considered viral nucleocapsids, their viral identification remains somewhat speculative. Gherardi (1981) has found nuclear microfilaments to be slightly argyrophylic, 111-311 µm long, packed parallel to form bundles. These intranuclear and intracytoplasmic inclusions are similar to myxo- and paramyxoviruses, among which are measles, mumps, respiratory syncytial virus, and the parainfluenza viruses. Revel et al (1975) used immunofluroescence and immunoperoxidase staining to demonstrate measles virus antigen in osteoclasts from Paget's disease. Subsequently, Mills et al (1981) reported fluorescent antibody studies which identified respiratory syncytial virus. Later, positive reaction towards both respiratory syncytial and measles virus were obtained with affected osteoclasts. The finding of both viruses is unexplained (Mills et al, 1984). Howatson and Fornasier (1982) compared osteoclast microtubules in Paget's disease to nucleocapsids in cells infected with measles virus and respiratory syncytial virus. While the distribution of microtubules in Paget's disease was similar to that in cells infected with measles' nucleocapsids, they differed in conformation and location. These authors suggested that the inclusions simulated a pneumovirus (respiratory syncytial) rather than measles virus. Although immunofluorescence has been positive with bone cells in tissue culture, inclusion bodies have not been identified in cells passed in tissue culture.

Familial Clustering in Osteitis deformans

The prevalence of familial osteitis deformans has increased within the past few years, perhaps due to increased awareness of this disease. The tendency of Paget's disease to recur within certain families exceeds random distribution. Singer reported a familial distribution with autosomal dominant inheritance in 15% of cases, while Siris et al observed that nearly 31% of affected individuals had a positive family history (Singer et al, 1978; 1985; Siris et al, 1981). However, the incidence among identical twins is less than expected.

The presence of shared HLA antigens in Paget's disease has been uncertain. Singer et al (1985) have demonstrated that both familial and sporadic Paget's disease have an increased incidence of HLA-DQW 1 antigens, and increased incidence of the DQW 1 associated antigens DR1, DR2 and DRW 6. Thus, immunoregulatory factors could play a role in determining susceptibility to a putative viral agent.

Spontaneous Flares and Remissions: Pathophysiology

The primary event in osteitis deformans is excessive bone resorption; osteoclasts increase in activity and number. Presumably, an intact mechanism coupling bone formation and resorption invokes compensatory osteoblastic activity, visible adjacent to areas of resorption. The trigger, as noted above, may be linked to preexisting viral infection. However, if virus infection is involved, then questions arise regarding factors which modify the expression of that infection, the manner by which certain bones are involved more frequently than others, the nature of factors which moderate flares and remissions, or the eventual inactivity (sclerotic phase) of the pagetic process in some patients.

Three phases have been recognized in the evolution of Paget's disease: 1) the initial osteolytic phase, which involves resorption of previously normal bone; 2) the active, or mixed -lytic and -blastic phase, which is associated with increased vascularity in the involved areas; and 3) an inactive or sclerotic phase in which both osteoclastic and osteoblastic activity has ceased (Handy, 1981). In fact, these are not distinct in time but tend to overlap. Total inactivity of the disease is rarely seen; some activity almost always persists. Indeed, bone adjacent to involved areas may not be morphologically normal.

Variables of Disease Activity

Variables of the disease process useful in determining the current activity of Paget's disease include the following: serum alkaline phosphatase activity (heat labile fraction); urinary hydroxyproline and hydroxylysine excretion; the measurement of serum osteocalcin and urinary Gla protein; and the uptake of bone-seeking isotopes. Determination of serum collagen propeptides has been applied to Paget's disease but is still a research tool. The following limitations apply to these clinical tests of disease activity:

Serum alkaline phosphatase activity, a composite of several isoenzymes, reflects osteoblastic not osteoclastic function, and is therefore only an indirect measure of disease activity. The bone - derived fraction is approximately 51% of total serum enzyme activity; hepatic, intestinal, placental, or neoplastic isoenzymes make up the remainder (Van Lente, 1979). Bone-derived enzyme is usually identified by its inactivation by heat at 56 degrees, or inactivation with urea, or phenylalanine. Skeletal alkaline phosphatase is heterogenous, and attempts to characterize the enzyme with monoclonal antibodies have proved incomplete (Mulivor et al, 1985). The correlation between rates of bone turnover and serum alkaline phosphatase activity approximates only 51%.

Measurement of *urinary hydroxyproline* is more reflective of osteoclastic activity in Paget's disease. Due to further degradation, however, hydroxyproline in urine is only about 25% of that actually metabolized in bone; it is, therefore, only an indirect measure of disease activity. Nevertheless, correlation with rates of bone turnover appears to be higher than that for alkaline phosphatase -- approximately 61%. One problem of frequent measurement of hydroxyproline has been the need to ingest a meat- and gelatin-free diet for three days before 24 hour urine collection. Studies by Niell et al (1981) suggest that because ingested hydroxyproline is cleared rapidly, a 12-hour fast followed by determination of the hydroxyproline/creatinine ratio on a fasting urine sample may provide a clinically useful and more convenient estimate of collagen turnover in bone.

Hydroxylysine, also a collagen amino acid, provides a more accurate measure of collagen turnover than hydroxyproline because it is not degraded; however, it is present in one-tenth the quantity of hydroxyproline and tests are not available on a routine basis (Krane et al, 1977).

Osteocalcin is a vitamin K-dependent, calcium-binding protein found in bone and distinguished by the presence of 3 gamma carboxy-glutamic acid (Gla) residues. Measurable in serum by radioimmunoassay, osteocalcin is considered to mirror the rate of bone turnover. The urinary excretion of breakdown products of osteocalcin and other Gla-containing proteins, mostly clotting factors, less accurately reflects bone turnover. Gundberg et al (1983) have found serum osteocalcin measurement increased three-fold in Paget's disease; urinary Gla excretion was consistently normal regardless of disease activity. The measurement of serum osteocalcin, when commercially available, should provide an accurate evaluation of bone turnover in Paget's disease.

The *uptake of bone-seeking isotopes* (Tc-99m disphosphate) is useful in the initial evaluation of Paget's disease. Vellenega et al (1984) have evaluated scintigraphy in the untreated pagetic patient with the following results: 16% of lesions visualized on scan showed no radiologic abnormalities. Radiographic deformation and scintigraphic score were associated with increased symptomatology, and biochemical measurements of activity were positively correlated with scintigraphic indices. The whole body retention of Tc-99m diphosphonate has been suggested for the quantitative assessment of bone turnover, but its usefulness, particularly during diphosphonate therapy, has been questioned. Smith et al (1984) found whole bone retention of radiolabeled diphosphonate to correlate well with serum alkaline phosphatase and urinary hydroxyproline excretion, during, and for 13 months following oral diphosphonate therapy.

The triple helical collagen precursor, *procollagen*, contains both N- and C-terminal propeptide extensions which are cleaved by specific proteases once procollagen is secreted into the extracellular space. A radioimmunoassay for procollagen C-terminal propeptide in serum was initially developed by Taubman, who demonstrated abnormally high levels of the procollagen protein in the serum of patients with Paget's disease (Taubman et al, 1976). Simon et al (1984) have also found determination of type I procollagen C-terminal propeptide to be a potentially useful marker of bone collagen turnover in Paget's disease.

Treatment

Effective medical and surgical therapies are available for the treatment of Paget's disease. However, their proper use, either singly or in combination, must be individualized and depends on the patient's symptoms, the activity of the disease, and the expected outcome of therapy. Some patients need not be treated, while others require therapy regardless of biochemical evidence of activity; eg, the decision to treat should not be based solely on the level of serum alkaline phosphatase or the radiologic extent of skeletal involvement.

Indications for pharmacotherapy in Paget's disease as defined by Merkow and Lane (1984) include:

1) pain, chronic and debilitating;
2) significant deformity which may presage fracture;
3) compression syndromes: vertebral overgrowth with radiculopathy or cranial nerve compression;
4) pathologic fractures requiring immobilization or to facilitate healing;
5) high output congestive cardiac failure;
6) preoperative -- osteotomy or arthroplasty -- for three months if possible;
7) immobilization hypercalcemia;
8) alkaline phosphatase elevation, if at least twice normal and associated with significant symptoms.

Treatment is not indicated in mildly symptomatic patients or those with osteoarthritic complaints whose pain may be controlled with salicylates or nonsteroidal anti-inflammatory drugs. There is no set level of elevation in alkaline phosphatase which requires treatment. Conversely, in certain subjects the level of chemical tests does not accurately match the activity of disease. In addition, therapy with bone-specific agents will not be effective for the following complications:

- VIII nerve palsy with deafness;
- coxa vara deformities of the hip;
- long bone deformities;
- symptoms primarily due to osteoarthritis;
- osteosarcoma.

Opinion is divided about the use of salmon calcitonin or diphosphonate as initial therapy. The choice is frequently a cost factor, and whether the patient or family can handle parenteral administration of calcitonin.

Calcitonin

Calcitonin modifies the activity of Paget's disease by inhibiting osteoclastic bone resorption, and is most effective where bone turnover is elevated. Salmon calcitonin is useful because its clearance in serum is prolonged compared with porcine or human analogues. Human calcitonin, which should be nonantigenic, is not commercially available.

Where feasible, I recommend initiating therapy with salmon calcitonin, particularly for those with osteolytic lesions. Evidence is conflicting whether diphosphonates aggravate osteolytic disease and increase the risk of fracture. Johnston et al (1983) did not find an increase of fractures in diphosphonate-treated patients. Subcutaneous, compared with intramuscular injection of calcitonin, lessens annoying side effects of nausea and flushing, both of which are transient. Most patients tolerate a dose of 111 MRC units, or 1.1 mg protein, three or four times weekly with minimal nausea. MacIntytre et al (1980) recommend using calcitonin twice weekly for six months, after which, if symptoms have been relieved, medication can be taken intermittently. Biochemical relapse, if significant, can be treated with twice weekly injections, while radiologic or clinical relapse may require more frequent, or even daily injections. Retreatment will usually result in a prompt fall in urinary hydroxyproline and serum alkaline phosphatase levels. Calcitonin promotes a 51-85% fall in baseline alkaline phosphatase levels. Resistance to calcitonin occurs for various reasons, including the formation of antibodies -- in 61% of patients -- but only 11% become clinically resistant. Patients may exhibit a plateau in biochemical response, or they may demonstrate complete escape from inhibition of osteoclast activity; however, the presence of anticalcitonin antibodies does not necessarily signify resistance, and a clinical response may persist in spite of a biochemical relapse (Singer et al, 1977). The duration of remission varies once therapy is stopped. Recurrence is signaled by an increase in alkaline phosphatase followed by an increase in urinary hydroxyproline.

Diphosphonates

Diphosphonates are structural analogues of pyrophosphate which contain the P-C-P rather than the P-O-P backbone. Three have been investigated clinically, but only etidronate disodium (EHDP) is marketed. The potent agent dichloromethylene diphosphonate is not available, while a newer and reportedly highly effective compound, APD (3-amino-1-hydroxypropylidene), is being tested overseas (Frijlink et al, 1979). Diphosphonates act both to decrease bone resorption and inhibit mineralization. The former is a result of direct ingestion of the agent by osteoclasts resulting in a toxicity to those cells, while the latter effect is the result of EHDP binding to the surface of hydroxyapatite crystals causing inhibition of crystal growth and dissolution. Diphosphonate therapy has several advantages compared with calcitonin: it is given orally, costs less, and has few side effects other than a rise in serum phosphate and mild gastrointestinal upsets. The conventional dosage of EHDP, not associated with a significant mineralization defect, is 5 mg/kg/day, or approximately 411 mg in an adult. Higher dosages may be warranted, but these incur the risk of inducing the mineralization defect. With treatment, bone turnover falls, pain is diminished, and isotope scans show improvement within six months of therapy.

Alexandre et al found a reduction of about 70% in alkaline phosphatase and urinary hydroxyproline levels associated with a significant reduction in the number of osteoclasts. Therapy is usually limited to cycles of six months to limit the development of abnormal, uncalcified matrix.

As to the failure of lesions to improve radiologically, de Deuxchaisnes (1984) found that at a dose of 7 mg/kg/day, osteolytic lesions were negatively affected in 56% of patients; no effect was seen in 11%, while a dissociated effect with both positive and negative signs occurred in 33%. Overall, prolonged clinical remission has been noted in approximately one-third of patients following therapy with diphosphonates.

Bijvoet et al (1978) and Mautalen (1983) have published results of therapy with APD. Biochemical remission as a consequence of inhibition of bone resorption was rapidly achieved in the majority; in some instances remission was prolonged. A lessened formation of osteoid may be an important feature of APD.

Combination therapy: calcitonin and EHDP

Bijvoet et al (1980) reported that 25 of 31 patients given 111 MRC units of calcitonin and 7.5 mg/kg/day of EHDP concurrently experience complete biochemical remission after 6-12 months of therapy. Sustained remission occurred in 11 patients, including those with active and widespread disease. However, de Deuxchaisnes (1980) has observed EHDP-related osteolytic lesions appearing once combination therapy was discontinued, presumably due to the continued presence of the agent in bone. Perry et al (1984) have administered calcitonin and etidronate alternately to 37 patients with Paget's disease. They concluded that the patients showed better biochemical and symptomatic response when treatment was initiated with EHDP for the first six months. No difference in bone scan appearance was seen between the two regimens. This study suggests that calcitonin should be considered as follow-up therapy in patients treated for six months with etidronate.

Mithramycin

Ryan, who has extensive experience with this drug, states that mithramycin must be considered a second-line agent in the treatment of Paget's disease because of its toxicity (Ryan, 1983). Mithramycin should be reserved for patients who have not responded to other agents or in whom a rapid response is essential, as in the presence of spinal cord compression. The drug has several disadvantages. It must be administered intravenously over several hours, which is very costly, and is irritating if leaked into soft tissues. It may be administered by indwelling intravenous catheter in patients requiring prolonged therapy. Careful monitoring of hepatic enzymes, serum creatinine and white blood cell and platelet counts are essential before each treatment. Therapy must be withheld when hepatic enzymes rise to ten times normal. While a ten-day course of therapy is customary, twice or thrice-weekly outpatient treatments may be useful in suppressing disease activity. A ten-day course of therapy may result in 61% reduction in alkaline phosphatase for one month, followed by a 25% reduction which may last for several months. While complete remission for two years has been observed, remissions are usually of shorter duration. Combination therapy with a six-month course of EHDP followed by 11 days of IV mithramycin has been suggested for unusually resistant patients (Ryan, 1980).

Conclusion

The patient with Paget's disease requires therapy for a variety of symptoms and signs: pain, osteoarthritis, erosive joint disease, deformities, fractures, and in about 1% of patients, osteosarcoma. Osteolytic and/or osteoblastic lesions may be due to osteitis deformans, to prostatic cancer or other neoplasms. Should a bone biopsy be performed for diagnosis, or will a bone scan suffice? If confirmed Paget's disease, do symptoms or biochemical variables require therapy, with which agent, and for how long? How much of the back or joint pain is due to osteoarthritis, and how much is the result of pagetic involvement? When is joint replacement, or laminectomy for spinal compression indicated? These are all too common questions in the management of Paget's disease; no set answers are applicable to all patients. It is clear, however, that most patients will gain maximum benefit if medical and surgical therapy are individualized and coordinated.

REFERENCES

1. Alexandre: Personal communication

2. Barker, D.J., Chamberlain, A.T., Guyer, P.B., Gardner, M.J.: Paget's disease of bone in 14 British towns. Brit.Med.J. 1, 1181, 1981.

3. Bijvoet, O.L.M.: Bisphosphonate treatment for Paget's disease of bone. In, Clinical Disorders of Bone and Mineral Metabolism. Eds: Frame, B. and Potts, J.T. Excerpta Medica, Amsterdam, 1984. pp 389-393.

4. Bijvoet, O.L.M., Frijlink, W.B., et al: APD in Paget's disease of bone. Arthritis Rheum. 23, 1193, 1980.

5. de Deuxchaisnes, C.N.: Do calcitonins help Paget's disease. In, Clinical Disorders of Bone and Mineral Metabolism. Eds: Frame, B. and Potts, J.T. Excerpta Medica, Amsterdam, 1984. pp 384-388.

6. de Deuxchaisnes, et al: Therapeutic regimens in Paget's disease of bone. Arthritis Rheum. 23, 1225, 1980.

7. Frijlink, W.B., TeVelde, J., Bijvoet, O.L., and Heynen, G.: Treatment of Paget's disease with (3-amino-1-hydroxypropylidene)-1, bisphosphonate (APD). Lancet 1, 799, 1979.

8. Gherardi, G., Lo Cascio, V., and Bonucci, E.: Fine structure of nuclei and cytoplasm of osteoclasts in Paget's disease of bone. Histopathology 4, 63, 1981.

9. Gundberg, C.M., Lian, J.B., Gallop, P.M., and Steinberg, J.J.: Urinary gamma carboxyglutamic acid and serum osteocalcin as bone markers: Studies in osteoporosis and Paget's disease. J.Clin.Endo.Metab. 57, 1221, 1983.

10. Handy, R.C.: Paget's Disease of Bone. Assessment and Management. Praeger Publ., Great Britain, 1981.

11. Howatson, A.F. and Fornasier, V.L.: Microfilaments associated with Paget's disease of bone: Comparison with nucleocapsids of measles virus and respiratory syncytial virus. Intervirology 18, 151, 1982.

12. Johnston, C.C., Altman, R.D., Canfield, R.E., Finerman, G.A.M., Taulbee, J.D., and Ebert, M.L.: Review of fracture experience during treatment of Paget's disease of bone with etidronate disodium (EHDP). Clin. Orthop. 172, 186 , 1983.

13. Krane, S.M., Kantrowitz, F.G., Byrne, M., Pinnell, S.R., and Singer, F.R.: Urinary excretion of hydroxylysine and its glycosides as an index of collagen degradation. J.Clin.Invest. 59, 819, 1977

14. MacIntyre, I., Evans, I.M., Hobitz, H.H.G., Joplin, G.F., and Stevenson, J.C.: Chemistry, physiology and therapeutic applications of calcitonin. Arthritis Rheum. 23, 1139, 1980

15. Mautalen, C.A.: Treatment of Paget's bone disease with bisphosphonate APD. Henry Ford Hosp.Med.J. 31, 244, 1983.

16. Merkow, R.L. and Lane, J.M.: Current concepts of Paget's disease of bone. Ortho.Clin.N.A. 15, 747, 1984

17. Mills, B. and Singer, F.: Nuclear inclusions in Paget's disease of bone. Science 194, 211, 1976.

18. Mills, B.G., Singer, F.R., Weiner, L.P., and Holst, P.A.: Immunohistological demonstration of respiratory syncytial virus antigens in Paget's disease of bone. Proc.Nat.Acad.Sci. 78, 1219, 1981.

19. Mills, B.G., Singer, F.R., Weiner, L.P., Suffin, S.C., Stabile, E., and Holst, P.: Evidence for both respiratory syncytial virus and measles virus antigens in the osteoclasts of patients with Paget's disease of bone. Clin. Orthop. 183, 313, 1984.

20. Mulivor, R.A., Boccelli, D., and Harris, H.: Quantitative analysis of alkaline phosphatases in serum and amniotic fluid: Comparison of biochemical and immunologic assays. J. Lab. Clin. Med. 115, 342, 1985.

21. Niell, H.B., Palmieri, G.M., Neely, C.L., and McDonald, M.W.: Postabsorptive urinary hydroxyproline test in patients with metastatic bone disease from breast cancer. Arch. Int. Med. 141, 1471, 1981.

22. Perry, H.M., Droke, D.M., and Avioli, L.V.: Alternate calcitonin and etidronate disodium therapy for Paget's bone disease. Arch. Int. Med. 144, 929, 1984.

23. Revel, A., Bregeon, C., Basle, M., and Malkani, K.: Is Paget's bone disease a viral infection? Calcif. Tiss. Res. 22, 283, 1975.

24. Ryan, W.G.: Pathophysiology and modern management of Paget's disease. Compreh. Therapy 9, 64, 1983.

25. Ryan, W.G. and Schwartz, T.B.: Mithramycin treatment of Paget's disease of bone. Arthr. Rheum. 23, 1155, 1980.

26. Simon, L.S., Krane, S.M., Wortman, P.D., Krane, I.M., and Kovitz, K.L.: Serum levels of type I and III procollagen fragments in Paget's disease of bone. J. Clin. Endo. Metab. 58, 110, 1984.

27. Singer, F.R. and Ahrne-Collier, I, L.: Salmon calcitonin therapy: antibodies and clinical resistance in patients with Paget's disease of bone. In, Proc. Conference on Molecular Endocrinology, Endocrinology '77. Eds: MacIntyre, I. and Szelke, M., Elsevier /North Biomedical Press, Amsterdam, New York, 1977, pp 207-213.

28. Singer, F.R., Mills, B.G., Park, M.S., Takemura, S., and Teraskai, P.I.: Increased HLA-DQW. Antigen pattern in Paget's disease of bone. Clin. Res. 33, 547A, 1985.

29. Singer, F.R., Schiller, A., Pyle, E.B., and Krane, S.M.: Paget's disease of bone. In, Metabolic Bone Disease, Vol. 2. Eds: Avioli, L. and Krane, S., Academic Press, New York, 1970, p. 492.

30. Siris, E.S., Jacobs, T.P., and Canfield, R.E.: Paget's disease of bone. Bull. N.Y. Acad. Med. 56, 285, 1981.

31. Smith, M.L., Fogelman, I., Ralston, S., Boyce, B.F., and Boyle, I.T.: Correlation of skeletal uptake of 99m-Tc-diphosphonate and alkaline phosphatase before and after oral disphosphonate therapy in Paget's disease. Metab. Bone Dis. Rel. Res. 5, 167, 1984.

32. Taubman, M.B., Kammerman, S., and Goldberg, B.: Radioimmunoassay of procollagen in serum of patients with Paget's disease of bone. Proc. Soc. Exp. Biol. Med. 152, 284, 1976.

33. Van Lente, R.: Alkaline and acid phosphatase determinations in bone disease. Orthop. Clin. N.A. 11, 437, 1979.

34. Vellenga, C., Pauwels, E.K., Bijvoet, O.L., Frijlink, W.B., Mulder, J.D., and Hermans, J.: Untreated Paget's disease of bone studied by scintigraphy. Radiology 153, 799, 1984.

Paget's Disease of Bone: Orthopedic Management

A. G. HADJIPAVLOU, P. H. LANDER, and I. P. ENKER

Introduction

Paget's disease of bone is a peculiar disorder of the bone modeling and remodeling processes. It is a relatively common condition after 45 years of age. While often an incidental finding on roentgenograms, it can be symptomatic and crippling, characterized by bone deformities, arthropathy, pathologic fractures, malignant transformation, cranial nerve compression, spinal stenosis, and back pain syndrome. Cranial nerve compression will not be dealt with in this review.

Pain in Paget's disease is derived from several sources such as bone hyperemia, mechanical factors, including bone deformity with periosteal stretching and microfractures, arthritis, nerve root compression or malignancy. Therefore, the choice of medical and/or surgical treatment is partly determined by the origin of the painful symptoms.

Conservative medical therapy for Paget's disease is the mainstay of management, with surgery reserved for specific indications. While medical therapy can control the disease process, it is not curative and significant side effects, such as osteopenia with pathologic fractures, highlight the hazards of medical therapy. The questions therefore are: a) when to initiate medical treatment; b) the end point of medical treatment; c) criteria for failure of medical treatment; d) indications for concurrent and/or subsequent surgical treatment; and e) monitoring lesions for potential complications, eg, malignant transformation and fractures.

We classify the remodeling disorders of Paget's disease into four phases: 1) osteolytic; 2) mixed; 3) osteoblastic; and 4) osteosclerotic. The first three phases are active, showing increased radioisotope uptake on scintillation scans, while the fourth phase is inactive with a reduced scintiscan uptake. Remodeling disorders, although usually generalized, can also present as a focal lesion (lytic or blastic) which may be confused with a metastatic tumor (Hadjipavlou and Lander, 1982).

Pagetic bone deformities are caused by modeling disorders of the periosteal and endosteal envelope with associated bone drift. These can display the following patterns:

1) periosteal apposition and endosteal absorption, resulting in an expanded bone with thin cortices;

Current Concepts of Bone Fragility

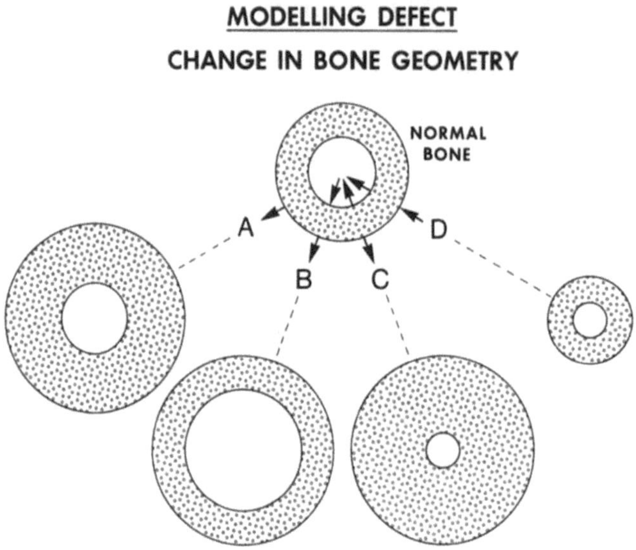

Fig. 1. Diagramatic representation of the different modeling patterns of envelope activity in Paget's disease.

2) periosteal and endosteal apposition, giving rise to an expanded bone with thick cortices and a narrow medullary canal; and

3) endosteal apposition associated with periosteal absorption, resulting in bone contraction (Fig. 1), which may be the most aggressive modeling disorder (Hadjipavlou and Lander, 1982).

As in the remodeling phases, the modeling disorder, usually generalized, can be focal, highlighted by the pumice-stone lesion, secondary to localized exuberant periosteal apposition (Jaffe, 1933).

Medical antipagetic therapy is indicated in symptomatic patients displaying in the scintiscan positive lesions in the osteolytic, mixed, or osteoblastic remodeling phases. The treatment objective is to accelerate progression through the phases of Paget's disease to reach the bone forming phase and, at least theoretically, avoid or minimize modeling disorders such as bone expansion with deformities.

Radionuclide bone blood flow studies can provide useful additional clinical information in the management of Paget's disease. The end point of medical therapy is symptomatic relief with normalization of bone blood flow of the affected region and normalization of biochemical variables such as serum alkaline phosphatase and urinary hydroxyproline (Boudreau et al, 1983; Hadjipavlou et al, 1984). We have shown that bone blood flow studies as an index of bone hyperemia correlate well with the patient's pain when compared with serum alkaline phosphatase levels. Changes in disease activity were more reliably demonstrable by bone blood flow than by conventional bone scan. Therefore, if pain persists inspite of normalization of bone blood flow (hyperemia resulting from an abnormal metabolic process), other mechanical causes should be sought such as stress microfractures, end stage arthritis, nerve compression, and malignancy.

Pain experienced in the osteoblastic phase is frequently secondary to microfracture and close attention should be paid to the radiographs to detect the appearance of visible incomplete or complete stress fractures, especially while on medical therapy. Finally, treatment should not be continued into the inactive osteosclerotic phase because the associated brittleness of bone may lead to an increased tendency to fracture.

Asymptomatic patients may require prophylactic antipagetic therapy if, on the basis of the assessment of the remodeling and modeling disorders, potential late complications are anticipated. Such complications may be vertebral involvement with a tendency for expansion which may lead to spinal stenosis with encroachment of nerve roots and/or the spinal cord; involvement of the base of the skull which may produce cranial nerve encroachment or basilar invagination with its catastrophic sequelae; and involvement of the weight bearing joints possibly resulting in pagetic arthritis.

Arthritis

Arthritis in Paget's disease of bone should not be considered a nonspecific arthritis (Frank et al, 1974) or a coincidental finding (Guyer and Dewbury, 1978), but rather a specific entity (Hadjipavlou and Lander, 1982).

Radiologically, pagetic arthritis of the weight bearing joints is characterized by: a) joint space narrowing; b) minimal osteophyte formation; c) bone expansion with incongruity; d) varus deformity with medial joint space narrowing of the hip and knee; e) *protrusio acetabuli*; f) subchondral and intraosseous radiolucencies and radiodensities reflecting bone resorption or formation respectively; g) true cysts or geodes; h) irregular, coarse, and thickened bone trabeculae and cortex. The predominant remodel-

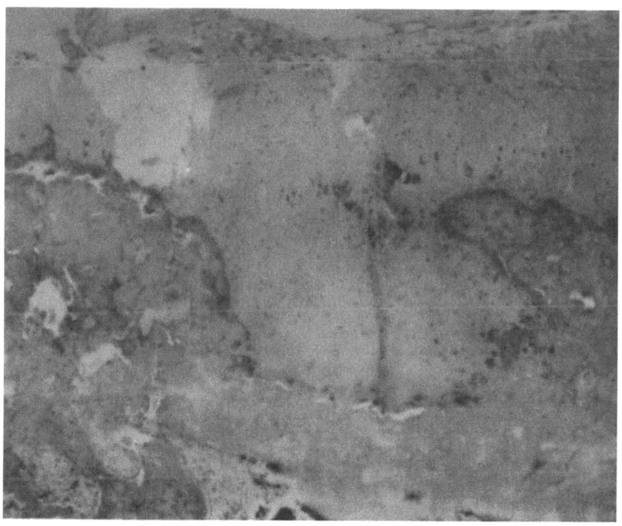

Fig. 2. Histologic section showing collapse of the articular cartilage through the subcondral bone.

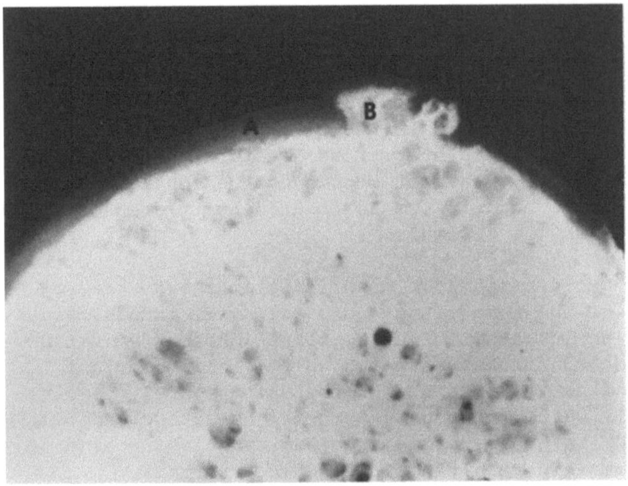

a)

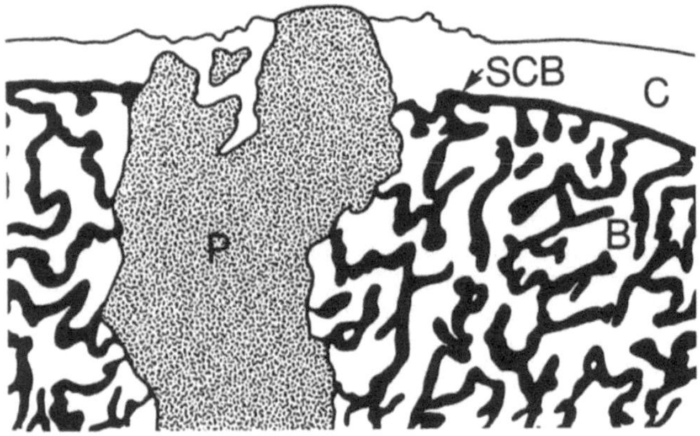

b)

Fig. 3. a) Radiograph of a coronal section of a pagetic femoral head, demonstrating the transgression of the articular cartilage by the pagetic process. b) Diagramatic illustration of the same: (P) - pagetic tissue; (SCB) - subcondral bone; (C) - cartilage; (B) - trabecular bone.

ing phase is the osteoblastic phase followed by the mixed phase (Hadjipavlou and Lander, 1982).

Several distinct pathologic processes contribute to articular cartilage degeneration and destruction. Jaffe, in 1933, stated that the pagetic process may erode subchondral bone. We have shown that, in certain regions, subchondral bone is replaced focally by active fibrovascular pagetic tissue (Hadjipavlou and Lander, 1982). This destruction of the supporting structure of the articular cartilage results in its collapse into the subchondral bone (Fig. 2) which, if large enough, can be seen on the radiograph as subchondral radiolucencies. These are distinct from the geodes of osteoarthritis caused by cartilage metaplasia of the bone marrow (Bombelli, 1983) that may also be seen in pagetic arthritis.

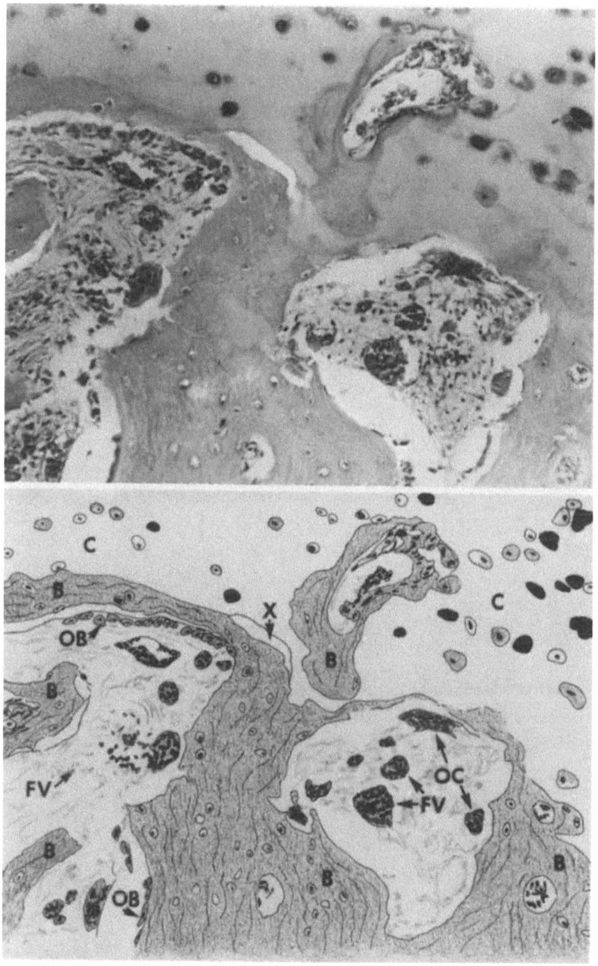

a)

b)

Fig. 4. a) Histologic section of articular cartilage showing invasion by the pagetic process.
b) Schematic representation: C - cartilage; B - subcondral bone; OB - osteoblasts; FV - fibrovascular tissue; OC - osteoclasts; X - artifact.

The articular cartilage can also be eroded. Goldman and coworkers (1977) attributed the erosion of the articular cartilage to accelerated endochondral ossification of subchondral bone. We have shown that the articular cartilage may be transgressed by invading pagetic tissue (Fig. 3 and 4) due to its tendency to expand. Resnick and Niwayamo (1981) have shown such invasion of the articular cartilage of the sacroiliac joints. Therefore, articular cartilage invasion should be considered a distinctive feature of pagetic arthritis (Hadjipavlou and Lander, 1982).

Bone expansion of one or both components of an involved joint is an invariable radiologic feature (Fig. 5). Such bone expansion may cause stretching and thinning of the overlying articular cartilage and, theoretically, could

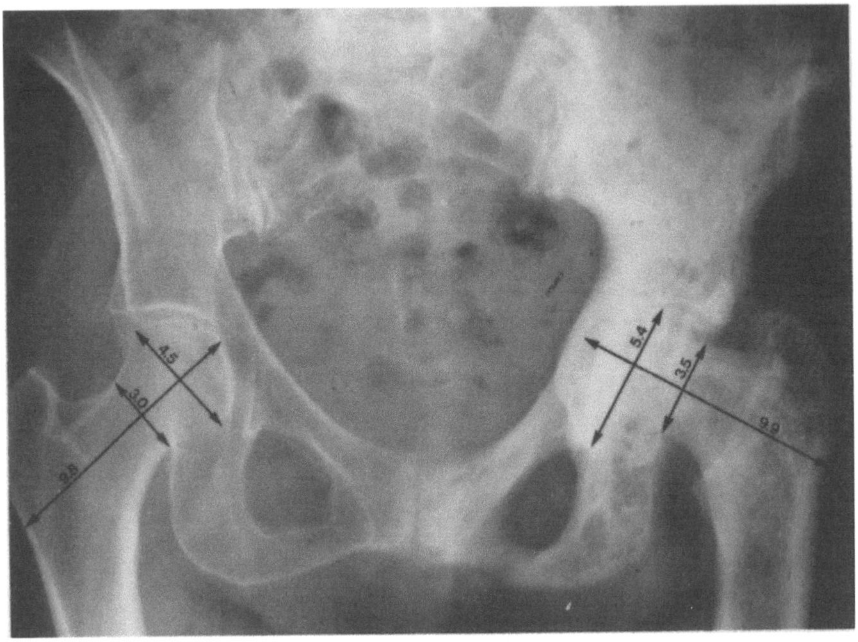

Fig. 5. Bone expansion of the left femoral head and neck, axial migration, joint space narrowing, and varus deformity in a blastic and mixed phase.

be another contributing factor to cartilage damage. Further investigation will be necessary to assess the role of this mechanism.

It can be postulated that the varus inclination of the femoral neck is a result of sequential trabecular microfractures occurring in brittle pagetic bone with reduced elasticity due to sclerosis. Support for this hypothesis was seen in our specimen radiographs, showing discontinuity and fusiform trabecular enlargement suggestive of healing fractures (Hadjipavlou and Lander, 1982). These microfractures, by weakening the bone architecture, may stimulate buttressing of the inferior cortex of the femoral neck which results in a thicker and wider neck in varus inclination (bone modeling abnormality) (Frost, 1973; Hadjipavlou and Lander, 1982).

The normalization of bone blood flow following antipagetic medical therapy and its relationship to pain relief has been previously documented (Boudreau et al, 1983; Hadjipavlou et al, 1977). Thus, it appears that engorgement of bone is one of the mechanisms contributing to arthritic pain. Failure of conservative therapy can only be considered if pain persists after an adequate course of medication; successful therapy normalizes bone blood flow and shows improvement on the bone scan and of biochemical variables. Non-responders can be considered to have reached the end stage of cartilage destruction, or to have developed stress microfractures within a pagetic femoral neck with concomittent varus deformity of the femoral neck (Fig. 6). As a corollary, the former group should be treated by total joint arthroplasty, and the latter group with valgus realignment surgery (Hadjipavlou and Lander, 1982) provided the medial articular cartilage of the femoral

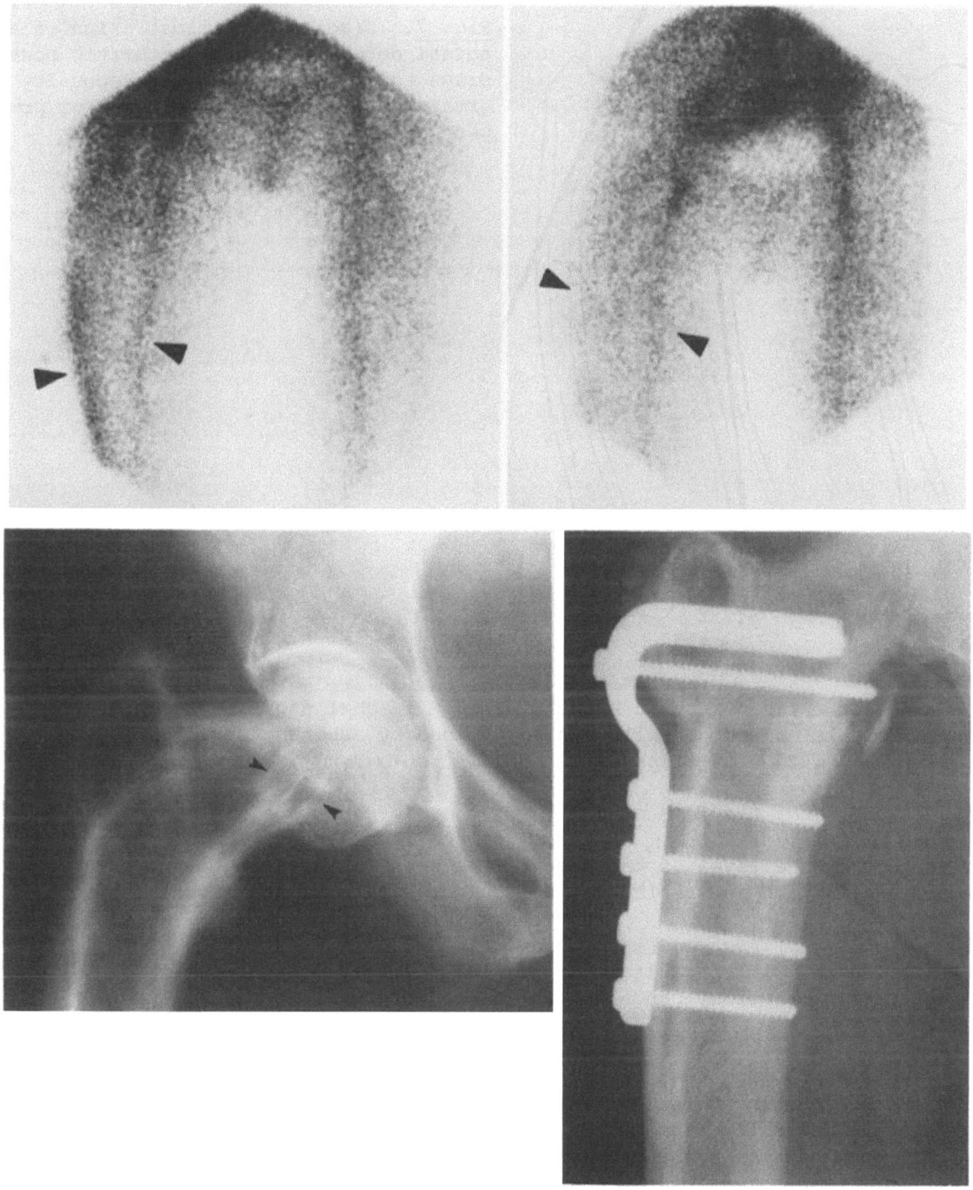

a) c) b) d)

Fig. 6. Example of a complete therapeutic cycle. Note the improvement of bone flow (a) before and (b) after therapy. Arrows point to the femoral arteries medially and the engorged pagetic bone laterally. Because of persistent pain, tomographic investigation revealed stress microfractures (c), treated successfully by valgus osteotomy (d)

head is preserved. In the knee joint, valgus realignment osteotomy is indicated in varus deformity with preservation of the lateral compartment articular cartilage. Varus osteotomy of the proximal femur is contraindicated in Paget's disease because the accentuation of the underlying varus inclination will result in impingement of the greater trochanter, and/or propagation of stress fractures.

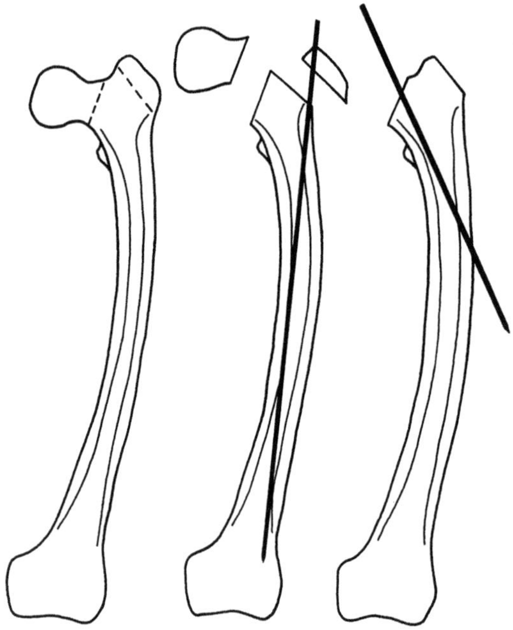

Fig. 7. Diagramatic illustration of an actual deformed femoral arthritic bone drawn to scale, showing the necessity of greater trochanteric osteotomy for proper centralization of the canal.

Total joint arthroplasty in Paget's disease is challenging. Serious technical difficulties and pitfalls can be avoided by adhering strictly to the following sequence of steps:

A. *Osteotomy of the femoral neck:* If the hip cannot be dislocated due to severe *protrusio acetabuli*, osteotomy of the femoral neck in situ is advised. Osteotomy at the level of the base of the neck will eliminate the pathologic varus inclination and replace it with a more anatomic neck shaft angle.

B. *Osteotomy of the greater trochanter*: An oblique osteotomy of the greater trochanter will facilitate its distal transfer and lateralization. Trochanteric osteotomy can also facilitate peroperative hip dislocation (Fig. 7).

C. *Canal centralization:* Because of the proximal varus deformity of the femur, the starting point for rasping should be as far lateral as possible to achieve centralization of the canal and to prevent placement of the prosthetic component in varus and its cortical penetration. With severe deformity, this rasping may even cut through the lateral proximal cortex (Fig. 8).

D. *Rasping:* 1) Opening of the medullary canal is done in routine fashion. 2) In obliterated canals, proper rasping consists of placing a guidewire down the obliterated medulla under biplane fluoroscopy. The canal is then widened to the appropriate size with graduated reamers, using standard intramedullary techniques.

E. *Choice of stem length:* This depends on the presence or absence of stress fractures. A prime consideration should be placement of the tip of the femoral component beyond the most distal stress fracture sufficiently distant to achieve stress shielding. Significant bowing of the femoral shaft may require concurrent osteotomy to avoid cortical penetration. The a)

b)

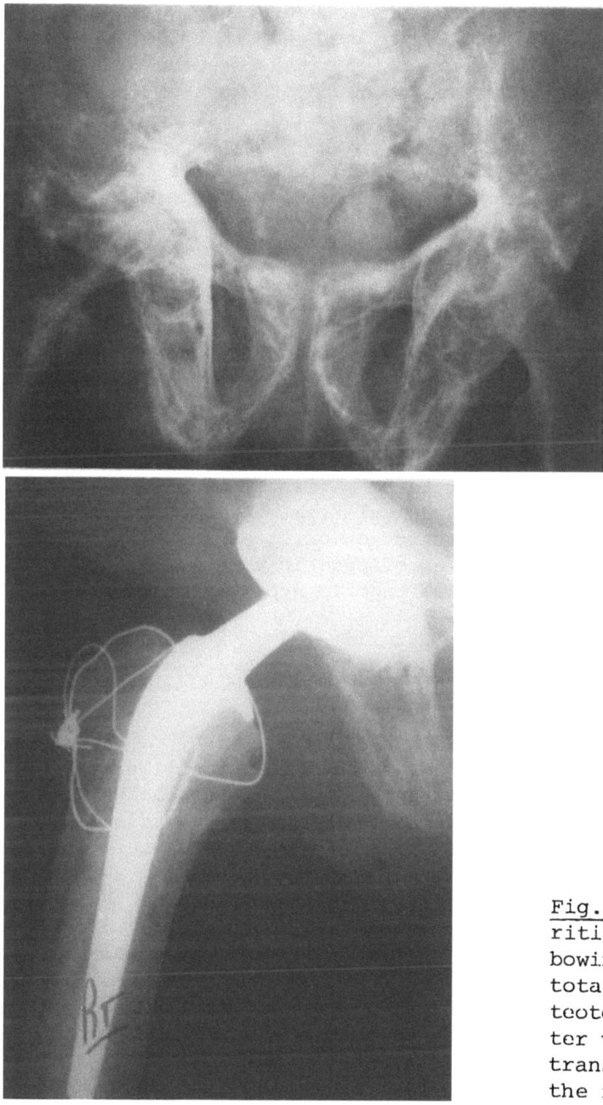

Fig. 8. a) Advanced pagetic arthritis with varus inclination and bowing of the femur. b) After total hip replacement. Note osteotomy of the greater trochanter with distal and lateral transfer, and centralization of the femoral stem.

consideration of stem length in this situation is the same as for revision arthroplasty in the presence of a femoral shaft fracture.

F. *Canal preparation and cement technique:* Because of the increased bleeding tendency in Paget's disease of bone, thorough irrigation of the canal should be carried out during the interval between canal preparation and component insertion with cement. This interval should be kept as short as possible.

G. *Acetabular component:* Most of the reaming should be peripheral with an expanding reamer due to the tendency of *protrusio acetabuli*. Medial wall grafting and use of a protrusio cup is indicated if during reaming the medial wall is deficient or inadvertently violated.

H. *Greater trochanter fixation:* The greater trochanter should be transferred distally and laterally: 1) to prevent impingement of the greater trochanter against the lateral wall of the ilium or the acetabular cup component (Fig. 7 and 8); 2) to minimize the incidence of extra-articular arthrodesis by ectopic bone formation.

I. *Increased bleeding:* Because of the increased incidence of bleeding in Paget's disease, treatment with antipagetic medication, preoperatively, is recommended to minimize vascularity. In our patients, we have found that osseous vascularity can be effectively assessed by radionuclide bone blood flow studies (Boudreau et al, 1983).

J. *Loosening of the prosthesis:* Expansion with endosteal absorption as depicted in Figure 1 (B) will lead to an enlarged medullary canal and predispose to loosening. It remains to be seen whether postoperative medical treatment in this pattern of modeling expansion can prevent loosening.

In conclusion, pain from pagetic arthritis should initially be treated with conservative therapy. A large number of these patients, even with impressive arthritic disease, will improve. Surgical treatment depends on distinguishing between end stage cartilage destruction or stress microfractures in the pagetic femoral neck from other causes of pagetic arthropathy, such as crystal synovitis (Singer, 1977), and true pagetic hypermetabolic activity resulting in bone engorgement.

Malignancies

The development of sarcoma is the most dreadful complication of Paget's disease of bone. Survival rates are low (Barry, 1969). In the early stage, sarcomas are extremely difficult to differentiate from Paget's disease because of subtle radiographic changes. Table I is a summary of the reported cases in the literature. Eight patients in our series came from a population group of 1,078 patients with a diagnosis of Paget's disease seen between 1970 and 1980 at four hospitals. The overall incidence of sarcomatous transformation in our series was 0.8%. Because the true population of Paget's disease is not known, the incidence of malignant transformation may be even smaller. Sarcoma commonly involves the pelvis, humerus, femur, and craniofacial bones (Barry, 1969; Huvos et al, 1983; Schatzki and Dudley, 1961; Smith et al, 1984; Wick et al, 1981). Generalized metastasis is found in 30% of patients at the time of diagnosis. This should not be confused with primary multifocal sarcomatous transformation (Choquette et al, 1983). The cause of death is most frequently from pulmonary metastasis (Barry, 1969).

The various forms of malignant transformation in Paget's disease of bone are osteogenic sarcoma, fibrosarcoma, fibrous histiocytoma, giant cell tumor and chondrosarcoma. These sarcomas are very aggressive (Barry, 1969; Grenditzer et al, 1983; Price and Goldie, 1969). The incidence of metastatic tumor in sarcoma is unknown. Over the age of 40, osteogenic sarcoma is mostly superimposed on a pagetic lesion.

In our series (Table II), we had five patients with osteogenic sarcoma, one patient with malignant fibrous histiocytoma, one patient with epitheloid cell sarcoma, and one patient with a reticulum lymphosarcoma. Case 6 illustrates a lymphosarcoma complicating Paget's disease of bone. We are aware

Table I. Literature review of malignancies in Paget's disease of bone

Author	Year	No. of patients with sarcoma
Paget	1889	5
Camp	1925	2
Bird	1927	7
Coley et al	1931	3
Davie et al	1937	2
Sumney et al	1946	3
Platt	1947	10
Poretta et al	1957	16
Freydinger et al	1963	7
McKenna	1964	33
Barry	1969	116
Price	1969	80
Milgram	1977	20
Greditzer et al	1983	41
Hadjipavlou et al	1983	8
Choquette et al	1983	
Huvos et al	1983	65
Smith et al	1984	85

of only two other cases reported in the world literature (Molle et al, 1983; Ryan and Schwartz, 1981).

Clinically, acute onset of pain (Choquette et al, 1973; Huvos et al, 1983), or change in the underlying nature of the pain was common in our patients who developed sarcoma. A fracture occurring in a pagetic bone, especially when associated with osteolysis, should alert the physician to a sarcomatous transformation (Huvos et al, 1983), even if it heals (Fig. 9). The tumors in our series occurred in all remodeling phases (Huvos et al, 1983).

Paget's disease of bone can also be associated with metastatic tumors of bone (Burgener and Perry, 1977; Epstein et al, 1970). Occasionally, benign focal remodeling pagetic lesions may be indistinguishable from metastatic lesions (Fig. 10). In our series, we had four patients with metastatic osteoblastic lesions. The diagnosis was made late in each of these patients, illustrating the difficulty in diagnosing metastatic osteoblastic tumors in pagetic bone. A definitive diagnosis can only be made by tissue biopsy.

Bleeding can be a major complication in Paget's disease of bone. We recommend assessment of the bone blood flow and, if increased, pretreatment with mithramycin before biopsy is instituted. One of our untreated patients

Table II. Malignant transformation in Paget's disease

No. Name	Age Sex	Site	Fracture	Histologic findings	Alkaline phosphatase		Treatment	Metastasis	Survival (months)	
					Preop	Postop			After onset of symptoms	After diagnosis
1 RM	42 M	Distal femur	No	Osteogenic sarcoma	250	110	Above elbow amputation; adriamycin	Lungs	8	6
2 RC	76 M	Proximal femur	Yes	Epitheloid cell sar-coma	225	115	En block resec-tion; Moore's arthroplasty; local radio-therapy	Lungs	12	6
3 DC	73 F	Distal femur	No	Osteogenic sarcoma	2520	110	Hip disarticu-lation; preop and postop calcitonin	Lungs Spine	29	23
4 AG	64 F	Middle femur	Yes	Malignant fibrous hystiocytoma	275	85	Hip disarticu-lation; preop and postop mithramycin	Lungs	16	4
5 LM	72 M	Pubis ilium	No	Osteogenic sarcoma	325	-	Biopsy exsan-guinated	Lungs Spine	1	0
6 DL	77 F	Distal femur	Yes	Reticulum cell lympho-sarcoma	150	150	Curettage; radiotherapy; chemotherapy	Inguinal region	60	48
7 LT	78 M	Skull	No	Osteogenic sarcoma	231	-	NIL	Lungs	1	1
8 TB	55 F	Humerus	Yes	Osteogenic sarcoma - lytic	168	170	Radiotherapy	Unknown	7	1

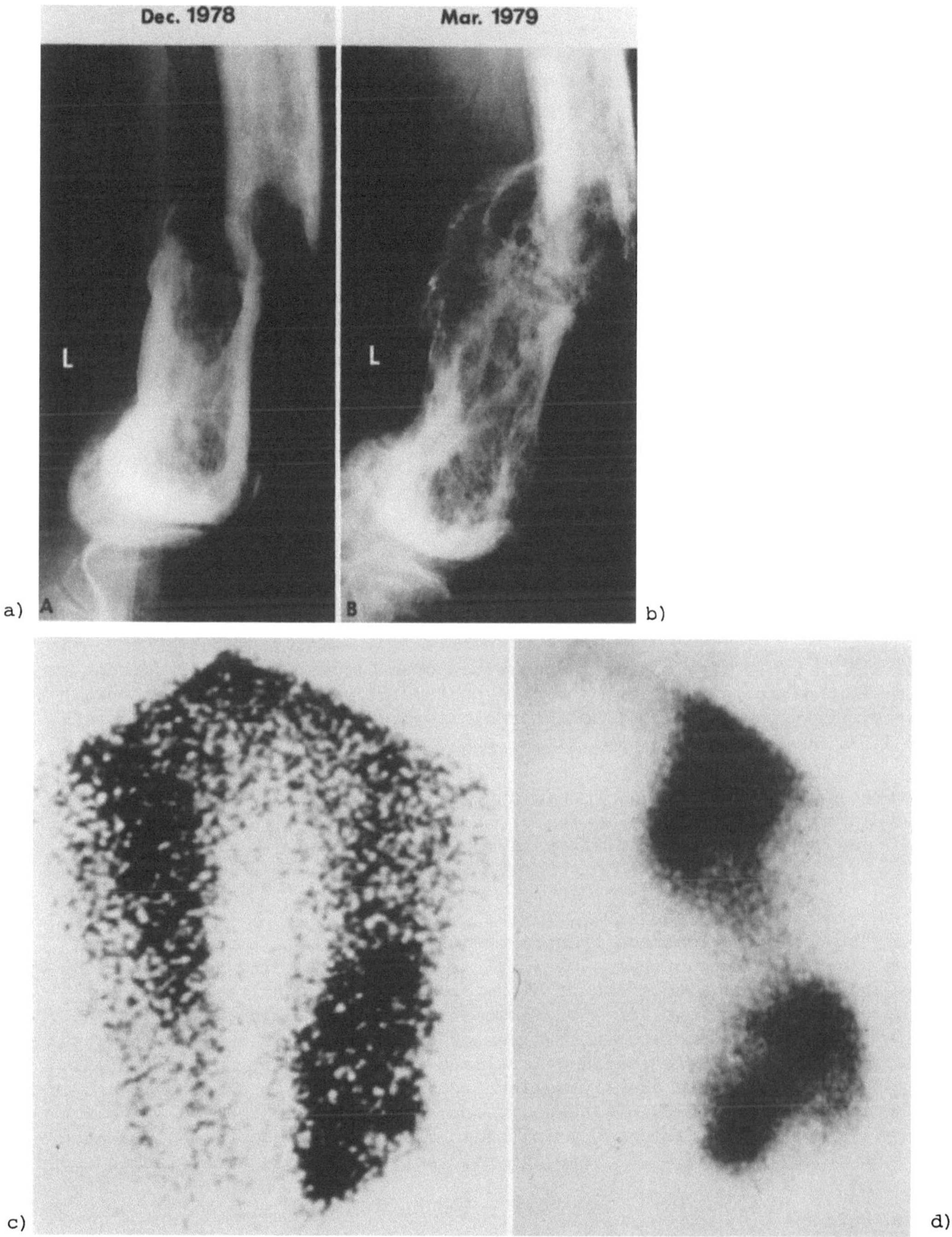

Fig. 9 a) Malignant transformation to fibrous histiocytoma, complicated by fracture. b) Fracture healed. c) Increased bone blood flow in the lytic region, corresponding to d) photonegative scintiscan, suggestive of nonosteoid forming sarcoma.

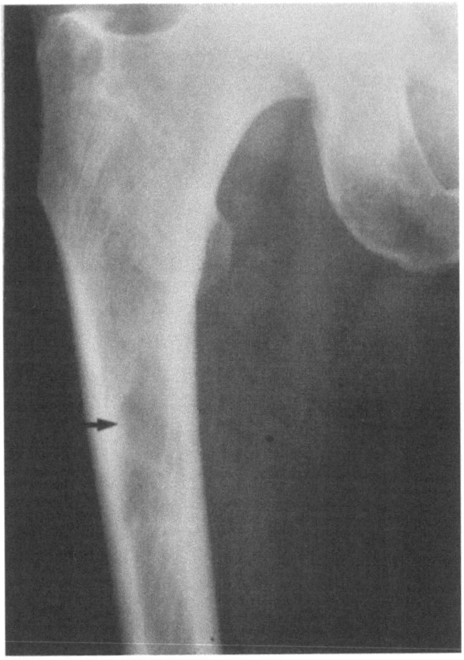

Fig. 10. Focal osteolytic remodeling lytic lesion, suggestive of metastatic lesion. (Courtesy of Dr. Robert Dusseault, Montréal, Canada)

(Case 5 in Table II), exsanguinated after open biopsy. Only the patient with lymphosarcoma is alive 64 months postoperative. The five-year survival rate is very low. In 1984, Smith et al reported a five-year survival rate of 3.5%; Huvos et al, in 1983, 4.6%; and Grenditzer et al, in 1983, 8%.

In all our patients, diagnosis was delayed and undoubtedly contributed to the poor outcome. The average survival in our series after the onset of symptoms was 14 months, and after tissue diagnosis was six to eight months.

Early stages of sarcomatous transformation are difficult to differentiate from Paget's disease of bone. A soft tissue mass expanding from an irregular and eroded periosteum should be regarded as malignant transformation. Figure 11 shows the evolution of sarcomatous transformation. However, a soft tissue mass associated with a pumice stone lesion is a benign process (Jaffe, 1933). This lesion is a localized focal extracortical periosteal expansion of bone with clearly delineated and circumscribed borders, and is a benign process. In this situation, one should refrain from ablative surgery. Biopsy under fluoroscopy is the most appropriate approach. Because of the gloomy prognosis of these tumors, early tissue diagnosis is mandatory.

Fractures

Pathologic fractures are a frequent complication of Paget's disease (Jaffe, 1933; Roberts and Cohn, 1926), and may even be the presenting manifestation. The incidence varies between 10% and 30% (Grundy, 1970; Merkow and Lane, 1984) and is difficult to determine accurately because many patients with Paget's disease remain asymptomatic and therefore undiagnosed.

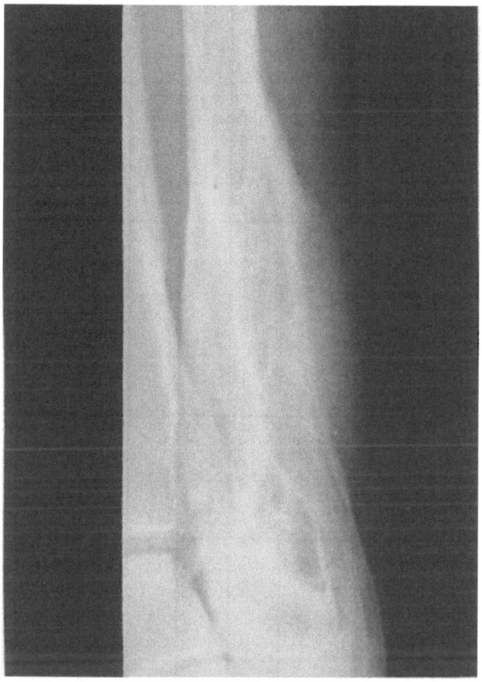

Fig. 11. a) Soft tissue extending from a pumice stone lesion, suggestive of a benign focal modeling process. b) In contrast to soft tissue extending from ragged borders, suggestive of osteosarcoma. c) Six months later, obvious transformation to osteosarcoma. (With permission: Resnick and Niwayama, Diagnosis of Bone and Joint Disorders, W.B. Saunders, 1981).

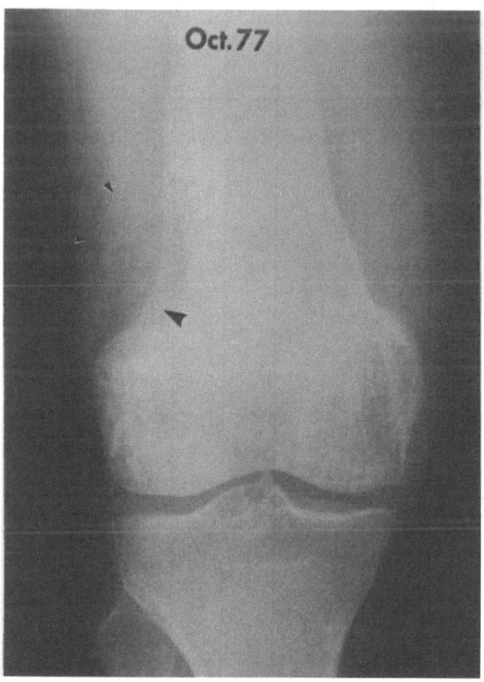

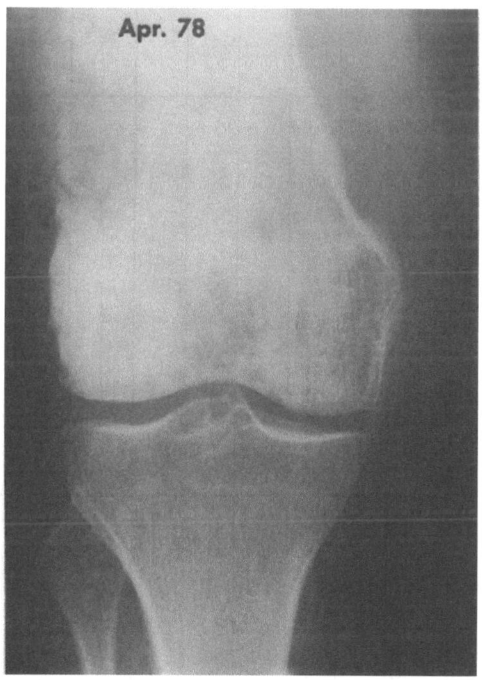

Reports in the literature are conflicting concerning the time to bone union in pagetic fractures (Table III). Part of this controversy stems from the fact that some authors have not related healing in Paget's disease to the remodeling phase at the time of fracture.

Table III. Time to bone union: Literature review

Author(s)	Phase	Duration to union of fracture			
		Decreased	Normal	Increased	Nonunion
Roberts & Cohen, 1926	Never in sclerotic stage		+		Exceptional
O'Reilly & Race, 1932	Decalcifying stage (vascular)		+		·
Jaffe, 1933				+	
Roger & Ulin, 1936			+		
Brailsford, 1938			+		Nil
Dickson et al, 1945	23/27 combined phase 4/27 sclerotic phase				1/77 cases
Lake, 1951	Commoner in vascular phase	Rapid in vascular phase		In sclerotic phase	6/45 cases
Lake, 1958	Commoner in vascular phase	1/3		2/3	14/78 in sclerotic bones
Barry, 1967	No correlation with phase in this series		+		10/70
Barry, 1969	Commonest in sclerotic phase		73%		Small growth - either porotic or sclerotic
Grundy, 1970			+		
Beyer & Paul, 1972			+		
Lemaire, 1974			+		
Rauis, 1974	No particular phase incidence		+		
Dove, 1980					40%

Table IV. Distribution of fractures according to remodelling phase and treatment

Region	No. fractures	Lytic phase						Mixed phase						Blastic phase					
		Union		Delayed union		Nonunion		Union		Delayed union		Nonunion		Union		Delayed union		Nonunion	
		Tx	NTx	Tx	NTx	Tx	NTx	Tx	NTx	Tx	NTx	Tx	NTx	Tx	NTx	Tx	NTx	Tx	NTx
Total bones	52																		
Femur	39																		
Shaft	23	2	2	1		1		1	2		2	1		1	5	1	1	2	1
Subtro-chanteric	8								2	1	2		1			1	1		
Intertro-chanteric	2		1					1											
Subcapital	3*																1		1
Supra-condylar	3	1	1								1								
Tibia	6								1			2					3		
Humerus	4	1	1								1								1
Clavicle	1	1																	
Radius	1								1										
Ulna	1								1										

* Prosthetic replacement
Tx = Patient treated with antipagetic medication at time of fracture.
NTx = Not on antipagetic therapy at time of fracture

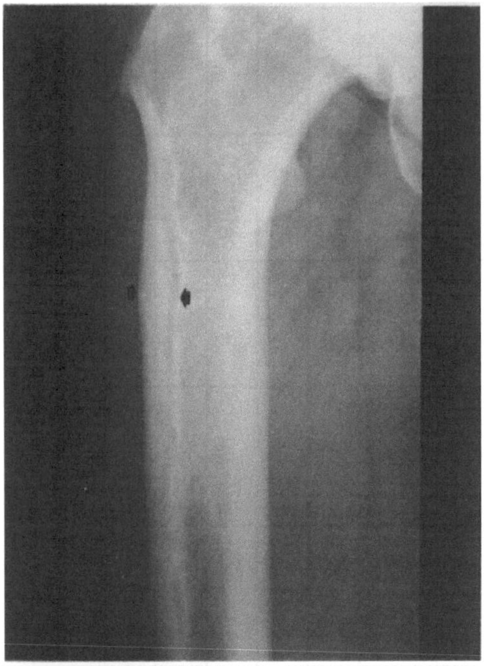

Fig. 12. a) Arrows to a stress fracture in an osteoblastic bone. b) Fracture completed and fixed with nail plate. c) Fracture healed and regressed to a mixed phase.

a)

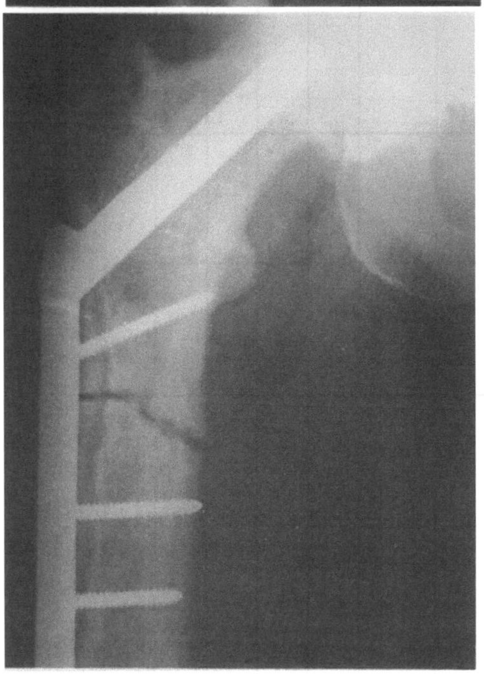

b)

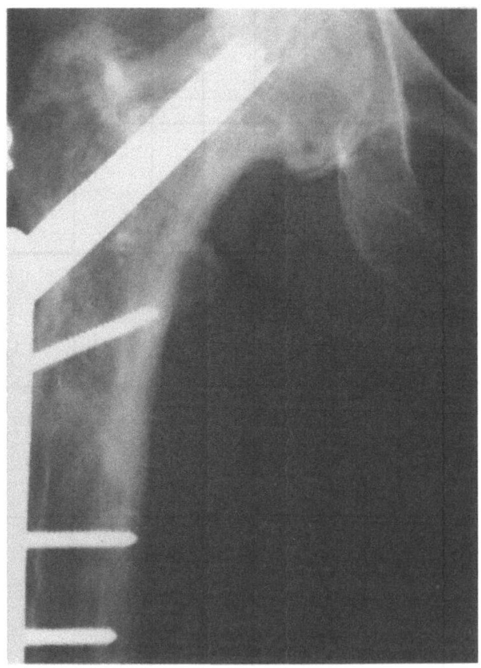

c)

Eighty-one pathologic fractures were identified in 55 patients in our review of 1,078 (symptomatic) pagetic patients in the Montréal area (incidence 7.5%). They occurred most frequently in the long bones of the lower extremities where the femoral shaft was the most common site of fracture (see Table IV).

Fractures of the long bones occurred in all remodeling phases, but were more common in the mixed and osteoblastic phases. Fractures in the osteolytic phase were seen at the junction of normal bone density and the radiolucent front.

We concur with Lake (1951, 1958) that fractures in the osteoblastic and mixed phases are associated with delayed union, whereas fractures in the osteolytic phase usually heal in the expected time. Union tends to be delayed and the incidence of nonunion increased in patients on antipagetic medical therapy (Krane, 1982).

Predisposing factors to complete fractures are incomplete stress fractures (Fig. 12); stress risers, particularly at bone-plate interfaces (5 cases in the femur); and possibly etidronate disodium therapy (Fig. 13) (9 cases -- 8 etidronate and 1 calcitonin in our series). Krane (1982) states that etidronate increases the incidence of fractures. We concur with Johnston (Johnston et al, 1983) that because of insufficient data of a control population of nontreated pagetic patients, we cannot substantiate our empirical observation that etidronate predisposes to fractures. However, because of delayed or nonunion of fractures in the mixed and blastic phases, we recommend that in patients with fractures medical antipagetic therapy with etidronate be discontinued or withheld until the fracture heals. Intramedullary nailing is the preferred treatment for stabilizing bone fractures to prevent stress risers.

Incomplete stress fractures arise mostly on the tension side of long bones where they may partially involve the cortex, either from the endosteal or periosteal surfaces. They occur mostly at the site of blastic and sclerotic phases within pagetic bones (lytic, 1; blastic-sclerotic, 12). Circumstantial evidence suggests that sclerotic bone is brittle (Jaffe, 1933; Lowry and Rutherford, 1937; Redden et al, 1981) and, therefore, predisposed to fracture. It remains to be shown whether the failure of these stress fractures to heal is due to a deficiency of BMU function within pagetic bone.

Incomplete stress fractures associated with pain and local tenderness are suggestive of impending complete fractures. Treatment in this situation depends on the remodeling phase. In the mixed phase, crutch walking with or without bracing is advisable whereas in the osteoblastic or sclerotic phase with an associated marked deformity, prophylactic realignment osteotomy and intramedullary fixation are the most appropriate treatments. In both situations, medical antipagetic therapy is not advisable and should be discontinued.

Fractures with pronounced bone deformities should be treated by open methods. Correction of the deformity will improve the adjacent joint mechanics and minimize stress riser formation. Fractures in otherwise nondeformed bone are amenable to closed treatment.

Fractures in the osteolytic phase usually heal as expected. Fracture healing can be associated with phase regression or osteopenia. We recommend that fractures in the osteolytic phase be treated with functional weight-bearing immobilization. Concurrent medical antipagetic therapy -- ie, calcitonin -- is also recommended to promote healing of the osteolytic phase by normalizing the metabolic state of the pagetic bone (Meyers and Singer, 1978). Fractures of the femoral shaft occurring in the osteoblastic and to a lesser extent in the mixed phase frequently had preexisting bone deformity. Open intramedullary nail is the treatment of choice. This allows for

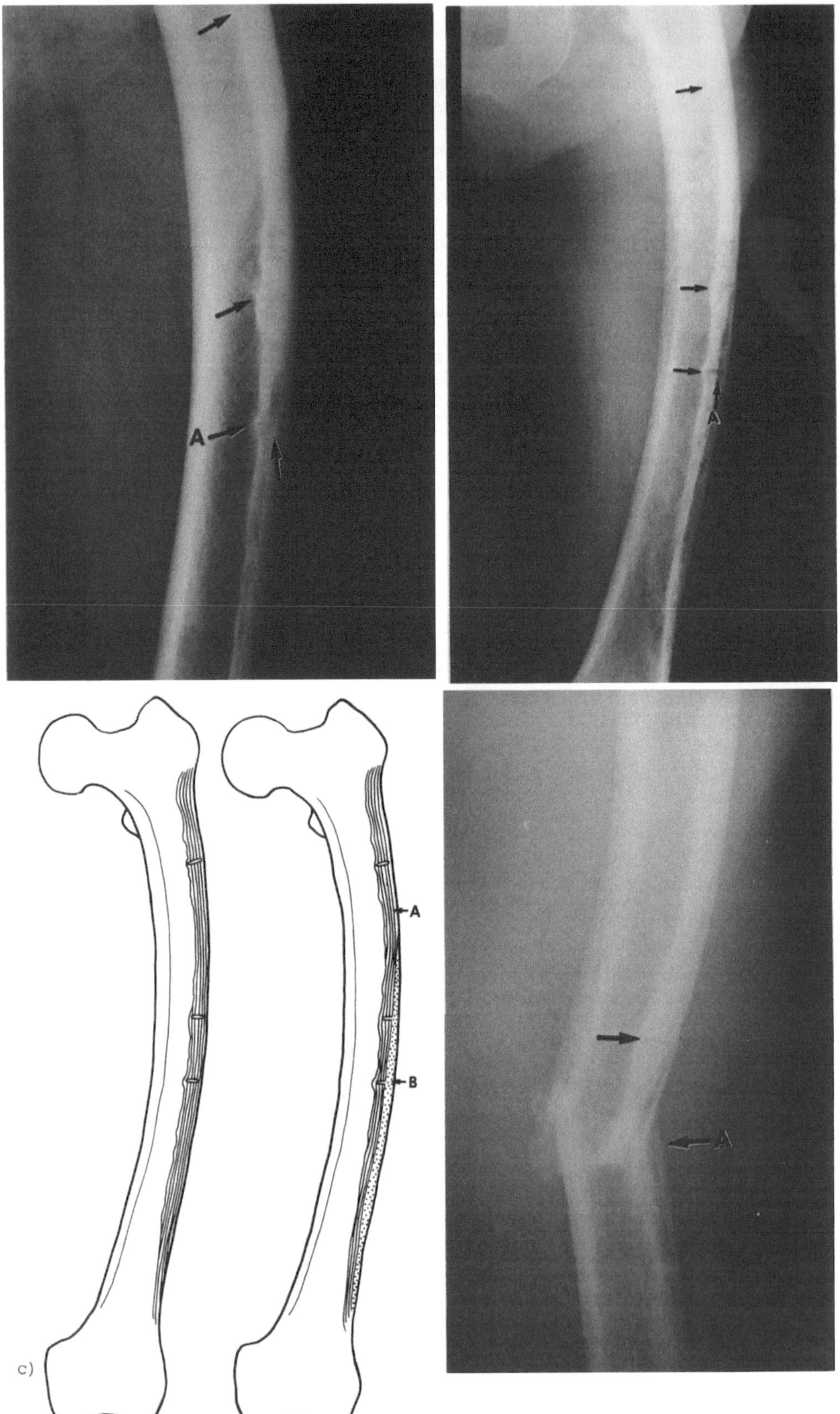

a) b) c) d)

correction of the deformity, a major contributing factor to refracture, affords better transient stabilization (because of the tendency for delayed union in the blastic phase) until union is achieved, and avoids stress risers. Patients treated with plate fixation are at risk of a fracture at the bone plate junction. We found that all patients treated with electrical stimulation and bone grafting (6 cases of femoral shaft fractures) healed with exuberant callus. We recommend their use for patients treated by open reduction.

Established nonunion responded well to discontinuation of antipagetic medication, internal fixation, bone graft, and internally implanted bone stimulator.

Back Pain and Spinal Stenosis

Back pain is the single most common complaint among patients with Paget's disease (Altman, 1980). This should be differentiated from coincidental mechanical or discogenic factors. Altman (1980) found that 46% of his patients with back pain had arthritis or disc disease not related to the pagetic process. In a group of 26 symptomatic patients out of 36 patients with known Paget's disease of the spine, we observed only one patient with significant symptoms of spondyloarthropathy of the spine unrelated to Paget's disease.

In the osteolytic phase, the vertebral body can be the cause of pain, either by microfracture or frank compression fracture. The pagetic process can invade across the adjacent vertebral disc.

The role of pagetic facet arthropathy in the generation of back pain is not clear as CT evidence of pagetic facet arthropathy was present in equal frequency in both the symptomatic and asymptomatic groups. However, severe arthropathy was considerably more frequent in the symptomatic group (Zlatkin et al, 1985), and was also present in symptomatic patients without CT evidence of spinal stenosis.

Spinal stenosis and compression syndrome due to Paget's disease has been known since 1923 (Smidek, 1977). Neurologic deficit with Paget's disease of the spine has been known for many years (Hartman and Dohn, 1966; Siegelman et al, 1968; Smidek, 1977; Weisz, 1983). Most authors conclude that bony compression of the spinal cord and nerve roots in the stenotic spine is the most likely etiology. This occurs as a result of significant modeling posterior expansion of the vertebral body, neural arch and facets, resulting in central canal narrowing, with or without subarticular canal or intervertebral foramen stenosis. However, other factors such as compression of the anterior central spinal cord artery (Mathé et al, 1973) by the pagetic process or vascular steal syndrome (Douglas et al, 1981) may also play a role.

◁ Fig. 13. a) Incomplete insufficiency type stress fracture and stress-induced fracture of the lateral cortex (arrows). Note that the fracture lines are buttressed medially and laterally by normal density cortical bone (arrow A). b) Demineralization of the lateral cortex (arrow A) after eight months of therapy with etidronate disodium. c) Diagramatic representation of the lateral cortical buttressing (arrow A) and demineralization contributing to the weakening of the buttress effect. d) Complete fracture occurred at the side of the previous stress fracture (arrow A) six months later.

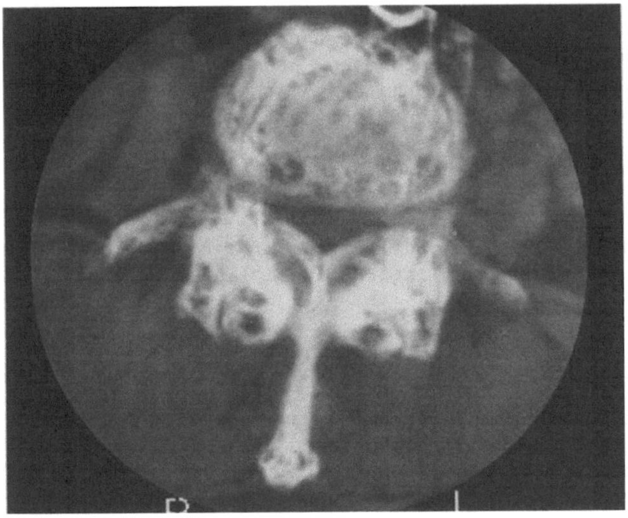

Fig. 14. CT scan shows a mixed phase of lumbar vertebra with central stenosis and facet arthroplasty.

Other evidence includes the dramatic response of pagetic spinal stenosis syndrome to medical antipagetic therapy (Hadjipavlou et al, 1977). Computed tomography is the most efficacious method of studying spinal canal narrowing (Dowart, 1984; Dowart et al, 1983). Computed tomographic evaluation in our series of patients shows a high incidence of moderate to severe spinal stenosis due to Paget's disease of bone among the symptomatic group (Fig. 14) and only two cases of mild stenosis due to Paget's disease alone in the asymptomatic group (Zlatkin et al, 1985). This points toward spinal stenosis as the most likely etiologic factor involved in the generation of these clinical manifestations. The presence of neurologic symptoms in four of our patients (4/26) without evidence of bony stenosis on CT is circumstantial evidence of pagetic steal syndrome. Hypermetabolic activity of the adjacent vertebra can deprive the spinal cord of blood supply. Direct compression of the neural elements by the large pagetic engorged vessels cannot be ruled out at this time. One specific case report will illustrate this point. A patient with significant clinical evidence of spinal stenosis, with myelographic evidence of block (no CT had been done at that time) responded dramatically to etidronate therapy and has had no recurrence of symptoms; however, a follow-up CT scan shows persistent evidence of significant bone spinal stenosis.

Antipagetic medical therapy is rewarding in treating pagetic back pain and spinal stenosis syndrome. Decompression for spinal stenosis should be instituted promptly after failure of a complete cycle of antipagetic medical therapy. In these circumstances, procrastination may lead to irreversible myelopathy or radiculopathy. In our series, one patient with central spinal stenosis from posterior expansion of the vertebral body failed to recover from spastic paraplegia and another patient with central spinal stenosis of the lumbar spine from facet joint hypertrophy failed to recover completely.

Acknowledgement

We sincerely thank Mr. David Saxe of the Department of Photography for his excellent work on the illustrations.

References

1. Altman, R.D.: Musculoskeletal complications of Paget's disease of bone. Arthritis Rheum. 23, 1121, 1980.
2. Barry, H.C.: Fractures in the femur in Paget's disease of bone in Australia. J. Bone Joint Surg. 49A, 1359, 1967.
3. Barry, H.C.: Paget's Disease of Bone. E.S. Livingstone, Ltd., Edinburgh and London, 1969.
4. Beyer, U., and Paul, D.: Frakturen bei Ostitis Deformans Paget. Zentralblatt für Chirurgie 97, 470, 1972.
5. Bird, C.E.: Sarcoma complicating Paget's disease of the bone. Arch. Surg. 14, 1187, 1927.
6. Bombelli, R.: Osteoarthritis of the Hip. 2nd Ed., Springer Verlag, New York, 1983. p. 8.
7. Boudreau, R.J., Lisbona, R., and Hadjipavlou, A.: Observation of serial radionuclide blood flow studies in Paget's disease. J. Nucl. Med. 24, 880, 1983.
8. Brailsford, J.F.: Paget's disease of bone. Its frequency, diagnosis and complications. Br. J. Radiol. 128, 507, 1938.
9. Burgener, F.A., and Perry, P.E.: Solitary renal cell carcinoma metastasis in Paget's disease simulating sarcomatous degeneration. AJR 128, 843, 1977.
10. Camp, J.D.: Sarcoma complicating osteitis deformans: A case report of two cases. Radiology 5, 495, 1925.
11. Choquette, D., Heraoui, B., Altman, D., and Pelletier, J.P.: Simultaneous multifocal sarcomatous degeneration in Paget's disease of bone. Clin. Orthop. 179, 308, 1983.
12. Coley, B.L. and Sharp, G.S.: Paget's disease predisposing factor to osteogenic sarcoma. Arch. Surg. 23, 918, 1931.
13. Davie, T.B. and Cooke, W.E.: Supervention of osteogenic sarcoma in Paget's disease. Br. J. Surg. 25, 299, 1937.
14. Dickson, D.D., Camp, J.D., and Ghormley, R.K.: Osteitis deformans, Paget's disease of bone. Radiology 44, 449, 1945.
15. Douglas, D.I., Duckworth, T., Kanis, J.A., Jefferson, A.A., Martin, J.G., and Russel, R.G.: Spinal cord dysfunction in Paget's disease of bone. Has medical treatment a vascular basis. J. Bone Joint Surg. 63B, 495, 1981.
16. Dove, J.: Complete fractures of the femur in Paget's disease of bone. J. Bone Joint Surg. 62B, 12, 1980.
17. Dorwart, R.H.: Fundamentals of the computed tomographic assessment of spinal stenosis. In, Spine Update, 1984. Perspective in Radiology, Orthopedic Surgery and Neurosurgery. Radiology Research and Education Foundation, 181, 1983.

18. Dorwart, R.H., Volger, J.B. III, and Helms, C.A.: Spinal stenosis. Radiol. Clin. North Am. 21, 301, 1983.

19. Epstein, L.T., Bixler, D., and Bennett, J.E.: An incidence of familial cancer including three cases of osteogenic sarcoma. Cancer 25, 889, 1970.

20. Frank, A.W., Bress, N.M., Singer, F.R., and Krane, S.M.: Rheumatic manifestations of Paget's disease of bone. Am. J. Med. 56, 592, 1974.

21. Freydinger, J.E., Dubig, J.T., and McDonald, I.: Sarcoma complicating Paget's disease of bone. Arch. Pathol. Lab. Med. 75, 496, 1963.

22. Frost, H.M.: Bone Remodeling and Skeletal Modeling Errors. Orthopaedic Lectures, Vol. IV. Charles Thomas, Springfield, 1973.

23. Goldman, A.B., Bullough, P., Kammeron, S., and Ambos, M.: Osteitis deformans of the hip joint. AJR 128, 601, 1977.

24. Greditzer, H.G., McLeod, R.A., Unni, K.K., and Beabout, J.W.: Bone sarcomas in Paget's disease. Radiology 146, 327, 1983.

25. Grundy, M.: Fractures of the femur in Paget's disease of bone. Their etiology and treatment. J. Bone Joint Surg. 52B, 252, 1970.

26. Guyer, P.B., and Dewbury, K.C.: The hip joint in Paget's disease (Paget's coxopathy). Br. J. Radiol. 51, 574, 1978.

27. Hadjipavlou, A., and Lander, P.: Unusual radiological manifestations and a dynamic classification of Paget's disease of bone. J. Bone Joint Surg. 64B, 258, 1982.

28. Hadjipavlou, A., Lisbona, R., and Boudreau, R.: Radionuclide bone blood flow in Paget's disease of bone. Orthopaedic Transactions. J. Bone Joint Surg. 8, 215, 1984.

29. Hadjipavlou, A., Tsoukas, G.M., Siller, T.N., Danais, S., and Greenwood, F.: Combination of drug therapy in treatment of Paget's disease of bone. J. Bone Joint Surg. 59A, 1045, 1977.

30. Hadjipavlou, A., and Zucker, J.: Sarcoma in Paget's disease of bone. In, Current Concepts of Diagnosis and Treatment of Bone and Soft Tissue Tumors. Eds: Uhthoff, H.-K., and Stahl, E.: Springer Verlag, Berlin-Heidelberg, 1983. pp 383-394.

31. Hartman, J.T., and Dohn, D.F.: Paget's disease of the spine with cord or nerve root compression. J. Bone Joint Surg. 48A, 1079, 1966.

32. Huvos, G.A., Butler, A., and Bretsky, S.: Osteogenic sarcoma associated with Paget's disease of bone. Cancer 52, 1489, 1983.

33. Jaffe, H.: Paget's disease of bone. Arch. Pathol. 15, 83, 1933.

34. Johnston, C.C., Altman, R.D., Canfield, R.E., Finerman, A.G., and Taulbee, J.D.: Review of fracture experience during treatment of Paget's disease of bone with etidronate disodium (EHDP). Clin. Orthop. 172, 183, 1983.

35. Krane, S.M.: Etidronate disodium in the treatment of Paget's disease of bone. Ann. Intern. Med. 96, 619, 1982.

36. Lake, M.: Studies of Paget's disease (osteitis deformans). J. Bone Joint Surg. 33B, 323, 1951.

37. Lake, M.: The pathology of fracture in Paget's disease. Aust. NZ J. Surg. 27, 307, 1958.

38. Lemaire, R.: Les fractures des os longs dans la maladie de Paget. Acta Orthop. Belg. 40, 4, 1974.

39. Lowry, A.M., and Rutherford, J.L.: Osteitis deformans (Paget's disease) fissure fractures - Their etiology and clinical significance. AJR 38, 109, 1937.

40. Mathé, J.F., Delobel, R., Resche, F., Cler, J.M., and Feve, J.R.: Syndrome medullaires au cours de la maladie de Paget. Rôle du facteur vasculaire. La Nouv. Presse Med. 39, 2619, 1976.

41. McKenna, R.J., Schwinn, C.P., Soong, K.Y., and Higinbotham, N.L.: Osteogenic sarcoma arising in Paget's disease. Cancer 17, 42, 1964.

42. Merkow, R.L., and Lane, J.M.: Current concepts of Paget's disease of bone. Orthop. Clin. North Am. 15, 747, 1984.

43. Meyers, M.H., and Singer, F.R.: Osteotomy for tibia vara in Paget's disease under cover of calcitonin. J. Bone Joint Surg. 60A, 810, 1977.

44. Milgram, J.W.: Orthopaedic management of Paget's disease of bone. Clin. Orthop. 127, 63, 1977.

45. Molle, D., Bord, H., Kuntz, D., Voisin, C., Farcet, J.P., Delepine, D., and Rychewaert, A.: Ostelyse rélévatrice d'un lymphome développé. Rev. Rhum. Mal. Osteoartic. 50, 217, 1983.

46. O'Reilly, T.J., and Race, J.: Osteitis deformans. Q. J. Med. 12, 471, 1932.

47. Paget, J.: Remarks on osteitis deformans. Illust. Med. News. 2, 181, 1889.

48. Platt, H.: Sarcoma in abnormal bones. Br. J. Surg. 34, 232, 1947.

49. Poretta, C.A., Dablin, D.C., and Jones, J.M.: Sarcoma in Paget's disease of bone. J. Bone Joint Surg. 39A, 1314, 1957.

50. Price, C.H.G., and Goldie, W.: Paget's sarcoma of bone. A study of eighty cases from the Bristol and Leeds Bone Tumor Registries. J. Bone Joint Surg. 51B, 205, 1969.

51. Rauis, A.: Étude statistique sur la maladie de Paget, ses complications et leur traitement. Acta Orthop. Belg. 40, 4, 1974.

52. Redden, J.F., Dixon, J., Vennart, W., and Hoskins, D.J.: Management of fissure fractures in Paget's disease. Int. Orthop. 5, 103, 1981.

53. Resnick, D., and Niwayama, G.: Diagnosis of Bone and Joint Disorders with Emphasis on Articular Abnormalities. W.B. Saunders, Philadelphia, 1981. p. 1738.

54. Roberts, R.E., and Cohen, M.J.: Osteitis deformans (Paget's disease of bone). Proc. Royal Soc. Lond. 19, 13, 1926.

55. Rogers, M.H., and Ulin, R.: Fractures in Paget's disease. J. Bone Joint Surg. 18, 914, 1936.

56. Ryan, W.C., and Schwartz, T.B.: Mithramycin and malignancy (Letter). Ann. Int. Med. 94, 279, 1981.

57. Schatzki, S.C., and Dudley, H.R.: Bone sarcoma complicating Paget's disease. Cancer 14, 517, 1961.

58. Siegelman, S.S., Levine, S.A., and Walpin, L.: Paget's disease with spinal cord compression. Clin. Radiol. 19, 421, 1968.

59. Singer, R.F.: Paget's disease of bone. Topics in Bone and Mineral Disorders Series. Ed: Avioli, L.V., Plenum Publishing Corporation, 1977. p. 112.

60. Smidek, H.H.: Neurologic and neurosurgical sequelae of Paget's disease of bone. Clin. Orthop. 127, 70, 1977.

61. Smith, J., Botel, F.J., and Yeh, S.D.J.: Bone sarcomas in Paget's disease: A study of 85 patients. Radiology 152, 583, 1984.

62. Sumney, T.J., and Pressley, C.L.: Sarcoma complicating Paget's disease of bone. Ann. Surg. 123, 135, 1946.

63. Weisz, G.M.: Lumbar spinal canal stenosis in Paget's disease. Spine 8, 192, 1983.

64. Wick, M.R., Siegel, G.P., Unni, K.K., McLeod, R.A., and Greditzer, H.G.: Sarcomas of bone complicating osteitis deformans (Paget's disease). Fifty years experience. Am. J. Surg. Pathol. 5, 47, 1981.

65. Zlatkin, B.M., Lander, P.H., Levine, J.H., and Hadjipavlou, A.: Computed tomography of Paget's disease of the spine. Presented at the 48th Annual Meeting of the Canadian Association of Radiologists, Toronto, Canada. June, 1985 - in program.

Reversible Osteopenias

Bone Fragility in Osteomalacia: Mechanisms and Consequences

A. M. Parfitt

Although traditionally related to vitamin D deficiency, osteomalacia is now commonly defined in histologic terms as significant replacement of normal lamellar bone by unmineralized osteoid, due to a defect in bone mineralization, without regard to etiology (Frame and Parfitt, 1978). An increase in relative osteoid volume must result from some combination of increased remodeling activation and increased mean mineralization lag time (MLT), ie, the time interval between synthesis and mineralization of an individual moiety of bone matrix (Parfit, 1984). The most satisfactory kinetic criteria for defective mineralization are a mean osteoid seam width (uncorrected for section obliquity) >15 µm and a mean MLT >100 days (Parfitt et al, 1981).

There are many other causes of osteomalacia, but intestinal malabsorption of vitamin D and calcium account for at least 75% of all adult cases in the USA. During the evolution of bone disease, as the result of depletion or impaired metabolism of vitamin D, the first stage is secondary hyperparathyroidism (Rao et al, 1983). This increases remodeling activation and bone formation rate, leading to increases in osteoid surface and volume but not thickness. Much later, this is followed by impaired mineralization which increases osteoid thickness with a substantial further increase in osteoid volume but little further increase in osteoid surface (Parfitt, 1984). Patients with impaired mineralization can be subdivided according to the presence or absence of some double tetracycline labeling (Rao et al, 1983), so that three stages in the evolution of hypovitaminosis D osteopathy can be recognized (Table I). In the less common forms of osteomalacia not due to

Table I. Histologic evolution of hypovitaminosis D osteopathy*

Grade	i	ii	iii
Osteoid seam width (µm)	7-15	15-25	> 25
Mineralization lag time (d)	< 100	> 100	∞
Double tetracycline labels	+	+	-
Bone formation rate	↑	N	0
Relative osteoid volume (%)	5-10	10-20	> 20

* Differences in osteoid measurements are approximate since there is significant overlap between grades.

Current Concepts of Bone Fragility

Table II. Iliac mineralized and unmineralized bone in osteomalacia - representative mean values*

	Cortical		Trabecular		Combined	
	N	OM	N	OM	N	OM
Tissue width (mm)	2.7	1.8	5.5	6.4	8.2	8.2
Relative osteoid volume (%TB)	0.4	6.0	2.0	30.0	0.9	15.5
Relative (%TT):						
Total bone volume	92.5	90.0	20.0	16.0	43.9	32.2
Osteoid volume	0.4	5.4	0.4	4.8	0.4	4.9
Mineralized bone volume	92.1	84.6	19.6	11.2	43.5	27.3
Absolute (mm^3/mm^2 periosteal area):						
Total bone volume	2.50	1.62	1.10	1.03	3.60	2.65
Osteoid volume	0.01	0.10	0.02	0.31	0.03	0.41
Mineralized bone volume	2.49	1.52	1.08	0.72	3.57	2.24

* Tissue width is measured perpendicular to the periosteum so that as cortical width declines trabecular width increases if there is no change in external dimensions. TB = total bone; TT = total tissue. Note that absolute values for cortical and trabecular bone can be combined by simple addition, but relative values cannot.

depletion or impaired metabolism of vitamin D, the natural history of osteoid accumulation is less well defined. An increase in osteoid surface probably precedes the increase in osteoid width, but the mechanism more likely relates to prolongation of sigma than to increase in remodeling activation (Jaworski, 1972).

Stage I hypovitaminosis D osteopathy, or preosteomalacia, is characterized by absence of symptoms, normal plasma calcium and phosphate levels, increased alkaline phosphatase, biochemical and histologic evidence of secondary hyperparathyroidism, accelerated loss of cortical and trabecular bone, increased fracture risk and need for treatment with some form of vitamin D. Osteoid accumulation, although of diagnostic and pathogenetic importance, does not become biomechanically significant until stages II and III are reached. In osteomalacia there is a mean increase in osteoid volume of about 15-fold in both cortical and trabecular bone, with a range of 5-30 fold, and an approximate 2-fold increase in remodeling space, manifested by an increase in cortical porosity (Table II). Assuming that cortical bone is 80% of the total for the whole body rather than about 70% as in the ilium, and that because of its higher rate of turnover relative deficits in the ilium are about twice as great as in the skeleton as a whole, this is equivalent to a reduction in total body calcium of about 5% that is potentially reversible (Table III).

The much larger irreversible reduction of about 25% is due to increased net endosteal resorption and cortical thinning, and is greater than would be predicted from the iliac measurements (Tables II and III) because of the

Table III. Skeletal mineral deficits in osteomalacia*

	Cortical	Trabecular	Combined
Reversible	- 2.5	- 2.5	- 5
Irreversible	- 22.5	- 2.5	- 25
Total	- 25	- 5	- 30

* Data expressed as percent of total body bone mineral. The reversible deficit includes osteoid accumulation and remodeling space; the irreversible deficit is due mainly to cortical thinning.

different behavior of cortical bone in the appendicular and axial skeleton (Parfitt et al, in press). As already mentioned and as discussed more fully elsewhere in this symposium (Parfitt, 1985), cortical thinning is most likely the result of prolonged secondary hyperparathyroidism. In osteomalacia due to various forms of primary hypophosphatemia not caused by secondary hyperparathyroidism, the magnitude of osteoid accumulation is similar, but the extent of cortical bone loss is less severe and more variable, and in some cases cortical thickness may even be increased.

The most characteristic expression of bone fragility in osteomalacia is the Looser zone, which begins as a stress fracture of the insufficiency type, but fails to undergo the usual mode of healing (McKenna et al, in press; Parfitt, 1977). Lesions that conform exactly to the classic description -- lucent bands that are multiple, symmetrical, perpendicular to the periosteum, with no visible abnormality of adjacent bone, and complete absence of adjacent sclerosis and visible callus -- occur only in osteomalacia (Table IV), but are nowadays quite rare. More commonly, the appearance is intermediate in one or more respects between this classic description and typical insufficiency fractures (McKenna et al, in press; Parfitt, 1977), and both individual lesions and groups of lesions in individual patients can be located anywhere on the spectrum between these two extremes. Such fractures are less specific and can occur in osteoporosis without osteoid accumulation

Table IV. Comparison of classic Looser zones and stress fractures

	Stress fractures	Looser zones
Lucent band	Absent	Present
Adjacent bone	Can be abnormal*	Normal
Number	Usually single	Multiple
	Asymmetric	Symmetric
Sclerosis	Present	Absent
Visible callus	Present	Absent
Healing	Rapid	Slow or absent

* eg, in Paget's disease

(McKenna et al, in press). Indeed, because of the much earlier diagnosis of osteomalacia with wider use of bone biopsy, even though the relative incidence is lower, the absolute frequency of atypical osteoporotic stress fractures resembling Looser zones is now greater than the absolute frequency of typical osteomalacic Looser zones. Histologic study of stress fractures of any type is still fragmentary and the pathogenesis of Looser zones is still obscure.

The most serious expression of bone fragility in osteomalacia is a hip fracture, but the nature of the relationship is complex and controversial. The frequent finding of subclinical vitamin D deficiency in patients with hip fractures (Parfitt et al, 1982) could be a marker for associated disease leading to inactivity and poor diet, or an etiologic factor for muscle weakness leading to more frequent falls and less efficient energy absorption during the fall. Because of the severity of cortical bone loss due to long-standing secondary hyperparathyroidism, it would be surprising if hip fracture risk were not thereby increased, but this remains to be conclusively demonstrated. Whether osteoid accumulation further increases fracture risk is unclear. Several investigators have reported an increased prevalence of histologic indices of osteomalacia in hip fracture patients (Aaron et al, 1974; Parfitt et al, 1982), but there is considerable geographic variation (Parfitt et al, 1982). With minimal additional trauma, a Looser zone can become a complete fracture with potential displacement or even separation of the bone ends, a sequence of events that, in the subtrochanteric region, is virtually confined to osteomalacia (Chalmers, 1970). The reported association between osteomalacia and subcapital rather than intertrochanteric fractures (O'Driscoll, 1973) might reflect an increased prevalence of the trabecular microfractures that are commonly found in the excised femoral head (Freeman et al, 1974). However, more recent studies have found either no difference (Aaron et al, 1974; Morris et al, 1984) or the opposite difference (Lawton et al, 1983) between the two fracture types.

In a study of 82 consecutive hip fractures at Henry Ford Hospital (Wixson et al, 1978), plasma 250HD levels, iliac bone biopsy, and photon absorptiometry of the radius were collectively performed only in 21 subjects. When

Table V. Vitamin D deficiency and hip fractures*

	250HD > 5 (n = 13)	250HD < 5 (n = 8)	p
Plasma 250HD (ng/mL)	14.3±2.0	3.4±0.4	-
Osteoclast surface (% NOS)	0.8±0.5	3.2±0.8	<0.01
Relative osteoid volume (% TB)	1.9±0.4	2.0±0.6	NS
Proximal BM/BW (z)	-0.6±0.5	-3.0±0.3	<0.001

* Comparison of histologic and densitometric indices between hip fracture patients subdivided according to plasma 250HD levels. NOS = non-osteoid surface; TB = total bone; BM/BW - bone mineral/bone width determined by single energy photon absorptiometry; data expressed as z scores, obtained by dividing the individual differences from age, sex and race predicted values by the population standard deviation. On this scale the normal range by definition extends from +2 to -2.

these were subdivided according to the plasma 25OHD level (Table V), those below 5 ng/mL had significantly higher osteoclast-covered surfaces and more severe cortical bone loss in the radius, but there was no difference in the degree of osteoid accumulation. These data are clearly preliminary, but support the presence of increased parathyroid hormone-mediated bone resorption in patients with hip fractures with subclinical vitamin D deficiency despite the absence of impaired bone mineralization (Lips et al, 1982; Wixson et al, 1978). Evidently much more study of this problem is needed because of its potential public health importance.

References

1. Aaron, J.E., Gallagher, J.C., Anderson, J., Stasiak, L., Longton, E.B., Nordin, B.E.C., and Nicholson, M.: Frequency of osteomalacia and osteoporosis in fractures of the proximal femur. Lancet 1, 229, 1974.

2. Chalmers, J.: Subtrochanteric fractures in osteomalacia. J. Bone Joint Surg. 52B, 509, 1970.

3. Frame, B., and Parfitt, A.M.: Osteomalacia: current concepts. Ann. Intern. Med. 89, 966, 1978.

4. Freeman, M.A.R., Todd, R.C., and Pirie, C.J.: The role of fatigue in the pathogenesis of senile femoral neck fractures. J. Bone Joint Surg. 56B, 698, 1974.

5. Jaworski, Z.F.G.: Pathophysiology, diagnosis and treatment of osteomalacia. In, The Orthopedic Clinics of North America, Vol. 3. W.B. Saunders, Philadelphia, 1972, pp 623-652.

6. Lawton, J.O., Baker, M.R., and Dickson, R.A.: Femoral neck fractures: two populations. Lancet 2, 70, 1983.

7. Lips, P., Netelenbos, J.C., Jongen, M.J.M., van Ginkel, F.C., Althuis, A.L., van Schaik, C.L., Van der Vijgh, W.J.F., Vermeiden, J.P.W., and van der Meer, C.: Histomorphometric profile and vitamin D status in patients with femoral neck fracture. Metab. Bone Dis. Rel. Res. 4, 85, 1982.

8. McKenna, M.J., Kleerekoper, M., Ellis, B.I., Rao, D.S., Parfitt, A.M., and Frame, B.: Insufficiency fractures confused with Looser zones of osteomalacia. In press.

9. Morris, H.A., Morrison, G.W., Burr, M., Thomas, D.W., and Nordin, B.E.C.: Vitamin D and femoral neck fractures in elderly South Australian women. Med. J. Aust. 140, 519, 1984.

10. O'Driscoll, M.: Subcapital fracture types and osteomalacia and vitamin D deficiency. J. Bone Joint. Surg. 55B, 882, 1973 (Abstr.)

11. Parfitt, A.M.: The clinical and radiographic manifestations of renal osteodystrophy. In, Perspectives in Hypertension and Nephrology: Calcium Metabolism in Renal Failure and Nephrolithiasis. Ed.: David, D.J. J. Wiley, 1977. pp 145-195.

12. Parfitt, A.M.: The cellular mechanisms of osteoid accumulation in metabolic bone disease. In, Mineral Metabolism Research in Italy, Vol. 4. Milano, Wichtig Editore, 1984. pp 3-9.

13. Parfitt, A.M.: Accelerated cortical bone loss in primary and secondary hyperparathyroidism. In, Bone Fragility in Orthopaedics and Medicine. Eds: Uhthoff, H.-K., and Stahl, E. Springer-Verlag, Berlin, New York, 1985.

14. Parfitt, A.M., Gallagher, J.C., Heaney, R.P., Johnston, C.C., Neer, R., and Whedon, G.D.: Vitamin D and bone health in the elderly. Am. J. Clin. Nutr. 36, 1014, 1982.

15. Parfitt, A.M., Mathews, C., Rao, D., Frame, B., Kleerekoper, M., and Villanueva, A.R.: Impaired osteoblast function in metabolic bone disease. In, Osteoporosis: Recent Advances in Pathogenesis and Treatment. Eds: DeLuca, H.F., Frost, H., Jee, W., Johnston, C., and Parfitt, A.M. University Park Press, Baltimore, 1981. pp 321-330.

16. Parfitt, A.M., Rao, D.S., Stanciu, J., Villanueva, A.R., Kleerekoper, M., and Frame, B.: Photon absorptiometry of the radius during treatment of osteomalacia: comparison with iliac bone histomorphometry and demonstration of irreversible bone loss. In press.

17. Rao, D.S., Villanueva, A., Mathews, M., Pumo, B., Frame, B., Kleerekoper, M., and Parfitt, A.M.: Histologic evolution of vitamin D depletion in patients with intestinal malabsorption or dietary deficiency. In, Clinical Disorders of Bone and Mineral Metabolism. Eds: Frame, B. and Potts, J.T., Jr. Excerpta Medica, Amsterdam, 1983. pp 224-226.

18. Wixson, R., Schock, C.C., Mathews, C.H.E., Kilates, M.C., and Parfitt, A.M.: The presence of osteomalacia and osteoporosis in patients with hip fractures. Orthopedic Transactions 1, 149, 1978. (Abstr.)

Drug-Induced Osteomalacia

J. A. BRUNET

Osteomalacia is a type of reversible osteopenia characterized by softening of bone due to impaired or inadequate mineralization. A surprisingly diverse spectrum of diseases can produce an osteomalacic process. However, from the point of view of pathogenesis, these disease entities can be classified into three broad categories: disorders of vitamin D metabolism; disorders related to hypophosphatemia; and miscellaneous conditions (Burtis and Lang, 1984).

Osteomalacia Due to Disorders of Vitamin D Metabolism

a) *Simple vitamin D deficiency*, secondary to either insufficient dietary intake or inadequate sunlight exposure, is an uncommon cause of osteomalacia. Susceptible individuals include poorly nourished groups; ethnic groups whose dressing habits allow little exposure to sunlight; chronically ill individuals who are unable to go out and are not receiving vitamin supplements; and breast-fed infants not receiving vitamin supplements.

b) *Intestinal malabsorption of vitamin D* as a cause of dietary vitamin D insufficiency is slightly more common, and includes primary biliary cirrhosis, pancreatic exocrine insufficiency, short bowel syndrome, and celiac sprue. In these conditions, interruption of the enterohepatic circulation of vitamin D metabolites leads to osteomalacia apparently in spite of adequate exposure to ultraviolet light.

c) *Impairment of vitamin D metabolism.* Hepatic causes of impaired vitamin D metabolism are rare since severe liver dysfunction must occur to produce 25-(OH)ase deficiency. Drug toxicity, especially phenytoin, may adversely affect the liver's handling of vitamin D metabolites; this contentious issue will be discussed later in this presentation.

Renal causes of impaired vitamin D metabolism include impaired renal production of 1,α(OH)ase enzyme, resulting in low serum levels of $1,25\text{-}(OH)_2D$. Vitamin D-dependent rickets of the Type I variety is thought to be a hereditary lack of the kidney enzyme 1,α(OH)ase. Low serum levels of $1,25\text{-}(OH)_2D$ characterize this disorder, and physiologic doses of this metabolite will reverse it. Finally, osteomalacia is also seen in some families whose members have elevated levels of $1,25\text{-}(OH)_2D$. This disease entity, known as Type II vitamin D-dependent rickets, has been attributed to possible end organ resistance to $1,25\text{-}(OH)_2D$, or to the requirement for a metabolite other than $1,25\text{-}(OH)_2D$ to correct the osteomalacic process.

Current Concepts of Bone Fragility

Osteomalacia Due to Hypophosphatemia

Osteomalacia also occurs in persons with a primary phosphate deficiency but with normal levels of vitamin D. Biochemically, these disorders are characterized by low serum phosphate, elevated alkaline phosphatase levels, and normal calcium levels (in contrast to the low or low-normal serum calcium levels seen in the vitamin D-related osteomalacias).

a) *Phosphate deficiency* caused by malnutrition or malabsorption is uncommon, but excessive use of aluminum hydroxide-containing antacids can lead to phosphate depletion and osteomalacia in some patients.

b) *Renal tubular loss of phosphate.* Phosphate depletion secondary to a renal leak is a very common cause of rickets and osteomalacia. Familial hypophosphatemic rickets, also termed vitamin D-resistant rickets, is the most common type of rickets today. This disease is characterized by a very low renal phosphate threshold (thus allowing phosphate to "spill" into the urine), and normal or slightly elevated iPTH levels. Levels of 1,25-$(OH)_2$D are low-normal. The condition is corrected in part by administering 1,25-$(OH)_2$ D and large doses of phosphate.

c) *Fanconi's syndromes* comprise a heterogenous group of disorders with varying degrees of impaired renal proximal tubular transport which may include renal phosphate wasting leading to osteomalacia.

d) *Oncogenic osteomalacia.* Rarely, osteomalacia can develop in the presence of a variety of benign or malignant tumors. The renal phosphate threshold is markedly depressed despite normal levels of serum iPTH; 1,25-$(OH)_2$D levels are low-normal. A tumor-derived humoral factor causing renal phosphate wasting is suggested by the fact that all biochemical and bone histologic measurements return to normal after resection of the tumor.

Miscellaneous Causes of Osteomalacia*

Other rare conditions which may cause rickets and osteomalacia include hypophosphatasia, fibrogenesis *imperfecta ossium*, amd axial osteomalacia.

Various drugs, including fluoride, disodium etidronate, and anticonvulsants, are known to cause osteomalacia. The moderate delay in mineralization observed in osteoporotic patients treated with fluoride is probably secondary to the increased osteoid production rather than due to fluoride toxicity (Lane et al, 1984). The morphologic bone changes seen during fluoride therapy appear to remodel toward normal after discontinuation of fluoride (Vigorita et al, 1984). In patients treated with the antipagetic agent etidronate, the incidence of an osteomalacic lesion developing in the normal portion of their bone tissue appears to be time- and dose-related. After discontinuing this drug, mineralization of the osteomalacic lesion proceeds normally.

Anticonvulsant-Induced osteomalacia

Research carried out on the mechanisms of osteopenia induced by exogenous glucocorticoids stimulated interest in the study of other metabolic bone

* For *aluminum osteopathy*, see "Skeletal problems in chronic renal disease", by Dr. M. Kaye.

diseases possibly related to chronic drug intake. The importance of accurately defining and understanding these disorders stemmed from the widespread use of these drugs and their essential role in controlling many disease states. Among these drugs, anticonvulsants were found to be related to a syndrome characterized by biochemical and occasionally histologic evidence suggestive of an osteomalacic process (Bouillon et al, 1975; Christiansen et al, 1981; Hahn et al, 1975; Melsen and Mosekilde, 1976).

The earliest descriptions of this new syndrome were contained in reports from Europe, where mild vitamin D deficiency is not uncommon. Although they dealt with epileptics living in northern European communities (and thus patients likely to receive less sunlight), subsequently, the same findings were discovered in patients on phenobarbital (PB) or diphenylhydantoin (DPH) treatment living in North America (Dent et al, 1970; Murchison et al, 1975; Richens and Rowe, 1970). In addition, although the condition was initially shown to affect predominantly institutionalized epileptic patients receiving long-term anticonvulsants, later all epileptic inpatients and outpatients of all age groups were found to be at risk of developing the syndrome (Hahn et al, 1972b; Lifshitz and MacLaren, 1973). However, the clinical spectrum was soon discovered to be extremely broad, with large variations in the degree of hypocalcemia, hypophosphatemia, raised alkaline phosphatase levels, and reduced bone mass (Christiansen et al, 1981; Hahn et al, 1972b, 1975; Lifshitz and MacLaren, 1973). Some of the severe cases described had obvious concomitant diseases and nutritonal hypovitaminosis D (Bouillon et al, 1975).

Over the years, careful epidemiologic assessment of the different series from various parts of the world helped to identify a number of risk factors shared by most of the affected epileptics. A few of these variables were subsequently shown to correlate well with either the severity of the biochemical or radiologic characteristics of the syndrome, whereas many other observed features were found to be simply associated with, or possibly predisposing to the development of the syndrome. These risk factors included:

a) multiple anticonvulsant drug regimens (Hahn et al, 1972b, 1975; Richens and Rowe, 1970);

b) total daily dose of the drug received and duration of therapy (Bouillon et al, 1975; Lifshitz and Maclaren, 1973);

c) type of anticonvulsant drug prescribed;

d) reduced dietary intake of D_2 or D_3 and reduced sunlight exposure leading to a state of relative hypovitaminosis D (Haddad and Hahn, 1973; Hahn et al, 1972b);

e) decreased physical activity, either because of the sedative effects of some anticonvulsants, or because of the physical limitations imposed by associated neurologic disorders, thereby compounding the osteopenic state of affected individuals (Dymling et al, 1979; Murchison et al, 1975);

f) interactions between nutritional factors and vitamin D biotransformation (Alvares et al, 1976). Since many institutionalized epileptics do not receive balanced nutritious diets, it is possible that dietary factors may alter their vitamin D metabolism;

g) the additive effects of many other drugs, taken concomitantly (ie, tranquilizers, oral hypoglycemic agents, etc), known to induce hepatic microsomal enzyme activity which in turn may affect vitamin D metabolism (Conney, 1967).

Pathogenesis of anticonvulsant-induced osteomalacia

With the advent of sensitive diagnostic laboratory techniques, attempts were made to shed light on the mechanisms of drug-induced hypocalcemia in epileptic patients receiving anticonvulsants. The interest and research were thus concentrated in two main areas: altered vitamin D metabolism and intestinal calcium malabsorption.

Effects of anticonvulsants on the hepatic metabolism of drugs and hormones

Almost all anticonvulsants are capable of increasing biliary flow (Roberts and Plaa, 1966) and of inducing cytochrome P-450-dependent hepatic microsomal, mixed function oxidase activity (Conney, 1967). These enzymes as a group are known to be involved in degradative or anabolic reactions of many hormones and of many drugs. An increased activity of these enzymes results in accelerated biotransformation of drugs *in vivo* with an increased production of polar, hydroxylated and biologically-inactive compounds which are eliminated in the bile and urine (Conney, 1967). This phenomenon of hepatic microsomal enzyme induction by drugs, resulting in significantly reduced duration and intensity of the activity of drugs or hormones, has been particularly well documented in the case of exogenous estrogen, progesterone, or corticosteroids administered concurrently with PB and DPH (Jubiz et al, 1970; Levin et al, 1967).

Effects of anticonvulsant medication on vitamin D metabolism

Lower serum levels of the 25-(OH)D metabolite was the first observed alteration in vitamin D metabolism seen in up to one-third of epileptics receiving long-term anticonvulsants (Hahn et al, 1972b). Early experimental studies demonstrated accelerated disappearance of vitamin D in rats and humans by an anticonvulsant-induced increase in hepatic production of more polar and hydroxylated (presumably inactive) vitamin D metabolites (Gascon-Barré and Côté, 1978; Hahn et al, 1972b; Silver et al, 1974). Increased bile flow and increased excretion of vitamin D metabolites were thus proposed as important pathogenetic mechanisms leading to reduced circulating levels of 25-(OH)D.

As the technology for measuring the activated form of vitamin D (1,25-$(OH)_2$D) became available, many studies reported normal or elevated levels in epileptic patients (Jubiz et al, 1977). These findings suggested either end organ unresponsiveness to the effects of 1,25-$(OH)_2$D, or that the observed hypocalcemia was independent of the effect of the drugs on vitamin D metabolism (Hahn, 1980).

The understanding of the pathogenesis of the syndrome continued to evolve as other more recent studies demonstrated normal levels of 25-(OH)D and of 1,25-$(OH)_2$D. In 31 ambulatory Israeli children and adolescents receiving DPH or PB for over one year, Weissman et al (1979) found that serum 25-(OH)D concentrations were similar to those of healthy, age-matched controls, presumably because of the abundant ultraviolet radiation prevalent in Israel.

In a group of noninstitutionalized, nonepileptic, cardiac patients receiving DPH for two years, Wark et al (1979) found normal 25-(OH)D levels, normal serum calcium and hepatic isoenzyme alkaline phosphatase levels compared to age-matched controls. Moreover, in a double-blind series performed in 74 children receiving either PB or placebo for 5 to 12 months for the control of single febrile seizures, Camfield et al (1981) did not find any significant alterations in serum 25-(OH)D levels. Finally, Weinstein et al (1984) found normal 25-(OH)D and 1,25-$(OH)_2$D levels in 120 adult outpatient-treated epileptics with ample solar exposure.

Anticonvulsant impairment of intestinal calcium absorption

Many experimental and clinical studies have demonstrated reduced or normal calcium intestinal absorption in a large proportion of patients treated with PB or DPH (Caspary et al, 1975; Corradino, 1972; Shafer and Nuttall, 1975). Unfortunately, in these studies, carried out in the 1970s, 1,25-$(OH)_2$D serum values were not measured, and thus a clear interpretation of these results was not possible. In a more recent study, increased calcium intestinal absorption was documented in treated epileptics, but the observed high 1,25-$(OH)_2$D serum levels may be responsible for this increased intestinal absorption of calcium (Bell et al, 1979).

Effects of anticonvulsants on bone tissue

In contrast to the numerous reports detailing the biochemical changes related to antiepileptic treatment, only a few descriptions pertaining to the histomorphologic changes have been published. Experimental animal models were developed to study this effect, but the data have been difficult to extrapolate to humans because of the inappropriate protocols in which osteomalacia and rickets were produced only after massive doses of the drugs had been administered to animals often maintained on rachitogenic diets (Harris et al, 1978; Villareal et al, 1978). Clinical histologic data, which have been sparse, were obtained from reviews of patients receiving principally DPH alone or combined with other anticonvulsants. One study simply described excessive osteoid and increased osteoclastic activity (Dent et al, 1970); others have reported more information in terms of static histologic measurements of increased osteoid seam thickness, diminished calcification front, and also increased osteoclastic resorption surfaces with increased mean volume of periosteocytic lacunae, suggesting secondary hyperparathyroidism (Eastwood et al, 1980; Johnell et al, 1979; Melsen and Mosekilde, 1976).

However, more recent studies have provided measurements with more meaningful data. Melsen and Mosekilde (1980) have presented histomorphometric data revealing normal mineralization lag times in bone biopsies obtained from 20 epileptics receiving DPH alone or in combination with other anticonvulsants for at least 10 years (ie, no mineralization defect despite increased osteoid width). Similarly, Weinstein et al (1984) reported that bone biopsies of 20 treated epileptics exhibiting severe osteopenia revealed increased osteoid but normal calcification front formation, accelerated mineralization rate, and decreased mineralization lag time, ie, histomorphometric data indicative of increased skeletal turnover rather than osteomalacia. These findings are seen in other conditions of increased skeletal turnover such as primary hyperparathyroidism, Paget's disease, and uremic osteitis.

Effects of anticonvulsants on the action of parathyroid hormone (PTH)

Various studies have reported elevated serum immunoreactive PTH levels in treated epileptics, produced in response to hypocalcemia (Bouillon et al, 1975; Hahn et al, 1972; Weinstein et al, 1984). It has been proposed that the failure of the secondary hyperparathyroidism to compensate for hypocalcemia, the relative paucity of osteoclasts in these patients' bone biopsies, and the histomorphometric data similar to those seen in hyperparathyroidism all suggest that anticonvulsants may indeed cause resistance to the action of PTH (Weinstein et al, 1984).

Summary

In summary, osteopenia of variable severity frequently occurs due to long-term administration of anticonvulsants. Biochemical changes appear to be more frequent than bone tissue changes. Many factors are known to be associated with the development of this syndrome, but the exact pathogenesis remains unclear.

Long-term anticonvulsant therapy seems to affect vitamin D metabolism at the hepatic level, in some cases leading to lower serum values of 25-(OH)D. However, in many instances, the serum levels of this metabolite remain unaffected by the antiepileptic medications.

Despite usually sufficient or elevated levels of the activated form of vitamin D [1,25-$(OH)_2$D], hypocalcemia, hypophosphatemia, and osteopenia are often present. This suggests that hypocalcemia is independent of the effects of the drugs on vitamin D metabolism. Possibly other vitamin D metabolites affected by anticonvulsant medications may be responsible for the observed biochemical abnormalities.

Anticonvulsant drugs may cause resistance to the action of PTH.

Dynamic morphometric analysis of bone biopsies of treated epileptics suggests increased skeletal turnover rather than osteomalacia.

The biochemical and bone tissue alterations induced by long-term anticonvulsant therapy are probably multifactorial. Further investigative work is required to elucidate the importance and the impact of this problem before recommendations for prophylactic supplementary vitamin D therapy are endorsed for treated epileptics.

References

1. Alvares, A.P., Anderson, K.E., and Conney, A.H.: Interactions between nutritional factors and drug biotransformations in man. Proc. Natl. Acad. Sci. USA 73, 2501, 1976.

2. Bell, R.D., Pak, C.Y.C., Zerwekh, J., et al: Effect of phenytoin on bone and vitamin D metabolism. Ann. Neurol. 5, 374, 1979.

3. Bouillon, R., Reynaert, J., Claes, J.H., et al: The effect of anticonvulsant therapy on serum levels of 25-hydroxy-vitamin D, calcium and parathyroid hormone. J. Clin. Endocrinol. Metab. 41, 1130, 1975.

4. Burtis, W.J., and Lang, R.: Chemical abnormalities. Orthop. Clin. North Am. 15, 653, 1984.

5. Camfield, C.S., Delvin, E.E., Glorieux, F.H., et al: Normal serum 25-hydroxyvitamin D levels in phenobarbital treated toddlers. Unpublished data.

6. Caspary, W.F., Hesch, R.D., Matte, R., et al: Intestinal calcium absorption in epileptics under anticonvulsant therapy. In, Vitamin D and Problems Related to Uremic Bone Diseases. Eds, Norman, A.W., Schaefer, K., Coburn, J.W., et al. Walter de Gruyter, Berlin, New York, 1975. pp 737-742.

7. Christiansen, C.K., Bi Lund, B.J., Lund, O.H., et al: Reduced 1,25-dihydroxyvitamin D and 24,25-dihydroxyvitamin D in epileptic patients receiving chronic combined anticonvulsant therapy. Metab. Bone Dis. Rel. Res. 3, 17, 1981.

8. Conney, A.H.: Pharmacological implications of microsomal enzyme induction. Pharmacol. Rev. 19, 317, 1967.

9. Corradino, R.A.: Diphenylhydantoin: direct inhibition of the vitamin D_3-mediated calcium absorption mechanism in organ-cultured duodenum. Biochem. Pharmacol. 25, 863, 1976.

10. Dent, C.E., Richens, A., Rowe, D.J.F., et al: Osteomalacia with long-term anticonvulsant therapy in epilepsy. Brit. Med. J. 4, 69, 1970.

11. Dymling, J. F., Lindgren, L., and Wallöe, A.: Biochemical variables related to calcium metabolism in epileptics. Acta Med. Scand. 205, 401, 1979.

12. Eastwood, J.B., Phillips, M.E., and DeWardener, H.E.: Effect of vitamin D_3 (cholecalciferol) in anticonvulsant osteomalacia. Metab. Bone Dis. Rel. Res. 2, 83, 1980.

13. Gascon-Barré, M., and Côté, M.G.: Effects of phenobarbital and diphenylhydrantoin on acute vitamin D_3 toxicity in the rat. Toxicol. Appl. Pharmacol. 43, 125, 1978.

14. Haddad, J.G., Jr., and Hahn, T.J.: Natural and synthetic sources of circulating 25-hydroxyvitamin D in man. Nature 244, 515, 1973.

15. Hahn, T.J.: Drug-induced disorders of vitamin D and mineral metabolism. Clin. Endocinrol. Metab. 9, 107, 1980.

16. Hahn, T.J., Birge, S.J., and Scharp, C.R.: Phenobarbital-induced alterations in vitamin D metabolism. J. Clin. Invest. 51, 741, 1972a.

17. Hahn, T.J., Hendin, B.A., Scharp, C.R., et al: Effect of chronic anticonvulsant therapy on serum 25-hydroxycalciferol levels in adults. New Engl. J. Med. 287, 900, 1972b.

18. Hahn, T.J., Hendin, B.A., Scharp, C.R., et al: Serum 25-hydroxycholecalciferol levels and bone mass in children on chronic anticonvulsant therapy. New Engl. J. Med. 292, 550, 1975.

19. Harris, M., Rowe, D.J.F., and Darby, A.J.: Anticonvulsant osteomalacia induced in the rat by diphenylhydantoin. Calcif. Tissue Res. 25, 13, 1978.

20. Johnell, O., Nilsson, B.E., Wallöe, A., et al: Bone morphology in epileptics. Calcif. Tissue Int. 28, 93, 1979.

21. Jubiz, W., Haussler, M.R., and McCain, T.A.: Plasma 1,25-dihydroxyvitamin D levels in patients receiving anticonvulsant drugs. J. Clin. Endocinrol. Metab. 44, 617, 1977.

22. Jubiz, W., Meikle, A.W., and Levinson, R.A.: Effect of diphenylhandantoin on the metabolism of dexamethasone: Mechanism of the abnormal dexamethasone suppression in humans. New Engl. J. Med. 283, 11, 1970.

23. Lane, J.M., Healey, J.H., Schwartz, E., et al: Treatment of osteoporosis with sodium fluoride and calcium: Effects on vertebral fracture incidence and bone histomorphometry. Orthop. Clin. North Am. 15, 729, 1984.

24. Levin, W., Welch, R.M., and Conney, A.H.: Effect of chronic phenobarbital treatment on the liver microsomal metabolism and uterotrophic action of 17β-estradiol. Endocrinology 80, 135, 1967.

25. Lifshitz, F., and Maclaren, N.K.: Vitamin D-dependent rickets in institutionalized mentally retarded children receiving long-term anticonvulsant therapy. I. A survey of 288 patients. J. Pediatr. 83, 612, 1973.

26. Melsen, F., and Mosekilde, L.: A quantitative analysis of bone changes following anticonvulsant therapy. Calcif. Tissue Res. 21, 247, 1976.

27. Murchison, L.E., Bewsher, P.D., Chesters, M., et al: Effects of anticonvulsants and inactivity on bone disease in epileptics. Postgrad. Med. J. 51, 18, 1975.

28. Richens, A., and Rowe, D.J.F.: Distrubance of calcium metabolism by anticonvulsant drugs. Brit. Med. J. 4, 73, 1970.

29. Roberts, R.J., and Plaa, G.L.: Effect of norethandrolone, acetohexamide and Enovid on α-naphthylisothiocyanate-induced hyperbilirubinemia and cholestasis. Biochem. Pharmacol. 15, 333, 1966.

30. Shafer, R.B., and Nuttall, F.Q.: Calcium and folic acid absorption in patients taking anticonvulsant drugs. J. Clin. Endocrinol. Metab. 41, 1125, 1975.

31. Silver, J., Neale, G., and Thompson, G.R.: Effect of phenobarbitone treatment on vitamin D metabolism in mammals. Clin. Sci. Mol. Med. 46, 433, 1974.

32. Villareale, M.E., Chiroff, R.T., Bergstrom, W.H., et al: Bone changes induced by diphenylhydantoin in chicks on a controlled vitamin D intake. J. Bone Joint Surg. 60A, 911, 1978.

33. Vigorita, V.J., Suda, M.K., and Schwartz, E.: Unpublished data, 1984.

34. Wark, J.D., Larkins, R.G., and Perry-Keene, D.: Chronic diphenylhydantoin therapy does not reduce plasma 25-hydroxy-vitamin D. Clin. Endocrinol. 11, 267, 1979.

35. Weisman, Y., Fartal, A., Eisenberg, Z., et al: Decreased serum 24,25 dihydroxyvitamin D concentrations in children receiving chronic anticonvulsant therapy. Brit. Med. J. 2, 521, 1979.

36. Weinstein, R.S., Bryce, G.F., Sappington, L.J., et al: Decreased serum ionized calcium and normal vitamin D metabolite levels with anticonvulsant drug treatment. J. Clin. Endocrinol. Metab. 58, 1003, 1984.

Accelerated Cortical Bone Loss: Primary and Secondary Hyperparathyroidism

A. M. Parfitt

The loss of cortical bone with age occurs by thinning due to increased net resorption from the cortical endosteal surface with little or no increase in porosity (Laval-Jeantet et al, 1983; Parfitt, 1984; Thompson, 1980). Acceleration of this process in primary hyperparathyroidism has been demonstrated repeatedly by a variety of methods in the last 15 years (Dalen and Hjern, 1974; Dequeker, 1972; Gryfe, 1973; Hossain et al, 1970; Meema and Meema, 1982; Pak et al, 1975; Parfitt, 1976a; 1977). Nevertheless, current authoritative texts either ignore the fact altogether (Arnaud and Strewler, 1984; Aurbach et al, 1981) or mention it only in vague terms lacking anatomic specificity (Broadus, 1981; Habener and Potts, 1979; Turek, 1984). Furthermore, it was concluded from a recent comparison of single energy and dual energy photon absorptiometry that hyperparathyroidism increases the loss of trabecular but not of cortical bone (Seeman et al, 1982).

To settle this issue, we carried out single energy photon absorptiometry by the Norland-Cameron method in 115 white women with surgically verified primary hyperparathyroidism. The series included more than 80% of all patients operated on at Henry Ford Hospital during a consecutive five year period. These patients did not differ in age or disease severity from those in whom bone measurements were not performed. Consequently, our study population is more representative of the disease than those reported in publications which fail to mention why particular patients were selected for bone measurement (Hossain et al, 1970; Pak et al, 1975; Seeman et al, 1982). The results were compared with those obtained in 284 white women attending a general medical clinic, who had no evidence of any disease or drug exposure known to affect bone. The hyperparathyroid patients and controls did not differ significantly in age, menopausal status, height or weight (Kleerekoper et al, 1983).

The bone mineral content (g/cm) was about 13% lower in the patients than in the controls at both proximal and distal sites. This difference was not due to an error in measurement sites or to a reduction in bone width at the sites of measurement, since bone width was not significantly different at the distal site and slightly but significantly increased in the hyperparathyroid patients at the proximal site. The relative magnitude of loss was similar to that found by metacarpal radiogrammetry (Parfitt, 1977), a method that, although less precise than photon absorptiometry, provides a direct rather than an indirect demonstration of increased net endosteal resorption and resultant cortical thinning. Serial measurements after successful parathyroid surgery showed that only about 10-20% of the deficit was reversible,

Current Concepts of Bone Fragility

presumably because of increased cortical porosity and osteoid accumulation (Parfitt, 1980; Parfitt et al, 1979).

Whether primary hyperparathyroidism also increases loss of trabecular bone is unclear. In the spine, this has been inferred from measurements by dual energy photon absorptiometry (Seeman et al, 1982), by computed tomography (Pozzi-Mucelli et al, 1983), and from an apparent increased incidence of vertebral compression fractures (Dauphine et al, 1975). However, the amount of trabecular bone in the ilium determined by histomorphometry is either normal (Kleerekoper et al, 1983; Mosekilde and Melsen, 1978; Parfitt et al, 1979), increased (Broadus et al, 1983), or slightly reduced in women <50 years of age and normal in older women and in men (Charhon et al, 1982). The reasons for the discrepancy between different sites in the axial skeleton is unclear. The histologic method is more direct, but preferential loss of vertebral rather than iliac trabecular bone in hyperparathyroidism is possible. None of the papers cited has shown the patients selected for study to be representative of the disease. Whatever the explanation, the uncertainty and variability of axial trabecular bone status in primary hyperparathyroidism is in striking contrast to the constancy of increased loss of appendicular cortical bone.

Accelerated cortical bone loss of similar or greater severity and similar irreversibility has also been demonstrated in every form of secondary hyperparathyroidism where appropriate measurements have been made. For example, in 24 patients with status postgastrectomy, or some other form of intestinal malabsorption (Parfitt et al, 1985; Rao et al, 1984a; 1984b), selected for study because of suspected skeletal symptoms and raised alkaline phosphatase, and who had biochemical evidence of secondary hyperparathyroidism [increased immunoreactive parathyroid hormone (PTH) or NcAMP], low plasma calcidiol (<10 ng/mL), absence of osteomalacia shown by iliac bone histomorphometry after double tetracycline labeling, and (to minimize selection bias) absence of fracture history, the even greater cortical bone deficit determined in the same manner was 24% at the proximal and 25% at the distal site (Kleerekoper et al, 1983).

To further emphasize the role of increased PTH secretion, similar bone deficits were found in 10 patients similar in every respect to the larger group but with normal plasma calcidiol levels (≧10 ng/mL). In both groups the patients are presumed to have secondary hyperparathyroidism due to some combination of reduced intake of calcium and intestinal malabsorption of calcium. In the former group this was a consequence of vitamin D depletion, but in the latter group calcium malabsorption must have been a direct result of the primary disease unrelated to depletion of vitamin D. Whether the greater magnitude of cortical bone loss in secondary than in primary hyperparathryoidism was the result of a greater increase in PTH secretion, longer duration, or some additional effect of decreased rather than increased net intestinal absorption of calcium, unrelated to PTH, was not determined.

Other causes of secondary hyperparathyroidism in which accelerated cortical bone loss has been demonstrated (either by metacarpal morphometry, single energy photon absorptiometry of the radius, or both) include anticonvulsant therapy (Hahn et al, 1975), chronic renal failure (Parfitt, 1977; Parfitt et al, 1980), pseudohypoparathyroidism (Breslau et al, 1983; Parfitt, 1979), and Paget's disease (Chapuy et al, 1981; Toh et al, 1983). Since these conditions collectively encompass all possible directional changes of plasma calcium, phosphate and calcitriol (Table I), it may reasonably be concluded

Table I. Cortical bone loss in hyperparathyroidism*

Form of hyperparathyroidism	CT	SPA	TTBV	Ca	P	1,25
Primary	↓	↓	N	↑	↓	↑
Secondary						
Intestinal malabsorption	↓	↓	↓	↓	↓	↓
Anticonvulsant therapy	ND	↓	N	↓	N	↑
Chronic renal failure	↓	↓	↑	↓	↑	↓
Pseudohypoparathyroidism	↓	↓	ND	↓	↑	↓
Paget's disease	ND	↓	↑	N	N	↑

* CT = cortical thickness, determined by metacarpal radiogrammetry
SPA = single energy photon absorptiometry of the radius
TTBV = trabecular total bone volume by iliac bone histomorphometry
Ca, P and 1,25 = plasma levels of calcium, inorganic phosphate and calcitriol.
For usual direction change: ↑ = increased, ↓ = decreased, N = normal, ND - not determined.

that the increased cortical bone loss is a direct consequence of the only common factor, ie, a sustained chronic increase in parathyroid hormone secretion. As in primary hyperparathyroidism, the uniformity of accelerated loss of cortical bone in secondary hyperparathyroidism is associated with considerable variability in the amount of trabecular bone (Table I), which is reduced in intestinal malabsorption (Kleerekoper et al, 1983; Parfitt et al, 1985), normal in anticonvulsant treated patients (Mosekilde and Melson, 1980), and frequently but not invariably increased in chronic renal failure (Frost et al, 1981; Melsen et al, 1977; Parfitt, 1976; Seeman et al, 1982) and Paget's disease (Meunier, 1975).

It has been clearly established that age-related loss of cortical bone is a major contributory factor to the age-related increase in long bone fracture (Horsman et al, 1981; 1984; Melton and Riggs, 1983; Smith et al, 1975). Given the magnitude of the acceleration of cortical bone loss by hyperparathyroidism, it is almost certain that the risk of long bone fractures is thereby increased, although not yet demonstrated by rigorous epidemiologic studies. This is most likely one reason for the association between subclinical vitamin D deficiency and hip fractures found in most, but not all, studies that have addressed this issue (Parfitt et al, 1982). The validity of the association is unrelated to the presence of osteomalacia at the time of fracture; its significance is further discussed elsewhere in this symposium (Parfitt, 1985). The role of the age-related increase in parathyroid hormone secretion in normal age-related loss of cortical bone is unclear (Marcus et al, 1984), but the demonstrated relationship between increased PTH secretion and cortical bone loss provides further support for the concept of Type II versus Type I osteoporosis (Riggs, 1984).

References

1. Arnaud, C.D., and Strewler, G.J.: Parathyroid hormone and primary hyperparathyroidism. In, Hypercalciuric States: Pathogenesis, Consequences and Treatment. Ed: Coe, F.L.; Grune and Stratton, Orlando, 1984.

2. Aurbach, G.D., Marx, S.J., and Spiegel, A.M.: Parathyroid hormone, calcitonin and the calciferols. In, Textbook of Endocrinology, 6th Ed. Ed: Williams, R.D.; W.B. Saunders, Philadelphia, 1981.

3. Breslau, N.A., Moses, A.M., and Pak, C.Y.C.: Evidence for bone remodeling but lack of calcium mobilization response to parathyroid hormone in pseudohypoparathyroidism. J. Clin. Endocrinol. Metab. 57, 638, 1983.

4. Broadus, A.E.: Mineral metabolism. In, Endocrinology and Metabolism. Eds: Felig, P., et al; McGraw Hill, New York, 1981.

5. Broadus, A.E., Magee, J.S., Mallette, L.E., Horst, R.L., Lang, R., Jensen, P.S., Gertner, J.M., and Baron, R.: A detailed evaluation of oral phosphate therapy in selected patients with primary hyperparathyroidism. J. Clin. Endocrinol. Metab. 56, 953, 1983.

6. Chapuy, M.-C., Zucchelli, P., and Meunier, P.J.: Parathyroid function in Paget's disease of bone. Mineral Electrolyte Metab. 6, 112, 1981.

7. Charhon, S.A., Edouard, C.M., Arlot, M.E., and Meunier, P.J.: Effects of parathyroid hormone on remodeling of iliac trabecular bone packets in patients with primary hyperparathyroidism. Clin. Orthop. 162, 255, 1982.

8. Dalen, N., and Hjern, B.: Bone mineral content in patients with primary hyperparathyroidism without radiological evidence of skeletal changes. Acta Endocrinol. 75, 297, 1974.

9. Dauphine, R.T., Riggs, B.L., and Scholz, D.A.: Back pain and vertebral crush fractures: An unemphasized mode of presentation for primary hyperparathyroidism. Ann. Intern. Med. 83, 365, 1975.

10. Dequeker, J.: Bone Loss in Normal and Pathological Conditions. Leuven University Press, Leuven, 1972.

11. Frost, H.M., Griffith, D.L., Jee, W.S.S., Kimmel, D.B., McCandlis, R.P., and Teitelbaum, S.: Histomorphometric changes in trabecular bone of renal failure patients treated with calciferol. Metab. Bone Dis. & Rel. Res. 2, 285, 1981

12. Gryfe, C.L.: Bone loss in primary hyperparathyroidism. Can. Med. Assoc. J. 109, 479, 1973.

13. Habener, J.F., and Potts, J.T.: Clinical features of primary hyperparathyroidism. In, Endocrinology, Vol. 2. Eds: De Groot, L.J., et al; Grune and Stratton, New York, 1979.

14. Hahn, T.J., Hendin, B.A., Scharp, C.R., Boisseau, V.C., and Haddad, H.G., Jr.: Serum 25-hydroxycalciferol levels and bone mass in children on anticonvulsant therapy. N. Engl. J. Med. 292, 550, 1975.

15. Horsman, A., Marshall, D.H., and Peacock, M.: Age-related bone loss and osteoporosis. In, Osteoporosis. Proc. Copenhagen International Symposium on Osteoporosis. Eds: Christiansen, C., Arnaud, C.D., Nordin, B.E.C., Parfitt, A.M., Peck, W.A., Riggs, B.L., 1984.

16. Horsman, A., Nordin, B.E.C., Aaron, J., and Marshall, D.H.: Cortical and trabecular osteoporosis and their relation to fractures in the elderly. In, Osteoporosis. Recent Advances in Pathogenesis and Treatment. Eds: DeLuca, H.F., Frost, H.M., Jee, W.S.S., Johnston, C.C., Parfitt, A.M.; University Park Press, Baltimore, 1981. pp 175-184.

17. Hossain, M., Smith, D.A., and Nordin, B.E.C.: Parathyroid activity and postmenopausal osteoporosis. Lancet 1, 809, 1970.

18. Kleerekoper, M., Villanueva, A.R., Mathews, C.H.E., Rao, D.S., Pumo, B., and Parfitt, A.M.: PTH medicated bone loss in primary and secondary hyperparathyroidism. In, Clinical Disorders of Bone and Mineral Metabolism. Eds: Frame, B., and Potts, J.T., Jr.; Excerpta Medica, Amsterdam., 1983. pp 200-208.

19. Laval-Jeantet, A.-M., Bergot, C., Carroll, R., and Garcia-Schaefer, F.: Cortical bone senescence and mineral bone density of the humerus. Calcif. Tissue Int. 35, 268, 1983.

20. Marcus, R., Madvig, P., and Young, G.: Age-related changes in parathyroid hormone and parathyroid hormone action in normal humans. J. Clin. Endocrinol. Metab. 58, 223, 1984.

21. Meema, S., and Meema, H.E.: Evaluation of cortical bone mass, thickness and density of z-scores in osteopenic conditions and in relation to menopause and estrogen treatment. Skeletal Radiol. 8, 259, 1982.

22. Melsen, F., Nielsen, H.E., and Christensen, M.S.: Bone histomorphometry in patients with chronic renal failure: Effect of 1-α-hydroxyvitamin D_3. Clin. Endocrinol. 7 (Suppl.): 39S, 1977.

23. Melton, L.J., III, and Riggs, B.L.: Epidemiology of age-related fractures. In, The Osteoporotic Syndrome. Detection, Prevention, and Treatment. Ed: Avioli, L.V.; Grune and Stratton, New York, 1983. pp 45-72.

24. Meunier, P.: La maladie osseuse de Paget: histologie quantitative, histopathogenie et perspectives thérapeutiques. Lyon Médicale 233, 839, 1975.

25. Mosekilde, L., and Melsen, F.: A tetracycline-based histomorphometric evaluation of bone resorption and bone turnover in hyperthyroidism and hyperparathyroidism. Acta Med. Scand. 204, 97, 1978.

26. Mosekilde, L., and Melsen, F.: Dynamic differences in trabecular bone remodeling between patients after jejuno-ileal bypass for obesity and epileptic patients receiving anticonvulsant therapy. Metab. Bone Dis. & Rel. Res. 2, 77, 1980.

27. Pak, C.Y.C., Stewart, A., Kaplan, R., Bone, H., Notz, C., and Browne, R.: Photon absorptiometric analyses of bone density in primary hyperparathyroidism. Lancet 2, 7, 1975.

28. Parfitt, A.M.: The actions of parathyroid hormone on bone. Relation to bone remodelling and turnover, calcium homeostasis and metabolic bone disease. III. PTH and osteoblasts, the relationship between bone turnover and bone loss, and the state of the bones in primary hyperparathyroidism. Metabolism 25, 1033, 1976a.

29. Parfitt, A.M.: The actions of parathyroid hormone on bone. Relation to bone remodelling and turnover, calcium homeostasis and metabolic bone disease. IV. The state of the bones in uremic hyperparathyroidism. The mechanisms of skeletal resistance to PTH in renal failure and pseudo-

hypoparathyroidism and the role of PTH in osteoporosis, osteopetrosis and osteofluorosis. Metabolism 25, 1157, 1976b.

30. Parfitt, A.M.: Metacarpal cortical dimensions in hypoparathyroidism, primary hyperparathyroidism and chronic renal failure. Calc. Tissue Res. 22 (Suppl.): 329, 1977.

31. Parfitt, A.M.: Target cell resistance in pseudohypoparathyrodism. Single or multiple? In, Vitamin D: Basic Research and Its Clinical Application. Eds: Norman, A.W., et al; Walter de Gruyter, Berlin, 1979. pp 949-950.

32. Parfitt, A.M.: The morphologic basis of bone mineral measurements. Transient and steady state effects of treatment in osteoporosis. Mineral Electrolyte Metab. 4, 273, 1980.

33. Parfitt, A.M.: Age-related structural changes in trabecular and cortical bone: Cellular mechanism and biomechanical consequences. a) Differences between rapid and slow bone loss. b) Localized bone gain. Calcif. Tissue Int. 36, S123, 1984.

34. Parfitt, A.M.: Bone fragility in osteomalacia. Mechanisms and consequences. In, Current Concepts of Bone Fragility in Orthopaedics and Medicine. Eds: Uhthoff, H.-K. and Stahl, E.; Springer-Verlag, Berlin, 1985.

35. Parfitt, A.M., Gallagher, J.C., Heaney, R.P., Johnston, C.C., Neer, R., and Whedon, G.D.: Vitamin D and bone health in the elderly. Am. J. Clin. Nutr. 36, 1014, 1982.

36. Parfitt, A.M., Pødenphant, J., Villanueva, A.R., and Frame, B.: Metabolic bone disease with and without osteomalacia after intestinal bypass surgery. A bone histomorphometric study. Bone 6, 193, 1985.

37. Parfitt, A.M., Rao, D.S., Crouch, M., Frame, B., Matkovic, V., Villanueva, A.R., Walczak, N., Kleerekoper, M.: Iliac histomorphometry and radial photon absorptiometry in primary hyperparathyroidism. Calc. Tissue Int. 28, 170, 1979. (Abstr.)

38. Parfitt, A.M., Rao, D.S., Kleerekoper, M., Walczak, N., Levin, N., Oliver, I., and Frame, B.: Midshaft and distal radius bone mineral in primary and secondary hyperparathyroidism: Diagnostic value and response to treatment. In, Proc. Fourth International Conference on Bone Measurement. US Dept. HHS NIH 80-1938, Bethesda, 1980. pp 183-190.

39. Pozzi-Mucelli, R.S., Kanter, A.S., Genant, H.K., Cann, C.E., Ettinger, B., and Kolb, F.O.: Quantitative bone mineral analyses in primary hyperparathyroidism. J. Comput. Assist. Tomogr. 7, 555, 1983. (Abstr.)

40. Rao, S.D., Kleerekoper, M., Rogers, M., Frame, B., and Parfitt, A.M.: Is gastrectomy a risk factor for osteoporosis: In, Osteoporosis. Proc. Copenhagen International Symposium on Osteoporosis. Eds: Christiansen, C., Arnaud, C.D., Nordin, B.E.C., Parfitt, A.M., Peck, W.A., and Riggs, B.L.; 1984a, pp 775-777.

41. Rao, D.S., Marel, G., Wong, K., Zonca, M., Kleerekoper, M., Frame, B., Parfitt, A.M.: Reversible and irreversible skeletal disease in adult coeliac disease. In, Endocrine Control of Bone and Calcium Metabolism. Eds: Cohn, D.V., Potts, J.T., Jr., and Fujita, T.; Elsevier Science Publishers B.V., 1984b. pp 279-280.

42. Riggs, B.L.: Abnormal vitamin D metabolism in involutional osteoporosis. In, Osteoporosis. Proc. Copenhagen International Symposium on Osteoporosis. Eds: Christiansen, C., Arnaud, C.D., Nordin, B.E.C., Parfitt, A.M., Peck, W.A., Riggs, B.L., 1984. pp 743-750.

43. Seeman, E., Wahner, H.W., Offord, K.P., Kumar, R., Johnson, W.J., and Riggs, B.L.: Differential effects of endocrine dysfunction on the axial and the appendicular skeleton. J. Clin. Invest. 69, 1302, 1982.

44. Smith, D.M., Khairi, M.R.A., and Johnston, C.C. Jr.: The loss of bone mineral with aging and its relationship to risk of fracture. J. Clin. Invest. 56, 311, 1975.

45. Thompson, D.D.: Age changes in bone mineralization. Cortical thickness, and haversian canal area. Calcif. Tissue Int. 31, 5, 1980.

46. Toh, S.H., Claunch, B.C., and Brown, P.H.: Effect of calcitonin treatment on the natural course of bone demineralization in Paget's disease. J. Clin. Endocrinol. Metab. 56, 405, 1983.

47. Turek, S.L.: Orthopaedics, 4th Ed., J.B. Lippincott, Philadelphia, 1984.

Skeletal Problems in Chronic Renal Diseases

M. KAYE

In this paper the common manifestations of bone involvement in chronic renal failure will be reviewed and the cellular changes responsible for and resultant from these abnormalities examined. Most of the data come from percutaneous iliac crest bone biopsies of patients with end stage renal disease.

Recent studies have clearly demonstrated that abnormalities of mineral metabolism start early in the course of chronic renal failure. Furthermore, elevated levels of immunoassayable parathyroid hormone (PTH) can be measured when the glomerular filtration rate (GFR) is reduced from one-third to one-half of normal (Chesney et al, 1982; Mallouche et al, 1975; Portale et al, 1982, 1984; Wilson et al, 1985). While the classic Bricker hypothesis suggested that the cause of secondary hyperparathyroidism was phosphate retention and hypocalcemia (Bricker et al, 1969), this explanation is only partially correct since hypophosphatemia is frequently present in early renal failure but ionized and total calcium levels are normal (Portale et al, 1984; Wilson et al, 1985). Lopez et al (1984) have suggested that, in the dog, the small reductions in 1,25 dihydroxycholecalciferol levels may be responsible for this early stimulation of the parathyroid glands, presumably by altering the sensing levels at which hormone secretion is stopped (Brown et al, 1982). Portale (1984) has shown in children that those changes are reversible by phosphate restriction. Wilson (1985) has shown elevated PTH levels and decreased calcium mobilization in adults with mild renal failure. We can summarize these early changes as shown in Figure 1.

30-60% Reduction in GFR

↓

↓ Renal Production $1,25(OH)_2D_3$

↓

? Change in PTG set point
? ↓ Calcemic response to PTH

↓

↑ Secretion PTH

↓

↓ Serum Pi. Early bone changes

Fig. 1. Early renal failure.

Current Concepts of Bone Fragility

Table I. Serum changes*

Hypocalcemia
Hyperphosphatemia
iPTH elevated
Alkaline phosphatase elevated

* GFR <30% normal

As renal function declines further, more striking abnormalities begin to appear and become increasingly prominent with time when the filtration rate is below one-third of normal. The serum changes are shown in Table I. These are, for the most part, the direct result of loss of renal parenchymal function so that fractional phosphate excretion has increased maximally, and further increments in phosphate excretion can only be achieved by increased serum phosphorus levels. The hypocalcemia is related to the more drastic lowering of $1,25(OH)_2D_3$ levels, leading to intestinal calcium malabsorption (Fig. 2). Moreover, hyperphosphatemia has a direct effect on the transfer or flux of calcium from the bone pool to the extracellular fluid and plasma and will directly lead to hypocalcemia. Both mechanisms will therefore lead to further parathyroid stimulation (Fig. 3).

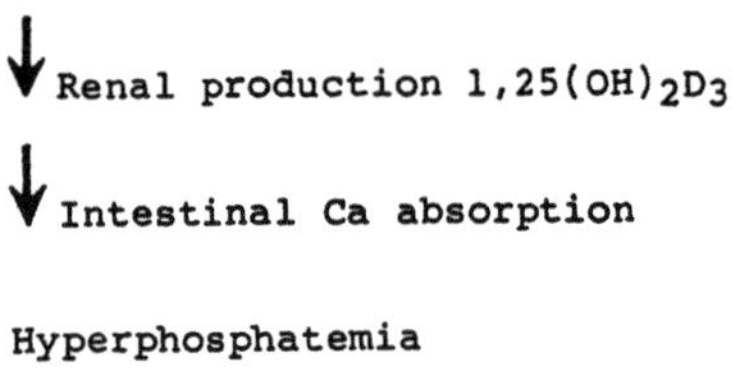

Fig. 2. Causes of hypocalcemia.

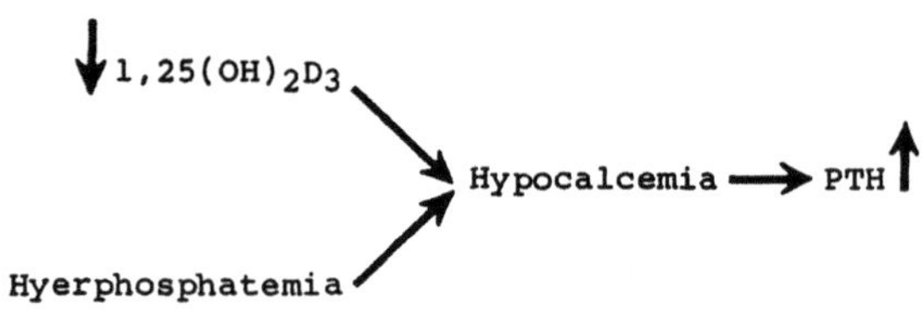

Fig. 3. Secondary hyperparathyroidism.

Thus, by the time the patient is in need for dialysis, all the markers of severe hyperparathyroidism are present after an interval of months but more commonly after years of chronic renal failure. The size of the parathyroid glands -- a rough index of the severity of the hyperparathyroidism -- correlates best with the duration of renal failure. It is therefore not surprising that patients with slowly progressive forms of renal disease, such as polycystic kidneys or chronic interstitial nephritis, tend to have the most severe hyperparathyroidism (Malmaeus et al, 1984).

What are the effects of persistent high levels of parathyroid hormone on bone and bone cells? Because the turnover of bone is relatively slow, particularly in adults, these changes take months and usually years to become apparent, this process being speeded up in children. However, this survey will be confined to adults only.

What are the changes to be found when we examine bone using conventional histologic techniques? The qualitative changes are shown in Table II. The most consistent of these changes are the increase in number and size of both osteoblasts and osteoclasts and the corresponding resorption areas produced by osteoclastic activity. Although the link between high levels of iPTH and

Table II. Histology in 2° hyperparathyroidism

Osteoclasts increased
Osteoblasts increased
Resorption areas increased
Marrow fibrosis

increased osteoclast numbers is firmly established, this does not necessarily mean that PTH stimulates the osteoclast directly. First, the evidence suggests instead that this stimulation is indirect having been reported by several observers who failed to find PTH receptors on osteoclasts while they are present on osteoblasts; second, investigators have shown that isolated osteoclasts are totally unresponsive to PTH although very responsive to certain other agents, particularly calcitonin (Chambers and Dunn, 1983; Silve et al, 1982). Presumably, PTH stimulates osteoblasts directly and these, in some unknown way, lead to osteoclast production, differentiation, and enlargement.

How can we be sure these changes are due to parathyroid hormone? Perhaps most convincing is the effect of parathyroidectomy. If the bone changes are quantitated using standard histomorphometric techniques, we see the following changes in a dialysis patient before and one year after parathyroidectomy (Table III). The values following surgery are within the range for normal subjects.

Table III. Static histomorphometry

	Before PTX	One year after PTX
Bone as % section	54.4	44.9
% osteoid	19.6	7.3
Osteoid with µm	17.5	10.0
% resorptive surface	14.9	1.0
Osteoclasts/mm	1.5	0.1
Osteoblasts/mm	7.4	3.1

PTX = parathyroidectomy

Static histologic variables of this type, while useful diagnostically, give little insight into the speed or rate at which things are happening in the bone, necessitating double tetracycline markers. Table IV shows the changes before and after parathyroidectomy at which time all values are normal. Clearly, secondary hyperparathyroidism markedly increases the number of sites at which mineralization is taking place and, furthermore, the mineralization process is not delayed; in fact, it may be slightly accelerated --

Table IV. Dynamic histomorphometry

	Before PTX	One year after PTX
% surface tetracycline labelled	21.1	2.2
% surface with two labels	10.9	0.5
Mineralization lag time - days	12.4	6.5
Bone formation rate $\mu^2/d/mm^2$	962.3	141.2

PTX = parathyroidectomy

Table V. Cellular results of 2° hyperparathyroidism

Increase in number and size of osteoblasts and osteoclasts
Increase in number of formation and resorption sites
Increase in overall bone formation and resorption
Marrow fibrosis
Net balance tilted toward resorption

that is to say, no osteomalacia is observed. The increased quantity of osteoid seen on the biopsies is due to the increase in number of sites where bone is being formed and is not due to any problem with mineralization.

These findings of secondary hyperparathyroidism may, therefore, be summarized as shown in Table V. It is possible to say that the net effect is more resorption because of the radiologic changes (Fig. 4). The roentgenogram was taken of the same patient before parathyroidectomy and 1-1/2 years later. The replacement of the lost bone is quite striking.

Within the last few years, it has become apparent that this picture -- which I might term pure hyperparathyroidism -- is frequently confused by the superimposition of another form of bone disease, such as that induced by aluminum. In its classical and most typical form it looks histologically like severe osteomalacia. The major change is that of a striking excess of osteoid without evidence of hyperparathyroidism. Rates of bone mineralization, measured using tetracycline labelling, are markedly reduced confirming that this is true osteomalacia.

Much of the original data collected several years ago on aluminum intoxication came from dialysis units in the United Kingdom and Denver, USA, among others where the dialyzate solution was contaminated with aluminum resulting in massive transfers of the metal from dialyzate to blood with each dialysis. The resulting clinical picture was a severe disease involving bone and brain (Dunea et al, 1978; Kaehny et al, 1977; McDermott et al, 1978; Ott et al, 1982; Pierides et al, 1980; Walker et al, 1982). In recent years, the picture has changed. The source of aluminum is now oral phosphate binders -- aluminum hydroxide and carbonate. Accumulation in the body

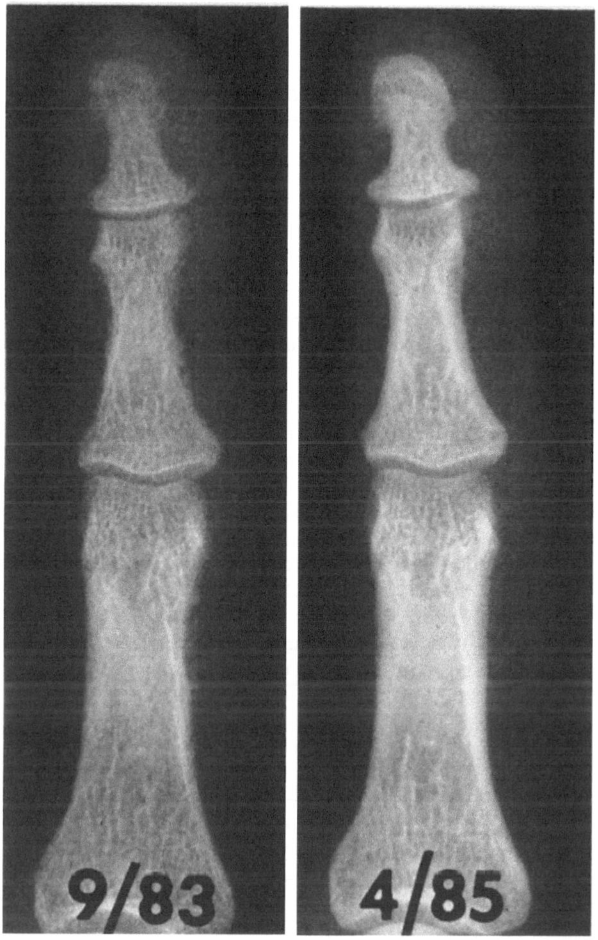

Fig. 4. Before (on the left) and after parathyroidectomy (on the right).

is much slower, more insidious, and bone disease frequently less obvious. In our series of 75 patients, we found that 72% had aluminum present on their bone biopsies. As Montreal has never had aluminum in the water used for dialyzate preparation, this shows the pervasiveness of the problem. We took a group of patients on dialysis without aluminum in their bone biopsy and compared them with a matched group who had quite high quantities. The findings are shown in Table VI. It can be seen that the standard static morphometric data appear surprisingly similar between the two groups. However, when we look at the time-related or dynamic variables, the differences are striking because these patients have virtually ceased to form bone. It is interesting that this bone looks so similar to that of a standard dialysis patient; without specifically staining it for aluminum the extent of the intoxication would never be appreciated. The end result of this process is either what others have called aplastic bone, which looks inactive with little osteoid and can only be distinguished from normal bone by tetracycline labelling and/or aluminum staining, or gross osteomalacia.

Table VI. Bone histomorphometry in renal failure

	Control	Renal failure <2% Al surface	Renal failure >30% Al surface
Number of cases	14	12	12
% surface Al	0	0.3	53.0
% osteoid	5.3	36.0	41.0
Osteoblasts/mm	2.3	7.4	3.3*
Osteoclasts/mm	0.1	1.0	0.4*
% tetracycline	13.0	25.0	4.0*

* Significant difference ($p < 0.05$) between renal failure groups

One important question is how the aluminum is affecting mineralization. Are the osteoblasts poisoned or is this an effect on the mineralization front inhibiting the deposition of calcium and phosphorus? We have examined this by looking at the amount of new protein synthesized by human osteoblasts when bone fragments are incubated in a medium containing a radioactive amino acid such as ^{3}H-leucine. Autoradiographs are prepared and the grains per cell counted to get an index of the metabolic activity of the osteoblasts. Using this technique, we have examined biopsies taken from normal subjects, patients with end stage renal disease but without aluminum accumulation, and finally patients with marked aluminum storage in their bones. The results are shown in Table VII.

Table VII. New protein synthesis from ^{3}H-leucine*

	Control	Renal failure <2% Al surface	Renal failure >30% Al surface
No. of cells	1016	1907	1328
Mean value ± SEM	1.56±0.2	3.21±0.2§	2.6±0.2†

* Mean square root of grain per osteoblast
Difference from control: $^§p < 0.001$, $^†p < 0.01$

It can be seen that in patients without aluminum storage osteoblastic activity is increased twofold due to the hyperparathyroidism, confirming the increased tissue labelling with tetracycline mentioned earlier. In patients with aluminum storage, the osteoblastic activity is reduced but is still above normal. We would infer from these data, therefore, that the striking arrest of new bone formation cannot be due to osteoblast poisoning directly, as these cells are still as active or more active than normal osteoblasts. Rather, it is due to a direct effect of aluminum at the mineralization front which inhibits calcification; or, less likely but possible, an effect on a subsection of the process such as, for example, the function of matrix vesicles.

We may now summarize the major changes found in end stage renal disease (Fig. 5). Good evidence is now available showing that in addition to the effect of aluminum on bone, it also has a direct inhibitory effect on the

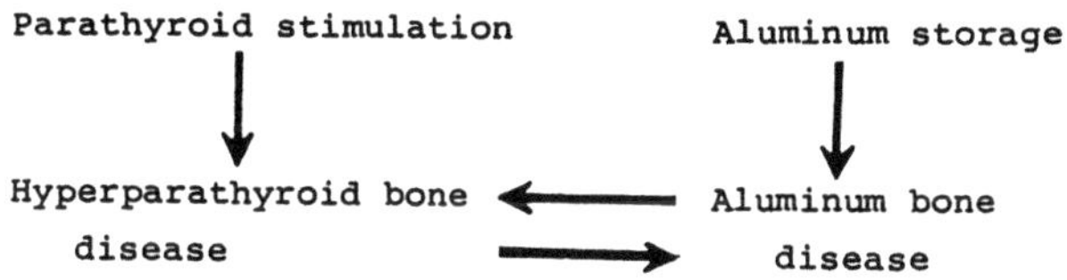

Fig. 5. Bone findings in ESRD (end stage renal disease)

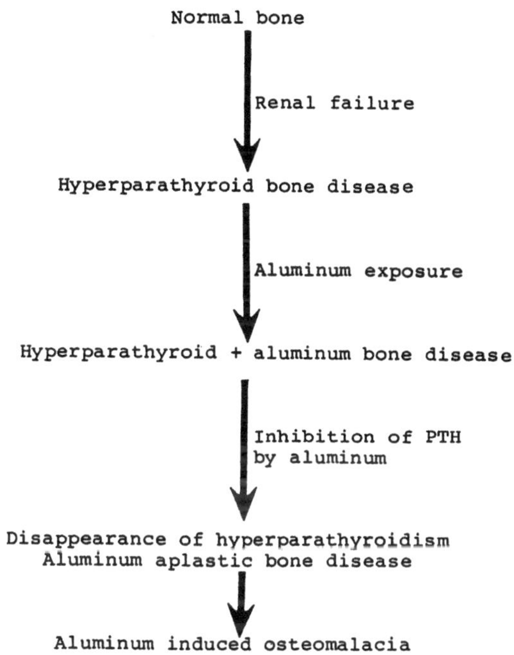

Fig. 6. Possible sequential bone changes.

parathyroid gland and accumulates in this tissue leading to secretory inhibition (Morrissey et al, 1983). We can end up, therefore, in any individual patient with a spectrum depending on which stage of the process the patient is undergoing (Fig. 6). Most patients will not go through all these stages and where any patient is at any one time will depend on the duration and severity of their renal failure and degree of aluminum exposure.

References

1. Bricker, N.S., Slatopolsky, E., Reiss, E., and Avioli, L.V.: Calcium, phosphorus and bone in renal disease and transplantation. Arch. Int. Med. 123, 543, 1969.

2. Brown, E.M., Wilson, R.E., Eastman, R.C., Pallotta, J., and Marynick, S.P.: Abnormal regulation of parathyroid hormone release by calcium in secondary hyperparathyroidism due to chronic renal failure. J. Clin. Endocrinol. Metab. 54, 172, 1982.

3. Chambers, T.J., and Dunn, C.J.: Pharmacological control of osteoclastic motility. Calcif. Tissue Int. 35, 566, 1983.

4. Chesny, R.W., Hamstra, A.J., Mazess, R.B., Rose, P., and DeLuca, H.F.: Circulating vitamin D metabolite concentrations in childhood renal disease. Kidney Int. 21, 65, 1982.

5. Dunea, G., Mahurkar, S.D., Mamdani, B., and Smith, E.C.: Role of aluminum in dialysis dementia. Ann. Int. Med. 88, 502, 1978.

6. Kaehny, W.D., Alfrey, A.C., Holman, R.E., and Shorr, W.J.: Aluminum transfer during hemodialysis. Kidney Int. 12, 361, 1977.

7. Lopez, S., Galceran, T., Chan, W., Rapp, N., Martin, K., and Slatopolsky, E.: Hypocalcemia may not be the cause of the development of secondary hyperparathyroidism. Proc. Am. Soc. Nephrol., 24A, 1984.

8. Mallouche, H.H., Ritz, E., Hodgson, M., Kutschera, J., Krause, G., Seiffert, U., Gati, A., and Lange, H.P.: Skeletal lesions and calcium metabolism in early renal failure. Proc. Europ. Dial. Transpl. Assoc. 11, 443, 1975.

9. Malmaeus, J., Grimelius, L., Johansson, H., Akerstrom, G., and Ljunghall, S.: Parathyroid pathology in hyperparathyroidism secondary to chronic renal failure. Scand. J. Urol. Nephrol. 18, 157, 1984.

10. McDermott, J.R., Smith, A.L., Ward, M.K., Parkinson, I.S., and Kerr, D.N.S.: Brain-aluminum concentration in dialysis encephalopathy. Lancet 1, 901, 1978.

11. Morrissey, J., Rothstein, M., Mayor, G., and Slatopolsky, E.: Suppression of parathyroid hormone secretion by aluminum. Kidney Int. 23, 699, 1983.

12. Ott, S.M., Maloney, N.A., Coburn, J.W., Alfrey, A.C., and Sherrard, D.J.: The prevalence of bone aluminum deposition in renal osteodystrophy and its relation to the response to calcitriol therapy. New Eng. J. Med. 307, 709, 1982.

13. Pierides, A.M., Edwards, W.G., Cullum, U.X., McCall, J.T., and Ellis, H.A.: Hemodialysis encephalopathy with osteomalacic fractures and muscle weakness. Kidney Int. 18, 115, 1980.

14. Portale, A.A., Booth, B.E., Tsai, H.C., and Morris, R.C.: Reduced plasma concentration of 1,25-dihydroxyvitamin D in children with moderate renal insufficiency. Kidney Int. 21, 627, 1982.

15. Portale, A.A., Booth, B.E., Halloran, B.P., and Morris, R.C.: Effect of dietary phosphorus on circulating concentrations of 1,25-dihydroxyvitamin D and immunoreactive parathyroid hormone in children with moderate renal insufficiency. Am. Soc. Clin. Invest. 73, 1580, 1984.

16. Silve, C.M., Hradek, G.T., Jones, A.L., and Arnaud, C.D.: Parathyroid hormone receptor in intact embryonic chicken bone: Characterization and cellular localization. J. Cell. Biol. 94, 379, 1982.

17. Walker, G.S., Aaran, J.E., Peacock, M., Robinson, P.J.A., and Davison, A.M.: Dialysate aluminium concentration and renal bone disease. Kidney Int. 21, 411, 1982.

18. Wilson, L., Felsenfeld, A., Drezner, M.K., and Llach, F.: Altered divalent ion metabolism in early renal failure: Role of $1,25(OH)_2D$. Kidney Int. 27, 565, 1985.

Glucocorticoid-Induced Osteoporosis

C. V. Odvina, J. E. Wergedal, and D. J. Baylink

Introduction

Glucocorticoids, in supraphysiologic doses, exert both anti-inflammatory and immunosuppressive actions which have made them useful in the treatment of rheumatoid arthritis, asthma, and systemic lupus erythematosus (SLE). Unless these conditions can be prevented, we will continue to depend on glucocorticoids and related compounds to alleviate symptoms and to slow down the progression of the disease. Unfortunately, long-term administration of these compounds often leads to untoward effects involving cardiovascular, gastrointestinal, and musculoskeletal systems. The most disabling of these adverse effects is the development of osteopenia. Bone loss secondary to glucocorticoid administration is known to have a characteristic distribution. It is more severe in the regions with high trabecular bone content (spine and ribs), and less striking in predominantly cortical bone areas (Hann et al, 1979). Consequently, rib fractures and compression deformities of the vertebrae frequently occur.

Although this potential complication of long-term glucocorticoid administration has long been recognized, ideal management of the condition still has to be established. In this paper, we discuss the rational approach to the treatment and prevention of glucocorticoid-induced osteoporosis, based on the currently accepted pathogenetic mechanisms (Fig. 1). In addition, we

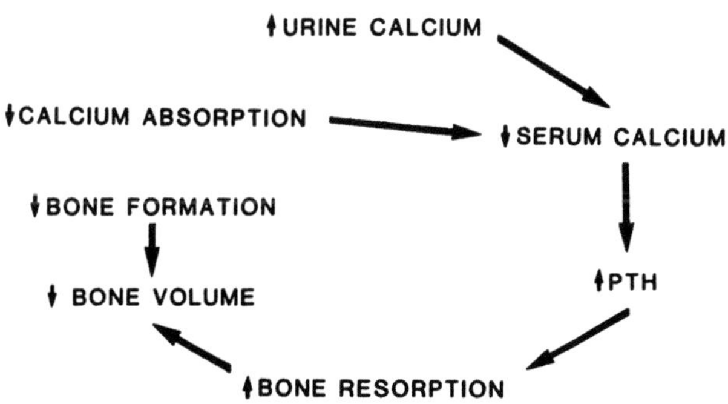

Fig. 1. Summary of the pathogenetic mechanisms in the development of glucocorticoid-induced osteoporosis.

Current Concepts of Bone Fragility

discuss the role of fluoride in the management of this condition by presenting the histories of five glucocorticoid-treated patients who are currently on fluoride therapy for osteoporosis.

Case Reports

Patient 1

A 61-year old woman was referred to our clinic by her primary physician for the management of osteoporosis. A year before consultation, the patient was given prednisone, 85 mg/day, which was later reduced to 50 mg every other day, for the treatment of granulomatous myopathy. During that time, the patient lost approximately 2 cm in height, associated with a feeling of tiredness in the back but no definite pain. The patient had been taking a thiazide diuretic once a day for hypertension for several months when she first consulted our Osteoporosis Clinic.

Thoracic and lumbar spine roentgenograms were done which showed marked demineralization of the skeletal structures without obvious wedge deformity. Spinal bone density, using the quantitative computed tomography scan (QCTS), showed values ranging from 47-61 mg/cm³, with a mean density of 55 mg/cm³. This was lower than our computed fracture threshold of 87 mg/cm³ (Odvina et al, 1984). Pretreatment biochemical data are summarized in Table I.

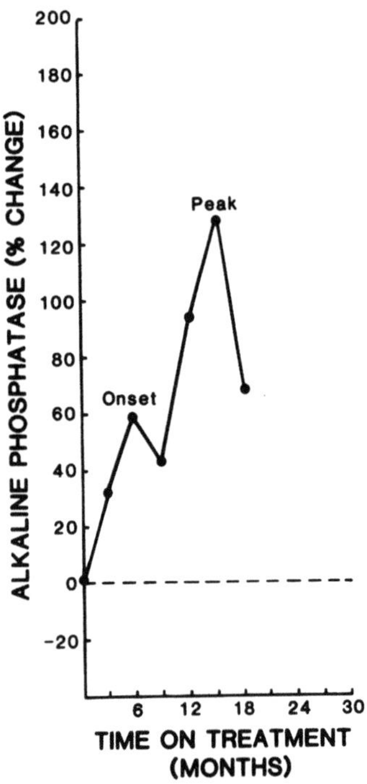

Fig. 2. Percent change in the total serum alkaline phosphatase activity with fluoride treatment in patient 1.

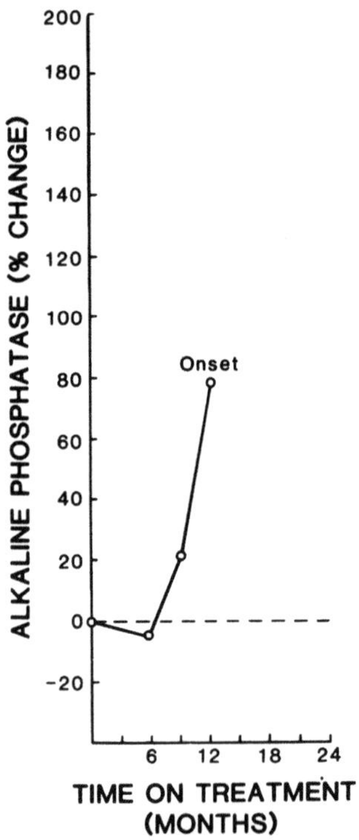

Fig. 3. Percent change in the total serum alkaline phosphatase activity with fluoride treatment in patient 2.

Table 1. Steroid dose, duration of steroid treatment, pretreatment serum and urinary biochemical data

Patient	Steroid dose	Duration of treatment	Serum calcium (2.2-2.7 mm/l)	Serum phosphorus (0.8-1.6 mm/l)	Serum alkaline (37-132 U/l)	Urine calcium*	Urine OH-proline**
1	50-80 mg Prednisone†	2 years	2.40	1.20	83	55	21
2	40µ ACTH per week	10 years	2.37	0.99	58	177	11
3	10-20 mg Prednisone†	2 years	2.30	1.20	126	125	17
4	5-10 mg Prednisone§	5 years	2.40	1.56	94	54	10
5	5-10 mg Prednisone†	2 years	2.35	0.83	63	113	22

( ) Normal range

* Normal range: 50-250 mg/24 hours for females; up to 300 mg/24 hours for males

** Normal range: 22-77 mg/24 hours

† Every other day

§ Every day

With these findings, the patient was started on the following program: sodium fluoride, 88 mg/day; vitamin D, 50,000 units per day; 1,500 mg of calcium; and stanozolol, 4 mg/day. Vitamin D and calcium were given to correct the negative calcium balance expected in this type of patient while fluoride and stanozolol were given for their anabolic effects. Response to treatment was measured by serial serum alkaline phosphatase* and spinal bone density measurements. A significant increase in alkaline phosphatase (>34% change from the baseline value**) was noted at six months, and peaked at 15 months after initiation of therapy (Fig. 2). Other measures of liver function (SGOT, SGPT, GTTP, SLDH, bilirubin) were all within normal limits. Spinal bone density was also noted to increase to 71 mg/cm³ at nine months. All these changes were associated with decreased back tiredness as reported by the patient. Serial serum calcium determinations were also done while the patient was on thiazide and vitamin D to insure that hypercalcemia would not develop, and no significant change was noted. This aspect of therapy will be further discussed below.

Patient 2

A 65-year old woman consulted the clinic because of chronic back pain. Osteoporosis had been diagnosed several years before consultation. Medical history revealed that the patient had received different synthetic glucocorticoids (methylprednisolone, dexamethasone, prednisone) for approximately 10 years for neurodermatitis. At the time of consultation, she was receiving ACTH injections, 40 units every week. The patient had dorsal kyphosis and had lost approximately 5 cm in height. She could not remember her age at menopause but had been taking diethylstilbestrol, 0.5 mg, for several years for hot flashes.

Initial biochemical studies are shown in Table I. Thoracic and lumbar spine roentgenograms showed generalized osteopenia with compression fractures at T_{10} and T_{11}, and mild anterior wedging at T_7 and T_8. Spinal bone density values ranged from 78-94 mg/cm³, with mean density of 84 mg/cm³. The average density for this patient's age and sex was 90 mg/cm³.

She was subsequently started on sodium fluoride, 88 mg/day; calcium, 1,700 mg per day, and was advised to continue taking the stilbestrol. Follow-up laboratory examinations showed a slight increase in serum alkaline phosphatase (71 U/l compared with a baseline value of 54) nine months after starting the therapy, with a significant increase seen after 12 months of treatment (Fig. 3). Repeat spinal bone density done at nine months was unchanged, and urinary calcium excretion increased to 204 mg/24 hours from a baseline value of 117 mg/24 hours.

---

* Serum alkaline phosphatase levels are an indirect measure of bone formation rate. We have recently shown that serial measurements of serum alkaline phosphatase are a convenient method of measuring response to fluoride therapy in osteoporotics.

** When we evaluated the repeat serum alkaline phosphatase measurements within two months or less in 37 untreated osteoporotics, we found that the standard deviation of repeat measurements was ±17% throughout the normal range. We therefore defined the minimim significant increase in alkaline phosphatase as >2 SD, or 34% above the baseline value.

Patient 3

A 63-year old man was diagnosed in 1977 as having chronic obstructive pulmonary disease secondary to emphysema. His condition became progressively worse, and he was subsequently started on prednisone three years after the diagnosis. He was maintained on an average dose of 15-20 mg/day, although this was frequently increased to as much as 60 mg/day because of acute exacerbations. Approximately four months after starting the steroid therapy, he fractured his ribs: first the 10th left rib, later the 11th. Rib roentgenograms showed osteopenia. With these findings, his primary physician started him on calcium as calcium lactate 100 mg, four tablets a day, and calciferol 50,000 units, one tablet every morning.

The patient continued to develop spontaneous rib fractures during the next two years. He also complained of upper and lower back pain. Due to the recurrent fractures, the patient was referred to the Osteoporosis Clinic. The results of his workup are shown in Table I. QCTS values ranged from 52-62 mg/cm^3 with a mean density of 60 mg/cm^3. Thoracic and lumbar spine roentgenograms revealed compression fractures of T_5, T_7, T_8. Bone scan findings were consistent with the history of rib and vertebral fractures. Sodium fluoride, 88 mg/day; vitamin D, 50,000 units per day; nandrolone, 100 mg every other week; and 1,500 mg calcium supplementation were started. The prescribed dosages of oral vitamin D and calcium increased the urine calcium to a maximum of 285 mg/24 hours from a pretreatment level of

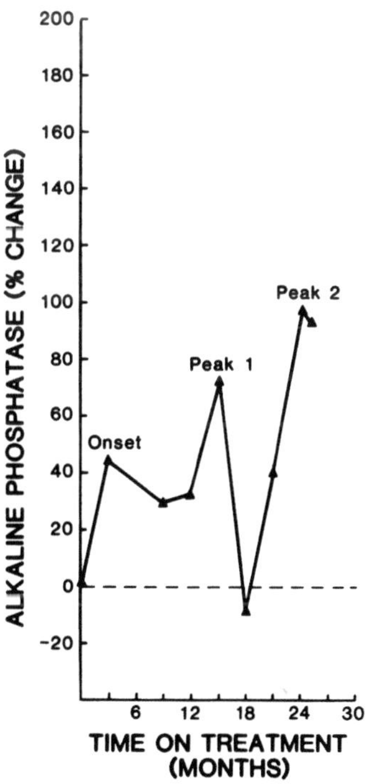

Fig. 4. Percent change in the total serum alkaline phosphatase activity with fluoride treatment in patient 3.

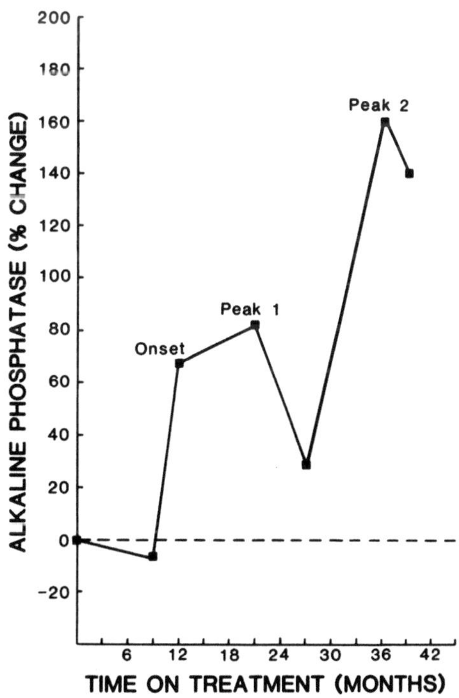

Fig. 5. Percent change in the total serum alkaline phosphatase activity with fluoride treatment in patient 4.

125 mg/24 hours. We presumed that this was indicative of improved calcium absorption.

The patient showed a cyclic serum alkaline phosphatase response to fluoride as noted in Figure 4. An initial increase was noted at three months, followed by a slight drop. Eventually there was a progressive increase, peaking at 24 months of therapy. A progressive increase in spinal bone density at 24 months was also noted (132 mg/cm³ compared with a baseline value of 60 mg/cm³). These changes were associated with symptomatic relief (cessation of rib fractures) after 15 months of treatment. The patient has had no new fractures in the past 10 months despite increased physical activity.

Patient 4

A 51-year old woman was referred to the Osteoporosis Clinic. She was diagnosed as having rheumatoid arthritis and had been on an average dose of prednisone 5-10 mg/day, for approximately five years. She had been complaining of upper back pain for approximately three years. Thoracic and lumbar spine roentgenograms showed marked demineralization without wedge or codfish deformity. Initial serum and urine evaluations are summarized in Table I. Bone mineral density of the radius was low at both proximal and distal sites: 0.502 mg/cm² and 0.374 mg/cm², respectively. QCTS was not available at that time; however, from the equation describing the relationship between the spinal bone density and density of the radius, we estimated her pretreatment CT value to be 43 mg/cm³ (Farley et al, 1985).

After her initial workup, the patient was started on fluoride treatment at a dose of 66 mg/day, which was subsequently increased to 88 mg/day. In addition, this patient was given conjugated estrogens, 0.625 mg/day in a 28-day cycle; methandrostenolone, 2.5 mg/day; vitamin D, 50,000 units every week; and she was advised to take 1,500 mg of calcium per day. Urine calcium was noted to increase to 262 mg/24 hours four months after initiation of treatment and has remained essentially unchanged. Alkaline phosphatase response is summarized in Figure 5. An initial, significant increase was noted at 12 months and a maximum increase at three years. Subjective improvement in terms of pain was noted at 12 months, and spinal bone density was 284 mg/cm³ at 96 months after initiation of treatment.

Patient 5

A 74-year old woman consulted our Osteoporosis Clinic with complaints of chronic back pain. Two years before consultation, the patient was diagnosed as having osteoporosis and was advised to take supplementary calcium.

Her main medical problem was chronic obstructive pulmonary disease, probably secondary to sarcoidosis, which was treated with prednisone at an initial dose of 60 mg/day. This was slowly tapered off to her current dose of 5 mg every other day. Menopause occurred at age 53, and she had been taking conjugated estrogens, 1.25 mg five times a week. At that time, the patient was also taking furosemide 40 mg/day for hypertension.

The chemistry profile, including urinary calcium and hydroxyproline determinations, is summarized in Table I. Physical examination revealed marked dorsal kyphosis. Thoracic roentgenograms showed multiple compression fractures in the mid and lower thoracic spine. Wedging of L_1 and L_4 vertebrae

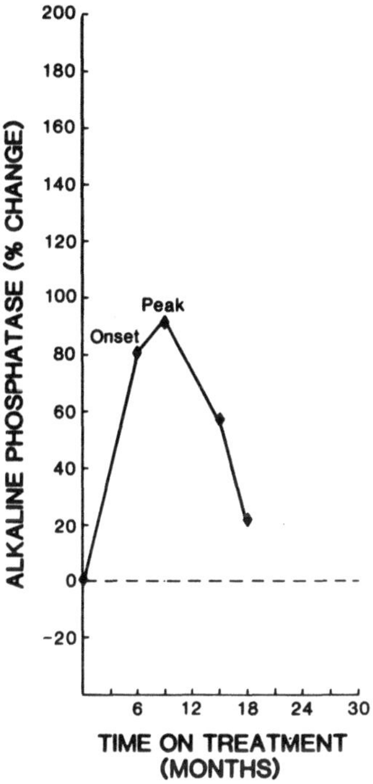

Fig. 6. Percent change in the total serum alkaline phosphatase activity with fluoride treatment in patient 5.

was also noted. Bone scan showed increased radioactive uptake by T_9-T_{11}, as well as by the costochondral junction of the right third and fourth ribs, suggesting fractures. QCTS showed values ranging from 24-36 mg/cm³, with a mean density of 30 mg/cm³.

After the baseline diagnostic studies, she was started on sodium fluoride, 88 mg/day; vitamin D, 50,000 units/day; and 1,500 mg calcium daily. To avoid further urinary calcium loss due to furosemide, this was discontinued and replaced by hydrochlorthiazide, 100 mg/day. Serum alkaline phosphatase, QCTS, serum and urinary calcium levels were monitored at regular intervals. Serum alkaline phosphatase showed a significant increase at six months, peaked at nine months, and gradually declined thereafter (Fig. 6). Mean spinal bone density increased to 49 mg/cm³ at 15 months; repeat serum calcium determinations were all within normal limits.

Discussion

Pharmacologic amounts of glucocorticoids commonly used in the long-term treatment of various disorders are known to have a pronounced effect on bone metabolism. Inhibition of growth in children with Cushing's syndrome and in children on chronic exogenous glucocorticoid treatment is widely recognized (Blodgett et al, 1956; Follis, 1951). Presumably, this is, at least partly, due to the antagonistic effect of glucocorticoids on the action of growth hormone (Blodgett et al, 1956). Abnormal secretion of growth hormone has also been proposed as an etiologic factor in the diminished growth rate in children with Cushing's syndrome. Response of growth hormone secretion to insulin-induced hypoglycemia has been reported to be either decreased or absent in these patients (Frantz and Robkin, 1964;

Hartog et al, 1964; Krieger and Glick, 1972). In addition to growth retardation, Saville et al (1967) and Bradley et al (1960) have shown a high incidence of symptomatic osteopenia in children treated chronically with glucocorticoids.

In adults, the primary disturbance in mineral metabolism caused by glucocorticoid excess frequently causes osteoporosis, leading to fractures, particularly of the vertebrae and the ribs (Hann et al, 1979). Histologic studies of bone biopsy samples from patients with Cushing's syndrome and patients treated with synthetic cortisol analogues for prolonged periods have shown a decrease in bone formation rate and an increase in bone resorptive activity, manifested by increased osteoclasts and resorptive sites (Frost and Villanueve, 1961; Jowsey and Riggs, 1970). The decreased bone formation rate has generally been attributed to the direct inhibitory effect of glucocorticoids on osteoblast function. This is supported by the studies of Frost and Villanueve (1961) and Thompson et al (1972), which showed a significant inhibition of both the collagen synthesis by preexisting osteoblasts and the conversion of precursor cells to functioning osteoblasts. The marked reduction of protein synthesis with the addition of cortisol to bone cells in culture further supports the idea that glucocorticoids exert a direct inhibitory effect on osteoblasts (Peck et al, 1967).

The mechanism by which glucocorticoids stimulate bone resorption is more complex (Jee et al, 1970). It has previously been demonstrated that this enhanced bone resorption is mediated by parathyroid hormone (PTH), the osteoclastic response to glucocorticoid administration being completely abolished by parathyroidectomy (Fucik et al, 1972). Furthermore, it has been shown that chronic steroid administration in man results in the elevation of PTH levels (Fucik et al, 1972; Hann et al, 1979; Lukert and Adams, 1976). This effect results from the well-known suppression of intestinal calcium absorption by corticosteroids (Fischer and Hastrup, 1954; Hann et al, 1979) and from its hypercalciuric effect (Suzuki et al, 1983). Both actions result in a tendency toward hypocalcemia, with a subsequent compensatory increase in PTH secretion and stimulation of bone resorption.

As with most conditions, the optimum treatment of glucocorticoid-induced osteoporosis involves the removal of the cause. Unfortunately, complete discontinuation of the drug is usually difficult and often impossible. It has been suggested that administration of glucocorticoids at the lowest possible dose has a potential advantage, but this has not been proven. Sheagren et al (1977), on the other hand, showed that alternate day dosing produces less bone loss compared with a daily glucocorticoid regimen. Such measures can reduce the risk but will not totally prevent the development of secondary osteoporosis.

In addition to these measures, one would like to have a direct means of correcting the adverse effects of glucocorticoids on the skeleton by suppressing the increased rate of bone resorption and stimulating the bone formation rate. Based on available evidence that the increased resorptive activity in glucocorticoid-induced osteoporosis is a result of secondary hyperparathyroidism, several therapeutic measures to suppress PTH secretion have been suggested. For example, Hann et al (1978; 1979) demonstrated a significant decrease in iPTH levels and an increased calcium absorption after giving a combination of vitamin D (50,000 units three times/week) or its metabolite (25-OH vitamin D, 40-60 μg/day) and calcium to patients receiving at least 15 mg of prednisone daily). Concurrent with these biochemical changes, a significant decrease in osteoclastic activity and a higher trabecular mass were observed after 12-18 months' therapy compared with the nonsupplemented group of glucocorticoid-treated patients.

Suzuki et al (1983), on the other hand, showed that hypercalciuria, in addition to reduced calcium absorption, plays an important role in the development of secondary hyperparathyroidism in these patients and suggested the use of trichlormethiazide in situations where increased urine calcium loss is present. In this study, we were able to demonstrate a significant decrease in iPTH and cAMP levels with the use of thiazides. Thus, it appears that vitamin D metabolites and/or thiazides can prevent further deterioration or even effect improvement of the skeletal status of patients receiving pharmacologic doses of glucocorticoids.

Although it is possible that the above approach can correct the elevated bone resorption rate, it is doubtful that bone loss can be entirely prevented by such measures. As previously discussed, the osteopenia of chronic glucocorticoid treatment is also partly due to a depression of bone formation. Therefore, suppression of bone resorption may not be sufficient to prevent the development of osteoporosis or to treat patients with established osteoporosis. Furthermore, although an increase in trabecular bone mass has been shown with reduction of bone resorption, the long-term effect of vitamin D and calcium supplementation still needs to be determined. Under normal conditions, bone resorption and bone formation rates are coupled. That is, a change in resorption rate is usually followed by a parallel change in formation rate. Thus, it is possible that suppression of resorption rate may ultimately lead to a further decrease in bone formation and, therefore, continued bone loss. Optimal therapy may require the use of a bone anabolic agent such as fluoride.

Patient 3 is a good example of this situation. When he started developing rib fractures, his primary physician started him on vitamin D and calcium to prevent further deterioration of his skeletal status. However, rib fractures continued to develop, and vertebral fractures began to occur. Fluoride was added for its osteogenic effect. This resulted in a progressive increase in spinal bone density and a decreased occurrence of fractures, suggesting that fluoride therapy can be an important adjunct in the management of glucocorticoid-induced osteoporosis.

Earlier studies have shown that fluoride therapy can effectively increase bone mass and decrease fracture rates in postmenopausal osteoporotics (Farley et al, 1985; Riggs et al, 1980; 1982). Its role, however, in the treatment of glucocorticoid-induced osteoporosis has yet to be clarified. Most reports have suggested that fluoride exerts an anabolic effect on the skeleton of glucocorticoid-treated patients (Cass et al, 1966; Meunier et al, 1982; Rich et al, 1964); however, the recent study by Rickers et al (1982) showed a conflicting result. The failure of the latter investigators to show the effect of fluoride was probably related to the site (distal radius) used in evaluating bone loss.

It is now becoming clear that fluoride exerts a preferential effect on the axial over the appendicular skeleton. Several studies have described increases in bone density in axial skeleton in one-third to two-thirds of osteoporotic patients on long-term fluoride treatment with no parallel increase in appendicular bone density (Baylink et al, 1983; Bernstein and Cohen, 1967; Briancon and Meunier, 1981; Rich and Ivanovitch, 1965; Riggs et al, 1980; 1982; Vose et al, 1978). The same pattern of response was demonstrated by the five patients presented in this paper; that is, mean

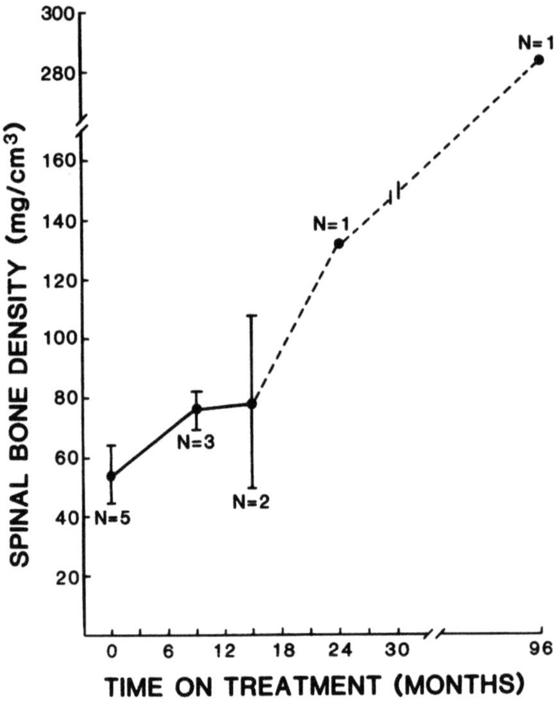

Fig. 7. Change in spinal bone density in mg/cm³ during fluoride treatment.

spinal bone density progressively increased with fluoride therapy (Fig. 7) while the bone density of the radius remained unchanged (Fig. 8a, 8b).

We believe that the osteoporosis in our patients is not entirely due to glucocorticoids, especially in patients 4 and 5. These two patients were on a relatively low dose of glucocorticoids (5-10 mg/day, and 5 mg every other day, respectively). It is possible that the administration of glucocorticoids resulted in an acceleration of the preexisting bone loss and, therefore, aggravated the condition. In these cases, it is clear that fluoride can still exert its osteogenic effect even in the presence of supraphysiologic levels of glucocorticoids. A significant increase in serum alkaline phosphatase (a measure of response to treatment) was noted as early as three months after initiation of therapy in one patient, and in 12 months in another. All five patients showed a significant alkaline phosphatase response. These changes are at least as rapid as those occurring in postmenopausal osteoporotics on fluordie treatment (Farley et al, 1984). Therefore, the combination of vitamin D, calcium, and fluoride seems to provide a rational approach to the treatment of patients with glucocorticoid-induced osteoporosis.

One further issue that has to be addressed is when to start therapy. The main goal of treatment, as with most diseases, is to prevent osteoporosis. Therefore, we are inclined to favor prophylactic therapy in high-risk individuals. Although available data suggest that the risk of developing osteoporosis increases with higher dosages and longer duration of glucocorticoid

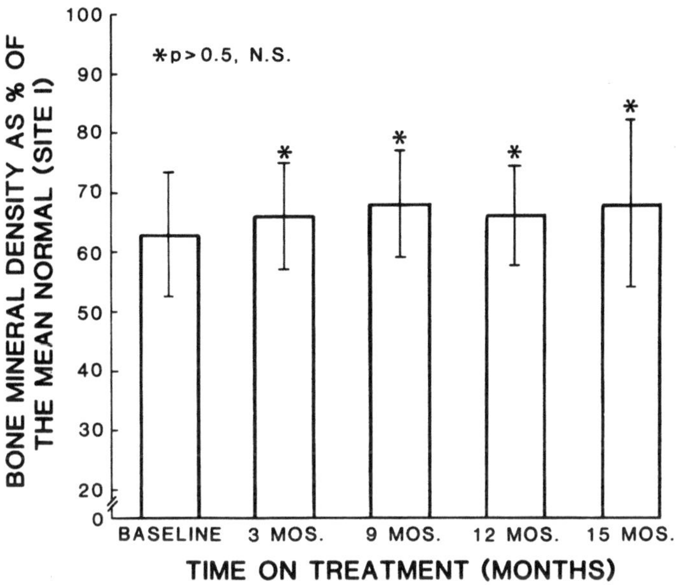

a)

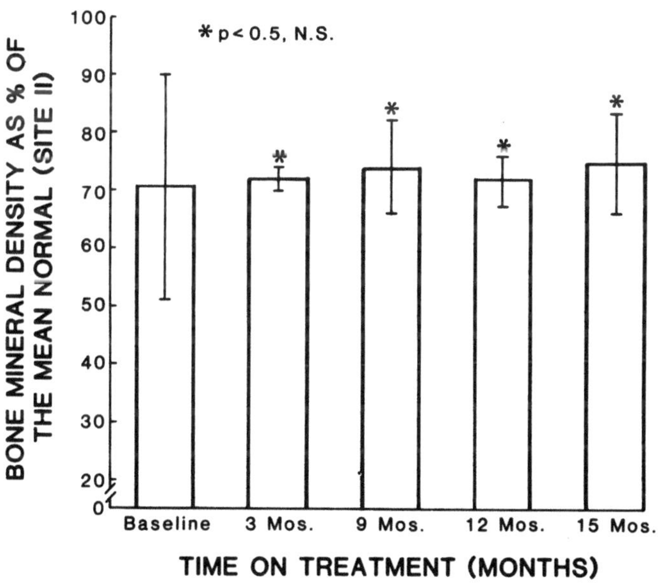

b)

Fig. 8. Bone density of the radius in sites 1 (a) and 2 (b) as percent of the mean before and during fluoride treatment.

treatment, we know that the response of individual patients is not entirely predictable. Moreover, it is not practical to apply preventive measures to all patients. It is important that patients at risk be identified so that preventive measures can be applied to them specifically.

The following is a rational approach for selection of patients for prophylactic therapy. Bone density (ideally measured in the spine by dual photon or quantitative CT scan, or of the radius by single photon absorptiometry) should be assessed at the start of glucocorticoid therapy and followed up every 6-12 months to determine the rate of bone loss. Preventive measures should be started if the rate is higher than one would expect as a result of the normal aging process -- eg, a QCT loss rate of >6% per year. Other risk factors to be considered when instituting treatment are as follows: 1) low baseline bone density (spinal bone density of <87 mg/cm^3, or density of the radius which is two standard deviations below that expected for age); 2) prednisone (or equivalent) dosage of 15 mg or more per day; 3) hypercalciuria; and 4) perimenopausal state in a woman with relatively low bone density and a family history of osteoporosis.

A prophylactic program for these patients should include vitamin D and supplemental calcium to improve calcium balance. One problem that may be encountered with this approach is determining the safe but effective dosage of vitamin D or its metabolites which will increase calcium absorption. Stimulation of intestinal calcium absorption by raising the serum concentration of 1,25 dihydroxy vitamin D (1,25$(OH)_2$) has been documented (Kaplan et al, 1977; Shen et al, 1977). Urinary calcium is increased as well. Since urinary calcium excretion is directly related to the increase in calcium absorption and 1,25 $(OH)_2$ vitamin D level in the serum (Adams et al, 1982), our approach is to give sufficient amounts of vitamin D or its metabolites to increase urinary calcium levels to the upper limits of normal (250 mg per 24 hours for women and 300 mg per 24 hours for men).

In a patient whose baseline urine calcium is elevated, it is important that this be corrected with hydrochlorothiazide before vitamin D is administered. One should be aware that vitamin D and calcium supplementation, especially when combined with hydrochlorothiazide, carries a risk of causing hypercalcemia, which may result in renal and vascular damage if not corrected. We seldom see either hypercalcemia or hypercalciuria because we monitor both serum and urine calcium levels at least every two months, allowing us to intervene before serious complications occur.

Summary

The currently available data suggest that glucocorticoid-treated patients who are at risk of developing osteoporosis may benefit from a prophylactic program designed to improve calcium absorption and decrease urinary calcium loss. The long-term efficacy of this program, however, has not been proven. Therefore, we emphasize continuous follow-up care for patients who have to be maintained on glucocorticoid therapy. If bone loss persists while on prophylactic therapy, one should consider the use of a bone anabolic agent such as fluoride.

References

1. Adams, N.D., Gray, R.W., Lemann, J., and Cheung, H.S.: Effects of calcitriol administration on calcium metabolism in healthy men. Kidney Int. 21, 90, 1982.

2. Baylink, D.J., Farley, S.M., and Smith, L.: Characterization of skeletal response to fluoride in osteoporosis. Clin. Res. 31, 543A, 1983. (Abstract)

3. Bernstein, D.S., and Cohen, P.: Use of sodium fluoride in the treatment of osteoporosis. J. Clin. Endocrinol. 27, 197, 1967.

4. Blodgett, F.M., Burgin, L., Fezzoni, D., Gribetz, D., and Talbot, N.B.: Effects of prolonged cortisone therapy on the statural growth, skeletal maturation, and metabolic status of children. New Eng. J. Med. 254, 636, 1956.

5. Bradley, B.E., and Ansell, B.M.: Fractures in Still's disease. Ann. Rheum. Dis. 19, 135, 1960.

6. Briançon, D., and Meunier, P.J.: Treatment of osteoporosis with fluoride, calcium, and vitamin D. Orthop. Clin. North Am. 12, 629, 1981.

7. Cass, R.M., Croft, J.D., Perkin, P., Nye, W., Waterhouse, W., and Terry, R.: New bone formation in osteoporosis following treatment with sodium fluoride. Arch. Intern. Med. 118, 111, 1966.

8. Farley, S.M., Libanati, C.R., Schulz, E.E., Grunberg, C.M., Lian, J.B., Smith, L., and Baylink, D.J.: Fluoride therapy in osteoporosis has rapid effects on both the axial and peripheral skeleton which can be detected by increase in serum alkaline phosphatase. Calcif. Tissue Int. 36, A41, 1984. (Abstract)

9. Farley, S.M., Libanati, C.L., Smith, L., Eliel, L., Kilcoyne, R.L., Cann, C., Wakely, G.K., and Schulz, E.E.: Long-term fluoride therapy corrects the spinal bone density deficit in osteoporosis. Endocrine Society Meeting, June 1985. (Abstract)

10. Fischer, J.A., and Hastrup, B.: Cortisone and calcium balance (effect of calcium, vitamin D and methylandrostenediol). Acta Endocrinol. 16, 141, 1954.

11. Follis, R.H.: The pathology of osseous changes in Cushing's syndrome in an infant and in adults. Bull. Johns Hopkins Hosp. 88, 440, 1951.

12. Frantz, A.G., and Robkin, M.T.: Human growth hormone. New Eng. J. Med. 271, 1375, 1964.

13. Frost, H.M., and Villanueva, A.R.: Human osteoblastic activity: III. The effect of cortisone on lamellar osteoblastic activity. Henry Ford Hosp. Med. Bull. 9, 97, 1961.

14. Fucik, R.F., Kukreja, S.C., Hargis, G.K., Browser, E.N., Henderson, W.J., and Williams, G.A.: Effect of glucocorticoids on function of the parathyroid glands in man. J. Clin. Endocrinol. Metab. 40, 152, 1972.

15. Hann, T.J.: Corticosteroid-induced osteopenia. Arch. Intern Med. 138, 882, 1978.

16. Hann, T.J., Halstead, L.R., and Teitelbaum, S.L.: Altered mineral metabolism in glucocorticoid-induced osteopenia. Effect of 25-hydroxyvitamin D administration. J. Clin. Invest. 64, 655, 1979.

17. Hartog, M., Gaafar, M.A., and Frazer, R.: Effect of corticosteroids on serum growth hormone. Lancet, 2, 376, 1964.

18. Jee, W.S.S., Park, H.Z., Roberts, W.E., and Kenner, G.H.: Corticosteroid and bone. Am. J. Anat. 129, 477, 1970.

19. Jowsey, J., and Riggs, B.L.: Bone formation in hypercortisolism. Acta Endocrinol. 63, 21, 1970.

20. Kaplan, R.A., Haussler, M.R., Deftos, L.H., Bone, H., and Pak, C.Y.C.: The role of 1a, 25-hydroxyvitamin D in the mediation of intestinal hyperabsorption of calcium in primary hyperparathyroidism and absorptive hypercalciuria. J. Clin. Invest. 59, 756, 1977.

21. Krieger, D.T., and Glick, S.M.: Growth hormone and cortisol responsiveness in Cushing's syndrome. Am. J. Med. 52, 25, 1972.

22. Lukert, B.P., and Adams, J.S.: Calcium and phosphorous homeostasis in man. Arch. Intern. Med. 136, 1249, 1976.

23. Meunier, P.J., Dempster, D.W., Edouard, C., Chapuy, M.C., Arlot, M., and Charlon, S.: Bone histomorphometry in corticosteroid-induced osteoporosis and Cushing's syndrome. Calcif. Tissue Int. 34, A7, 1982.

24. Odvina, C.V., Wergedal, J.E., Libanati, C.R., Schulz, E.E., and Baylink, D.J.: Relationship between quantitative computerized tomography scan values and vertebral fractures in osteoporotics. Calcif. Tissue Int. 1984. (Abstract).

25. Peck, W.A., Brandt, J., and Miller, I.: Hydrocortisone-induced inhibition of protein synthesis and uridine incorporation in isolated bone cells *in vitro*. Proc. Natl. Acad. Sci. (USA) 57, 1599, 1967.

26. Rich, C., and Ivanovitch, P.: Response to sodium fluoride in severe primary osteoporosis. Ann. Intern. Med. 63, 1069, 1965.

27. Rich, C., Ensink, J., and Ivanovitch, P.: The effect of sodium fluoride on clacium metabolism of subjects with metabolic bone disease. J. Clin. Invest. 43, 545, 1964.

28. Rickers, H., Deding, A., Christiansen, C., Rodbro, P., and Neistoft, J.: Corticosteroid-induced osteopenia and vitamin D metabolism. Effect of vitamin D_2, calcium, phosphate, and sodium fluoride administration. Clin. Endocrinol. 16, 409, 1982.

29. Riggs, B.L., Hodgson, S.F., Hoffman, D.L., Kelly, P.J., Johnson, K.A., and Taves, D.T.: Treatment of primary osteoporosis with fluoride and calcium. Clinical tolerance and fracture occurrence. J.A.M.A. 243, 446, 1980.

30. Riggs, B.L., Seeman, E., Hodgson, S.F., Taves, D.R., and O'Fallon, M.O.: Effect of fluoride/calcium regimen on vertebral fracture occurrence in postmenopausal osteoporosis. New Eng. J. Med. 306, 446, 1982.

31. Saville, P.D., and Kharmosh, O.: Osteoporosis of rheumatoid arthritis: Influence of age, sex, and corticosteroids. Arthritis Rheum. 10, 423, 1967.

32. Sheagren, J.N., Jowsey, J., Bird, D.C., et al: Effects on bone growth of daily versus alternate-day corticosteroid administration: An experimental study. J. Lab. Clin. Med. 89, 120, 1977.

33. Shen, F.H., Baylink, D.J., Nielsen, R.L., Sherrard, D.J., Ivey, J.L., and Haussler, M.R.: Increased serum 1, 25-dihydroxyvitamin D in idiopathic hypercalciuria. J. Lab. Clin. Med. 90, 955, 1977.

34. Suzuki, Y., Ichikawa, Y., Saito, E., and Homma, M.: Importance of increased urinary calcium excretion in the development of secondary hyperparathyroidism of patients under glucocorticoid therapy. Metabolism 32, 151, 1983.

35. Thompson, J.S., Palmieri, G.M.A., and Crawford, R.L.: The effect of porcine calcitonin on osteoporosis induced by adrenal cortical steroids. J. Bone Joint Surg. 54A, 1490, 1972.

36. Vose, G.P., Keele, D.L., Miller, A.M., Rawley, R., Roach, T.L., and Sprinkle, E.E.: Effects of sodium fluoride, inorganic phosphate, and oxymetholone therapies in osteoporosis: a six-year progress report. J. Gerontol. 33, 204, 1978.

Etiological Spectrum of Avascular Necrosis

L. SOLOMON

Until recently, avascular necrosis (AVN) of bone was usually associated with injury or infection. During the last few decades, however, many other causes have come to light and, with the increasing use of corticosteroids and other immunosuppressive agents, drug-induced necrosis has assumed alarming proportions (Table I). Two questions are explored in this paper: 1) What links these apparently disparate conditions? 2) Is there a final common pathway leading to bone death?

Clinical Disorders Associated with AVN

During the 15-year period 1970-1985, 126 patients were treated for avascular necrosis. In most cases the femoral head was involved, but 13 patients presented with lesions in other sites: the head of the humerus in five, the

Table I. Causes of avascular necrosis of the femoral head in 126 patients

Clinical disorder	No.	Age	M:F	Complications
Femoral neck fracture	24	18-79	1:4	Osteoarthritis (9)
Dislocation of the hip	4	21-47	3:1	-
Slipped femoral epiphysis	4	16-21	1:1	Chondrolysis (2)
Gaucher's disease	9	8-37	1:2	Infection (3)
Tuberculous caseation	1	38	0:1	-
Caisson disease	3	21-40	3:0	-
Sickle cell disease	2	21-25	1:1	Infection (1)
Cushing's disease	1	29	1:0	-
High-dose corticosteroids	43	16-70	1:1.5	Osteoporosis(?) (43) Fracture (7)
Low-dose corticosteroids plus azothiaprine	3	37-54	1:2	-
SLE plus corticosteroids	4	31-49	0:4	Vasculitis (2)
Alcohol abuse	28	29-72	6:1	Osteoporosis(?) (9)

Current Concepts of Bone Fragility

femoral condyles in five, and the talus in three. The clinical disorders associated with AVN are shown in Table I.

Trauma

Trauma is still the commonest cause of osteonecrosis; the site most frequently affected is the femoral head, with an incidence of 27% after displaced fractures of the femoral neck (Barnes et al, 1976). Ischemia results from interruption of the intraosseous and capsular blood supply and necrosis may involve all or most of the femoral head. With time, fragmentation and collapse of the femoral head occurs.

A variation of the straightforward fracture is slipping of the proximal femoral epiphysis. These lesions occur in young adolescents and necrosis may be limited to a circumferential band of subchondral bone.

Posterior hip dislocation is complicated by femoral head necrosis in over 13% of patients (Epstein, 1973). This may be the result of direct vascular injury; in some cases, however, the capsular vessels are strangulated without being severed and ischemia may be secondary to venous engorgement and stasis (Shin, 1979).

Infiltrative Disorders of Bone

In Gaucher's disease, one observes an abnormal accumulation of glycocerebrocide in the macrophages of the reticuloendothelial system. Osteonecrosis is a well recognized sequel (Amstutz and Carey, 1966) and is attributed to compression of capillary sinusoids by the swollen "Gaucher cells" (Jaffe, 1972). Other infiltrative disorders, such as tuberculous osteitis and metastatic disease, could encroach more directly on either the arterial or the venous circulation in the femoral head.

Sickle Cell Disease

The abnormal Hb S gene, which accounts for the sickle cell phenomenon, is limited to people of Central and West African black descent. The condition is rarely seen in Southern Africa; the two cases in this series occurred in visitors to the subcontinent, one from Nigeria and one from the U.S.A. Red cell distortion is most marked in deoxygenated blood and the risk of bone infarction is increased under conditions of hypoxia. Ischemia is due to intravascular clumping of the sickle-shaped cells with reduced capillary blood flow (Rickles and O'Leary, 1974).

Caisson Disease

Decompression sickness occurs mainly in deep sea divers and in persons working in pressure chambers. In some of these cases (numbers vary from 4-50%) further complication of bone necrosis is encountered, affecting mainly the proximal ends of the humerus and femur (Elliott and Harrison, 1970; Ohta and Matsunaga, 1974). Two types of change are seen: the classical subchondral, segmental necrosis which is similar to other types of AVN; and intramedullary calcification which is secondary to marrow necrosis. The cause of bone ischemia is discussed below.

Drug-induced Necrosis

High dosage corticosteroid administration and alcohol abuse are nowadays among the more common causes of femoral head necrosis. The former occurs most likely in patients receiving immunosuppressive therapy after renal transplantation (Solomon and Erken, 1975); the latter is seen in healthy, unrestrained social drinkers rather than in severe alcoholics (Solomon, 1973). They are grouped together here not only because they are both drug-induced, but because the clinical and pathologic features are similar.

Hip pain usually appears insidiously and early radiographs may show no abnormality (Fig. 1). Segmental sclerosis is not very marked until late and occurs sometimes in a rather patchy fashion throughout the femoral head. Subarticular fractures are common and may lead to separation of the articular cartilage (Fig. 2). Many patients have an associated hyperlipidemia and fatty overload of the marrow is visible in the femoral head. Although

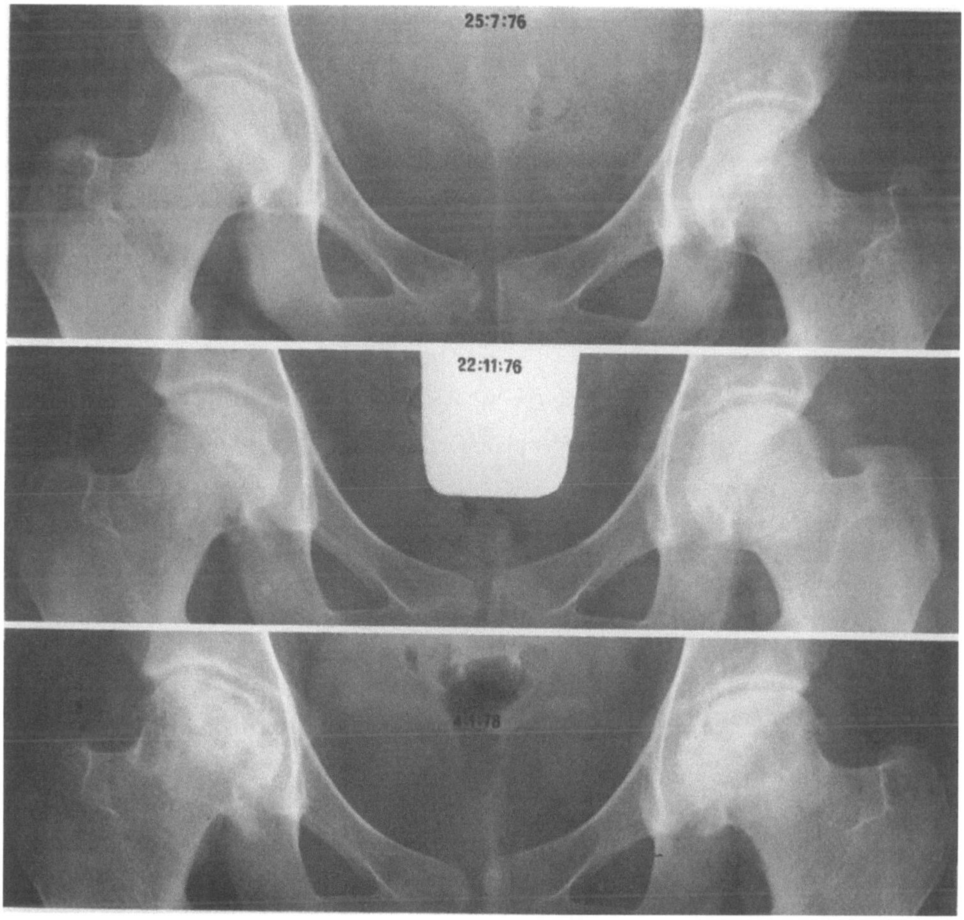

Fig. 1. Successive radiographs of a patient receiving high dosage cortico steroids. At the onset of symptoms x-rays appear to be normal; first the right and then the left femoral head develop signs of AVN.

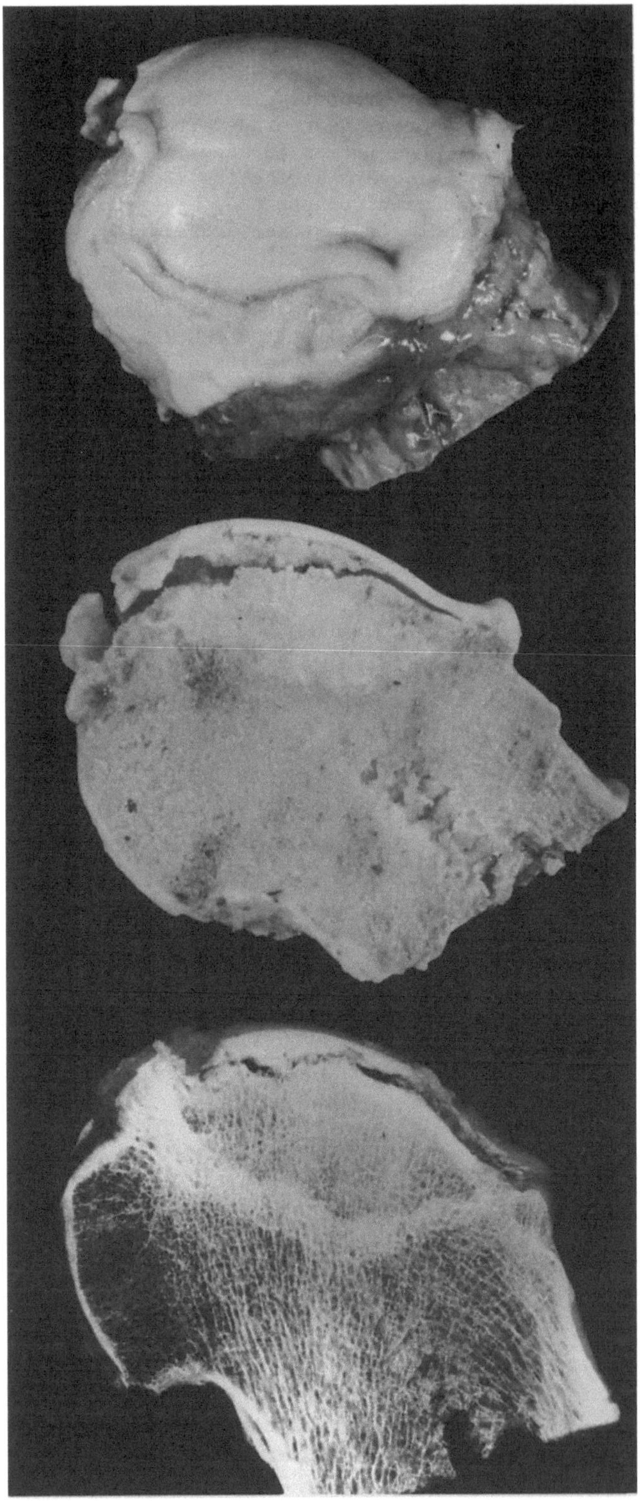

Fig. 2. Steroid-induced osteonecrosis of the femoral head. Distortion of the articular surface (a) is due to subarticular fracture through the necrotic segment (coronal section (b) and fine detail radiograph (c)).

the pathogenesis is disputed, it is generally agreed that fatty degeneration and hyperlipidemia are important concomitants.

The Mechanisms of Bone Death

Whatever the preceding disorder, the final common pathway in the pathogenesis of the various types of bone necrosis must be ischemia and infarction. When the details are unravelled, this can occur in only two ways: 1) arterial insufficiency and 2) venous or sinusoidal stasis.

AVN following a fracture clearly falls into the first category, and osteonecrosis associated with infiltrative disorders, like Gaucher's disease, almost certainly result from capillary stasis. What remains contentious is the mechanism of bone ischemia in disorders like hypercortisolemia and alcohol abuse. Two hypotheses vie for acceptance: a) circulatory insufficiency is caused by occlusion of end-arterioles by fatty emboli; and b) sinusoidal (capillary) bloodflow is impeded by the raised intramedullary pressure resulting from fatty replacement of myeloid tissue.

Fat gobules have been demonstrated in the haversian canals and subchondral arterioles in steroid-induced femoral head necrosis (Cruess et al, 1975). However, there is an inconstant relationship between fat embolization and osteonecrosis; I have found arteriolar fat globules in fresh fractures and in normal necropsy specimens (Fig. 3).

Several authors have reported raised intraosseous pressures associated with both alcohol-induced and steroid-induced femoral head necrosis (Arlet et al, 1972; Hungerford, 1979; Solomon, 1981). It has also been shown that marrow fat cell size is increased in these cases, not only in the affected femoral head but also in the apparently unaffected opposite hip (Solomon, 1981). Although neither of these observations constitute positive proof, taken together they strongly suggest a pathogenetic sequence: fatty infiltration of the marrow → increase in fat cell size and fat volume → intraosseous tamponade → capillary occlusion → vascular stasis → ischemia.

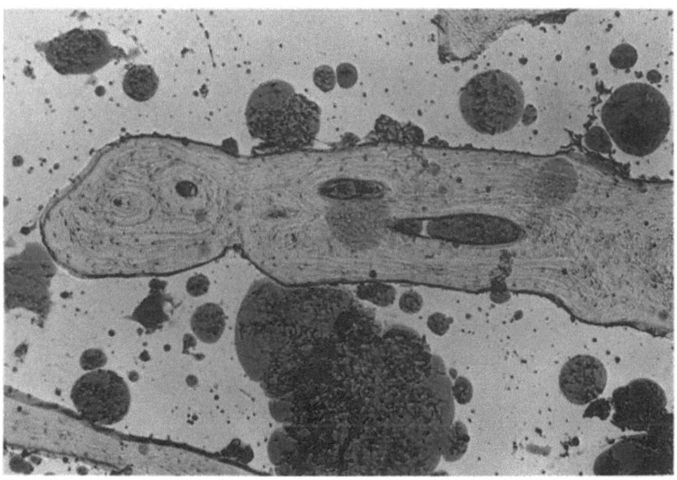

Fig. 3. Photomicrograph showing fat globules in haversian canals of the femoral head after a fracture. (Oil Red O fat stain. x 110)

Both corticosteroid and alcohol-induced necrosis appear to be dose related. Patients on low-dose steroids (eg, for rheumatoid arthritis) seldom develop AVN; however, osteonecrosis has been reported in patients receiving a combination of steroids and azothiaprine, as seen in three such cases in this series. If azothiaprine causes vascular thickening, this could tip the balance towards ischemia in patients on low steroid dosages.

The combination of vasculitis and corticosteroid therapy may, likewise, account for the relative frequency of AVN in patients with disseminated lupus erythematosus.

Changes in marrow fat have also been implicated in the AVN that follow: Caisson disease. Traditionally, infarction has been attributed to vascular occlusion by nitrogen bubbles which come out of solution on rapid decompression. However, it has now been shown that inert gases like nitrogen are taken up in the fatty marrow and may cause fat cell damage and swelling, leading to reduced sinusoidal blood flow (Thomas, 1983).

Among the patients in this series, 12 had advanced siderosis due to the ingestion of large quantities of iron in traditional alcoholic brews. Without doubt, the alcohol intake was the main cause of AVN, and the same bony changes have been encountered in those without overt iron overload. The possibility, however, that iron deposition in the marrow might further encroach on blood channels cannot be excluded.

Conclusion

A refinement of the etiologic spectrum of avascular necrosis brings out the following pathogenetic grouping:

Type 1 AVN - Arterial cutoff

1. Fracture
2. Slipped epiphysis
3. Dislocation
4. Massive arterial embolism

Type 2 AVN - Arteriolar occlusion

1. Sickle cell disease
2. Polycythemia
3. ? Caisson disease
4. ? Fat embolism

Type 3 AVN - Extraosseous venous occlusion (theoretical)

1. Capsular stretching due to effusion
2. Capsular strangulation

Type 4 AVN - Sinusoidal compression (tamponade)

1. Gaucher's disease
2. Corticosteroid-induced necrosis
3. Alcohol-induced necrosis

The implications for treatment are important. In types 1 and 2, the ischemia is irreversible. It is not known whether type 3 really occurs, but if it does it is potentially amenable to treatment; and type 4 is already being treated, with considerably success, by intraosseous decompression aimed at relieving sinusoidal stasis.

References

1. Amstutz, H.C., and Carey, E.J.: Skeletal manifestations and treatment of Gaucher's disease. J. Bone Joint Surg. 48A, 670, 1966.
2. Arlet, J., Ficat, P., Lartigue, G., and Tran, M.A.: Recherches cliniques sur la pression intra-osseuse dans la métaphyse et l'épiphyse fémorale supérieure chez l'homme. Application du diagnostic des ischémies et nécroses. Revue de Rhumatisme et des Maladies Ostéo-articulaires 42, 391, 1972.
3. Barnes, R., Brown, J.T., Garden, R.S., et al: Subcapital fractures of the femur. J. Bone Joint Surg. 58B, 2, 1976.
4. Cruess, R.L., Ross, D., and Crawshaw, E.: The etiology of steroid-induced avascular necrosis of bone. A laboratory and clinical study. Clin.Orthop. 113, 178, 1975.
5. Elliott, D.H. and Harrison, J.A.B.: Bone necrosis - an occupational hazard in diving. J.R.Nav.Med.Serv. 56, 140, 1970.
6. Epstein, H.C.: Traumatic dislocations of the hip. Clin.Orthop. 92, 116, 1973.
7. Hungerford, D.S.: Bone marrow pressure, venography and core decompression in ischemic necrosis of the femoral head. In, The Hip. Proc. 7th Open Scientific Meeting of the Hip Society. C.V. Mosby Co., St. Louis, 1979.
8. Jaffe, H.L.: Metabolic, Degenerative and Inflammatory Disease of Bones and Joints. Lea and Febiger, Philadelphia, 1972.
9. Ohta, Y., and Matsunaga, H.: Bone lesions. J. Bone Joint Surg. 56B, 3, 1974.
10. Rickles, F.R. and O'Leary, D.S.: Role of coagulation system in pathophysiology of sickle cell disease. Arch.Int.Med. 133, 635, 1974.
11. Shin, S.S.: Circulatory and vascular changes in the hip following traumatic hip dislocation. Clin.Orthop.Rel.Res. 140, 255, 1979.
12. Solomon, L.: Drug-induced arthropathy and necrosis of the femoral head. J.Bone Joint Surg. 55B, 246, 1973.
13. Solomon, L.: Idiopathic necrosis of the femoral head: pathogenesis and treatment. Can.J.Surg. 24, 573, 1981
14. Solomon, L., and Erken, E.H.W.: Osteonecrosis following renal transplantation. S.Afr.Med.J. 49, 1082, 1975.
15. Thomas, I.H.: Caisson disease of bone. The seed and the soil. J.Roy. Coll.Surg.Edinb. 28, 347, 1983.

Reversible Osteopenia: Orthopedic Aspects

J. P. MURNAGHAN

Introduction

Osteopenia, for clinical purposes, can be defined as any condition in which the bone mass is decreased below normal. For the orthopedic surgeon, osteopenia is usually evident by the presence of fracture.

The common sites of fractures are the distal radius, spine, humeral neck, and hip. Difficult fractures are seen in the lateral tibia plateau, diaphysis of long bones, especially in the diaphysis of the femur just below the tip of the femoral prosthesis.

The therapeutic goal, in this generally older population, is early return to the preinjury functional level. These patients rarely have the ability to walk with partial weight bearing. Internal fixation devices must, therefore, be able to withstand weight bearing stresses. To attain early ambulation is a major technical problem because of the poor quality of the bone. The usual internal fixation devices are not adequate since the fragile bone stock has poor holding power for the interfragmentary screws and the screws holding the plates.

As in all fracture management, the importance of bone grafting must not be overlooked. Autogenous bone grafts help to promote local fracture healing, and as such are a major benefit in fractures of the long bone. The harvesting of autogenous bone graft in the osteopenic population is sometimes difficult. The posterior iliac crest is often the only site where adequate bone can be obtained. Trying to harvest bone from the anterior iliac crest frequently results in a frustratingly inadequate 4-5 cc of poor quality bone graft.

The second role of the bone graft is mechanical support, especially in fractures of the tibial plateau where the metaphysis is often almost hollow in osteopenic patients. Without adequate support for the elevated tibial plateau fragments they will collapse back into their prereduction position. Packing cancellous bone, compressing the bone graft to 50% of its loose packed volume, has proven an excellent method in patients with moderate osteopenia.

Bone bank bone (allograft) may be very useful where only mechanical support is required. I prefer the cancellous bone of the femoral head for allo-

Current Concepts of Bone Fragility

grafts, recovered from total hip replacement, or pieces of cancellous bone harvested at the time of total knee arthroplasty.

Plates

During the past 20 years, internal fixation of fractures using interfragmentary screws and plates fixed to bone with screws has become popular in North America through the ASIF surgeons. The difficulty in patients with osteopenia is the poor purchase of the screw threads in the osteopenic bone. Where the bone stock is felt to be inadequate, supplementary fixation is necessary to obtain stable internal fixation.

Plates and Cement

Introducing methylmethacrylate into the femoral canal has become a straightforward procedure in total joint arthroplasty with the use of cement restric-

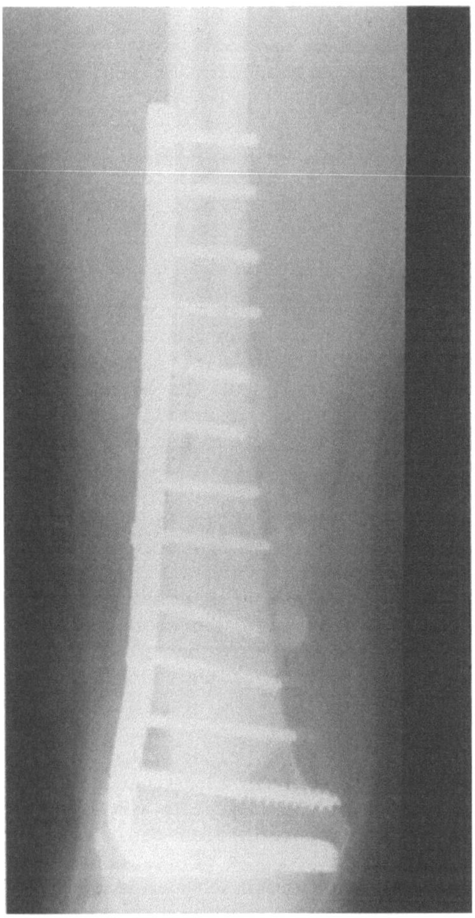

Fig. 1a. Fracture of the distal femur fixed with a blade plate supplemented with intramedullary methylmethacrylate.

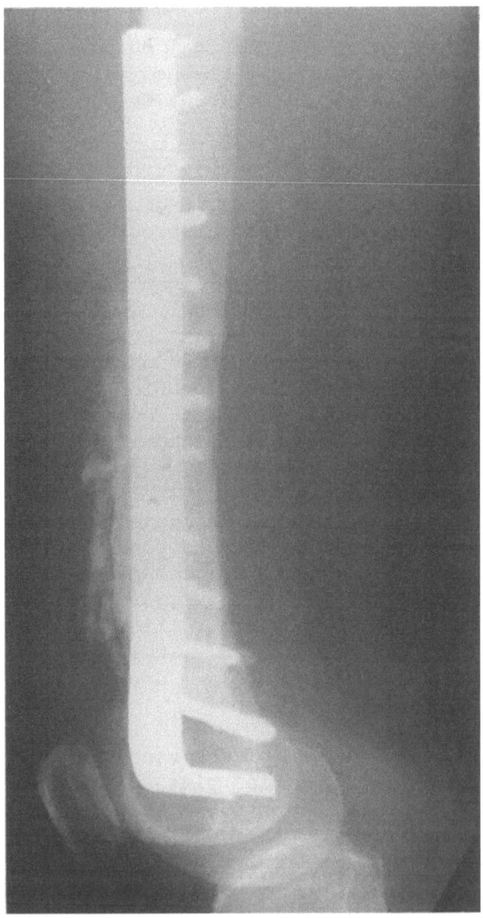

Fig. 1b. Fracture of the distal femur fixed with a blade plate, methylmethacrylate and supplemental bone graft.

tors, cement guns, and pressurizing devices. This technology can and should be applied when inserting cement as supplementary fixation with screws and plates. When bony purchase for the screws is adequate, the screw holes are drilled and tapped in the usual way. Screws of appropriate length are selected before injecting methylmethacrylate to fill the medullary canal. The medullary canal has to be cleared of soft tissue, and a bone curette or even a suction tip may be adequate for this purpose. The insertion of cement in a semiliquid state with a cement gun can greatly improve the filling of the medullary canal. If one does not curette out the cavity, the bone cement often stays pooled in one localized area. It is necessary to gauge the consistency of the cement between too liquid, which would run back out, and the later firm stage when it is impossible to get the cement distributed evenly.

If the screws are inserted while the cement is still soft, screw threads are moulded in the medullary canal as the cement sets around them. This greatly enhances screw fixation. Final tightening of the screws is done once the cement has polymerized (Fig. 1a, 1b).

In case of little or no bony purchase for the screws, Cameron (1975) has recommended methylmethacrylate cement, introduced through the screw hole, as

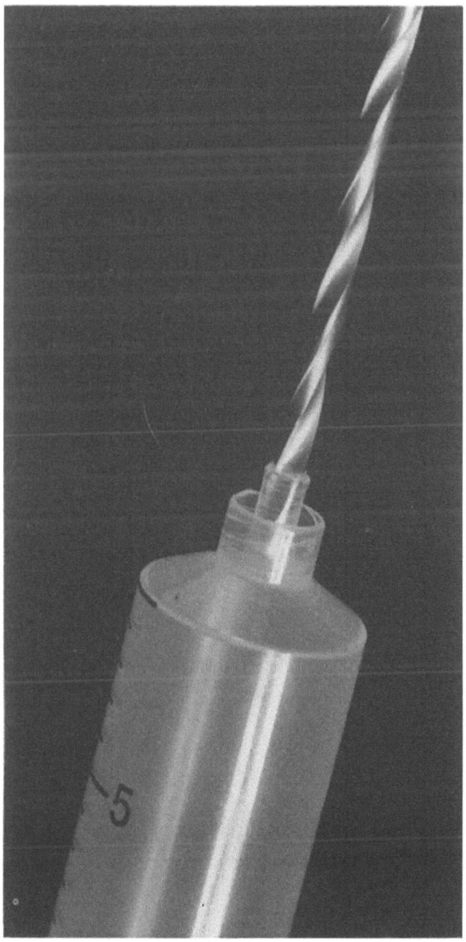

Fig. 2. Tip of a disposable 10 mL syringe enlarged by drilling out the tip with a 3.2 mm drill bit.

an intramedullary plug to increase screw fixation. Screw holes are drilled where possible. The bone may be too thin to tap any screw threads. The cement is introduced through an empty screw hole and the screw advanced through the soft cement.

The insertion of cement through the screw holes requires minor modifications to such readily available equipment as a plastic 10 mL disposable syringe. If one drills out the tip of the syringe with a 3.2 mm drill (Fig. 2), the cement, in a low viscosity phase early after mixing, will pass freely through the tip (Fig. 3). A slightly longer snout for the syringe can be achieved by using the plastic packaging tip that comes with the syringe. The packing cap is also drilled out with a 3.2 mm drill. When the cement is used early after mixing, methylmethacrylate can be inserted through the screw holes into the medullary canal (Fig. 4). The screws are then quickly inserted and left standing 1-2 mm proud without fully tightening them. When the cement in the intramedullary canal is set, the screws are then fully tightened down, giving excellent purchase for the screw threads. This method has the advantage of using smaller quantities of cement, localizing the methylmethacrylate to the sites where it is needed. The difficulty with this technique is to control the flow of the cement in the intramedullary canal restricting it to where it can be used to best mechanical advantage.

Care must be taken to avoid cement coming in contact with adjacent nerves and vessels, and to stop the cement from flowing into an adjacent joint. Totally occluding the medullary canal may have deleterious effect on the blood supply of the affected bone.

If it is not technically feasible to use methylmethacrylate in a liquid phase, then the cement may be drilled and tapped, after it has polymerized, for insertion of the screws using the same techniques as for bone. Such a procedure requires sharp cutting instruments, and several drills and tips which will have to be resharpened or discarded after the procedure.

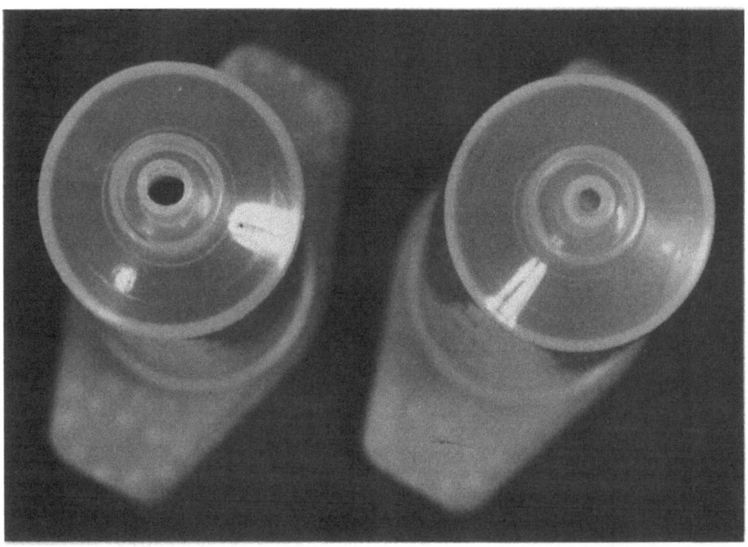

Fig. 3. Syringe tip enlarged for ease of passage of cement compared with the normal opening of a 10 mL syringe.

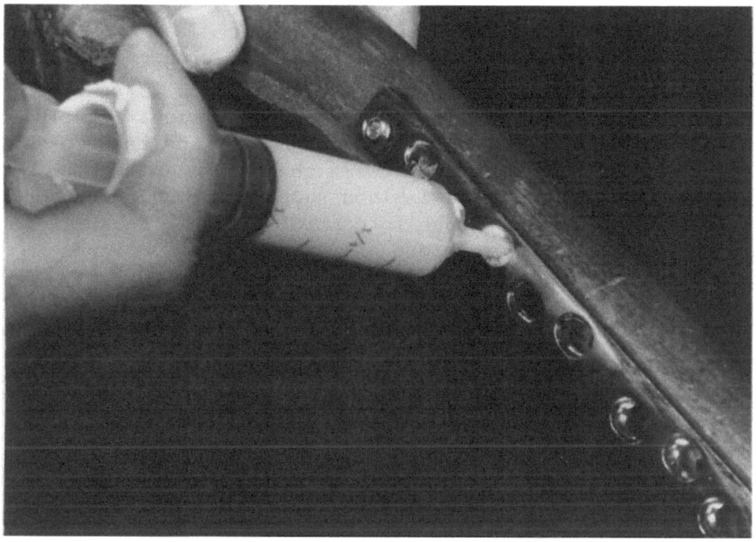

Fig. 4. Methylmethacrylate injected in an early dough phase into the screw hole with plate in situ before screw insertion.

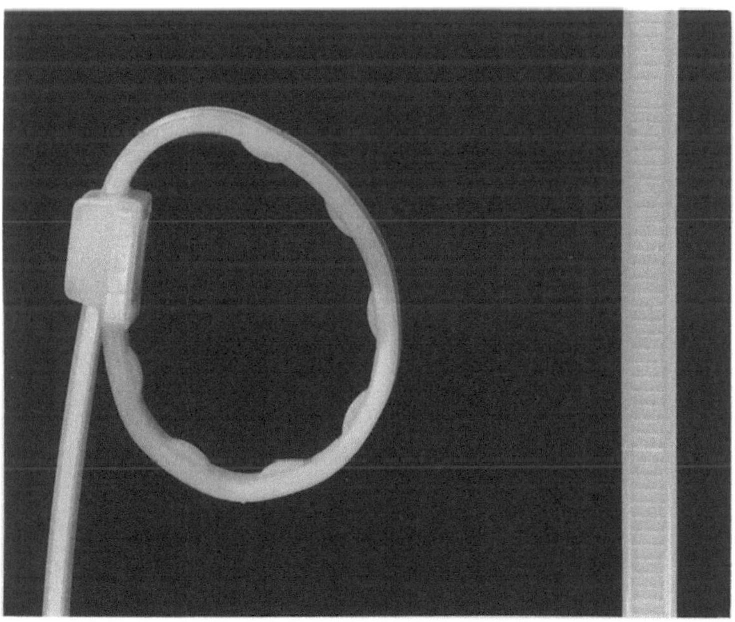

Fig. 5. Nylon Partridge band with ridges on the cortical surface to prevent total contact with bone. Cross ridges seen on the outer surface (right) are part of the self-locking mechanism.

Cerclage

Partridge, in 1981, developed a nylon band (Fig. 5) for cerclage fixation in diaphyseal fractures. The rationale of the Partridge bands is to reconstitute the cylindrical shape of the hollow bone and, thus, significantly restore its mechanical strength. The nylon band has ridges on its deep surface which allow only intermittent contact between the band and the bone, minimizing interference with the periosteal blood supply to bone. The Partridge bands alone are not strong enough to control oblique fractures without some form of external fixation unless an intramedullary device neutralizes the bending forces (Partridge, 1981). Where no intramedullary device can be used, Partridge recommended that two external plates be applied to the outer surface of the bone. The two special nylon plates are applied, separated by a quarter of the circumference of the bone and encircled with six Partridge bands (Fig. 6). Having special surgical instruments available for passing nylon bands or 1.2 mm wires around the bone greatly simplifies the cerclage (Fig. 7).

I have used cerclage and plate fixations on several occasions, primarily when screw fixation was not possible. Where the Partridge bands could be supplemented with an intramedullary device, fracture fixation was usually satisfactory. When plates were used with the bands but without an intramedullary device, patients were required to remain nonweight bearing over two to three months before proceeding to weight bearing. The cerclage bands and plates technique is a second best treatment choice in that the patients are freer than they would be in traction but still cannot start weight bearing.

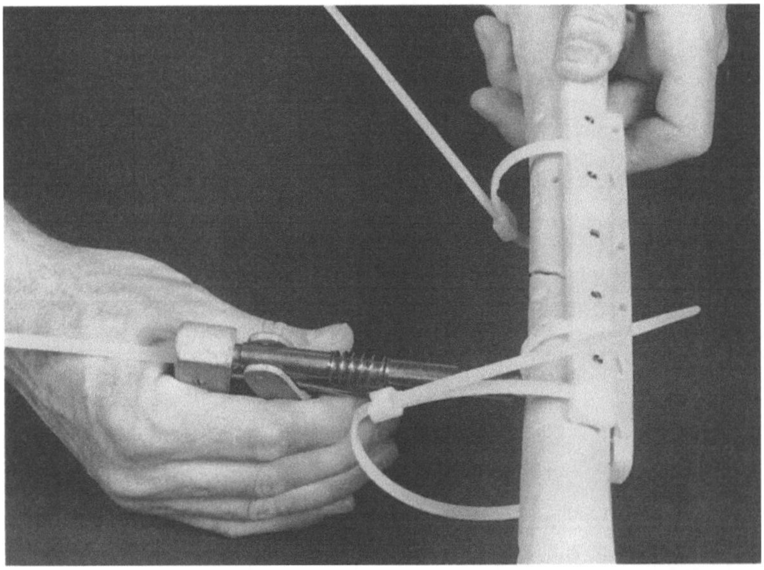

Fig. 6. Partridge bands inserted through two nylon Partridge plates that are positioned parallel to the long axis of the diaphysis and separated by one quarter of the bone's circumference. The tightening device allows individual adjustment of the Partridge bands.

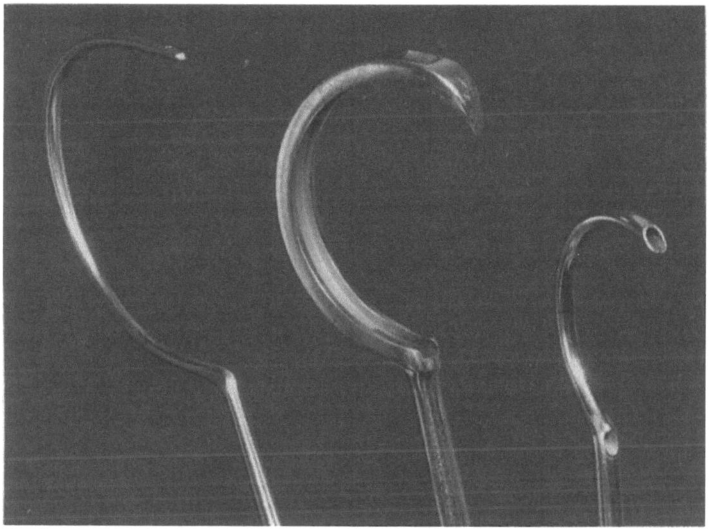

Fig. 7. A selection of instruments which facilitate the passage of cerclage bands and wires.

Intramedullary Devices

It is usually not possible to resort to an intramedullary device alone for fixation of long bone fractures in the elderly. In the occasional transverse diaphyseal fracture, a nail can be used alone with care not to split the bone. Occasionally, a large intramedullary nail supplemented with cerclage fixation may be appropriate for oblique or comminuted fractures. Ender nails can be used as an alignment device, but do not allow the same degree of walking as with a larger intramedullary nail.

When adequate bone stock is available, fractures of the proximal femur are treated with the usual nail-plate devices. Methylmethacrylate may be used to supplement the fixation, curetting out the neck and head of the femur as well as the medullary canal of the proximal shaft. If the patient is elderly, it is often necessary to decide which surgical technique will allow an early return to function. In certain fractures of the proximal femur, a total hip prosthesis is an excellent treatment, allowing early mobilization.

In fractures of the proximal femoral shaft below or around the stem of a femoral prosthesis, early return to function is often difficult. If the prosthesis is loose, removal of the prosthesis and cement by insertion of a long-stemmed femoral component with or without cerclage allows the best opportunity for early walking. If the prosthesis is solid and the fracture is at or just below the tip of the stem, internal fixation of the fracture with plates and screws, or plates and cerclage, allows bed-to-chair transfers but weight bearing must be deferred until fracture union.

Summary

Fractures in osteopenic individuals have to be observed for a long time. Protected weight bearing is advised until solid union has been achieved.

Long-term observation is necessary in conjunction with the medical treatment for the underlying cause of the osteopenia.

Osteopenia presents special problems to the orthopedic surgeon. With clear treatment goals, most of the problems can be overcome. The surgeon must always keep in mind the dynamic nature of the osteopenia and plan treatment in keeping with the patient's age and long-term outlook.

Selected Bibliography

1. Cameron, H.U., Jacob, R., MacNab, I., and Pilliar, R.M.: Use of polyurethylmethacrylate to enhance screw fixation in bone. J. Bone Joint Surg. 57A, 655, 1975.
2. Harrington, K.D., Sim, F.H., Enis, J.E., Johnston, J.O., Dick, H.M., and Gristina, A.G.: Methylmethacrylate as an adjunct in internal fixation of pathological fractures. J. Bone Joint Surg. 58A, 1047, 1976.
3. Partridge, A.J., and Evan, P.E.L.: The treatment of fractures of the shaft of the femur using nylon cerclage. J. Bone Joint Surg. 64B, 210, 1982.
4. Rhinelander, F.W.: The normal circulation of bone and its response to surgical intervention. J. Biomed. Mater. Res. 8, 87, 1974.

Osteoporosis

Pathogenic Mechanisms of the Osteoporoses

H. M. Frost

Introduction

To describe the pathogenetic mechanisms causing osteoporoses and bone fragility at the tissue and organ levels has become a complex task due to the discovery, since 1960, of the skeletal intermediary organization (IO) and some properties of its special systems. Prior to this, there was a huge gap in our knowledge of skeletal physiology. The idea that humoral agents acted directly on existing but independent osteoclasts and osteoblasts did not fit the evidence as seen in clinical practice, in the operating room, and under the microscope. Knowledge was lacking of nephron equivalents in skeletal tissue that are responsible for skeletal health and disease.

By 1960, a search for those mechanisms had begun and Table I shows steps in the discovery of the skeletal IO (intermediate organization). This concept has since become accepted by competent investigators (Arnold, 1964; Courpron, 1981; Duncan and Parfitt, 1975; Jaworski, 1984; Jee, 1983; Melsen et al, 1983; Meunier et al, 1979; Parfitt, 1984b). The special functions of the multicellular entities of the skeletal IO do indeed directly underlie health and pathologic features of the skeleton, including the osteoporoses. Moreover, many affections that seem unique in the clinical domain have their roots in the same IO functions (Frost, 1980; 1981a-b; 1983b-d; 1984; in press, a-f). As examples, the same IO mechanisms cause many clinically distinct features of Paget's disease of bone, osteomalacia (Frost, 1973a), shin splints (Frost, in press, c); osteoporosis (Frost, 1973a), osteogenesis imperfecta (Frost, in press, d), aseptic necrosis, stress fractures (Frost, 1973b), and fracture nonunions (Frost, in press, c). Finally, since approximately 1972 it has become possible to specify accurately the clinical effects of the middle and upper IO mechanisms causing osteoporoses and bone fragility and to specify more adequately the nature of these osteoporoses (Frost, 1981a; in press, c).

Definitions

Absolute bone volume (ABV): the volume of bone tissue, meaning volume of its organic bone matrix, left after subtracting the marrow and vascular channel spaces. Coined in 1963 (Frost, 1963b), the term replaces the "bone mass" expression sometimes used as the equivalent (Frost, 1981a). It is independent of the quality, composition, or degree of mineralization of that matrix. It directly measures the total past activities of the body's osteoclasts and osteoblasts.

Current Concepts of Bone Fragility

Table I. Skeletal IO features discovered since 1960*

Feature	Status	Year	Discovered by	Reference
Microdamage in bone	X	1960	Frost	Frost, 1960
Separate physiology of woven/lamellar bone	X	1960	Frost	" "
Osteoid lag time	X	1960	Frost	Frost, 1963b
On-Off states	X	1960	Frost	Frost, 1960
Remodeling BMU: R-F coupling and generality	X	1964	Frost	Frost, †
Sigma property	X	1964	Frost	" "
Transient-steady state distinction	X	1964	Frost	Frost, † Frost, 1973a
Remodeling space	X	1966	Frost	Frost, 1966
Modeling-remodeling distinction	X	1966	Frost	" "
Dependence of modeling on growth	X	1966	Frost	" "
Remodeling repairs MDx	X	1963	Frost	" "
Cell population dynamic basis remodeling and modeling	X	1964	Frost	Frost, † Frost, 1964
ΔB.BMU	XX	1966	Frost	Frost, 1966
Dynamic strain history controls remodeling, not stress	X	1964	Frost	Frost, §
Flexure-drift rules	XXX	1964	Epker/Frost	Frost, §
Flexural neutralization	XXX	1964	Frost	Frost, §
Chondral modeling laws	XX	1972-1979	Frost	Frost, 1973c
Fibrous tissue modeling laws	XX	1973-1985	Frost	" "
MES	X	1963-1981	Frost	Frost, 1961 Frost, 1983d
RAP	X	1966-1983	Frost	Frost, 1973a
Remodeling responses to MU	X	1960-1984	many	Frost, in press (c)
Modeling responses to MU	Xx	1964	Frost	Frost, §
Envelope independence	X	1962	Sedlin/Frost	Sedlin, 1964
Local control of remodeling ("L"-gated)	X	1966	Frost	Frost, 1966
Local control of modeling ("L"-gated)	X	1973-1979	Frost	Frost, §
Remodeling algebra and analytical scheme	X	1964-1976	Frost	Frost, †

(continued next page)

Table I. Skeletal IO features discovered since 1960* (continued)

Feature	Status	Year	Discovered by	Reference
The skeletal IO as a general concept	XX	1981	Frost	Frost, 1983c
The MCN, LBO, LOBO properties	XX	1982	Frost	Frost, 1983c; in press(c)
The Kro⁻ property	X	1964	Landeros/ Frost	Landeros, 1964
MU controls remodeling rate	X	1964	Frost	Frost, †
Streaming potentials and related effects	X	1969	Eriksson	Eriksson, 1976
Temporal coherence and incoherence	X	1979	Frost	Frost, 1981

* Properties (32) of skeletal physiology that arise uniquely in IO rather than in unassociated cells.
X = features generally accepted today by others with competent knowledge of the matter; XX = some which await "X" status; XXX = features proven by experimental data but not yet accepted as such by others.
These 32 features represent a major fraction of the conceptual base of tissue-level and organ-level skeletal physiology in 1985. They exclude cell- and molecular-level matters, but to use such knowledge effectively requires knowing first how it applies to IO. Moreover, understanding the role of renal cells in kidney physiology requires understanding first their roles in the economy of nephrons. None of these 32 features was known before 1960.
§ Laws of Bone Structure, C.C. Thomas, 1964.
† Mathematical Elements of Lamellar Bone Remodeling, C.C. Thomas, 1964.

Osteopenia (OPn): a skeleton with too little bone tissue, ie, with a bone-tissue-volume deficit, expressing the amount of ABV (Frost, 1973a-c; 1981a; 1983a). It assumes valid normal standards for comparison, and an OPn alone neither says nor implies anything about the quality or composition of the existing bone, which may be normal or abnormal. It is a sign, not a disease, and the term, reduced bone mass, in the clinical literature means, in fact, a reduced ABV rather than a true gravimetric measure. An OPn can exist without causing any disability, as explained in a companion article (Frost, 1985).

Mechanical incompetence (MIn): painful skeleton or bone fractures, or bone pain under normal mechanical use, whether or not it is osteopenic (Frost, 1981a; in press, c). It can also occur as a sign (not a disease) without osteopenia, as in stress fractures in healthy draftees and athletes, in aseptic necrosis, and in radiation necrosis. It can even occur when osteosclerosis exists, as in Paget's disease of bone and in osteopetrosis.

Bone balance: the state of any net gain/loss of bone tissue, preferably expressed in ABV terms. A net loss results from a negative bone balance, a net gain from a positive one. A negative bone balance is also a sign and is not evidence of increased bone resorption.

Osteoporosis (OPs): a disease that combines three essential features: an osteopenic skeleton; mechanical incompetence; and their underlying etiologic factor(s). Urist was among the first to report that an OPn alone need not cause clinical disease (Urist, 1960; 1963). It has become apparent since 1960 that in terms of their pathogenesis, pathologic findings and basic etiologic factors (Nordin, 1964) the OPs form a group of diseases rather than a single entity. Osteopenia and mechanical incompetence are the two direct major pathogenetic mechanisms of all OPs, espressed schematically as:

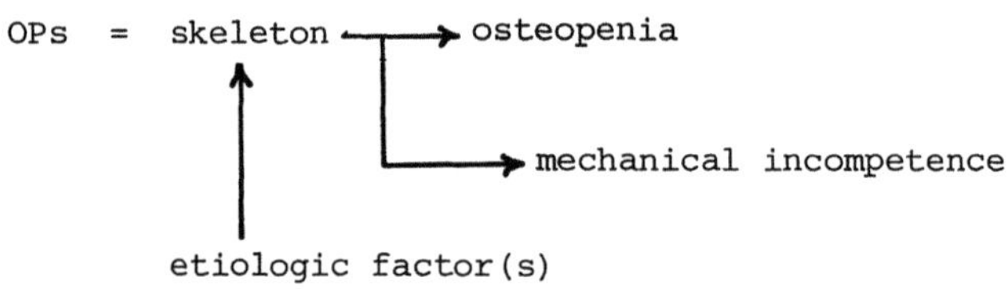

RELATION 1

Explaining a particular OPs requires explaining the pathogenesis of both its OPn and MIn. Frost related microdamage to MIn in 1966 before which most authorities attributed the MIn solely to the OPn. However, evidence as briefly outlined below now proves the proposal in Relation 1. Table II lists abbreviations and acronyms. (Frost, 1966; 1973; 1981; DeLuca et al, 1981).

Table II. Abbreviations and acronyms

ABV	absolute bone volume
ARF	activation-resorption formation
BMU	basic multicellular unit
BSU	basic structural unit
IO	intermediary organization
MDx	microdamage
MES	minimum effective strain
MIn	mechanical incompetence
OPn	osteopenia
OPs	osteoporosis
µE	Microstrain (10^{-6} unit strain)*

* See legend, Figure 3.

Intermediary Organization Mechanisms

The intermediary organization (IO)

Three major IO functions are discussed in this presentation: modeling, remodeling and microdamage physiology. Each arises uniquely in the IO; none exists in unassociated bone cells. Their explanations will use some of the terminology of the IO, some coined anew for its needs, and some borrowed but redefined from standard terminology (Frost, 1966; 1973a-c, 1983c-d; in press a-c; Jaworski, 1984; Melson et al, 1983; Meunier et al, 1979).

Generally speaking, any IO bridges unassociated cells to an organ. It fills what histologists call the tissue level of biologic organization, in which each level is an organizational domain that provides its own functions to higher levels according to its own rules:

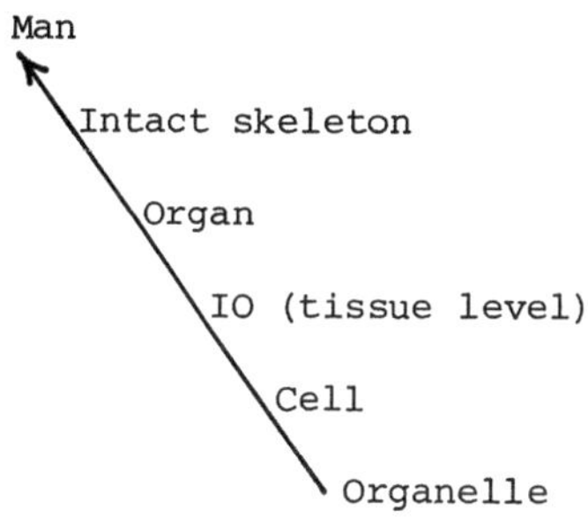

RELATION 2

Like the nephron, the skeletal IO organizes cells and intercellular materials in ways that create unique multicellular entities, mechanisms and functions. The IO term embraces the effector organ of lamellar bone physiology (Jaworski, 1984), but it also applies to all structures, activities, and functions that arise in the domain between the cell and the organ, and for chondral, dental, and fibrous tissues as well as bone. Its functions do not exist in isolated cells, yet without them mammalian life could not exist. However, the skeletal IO has at least three separate levels of its own, and is more complex than the renal one. It was first described in 1983 (Frost, 1983c) and is as important in skeletal physiology and disease as the nephrons are in kidney physiology (Frost, 1984).

Multicellular entities of that IO provide the three functions already named. Their properties concern two separate matters: their organ-domain functions (where function implies purpose as well as activity), and the IO-domain histologic mechanisms that provide those functions.

1) Modeling

As a general function or activity, modeling means shaping or sculpturing growing tissues and organs to produce the architecture visible in anatomical dissections, during surgery, and in roentgenograms. It acts by holding growth back in some places and directions, and allowing or even potentiating it in others. Since processes couple modeling closely to the growth process, it usually becomes ineffective after maturity (Frost, 1973c; Frost, in press, a; c). While modeling occurs in all growing organs, both soft and hard, and also in plants, the form known as bone modeling determines the outside and marrow cavity diameters as well as cortical thickness of growing bones. Therefore, among other factors, it influences how much compacta an animal or child accumulates in its ABV bone bank during growth (Fig. 1).

Two special multicellular IO units form the bone modeling mechanism, the resorption drift and the formation drift (Enlow, 1963; Jee, 1983; Putschar, 1960). The resorption drift marshalls an organized collection of osteoclasts, capillaries and supporting cells to erode some bone surfaces, while

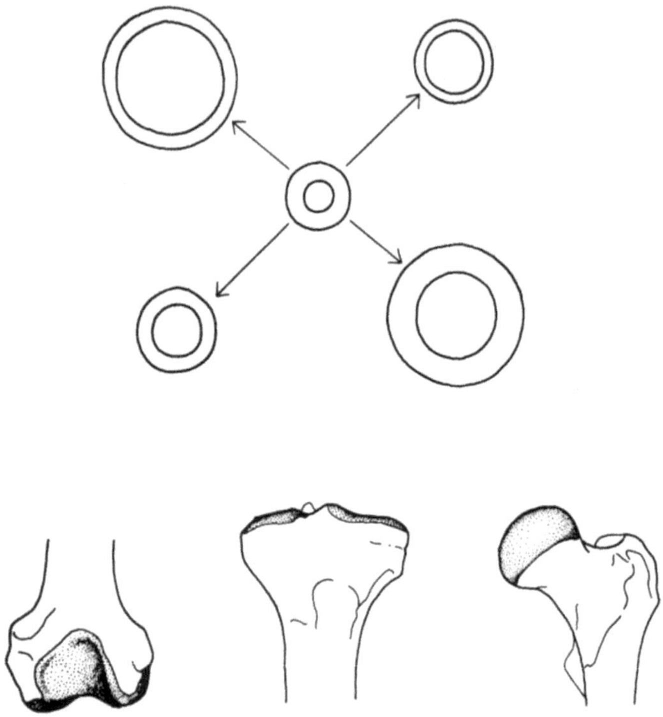

Fig. 1. Examples of modeling. Upper drawings: Given the original infant's diaphyseal cross-section in the middle, bone modeling can influence its subsequent growth to produce any of the surrounding configurations. It can also create elliptical, triangular or irregular cross-sections. Lower drawings: Similar control of articular cartilage growth -- chondral modeling -- can produce the different joint shapes shown. Thus, modeling (actually macromodeling as distinguished from micromodeling) is the process of creating and controlling shape and size by controlling growth. (Reproduced by permission, H.M. Frost, The Skeletal Intermediary Organization, C.R.C. Press, Boca Raton, 1985).

the formation drift uses organized collections of osteoblasts, capillaries and other supporting cells to build up other surfaces with new circumferential lamellar bone, as shown in Figure 2. Those drifts are not coupled, in that and the spatial sense each one occurs independently of all others (Frost, in press, a-c). However, at the organ level, they normally occur in sterotyped patterns over a bone's surfaces or envelopes, under the control at least in part of the mechanical strain patterns in the intact bone, thereby maintaining the shape of, for example, a femur as it increases from the fetal to the adult size (Jee, 1983; Rubin, 1984). There is evidence that the individual osteoclasts and osteoblasts of bone drifts have limited functional life spans (~3 weeks for the former, ~8 weeks for the latter) (Jaworski, 1984). Consequently, continuing modeling during the ~18 years humans take to mature requires continuing recruitment from precursor cell

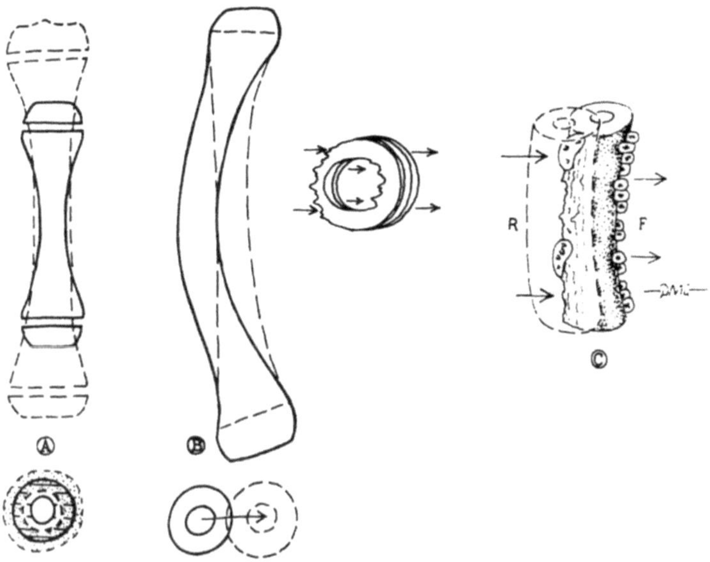

Fig. 2. Bone surface drifts. Left: As the infant bone (solid lines) grows to the size of the child's (dashed lines), the longitudinal and cross-sectional shapes of its periosteal and corticoendosteal surfaces are preserved by precisely controlled patterns of resorption and formation drifts on those surfaces. Middle: In normal children a postfracture deformity or malunion (solid lines) is also corrected by precisely patterned bone surface drifts. The cross-section of the right of this bone shows that drift pattern at midshaft. Right: A resorption drift on the left and a formation drift on the right moves this diaphyseal segment towards the right.
The above drifts are enabled and controlled, partly, by the patterns of strains generated in the intact bone, which in turn are generated by the loads applied to the bone and by its own shape and size. The game rules that govern those matters are now partly understood (Frost's macromodeling laws) and are described elsewhere. (Reproduced by permission, H.M. Frost, Osteogenesis imperfecta: the setpoint proposal)

reservoirs of new osteoclasts and osteoblasts, plus the other cells and IO-domain activities that support them (Frost, 1973c; 1983c; Jaworski, 1984; Parfitt, 1984a).

An apparent major purpose of bone modeling lies in fitting compact bone size, configuration and ABV to the needs of its mechanical usage to prevent and/or correct mechanical incompetence (Frost, in press, a). The mechanical strains caused by mechanical usage participate in a negative feedback mechanism(s) that controls where bone modeling will occur, what kind and how much (Fig. 3). Some of its mechanisms have been verified since 1980 (Carter, 1984; Cowin, 1984; Frost, 1980; 1983b, c; in press, a, c; Lanyon, 1984; Rubin, 1984).

First, remodeling determines the size and configuration of bone in a way that reduces the usual peak mechanical strains to or below a special thres-

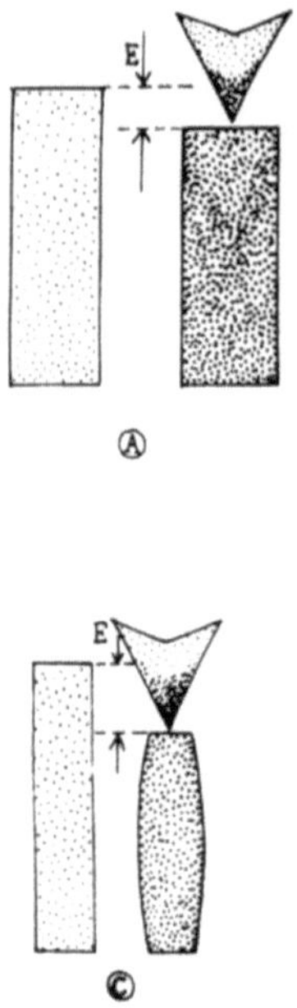

Fig. 3. Strain. Top: When a load is applied to the left hand bony column it will shorten as on the right. How much or little will depend on its materials properties (particularly its stiffness, usually measured as Young's modulus of elasticity), its size and shape, and the size of the load. That strain is signified by E in this text and is shown on the right. Bottom: When the same load is applied to a column of the same length and material but of smaller diameter, then the strain is greater, and approximately in inverse proportion to the reduction in cross-section area of the structure. The strain generates a stress within the material of the column that resists the deformation. 1,000 microstrain (μE) in compression is the same as a shortening under load of .1%, and a unit strain of .001. 2,000 μE in tension is the same as a stretching in length of .2%. 20,000 μE in tension therefore equals a 2% elongation or stretching.

hold range of values, termed the MES (Frost, 1983d), thus minimizing the production of mechanical fatigue damage in bone (Frost, in press, a). Second, increasing mechanical usage activates or turns modeling "on", which then enlarges and/or reshapes the bone, but inactivity renders it dormant, or makes it go "off" (Frost, in press, c). Like a car without a reverse gear, in most circumstances global modeling can only go forward (but at variable speeds) or stop. Third, in the steady state sense, most hormones, other humoral agents, nutrition and drugs have little direct influence on it (Frost, in press, c). Table III lists some major modeling properties.

Table III. Some properties of bone modeling

1)	Provided by resorption drifts and formation drifts.
2)	Dependent on growth; inactive in acults.
3)	Enabled by increasing mechanical usage.
4)	Inactive during mechanical disuse.
5)	Increases outside bone diameter and cortical thickness.
6)	Sizes and configures bones to fit mechanical usage.
7)	Under increasing activity it increases skeletal ABV by adding periosteal bone and conserving cortical-endosteal bone.

2) Remodeling

As an organ-level function or activity, this redefined term refers to turnover of bone or other tissue in discrete packets (Frost, 1966; 1969; in press, c; Jaworski, 1984; Melsen, 1983; Parfitt, 1984a). As a mechanism of

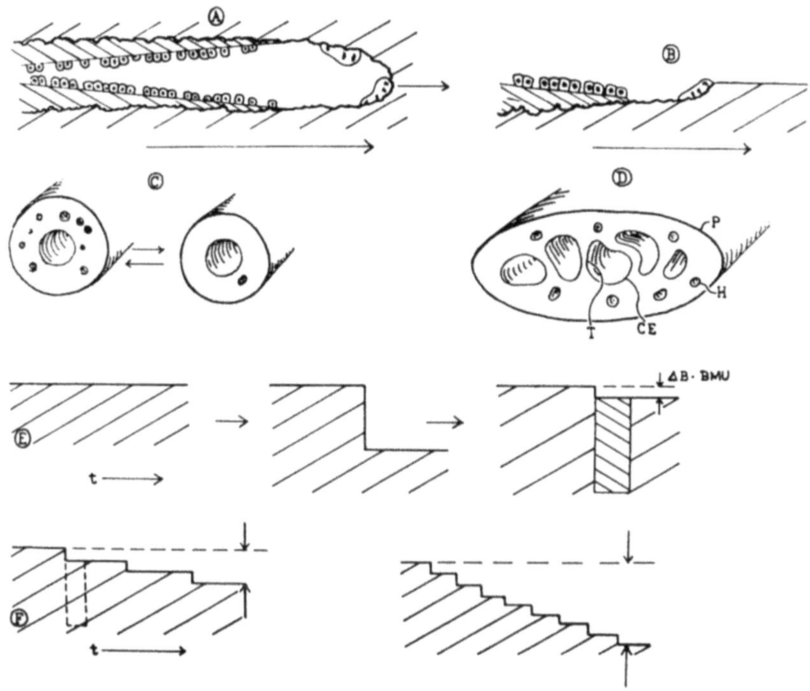

Fig. 4. Top: On the left, in longitudinal section, a newly forming secondary osteon is being made within compacta. The resorption process or cutting cone leads on and towards the right. The osteoblasts trail behind it on the left, and refill the cavity with new bone (capillary and supporting tissues omitted). On the right (B) a similar sequence or ARF occurs on a trabecular or corticoendosteal surface. C) The spots in the compacta of this diaphyseal cross-section represent active haversian remodeling foci or BMU. When mechanical use increases, that remodeling becomes inhibited, as on the right. On the other hand, acute disuse can change the right hand picture to that on the left. D) The 4 bony envelopes are defined: P = periosteal; H = haversian; CE = corticoendosteal; T = trabecular. They exhibit independent bone balances in health, in many diseases, and in response to some hormones and other humoral agents and to some drugs. E) The idea of a "BMU graph" is shown (after Frost). One looks in cross-section at some bone surface and follows the same locus, but in time only, towards the right. The resorption phase of a remodeling BMU (middle) excavates a hole or bay, and the following formation phase then refills it (right), here incompletely. The resulting net decrement equals the important ΔB.BMU parameter, which is a special new BMU function that can control bone balance independently of the rate of bone resorption or formation, and independently of the factors that control those rates. F) BMU activation effects. Given the same negative value of ΔB.BMU per typical completed BMU, when few new BMU are recruited or activated annually, only a minor net bone loss occurs; but when activation increases as on the right the net loss does too, in proportion (Reproduced by permission, H.M. Frost, Osteogenesis imperfecta: The setpoint proposal. In press)

the middle IO of bone, such packets, named basic multicellular units (BMU), begin when an activating event causes a batch of osteoclasts plus a supporting capillary and other cells to appear and resorb a predetermined amount of bone. The osteoclasts then disappear and osteoblasts replace them and fill the excavation with new bone nourished by the original capillary. Activation resorption formation (ARF) signifies that invariant activation-resorption formation sequence, which normally, in cross-sectional sense, consumes three to four months and turns over $\sim$.05-.1 mm^3 of bone (Fig. 4) (Courpron, 1981; Frost, 1973a; Jaworski, 1984; Parfitt, 1984a). Some 10^5-10^6 of BMU evolve at any one time in a healthy adult human skeleton (Frost, 1964; Parfitt, 1984a). The new moiety of bone produced by such BMU is referred to as a bone structural unit (BSU) (Jaworski, 1984), and the best known example is the secondary osteon or haversian system. This relation explains that terminology:

[activation-resorption-formation (BMU)] ⟶ (new BSU)

|⟵ $\sim$3-4 mos ⟶ | ⟵ $\sim$10 yr

RELATION 3

The sigma term means the time the BMU takes to run its completion as seen in a cross-section. That natural time period related to BMU's mean depth of erosion or its mean wall thickness has important effects on the global behavior of remodeling (Courpron, 1981; Frost, in press, c; Melson et al, 1983; Jee, 1983; Kimmel and Jee, 1980).

The remodeling BMU has further pertinent properties. Some are unusual and include the following:

a) BMU-based remodeling occurs throughout life in man and other large, long-living animals, and on all four skeletal envelopes (Fig. 4D), although relatively little occurs within compacta in infants and in small, short-living animals such as the rat, mouse, chick and rabbit.

b) Somewhat as the nephron creates the new functions of renal clearance, glomerular filtration and countercurrent flow, the remodeling BMU also creates three new functions.

i) It can turn bone over independently of changes in its amount or ABV, or in its macroarchitecture including shape and size (Frost, 1983c; in press, c). The BMU may change that amount and architecture as described below, but only slowly. That contrasts with modeling which changes size, the shape, and the amount of bone (usually by increasing it), and it can do so relatively quickly.

ii) When the typical completed BMU resorbs and forms equal amounts of bone, turnover occurs without local or global net gains or losses of bone, as on the normal haversian envelope. Unequal amounts, however, cause net gains or losses per completed BMU. The coupling of the R to the F in the BMU, described in 1964 (Frost, 1964), usually causes the amount of one to reduce when the other does, and likewise for increases, but not always equally. The resulting decrements/increments per typical completed BMU are termed the ΔB.BMU, and represent a second special BMU function (Fig. 4E and 5). The ΔB.BMU parameter controls bone balance, and thus much of the bone loss/gain features of the adult human skeleton (Frost, 1981a).

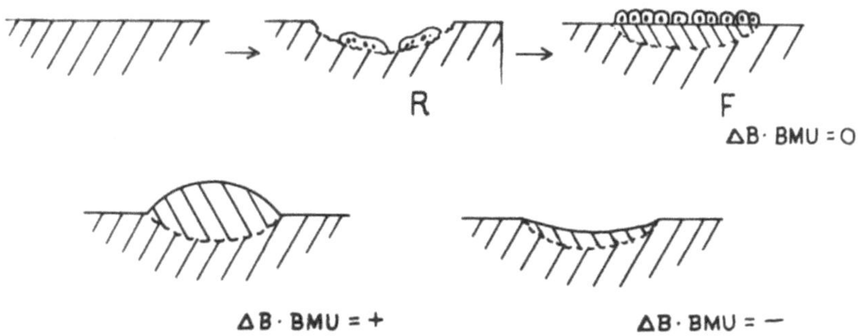

Fig. 5. BMU graphs and the ΔB.BMU. The ARF events diagrammed in Fig. 4E are redrawn here. Top: Here the bone formed by the completed BMU equals that resorbed so the ΔB.BMU has a value of zero: no net deficit or increment. Bottom left: A positive value, meaning a permanent increment of extra bone. Bottom right: A negative value. (Reprinted by permission, H.M. Frost, The Skeletal Intermediary Organization, C.R.C. Press, Boca Raton, in press)

In large part, local rather than systemic factors regulate the ΔB.BMU, and in a way that makes BMU, in touch with marrow, result in a negative ΔB.BMU; those on the haversian envelope a zero value, and those on the periosteal envelope a positive one (Frost, in press, b). Figure 5 illustrates those important envelope-specific effects (Frost, 1966; Sedlin, 1964). While, in 1964, it was generally believed that systemic agents control both bone balance and the turnover rate (Rasmussen and Bordier, 1974; Urist, 1963), it is now clear that local factors usually control bone balance, and both local and systemic factors can affect its turnover rate (Frost, in press, c). The evidence that the marrow cavity somehow weighs all bone turnover activities in contact with it in favor of net loss is voluminous; it goes back over 150 years. It took some time, however, to perceive its relation to matters discussed here (Frost, 1966; Johnson, 1964).

iii) The typical normal adult human BMU deposits ~29 parts of bone for every ~30 parts it removes (Frost, in press, c)*. Consequently, minor unequal changes in the absolute bone resorption or formation rates can cause large changes in net bone balance, and in some situations the bone resorption rate declines 50% or more while the net bone loss increases by 100%. Figure 6 illustrates some of the mechanisms of these effects, which have seemed paradoxical to many.

The ΔB.BMU function can control bone balance independently of the bone resorption (or formation) rate alone.

c) In a given bone, the amount turned over per typical completed BMU varies only some ±20% over man's life span (Frost, 1969), in spite of large changes in time the typical BMU takes to evolve (Landeros and Frost, 1964) which can vary from 3 months in healthy individuals to over 120 months in patients with certain kinds of osteoporosis, osteomalacia and rickets.

---

* Virtually all adult lamellar bone turnover is produced by BMU -- annual turnover rates ~15%-30% of the skeleton, especially in spongiosa; annual net bone losses ~.5%-1%; so the excess of R/F per BMU ~.5/15 = 1/30.

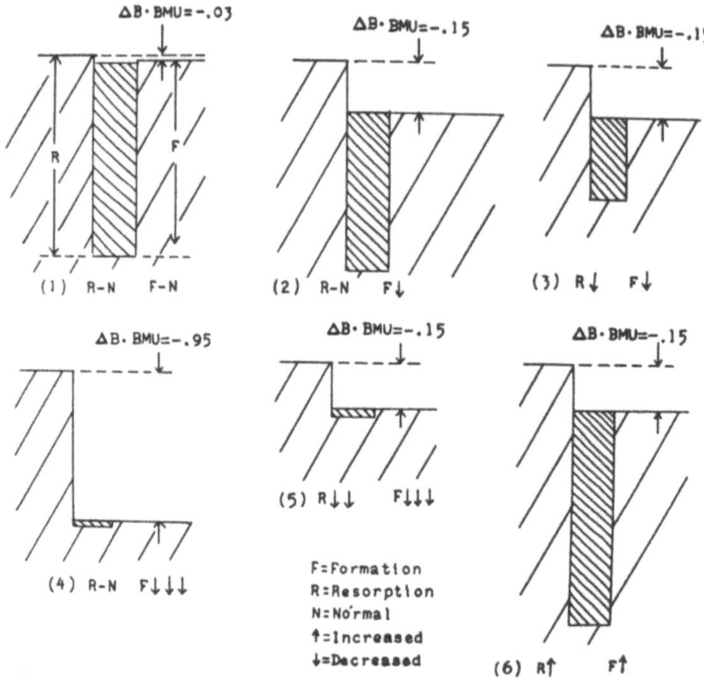

Fig. 6. ΔB.BMU effects. The "typical" adult human BMU resorbs ~30 and forms ~29 parts of bone, to leave a net decrement of ~.03 of the amount turned over. The insets illustrate how the net loss of bone can increase 5x while total resorption remains normal (#2), decreases (#3, 5) or increases (#6); #4 illustrates a 30x increase in the rate of net bone loss with no change in total bone resorption; #6 illustrates a 5x increase in net bone loss with only a 1.5x increase in total resorption. Each of the above situations probably occurs in life. The prevalent view that an increase in net loss is *prima facie* evidence of an equal increase, or even of any kind of increase, in resorption is, in my opinion, erroneous. (Reproduced by permission. H.M. Frost, The Skeletal Intermediary Organization, C.R.C. Press, Boca Raton, in press)

d) That property has a unique effect on the control of bone turnover and balance, many originally found particularly difficult to accept. In steady state, the number of new BMU activated in unit time determines the rate of bone turnover, independently of how slowly or quickly individual BMU (or osteoclasts or osteoblasts) resorb or make bone (Frost, 1964; 1969; 1983a). The graphs in Figure 7 illustrate that property (Villanueva and Frost, 1970). Also, the number of new remodeling BMU that arise annually can affect the rate of any net gains or losses of bone, by the mechanism shown in Figure 4F.

The above facts indicate that the poorly understood factors that control bone cell population dynamics (eg, precursor cell proliferation rate and

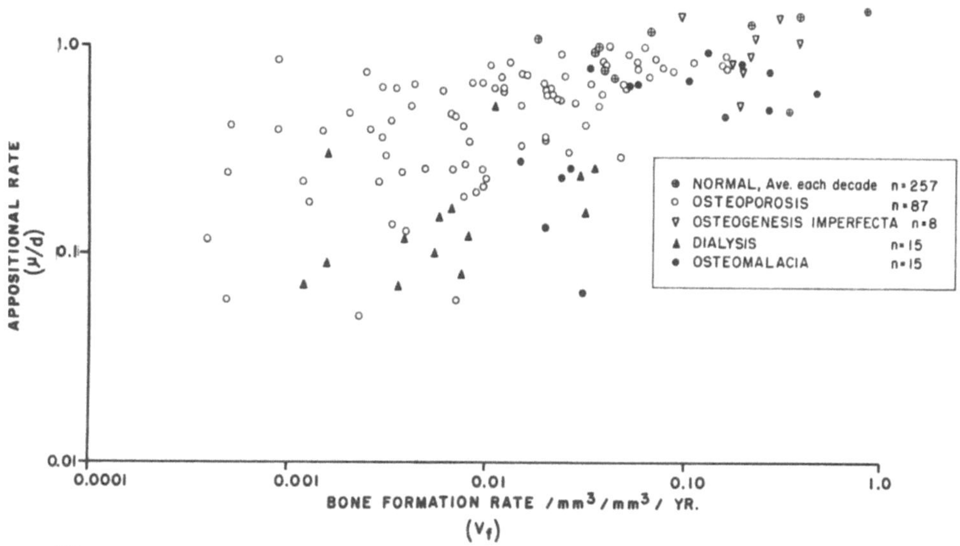

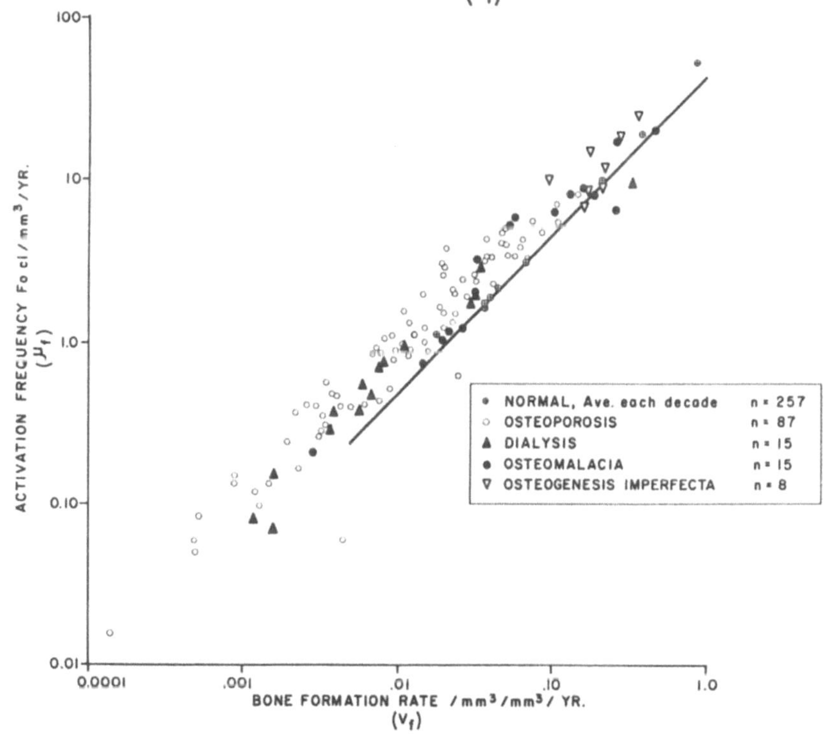

Fig. 7. Control of the bone remodeling rate. These graphs plot dynamic histomorphometric data obtained from 11th and 10th rib biopsies of over 350 patients after *in vivo* double tetracycline labelling. The boxes describe their diseases. The horizontal axes plot on a logarithmic scale their measured tissue-level bone formation rates in dimensions of mm^3 new bone formed, per mm^3 preexisting bone, annually. On a logarithmic

(caption continued on next page)

differentiation) have larger effects on global bone remodeling and modeling than the better understood factors that control already existing osteoclasts and osteoblasts. In other words, the factors that determine if, when, where, how many, and for how long new osteoclasts or osteoblasts will be produced, exert more control over global bone biodynamics than the more intensively studied factors that control the function of already existing cells (Frost, in press, c).

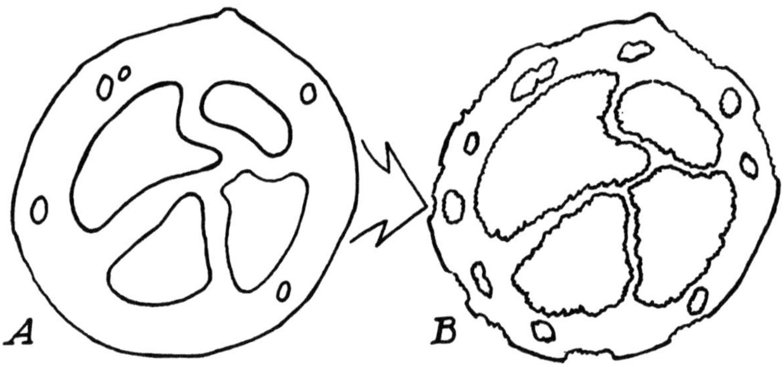

Fig. 8. The remodeling space. Left: A diagrammatic cross-section of bone, with a few active bone remodeling centers or BMU going on within the compacta. Right: A generalized large increase in the activation or recruitement of new remodeling BMU will pepper the compacta with resorption cavities, and the periosteal, corticoendosteal and trabecular surfaces with temporary resorption bays, leading to significant but transient losses of compacta and spongiosa. In part because of surface-to-volume ratio effects, the loss of spongiosa by that mechanism exceeds that of compacta. As long as the increased activation persists, the enlarged remodeling space and the bone loss it represents persist too, because for each BMU that completes its formation stage a new one begins its resorption stage. When the increased activation subsides, then new BMU do not replace those that finish their formation, so the situation shown in the right hand drawing then reverts to that in the left. (Reproduced by permission. H.M. Frost, The Skeletal Intermediary Organization, C.R.C. Press, Boca Raton, in press)

---

scale for the same patients and biopsies, and on the vertical axis, the upper graph plots the mean thickness of new bone deposited in microns per day (the radial closure rate). That thickness is a reliable index of the amount of new bone made by the typical osteoblast in unit time. Clearly, knowing either the radial closure rate or the tissue-level formation rate does not allow one to predict the other. They are independent functions. For the same patients, the lower graph now plots on the vertical axis the number of new BMU they recruited annually per mm^3 of preexisting bone, and clearly it is possible, given the value on either axis, to predict that on the other axis. (Reprinted by permission, A.R. Villanueva and H.M. Frost, Evaluation of factors determining the tissue level haversian bone formation rate in man. J. Dent. Res. 49, 836, 1970)

e) Another special bone balance effect also depends on the activation of new BMU. It concerns the remodeling space (Jaworski, 1984). The cavity or hole made by the typical BMU represents a temporary loss of $\sim$.03 mm^3 of bone ($\sim$1/2 the size of the completed resorption bay or cavity). When BMU activation increases greatly, those added temporary holes, collectively forming the remodeling space, can remove over 15% of the compacta and over 50% of the spongiosa within $\leq$8 weeks, as shown in Figure 8. Most of that loss is inherently reversible. When BMU activation returns to normal, the already ongoing BMU or holes fill up with new bone but are not replaced by new resorption cavities; thus, the "lost" bone returns to the system (Fig. 8).

f) Remodeling activity can respond to some hormones, other humoral and biochemical agents and some drugs (Frost, in press, c). It also responds to mechanical usage of bone and by becoming active during acute disuse situations (Jaworski et al, 1980; Meunier et al, 1979; Minaire, 1964; Uhthoff and Jaworski, 1978). In contrast, increasing mechanical usage (within its physiologic range) inhibits the bone loss (Jaworski et al, 1980; Minaire, 1964; Uhthoff and Jaworski, 1978). Thus, during inactivity, bone tissue is lost from the trabecular and corticoendosteal envelopes (and thus spongiosa and corticoendosteal bone), by mechanisms shown in Figures 4F and 8 (Frost, in press, c). Concerning its effects on bone balance and ABV, remodeling resembles a car with only a reverse gear. It can only stop, which tends to conserve existing bone, or go backwards, ie, remove bone, usually in contact with marrow (Frost, in press, c).

These relations summarize the important (but only recently clarified) responses of bone modeling and remodeling to mechanical usage (MU):

Increasing MU → enabled modeling
→ inhibited remodeling

Acute disuse → disabled modeling
→ active remodeling RELATION 4

BMU-based lamellar bone remodeling also repairs mechanical bone microdamage as described below (Frost, 1966; 1981b) and it participates in homeostasis, in the blood-bone exchange of certain ions (Rasmussen and Bordier, 1974), and in some other functions (Frost, in press, c).

Table IV summarizes some features of remodeling; Table V summarizes some bone balance and architectural responses of modeling and remodeling to mechanical usage.

The modeling-remodeling mechanism. The modeling-remodeling distinction was unknown before 1966, although Lacroix and his colleagues suspected that growth-related phenomena differed from those acting in adult bone disease. The remodeling term formerly described all features of what are now called modeling and remodeling. By 1966, however, dynamic histomorphometric as well as clinical and conventional pathologic data exposed modeling and remodeling as operationally distinct activities with their own properties, purposes and responses to controlling agents (see Relation 4), and also that their malfunctions caused different diseases. Like modeling in clay, modeling controls architecture; that term was therefore adopted, and re-

Table IV. Some properties of bone remodeling

1) Provided by BMU that couple resorption to formation.
2) Occurs in packets.
3) Provides the special ΔB.BMU function that determines the signs of the bone balance.
4) Continues throughout life; not dependent on growth.
5) Increasing mechanical usage inhibits it.
6) Acute disuse releases it so it increases.
7) Increases increase net bone loss where bone touches marrow.
8) Under increasing mechanical usage it decreases, which conserves spongy and corticoendosteal bone.
9) In acute disuse it increases, which discards spongy and corticoendosteal bone.

Table V. Bone modeling and remodeling responses to mechanical usage (MU)

Activity effects	
Increasing MU:	Modeling is enabled, more active
	Remodeling is inhibited, less active
Decreasing MU:	Modeling becomes less active or disabled
	Remodeling becomes derepressed, more active
Architectural effects	
Increasing MU:	Modeling increases outside diameter, cortical thickness
	Slowed remodeling retards expansion of marrow cavity and loss of spongiosa; decreases cortical porosity
Decreasing MU:	Modeling: outside bone diameter increases little, cortex thins.
	Increased remodeling removes spongiosa and enlarges marrow cavity, increases cortical porosity.
Bone balance effects	
Increasing MU:	Modeling adds new periosteal bone, retards loss of corticoendosteal bone
	Inhibited remodeling conserves spongiosa and cortico-endosteal bone; reduces remodeling space
Decreasing MU:	Slowed modeling retards addition of new periosteal bone
	Increased remodeling accelerates loss of bone in contact with marrow, and increases the remodeling space.

modeling was redefined to mean a piecemeal turnover of tissue in biologically and spatially coupled packets of resorption and formation. Many anatomists and clinicians still use the remodeling term in its earlier all inclusive -- and thus ambiguous -- sense, and that has caused some confusion.

3) Microdamage physiology

Mechanical microdamage (MDx) that arises in normal human bone during life was demonstrated in 1960 (Frost, 1960). A form of mechanical materials fatigue which can occur in all structural materials, both living and inanimate (Roth et al, 1961), it is usually caused by cyclic strains, as in the load-deload cycles associated with walking, lifting and running. The larger the strains and the number of strain cycles, the greater the amount of resulting MDx, but some occurs even when a structure is loaded well below a level that threatens to fracture it under a single load.

During 1960-1973, it was proposed that those properties apply to human bone too, and that BMU-based remodeling repairs MDx before it becomes mechanically serious (Frost, 1963b; 1966; 1973a-c). MDx weakens an intact bone without affecting its size or the amount of bone in it, and makes it more likely to fracture from mechanical loads or traumatic incidents that would not fracture normal bones. While significant MDx burdens probably also underlie the clinical phenomenon of bone pain (via the innervation of bone as described by Duncan and Shim (1979) and Miller and Kasahara (1963), they do not necessarily cause roentgenographic or serum biochemical evidence that they exist. It follows that increasing MDx burdens could cause complete fractures even during normal activity (Frost, 1973a). Clinicians recognize several kinds of such fractures, including stress fractures, spontaneous fractures, pathologic fractures, the asymptomatic vertebral partial collapses described by Briançon and Meunier (1979), and pseudofractures. These "MDx relations" can encode that situation:

a) repeat strain $\longrightarrow$ MDx;

b) MDx = microscopic mechanical fatigue;

c) MDx fragilizes bone;

d) Remodeling normally repairs MDx;

e) MDx burden = new MDx-repair RELATION 5

New MDx > repair = accumulating MDx burden RELATION 6

Accumulating MDx burden $\longrightarrow$ fatigue fracture RELATION 7

While first described between 1960-73 (Frost, 1960; 1963a, b; 1973a; Roth et al, 1961), the ideas and facts expressed by those relations remained dormant until others reported evidence of human bone microdamage, including Arnold (1964), Cameron et al (1975), Freeman et al (1974), Radin (1972), Todd et al (1972), and Watson (1975). Those ideas are now part of the conceptual base of skeletal biomechanics, as reflected in a recent review by Carter (1981), and they apply to problems which affect current dental, bone and joint endoprostheses (Frost, in press, c).

Among several causes of accumulating MDx burdens are biologic and mechanical factors, but a given MDx burden represents the state of the balance encoded

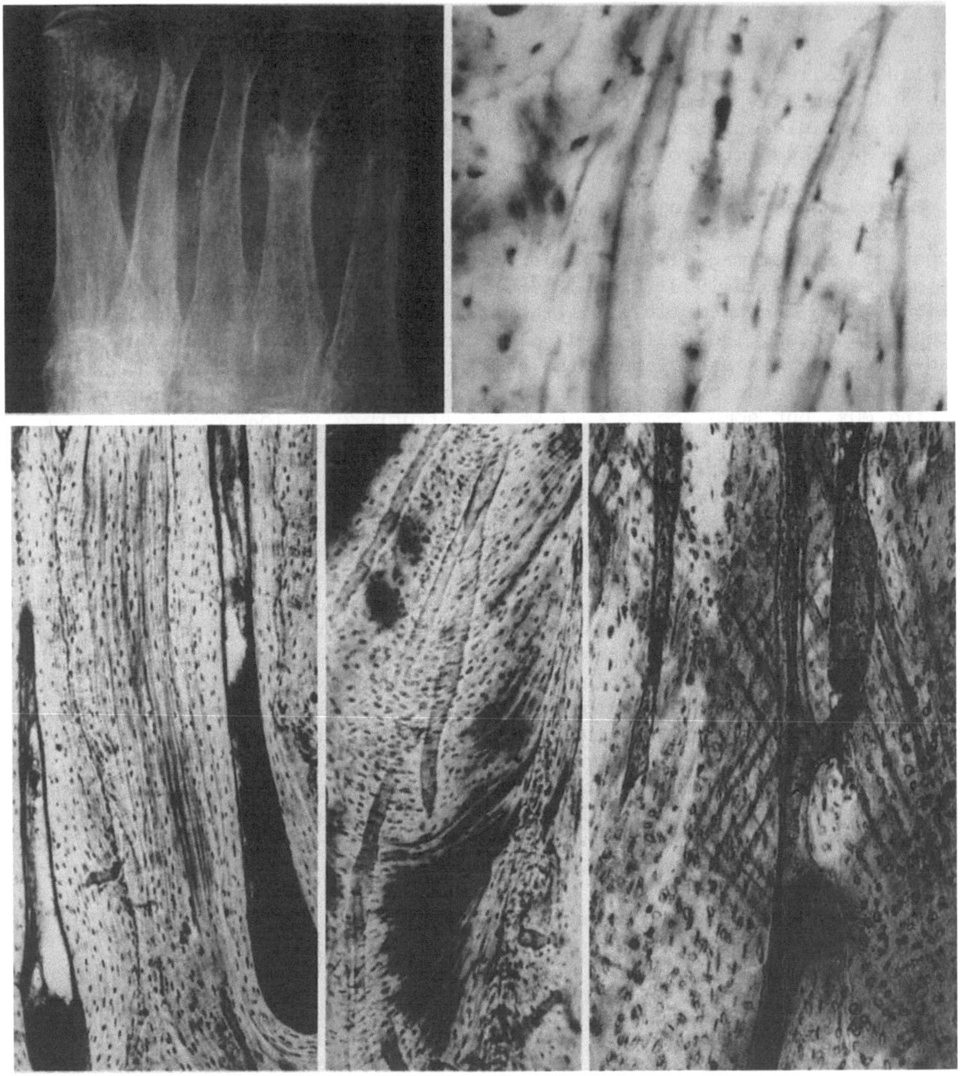

Fig. 9. Bone microdamage. Upper left: This elderly woman on adrenocortical steroids and engaged in a sedentary life because of cardiorespiratory disease has developed a new stress fracture in the distal 5th matatarsum, added to an earlier healing one in the 4th. Upper right: Undecalcified cross-section compacta, 10th rib, of a patient who died with chronic respiratory disease. About 60x. The bulk rib sample was stained with basic fuchsin for 4 months before sectioning and not stained after sectioning. The vertical lines represent microcracks that arose and existed during life. Lower left: Fuchsin-stained prefailure planes in an undecalcified section of tibial compacta of a child with severe *genu varum*. They are the dark vertical lines lying between the haversian canal on the right and the cement line on the left. Middle: More prefailure planes in a similar section of the tibia of another child with a similar problem. Lower right: Longitudinal undecalcified section of human compacta tested in the laboratory by impressing a 3 mm diameter ram into the surface of a fresh, wet cube of compacta ~1 cm on a side. The dark oblique lines represent prefailure planes stained with basic fuchsin, apparently paralleling the shearing strain planes produced by the test. (Reproduced by permission. H.M. Frost, The Skeletal Intermediary Organization: A synthesis. In, Bone and Mineral Research, Vol. II. Ed: Peck, W.; Excerpta Medica, New York, in press)

in Relation 5 (Frost, 1973a). The burden is the difference between the MDx produced less what was repaired. Essentially, mechanical factors cause MDx and biologic ones repair it. As applies to any balance situation, MDx burdens can accumulate if their production increases, if their repair decreases, if both occur, or if both increase but the former the most, or if both decrease but the latter the most (Frost, 1985).

Biologic factors: Inhibiting the activation of new BMU could reduce MDx repair, allowing normal amounts of new MDx to accumulate until a final, complete fracture occurs under normal or trivial mechanical usage. Inhibited activation does occur after radiation damage to bone, in many osteomalacias and OPs, in etidronate intoxication, in infarcted femoral heads or other ischemic bones, as well as in still unexplained cases.

Also, markedly retarding completion of an already activated BMU that is in its R-F stages would have the same effect. Most patients with senile and postmenopausal OPs show such retardations (eg, prolonged sigmas) on dynamic histomorphometric analysis of their bone biopsies (Frost, 1985). Similar retardations occur in osteomalacias (Frost, 1985) and in idiopathic aseptic necrosis of the femoral head (Arlot et al, 1983), although the histologic details differ from those found in the osteoporotics. What causes those prolonged sigma values remains obscure. Combinations of the depressed activation and prolonged sigma effects also may occur (Frost, 1985)(Fig. 9).

Mechanical aspect: Increasing MDx burdens can also follow increased MDx production. For example, this can be caused by suddenly escalated mechanical usage of the skeleton or of a part of it (Putschar, 1960). It can also occur in apparently healthy adolescents and adults who engage in some unaccustomed vigorous sport. In those situations, at least in part, new MDx creation increases so much and so rapidly that the remodeling system, which needs ~3 months to begin to cope, lacks enough time to handle it. Consequently, a stress fracture results (Frost, 1985). Increasing MDx burdens can also occur in bone of abnormal quality, even during normal usage. Yet, little is known about the fatigue properties of bone as a material or how age, sex, density, disease, drugs and BMU history affect them. Increased MDx production also occurs where metastases or other local disease has destroyed a major fraction of the preexisting bone (see below); they cause most pathologic fractures.

The Pathogenetic Mechanisms of the Osteoporoses

As mentioned above, OPs have two different pathologic elements: an osteopenia and mechanical incompetence. That deceptively simple statement represents a fundamental advance over previous dogma which held that the OPn was the major pathologic feature of the OPs skeleton and, therefore, its pathogenesis was the major problem in those diseases (Rasmussen and Bordier, 1974). That erred by omission, for what was viewed as a "pure" metabolic bone disease actually involves a major element of "pure" biomechanics.

The osteopenia

Figure 10 illustrates how the amount of bone in the whole skeleton changes during normal growth and aging (Eastell et al, 1984; Garn, 1970; Kanis, 1984; Keshawarz and Recker, 1984). Two situations in those graphs require explanation, the pre- and postmaturity changes.

1) Before skeletal maturity

Up to about age 20, the steady accumulation of bone in the body's bone bank adds two different activities (Jee, 1983; Weinmann and Sicher, 1955). Longitudinal growth adds both new spongiosa and new length to the compacta of a bone, while modeling adds new compacta transversely by increasing its outside diameter and cortical cross-section area, and in correct proportions relative to longitudinal bone growth, to growing body mass, and to growing muscle forces and usage. Defective modeling can add too little compacta during growth, and relative to bone length and general body growth, to cause an inadequate deposit of compacta. This type of large deficit can contribute to MIn during childhood, as in some cases of muscular dystrophy, biliary stenosis, cystic fibrosis and osteogenesis imperfecta. A small deficit, however, may not cause problems until adult life, when the separate and general age-related loss of bone further reduces that original deposit below the level needed to sustain normal mechanical usage (a level referred to as "fracture threshold" (Meunier et al, 1979)), and/or when particular remodeling impairments retard the repair of the MDx caused in part by that OPn (Fig. 10)(Frost, 1966; 1981a; in press, c).

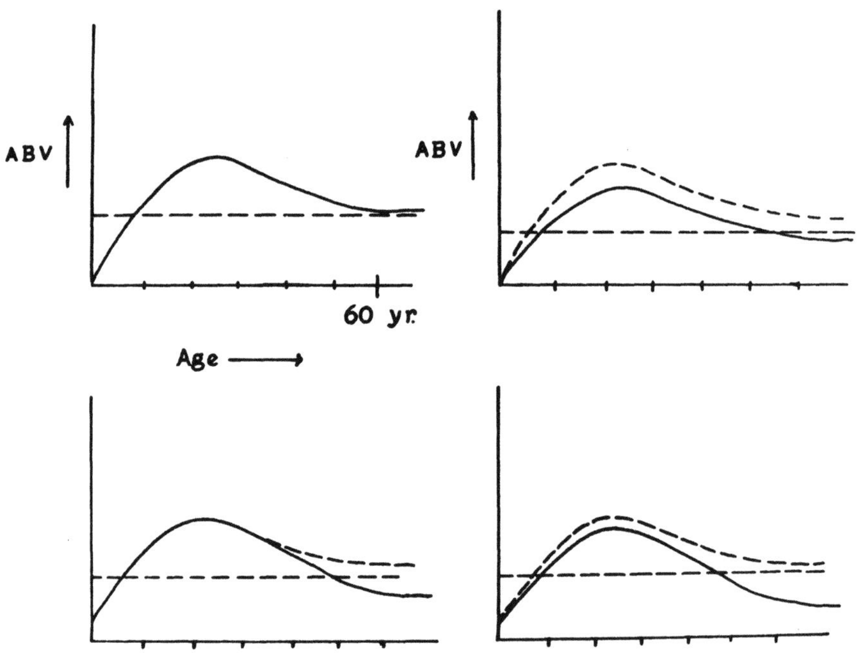

Fig. 10. (See Text)

Special forms of remodeling also occur in the spongiosa beneath growth plates (Jee, 1983; Kimmel, 1980; Putschar, 1960; Rubin, 1964). In various clinical conditions they, too, can remove growth-derived spongiosa more rapidly than normal to cause an osteopenia of trabecular bone in childhood, as in Gaucher's disease, osteogenesis imperfecta, muscular dystrophy and cystic fibrosis.

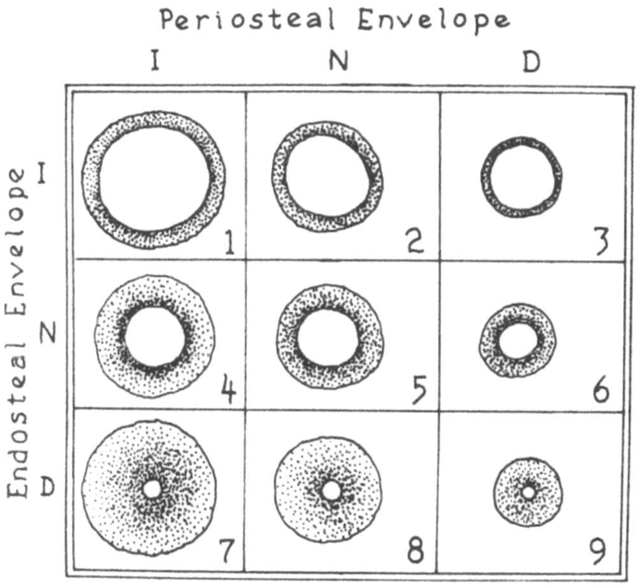

Fig. 11. See text.

Hence, the growth-modeling dependent OPn (Frost, 1981a) depends on mechanisms inherently associated with general growth. Since most of those mechanisms do not act in adult life, their malfunctions can only occur during growth and an adult may inherit but cannot acquire them in adult life. Since the trabecular, periosteal and corticoendosteal envelopes can show independent bone balances in health and in disease, and in response to some drugs (Frost, 1966; in press, c), several different bone cross-sectional configurations of such OPn are possible (Fig. 11).

2) After skeletal maturity

Two pathogentically different OPn can occur here: the naturally reversible, and the naturally irreversible.

Naturally reversible OPn represent enlarged remodeling spaces (Frost, 1966; Jaworski, 1984). They usually (but not invariably) follow increased lamellar bone turnover due to a proportionally increased activation of new remodeling BMU (Fig. 7)(Frost, 1984; Villanueva and Frost, 1970). Such OPn are naturally reversible because when the increased activation subsides, so does the remodeling, whereupon the temporary bone loss becomes restored (Fig. 8)(Frost, 1973a; 1981a; in press, b, c).

Naturally irreversible OPn combine the effects of

i) increased BMU activation, which increases the number of new ΔB.BMU "bites" usually taken out of the trabecular and corticoendosteal envelopes; and,

ii) the special ΔB.BMU parameter itself, which can change from positive to negative or become even more negative under the influence of some drug, hormone, marrow and mechanical use effects, and of still unknown factors (Frost, 1973; 1981a; 1983c; Lanyon, 1984).

Figures 4F and 5 illustrate those effects. Since, normally, the ΔB.BMU is negative only an trabecular and corticoendosteal surfaces (Frost, 1960; Kimmel, 1980), the irreversible bone losses it can cause usually affect only spongiosa and corticoendosteal bone, thereby removing spongiosa and enlarging the marrow cavity.

Hence, the remodeling-dependent OPn (Frost, 1981a) can occur in adult life, but in children can combine with growth-modeling malfunctions. Since such combinations have not been studied systematically, little published data are available. The lamellar bone balance and net losses of the remodeling-dependent OPn are controlled specifically, and exactly, by the following relation:

$$B = \mu \ (\Delta B.BMU) \qquad \text{RELATION 8}$$

where B is the bone balance, μ the number of new BMU activated annually, and ΔB.BMU (as previously defined) has the dual properties of sign (negative, positive, or zero), and quantity in ABV units. This too is discussed in more detail elsewhere (Frost, in press, c).

Mechanical incompetence

Recall that this means bone that hurts and/or fractures under normal usage. At least two different factors contribute to it but in different ways: the OPn and MDx.

1) Osteopenia (OPn)

When too little bone still carries normal mechanical loads it strains more in approximate proportion to the reduction in ABV (Carter, 1981; Currey and Butler, 1975; Hansson, 1977). Or, when half the usual amount of bone still carries usual loads, its strains increase twofold. Numerous studies of OPs patients show that they have from 80% to occasionally only 40% of normal bone amount, the relative reductions in spongiosa often exceeding those of compacta (Courpron, 1981; Eastell, 1984; Garn, 1970; Keshawarz and Recker, 1984; Minaire, 1973; Sedlin, 1964; Wakamatsu and Sissons, 1969). That reduction weakens an intact bone commensurately, as shown for example by a study by Hansson in 1979. That global bone loss can combine the contributions of four separate anatomic factors and in characteristic patterns in particular kinds of OPs. Those factors include cortical thinning, cortical porosity, trabecular thinning, and reduced number of trabeculae.

During normal physical activities, typical maximum strains in normal adult and elderly human bone approximate 500 με, in both spongiosa and compacta (Carter, 1981; 1984; Carter and Caler, 1981; Currey and Butler, 1975; Reilly and Burstein, 1974). Under extreme effort, the peak strains might increase to 1500-2000 με*. Consequently, in a woman with osteopenia who had, for example, only 50% of the normal amount of bone in her vertebrae, those exceptional loads might cause peak strains as large as 3000-4000 με. But even that larger value is only 1/5 the strain needed to fracture otherwise normal bone under a single load (the rupture strain of adult lamellar bone ~20,000 με, range 15,000-35,000 με). In other words, were osteopenic

---

* In normal adult lamellar bone a strain of 1000 με would correspond to a unit stress of ~800 psi.

Table VI. Materials properties of fresh wet human lamellar bone (approximate)

Fracture strain (single load)	15,000-25,000 μE
Fatigue life, <2000 μE	» 10^6-10^7 cycles
Fatigue life, ~2000 μE	~ 10^6-10^7 cycles
Fatigue life, ~4000 μE	< 20,000 cycles
Typical peak strain *in vivo*, adults, normal MU:	~1000-2000 μE
Fracture stress (unit)	~ 18,000 psi (124 MPa)
Fatigue life, <1800 psi (12.4 MPa)	» 10^6 cycles
Fatigue life, ~1800 psi (12.4 MPa)	~ 10^6-10^7 cycles
Fatigue life, ~3600 psi (24.8 MPa)	< 20,000 cycles
Typical peak stress *in vivo*, normal MU:	900-1800 psi (6.2-12.4 MPa)

μE = microstrain. 1000 μE in compression is the same as a shortening in length of 0.1%. MPa = megaPascal = 10^6 Newtons/M²

bone otherwise normal, it should still be ~5x stronger than needed to carry loads large enough to cause strains ~4000 μE. Consequently, it should not fracture spontaneously. Table VI summarizes pertinent material properties of human bone, taken from reports by Carter (1981; 1984), Carter and Caler (1981), Currey and Butler, 1975; Evans (1957), and Reilly and Burstein, 1974).

Yet, in OPs, fractures frequently occur under perfectly ordinary loads, where the strains in the spongiosa probably do not exceed 1000 μE, which is only 1/20 of the strain needed to fracture normal bone in the laboratory. Clearly, the fragility problem has more to it than the simple global reduction in the amount of bone. One such missing factor was encoded in the MDx relations earlier, and while the evidence for it remains indirect it has become compelling.

2) Microdamage (MDx)

Relation 5 shows that strain causes MDx, and Relation 6 that MDx burdens accumulate whenever MDx production exceeds its repair.

As to MDx production, in the laboratory fresh wet human bone subjected to cyclic strains of only 4,000 μE can fail in fatigue under the equivalent of less than two months' use by a normally active adult (eg, ~20,000 cycles) (Carter, 1981; 1984; Carter and Caler, 1981). Yet in the body, healthy bones are repeatedly strained up to 2,000 μE apparently indefinitely, except stress fractures which, however, are exceptions and become rare after an adequate training period. Such facts imply that doubling the typical peak strains of a bone from 2,000 to 4,000 μE (the latter number is only 1/5 of the normal fracture strain) increases new MDx production 4x or more. Thus, in living bone the general relationship between strain magnitude and history, and new MDx production, is probably exponential. Additional factors can also act here, including the "LOBO" phenomenon (Frost, in press, c) which can significantly reduce the number of trabeculae in a given cubic centimeter of spongiosa (Arnold, 1964; Parfitt, 1984b; Wakamatsu and Sissons, 1969). Such factors, however, do not really change the thrust of this argument.

Accordingly, the evidence currently available suggests that bone fragility and the propensity to fracture in OPs patients occur to a minor extent because one or more of the osteopenic mechanisms described above reduce their ABV. The osteopenic mechanisms moderately weaken their bones, to ~80%-40% of normal, but they also increase bone strains commensurately, which can increase the production of new MDx even more. That larger MDx burden further weakens their bones to 20% to less than 10% of normal strength, allowing fractures to occur during ordinary activities, which is one meaning of mechanical incompetence. Through normal innervation of bone (Duncan and Shim, 1979; Miller and Kasahara, 1963) that MDx (and the locally increased strains of adjacent undamaged bone that it causes (Frost, 1985)) may also cause bone pain without overt fracture, this being another meaning of mechanical incompetence.

The MDx repair factor. Some bone dynamic histomorphometric findings from the laboratory at Henry Ford Hospital now require pointed significance (Frost, 1985). By 1968, that laboratory had a respectable collection of rib biopsies of patients with various kinds of OPn and OPs who received double tetracycline labels before their biopsy and histomorphometric analysis (Courpron, 1981; Frost, 1969; 1983a; Melson et al, 1983; Meunier et al, 1979). Most patients with MIn had markedly prolonged sigma values (Jett et al, 1967; Wu and Frost, 1969; Wu et al, 1967). Such prolongations were uncommon in other patients (except those with osteomalacias but in which MIn is also usually present)(Frost, 1973a; Jett et al, 1967; Villanueva et al, 1966; Wu and Frost, 1969; Wu et al, 1967). Later similar findings in similar patients were observed in iliac spongiosa (Parfitt, 1973-1984; Recker, 1976-1983; Melson et al, 1983) and by several observers in osteomalacic patients (Frost, 1983a; 1985). Therefore, association of MIn and prolonged sigma values is not peculiar to compact bone or to OPs.

Sigma is the time the typical remodeling BMU, once activated, takes to progress through its R and F stages to completion in the cross-sectional observations (Frost, 1969; 1973a; in press, c). In normal adults aged 50 years and over, sigma equals three to four months, but in the above mechanical incompetence patients it exceeded two years (Wu and Frost, 1969; Wu et al, 1967). When BMU repair MDx at such a slow rate the latter could easily propagate through bone faster than its repair, so they could accumulate and fragilize bone (Frost, 1985).

3. Synthesis

The following picture of the OPs and their pathogenesis then emerges:

a) An OPs combines three essential elements: an OPn, MIn and etiologic cause.

b) The OPn can follow retarded bone deposits by bone modeling activity during growth, or pathologic loss of bone in adult life due to BMU activation and ΔB.BMU effects, or both.

c) The MIn reflects a minor structural weakening caused by the OPn, and (probably) a major fragilization by increased MDx burdens.

Table VII. IO mechanisms underlying osteoporoses

Osteopenia

Bone modeling: affects periosteal, corticoendosteal envelopes.

Bone remodeling: affects all 4 bone envelopes
Activation frequency (controls turnover and remodeling space)
ΔB.BMU (controls the sign of the bone balance)
Sigma (controls completion time of typical BMU)

Mechanical incompetence

MDx production (mechanical, depends on strain and bone quality)

MDx repair (biologic, depends on remodeling parameters)

OPn (increases strain and MDx)

Mechanical usage; increases increase MDx

Table VIII. Some architectural effects of changes in MES setpoint

Structural	State of Setpoint				
	Normal	I		D	
		$\bar{a}$SM	$\bar{p}$SM	$\bar{a}$SM	$\bar{p}$SM
Feature					
Outside bone diameter	N	D	N	I	N
Marrow cavity diameter, relative	N	I	I	D	N
Cortical thickness	N	D	D	I	N
Amount of spongiosa	N	D	D	I	I
Bone fragility	N	I	I	D	D
MDx production	N	I	I	D	D
MDx repair	N	D	D	I	I
Representative disease	N	OGIM	PMOPs	FDRk	AOMAL

$\bar{a}$SM = before skeletal maturity. $\bar{p}$SM = after skeletal maturity
N = normal I = increased D = decreased
OGIM = osteogenesis imperfecta PMOPs = postmenopausal osteoporosis
FDRk = familial vitamin D resistant rickets AOMAL = axial osteomalacia

d) That MDx arises from increased MDx production (a mechanical phenomenon) and retarded repair (a biologic phenomenon).

e) Increased MDx burdens occur because the moderately increased bone strains of an OPn skeleton increase MDx production, and because depressed activation and/or markedly slowed evolution of remodeling BMU allow that MDx to persist and accumulate.

f) Particular kinds of OPs (eg, Cushing's senile, postmenopausal, postparalytic, nutritional, hyperthyroid, hyperparathyroid, acromegalic) can combine the above pathogenetic elements in different but characteristic patterns (Tables VII and VIII).

Comment

1) Role of the MES in OPn

Bone modeling and remodeling respond to mechanical usage in ways that tend to conserve or add to vigorously-used bone but discard unused bone (but in ways that have special bone architectural effects described elsewhere (Frost, in press, c, d). *In vivo* strain gauge and other studies now confirm (Carter, 1984; Frost, 1963a; Lanyon, 1984; Rubin, 1984) that some threshold range of dynamic mechanical strain is involved in controlling those modeling and remodeling responses. The author has termed that threshold the minimum effective strain, or MES (Frost, 1983d). Setting aside the currently unresolved matter of exactly how to measure and express the MES, strains ~2,000 μE or greater appear to enable modeling, and strains ~200 μE or greater appear to inhibit remodeling-related bone loss (Frost, in press, c).

That IO-domain MES mechanism involves a load on bone that strains it, which generates a primary error signal or S_1 (probably the streaming potentials and related effects described by C. Eriksson (1976) and recently reviewed by others (Johnson, 1984; Pienkowski and Pollack, 1983). That signal may affect an intermediary receptor mechanism or cell, R_1, which may respond by generating a secondary error signal, S_2, that would make the final responding cells/systems (R_2) create modeling drifts or remodeling BMU (Frost, in press, c). That arrangement would look like this:

Load → bone → strain → S_1 → R_1 → S_2 → R_2

|← mechanical →|← biological →|

RELATION 9

Much catalogued clinical and anatomic pathologic evidence suggests that in some bone diseases the "setpoint" of that MES is too high, and in others too low (Fig. 12). If the bone modeling MES were set at, say, ~2,500 μE rather than ~2,000, the effects on bone architecture and ABV can now be predicted with useful accuracy for both children and adults (Frost, in press, d). Table VIII lists some of those effects (discussed in more detail elsewhere (Frost, in press, c, d). It shows that too high a setpoint from birth will cause a growth-modeling dependent OPn, while a previously normal setpoint that becomes too high in adult life should cause precisely the patterns of bone loss and fragility observed in many adult-acquired OPs.

The MES and its setpoint may form a real control mechanism, although not yet well understood. It can affect both bone ABV and MIn; it seems to explain many features of the OPn and OPs; and it is probably a site of action of many skeletally-active systemic and local humoral agents, drugs, and other factors.

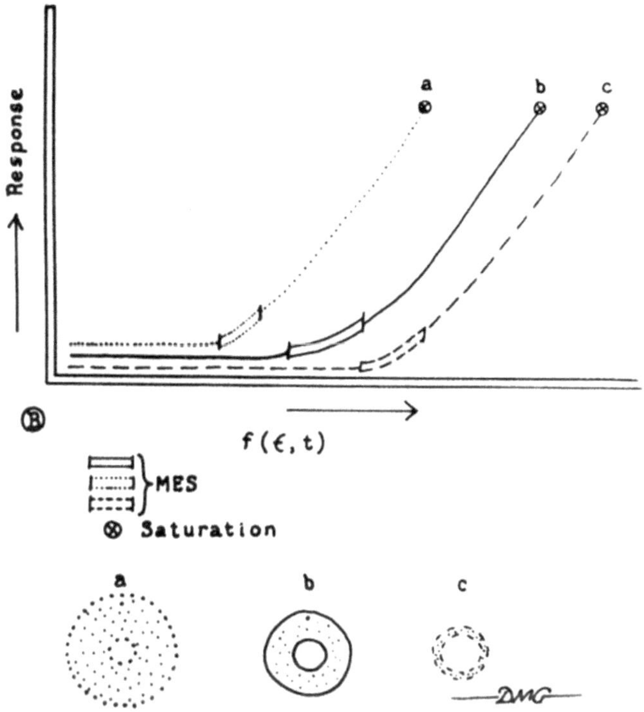

Fig. 12. See text.

That setpoint could be raised if the primary mechanical signal, S_1, generated by strained bone, were somehow defective, or if the subsequent cellular responses were defective, or by some combination of both. The first possibility would point to an abnormal mechanical-ultrastructural property of the bone itself as the primary cause, and circulating hormones and/or biochemical factors probably would not alter it directly, greatly and/or promptly. But the cellular responses could in principle readily respond to drugs, hormones and local, labile biochemical messengers in ways that would change the apparent setpoint. Those postulated mechanisms may hold some answers permitting the control of this system for medical needs, in part because the ultimate causes of the OPn and MIn may act through the MES mechanisms to produce many of their ultimate organ-level effects.

2) Further MDx problems

That MDx arises normally in human skeletal tissues is no longer a matter of legitimate controversy. Studying and understanding it should therefore address the following related matters:

a) How is MDx affected by strain rate, magnitude, frequency, range and duration of time; what is the relative importance of the three principal strains in relation to the grain of lamellar bone, and for spongiosa and compacta?

b) How does the quality and composition of bone affect its susceptibility to fatigue? Does that susceptibility vary in relation to age (including mean tissue age on the microscopic as well as the macrolevel), disease, mechanical usage history, bone composition, density and microstructure, and to certain drugs and hormones?

c) What are the origins of MDx at the molecular level, and does some degree of molecular-level repair occur independently of the histologic-level repair by remodeling?

d) What causes the dynamic remodeling abnormalities that retard MDx repair in most OPs and osteomalacias, and how could one restore them to normal?

e) A further salient fact concerns bone fragilization caused by the above mechanisms which does not usually affect equally either the whole skeleton, or even its entire axial or appendicular fractions. In most cases, additional local factors should explain why, for example, one particular vertebra collapses but not its neighbors, or why the right tibia develops a stress fracture in an athlete but no other bone does in the same patient.

Acknowledgements

The author would like to express his appreciation to Mrs. Betty Uhernik of Pueblo who typed the many drafts of this and its two companion articles, to Mr. David Gavin of Pueblo who prepared many of the drawings, to colleagues in the Southern Colorado Clinic in Pueblo who allowed the time and provided the facilities for preparing the text, to all the colleagues who provided encouragement and shared some of their experience and data, and to the medical staffs of Parview Episcopal and Saint Mary-Corwin Hospitals of Pueblo who also allowed the time needed to accomplish this work.

References

1. Arlot, M.E., Bonjean, M., Chavassieux, P.M., and Meunier, P.J.: Bone histology in adults with aseptic necrosis. J. Bone Joint Surg. 65A, 1319, 1983.

2. Arnold, J.S.: The quantitation of bone mineralization as an organ and tissue in osteoporosis. In, Dynamic Studies of Metabolic Bone Disease. Eds. Pearson, O.H. and Joplin, G.F. F.A. Davis Co., Philadelphia, 1964, pp 59-70.

3. Briançon, D., and Meunier, P.J.: Le Traitement de l'Ostéoporose par l'Association Fluore de Sodium, Calcium, Vitamine D. Univ. Claude Bernard, Lyon, 1979.

4. Cameron, H.V., and Fornasier, V.L.: Trabecular stress fractures. Clin. Orthop. Rel. Res. 111, 266, 1975.

5. Carter, D.R.: The relationship between *in vivo* strains and cortical bone remodeling. C.R.C. Critical Reviews of Biomechanical Engineering 8, 1, 1981.

6. Carter, D.R.: Mechanical loading histories and cortical bone remodeling. Calc. Tissue Int. Suppl. 36, S19, 1984.

7. Carter, D.R., and Caler, W.E.: Uniaxial fatigue of human cortical bone. The influence of tissue physical characteristics. J. Biomech. 14, 461, 1981.

8. Courpron, P.: Bone tissue mechanisms underlying osteoporoses. Orthop. Clin. N. Amer. 12, 513, 1981.

9. Cowin, S.C.: Mechanical modeling of the stress adaptation process in bone. Calc. Tissue Int. Suppl. 36, S98, 1984.

10. Currey, J.D., and Butler, G.: The mechanical properties of bone tissue in children. J. Bone Joint Surg. 57A, 810, 1975.

11. Duncan, C.P., and Shim, S.: The autonomic nerve supply of bone. J. Bone Joint Surg. 59B, 323, 1979.

12. Duncan, H., and Parfitt, A.M.: Metabolic bone disease of the spine. In, The Spine. Eds: Rothman, R.H., and Simeone, F.A.; W.B. Saunders Co., Philadelphia, 1975, pp 570-599.

13. Eastell, R., Kennedy, N.S.J., Smith, M.A., Simpson, J.D., Strong, J.A., and Tothill, P.: The assessment of postmenopausal osteoporosis by total body neutron activation analysis. J. Metab. Bone Dis. Rel. Res. 5, 65, 1984.

14. Enlow, D.H.: Principles of Bone Remodeling. Charles C. Thomas, Springfiled, 1963.

15. Eriksson, C.: Bone morphogenesis and surface change. Clin. Orthop. Rel. Res. 121, 295, 1976.

16. Evans, F.G.: Stress and Strain in Bones. Charles C. Thomas, Springfield, 1957.

17. Freeman, M.A.R., Todd, R.C., and Pirie, C.J.: The role of fatigue in the pathogenesis of senile femoral neck fracture. J. Bone Joint Surg. 56B, 698, 1974.

18. Frost, H.M.: The presence of microscopic cracks *in vivo*. Henry Ford Hosp. Med. Bull. 8, 25, 1960.

19. Frost, H.M.: An Introduction to Biomechanics. Charles C. Thomas, Springfield, 1963a.

20. Frost, H.M.: Bone Remodelling Dynamics. Charles C. Thomas, Springfield, 1963b.

21. Frost, H.M.: The dynamics of bone remodeling. In, Bone Biodynamics. Ed: Frost, H.M.; Little Brown and Co., Boston, 1964, pp 315-333.

22. Frost, H.M.: Bone Dynamics in Osteoporosis and Osteomalacia. Charles C. Thomas, Springfield, 1966.

23. Frost, H.M.: Tetracycline based histological analysis of bone remodeling. Calc. Tissue Res. 3, 211, 1969.

24. Frost, H.M.: Bone Remodeling and Its Relation to Metabolic Bone Disease. Charles C. Thomas, Springfield, 1973a.

25. Frost, H.M.: Orthopaedic Biomechanics. Charles C. Thomas, Springfield, 1973b.

26. Frost, H.M.: Bone Modeling and Skeletal Modeling Errors, Charles C. Thomas, Springfield, 1973c.

27. Frost, H.M.: A theory of lamellar bone modeling. In, Physiology and Pathology of Bone and Cartilage Metabolism. Japan Orthop. Res. Soc., Chukago, Tokyo, 1980, pp 571-628.

28. Frost, H.M.: Orthopedic Clinics of North America (Editor) 12, 1981a.

29. Frost, H.M.: Mechanical microdamage, bone remodeling and osteoporosis. An overview. In, Osteoporosis. Eds: DeLuca, H.F., Frost, H.M., Jee, W.S.S., Johnston, C.C. Jr., and Parfitt, A.M.; University Park Press, Baltimore, 1981b, pp 185-190.

30. Frost, H.M.: Bone histomorphometry. Analysis of trabecular bone dynamics. In, Bone Histomorphometry: Techniques and Interpretation. Ed: Recker, R.R.; C.R.C. Press, Boca Raton, 1983a, pp 109-132.

31. Frost, H.M.: Mechanical determinants of bone modeling. J. Metab. Bone Dis. Rel. Res. 4, 217, 1983b.

32. Frost, H.M.: The skeletal intermediary organization. A review. J. Metab. Bone Dis. Rel. Res. 4, 281, 1983c.

33. Frost, H.M.: A determinant of bone architecture: The minimum effective strain. Clin. Orthop. Rel. Res. 175, 286, 1983d.

34. Frost, H.M.: The ADFR concept revisited. Calc. Tissue Int. 36, 349, 1984.

35. Frost, H.M.: Microdamage : Factors that impair its repair. In, Current Concepts of Bone Fragility in Orthopaedics and Medicine. Eds: Uhthoff, H.K., and Stahl, E.; Springer-Verlag, Berlin-Heidelberg-New York, in press

36. Frost, H.M.: Mechanical determinants of skeletal architecture: Bone modeling. In, Basic Science in Orthopaedics, Vol. II. Eds: Albright, J.A. and Brand, R.A.; Appleton-Century-Crofts, New York. In press (a).

37. Frost, H.M.: The skeletal intermediary organization: A synthesis. In, Bone and Mineral Research, Vol. II. Ed.: Peck, W.; Excerpta Medica, New York. In press (b).

38. Frost, H.M.: The Skeletal Intermediary Organization. C.R.C. Press, Boca Raton. In press (c).

39. Frost, H.M.: Osteogenesis imperfecta: the setpoint proposal. A possible causative mechanism. In press (d)

40. Frost, H.M.: Pathogenesis of the osteoporoses in 1985: A review. Clin. Orthop. Rel. Res. In press (e)

41. Frost, H.M.: Mechanical determinants of skeletal architecture. II: Chondral modeling; III: Fibrous tissue modeling. In, Basic Science in Orthopaedics, Vol. II. Eds: Albright, J.A. and Brand, R.A.; Appleton-Century-Crofts, New York. In press (f)

42. Frost, H.M., Roth, H., and Villanueva, A.R.: Physical characteristics of bone. IV: Microscopic prefailure and failure patterns. Henry Ford Hosp. Med. Bull. 9, 163, 1961.

43. Garn, S.M.: The Earlier Gain and Later Loss of Cortical Bone. Charles C. Thomas, Springfield, 1970.

44. Hansson, T.: The Bone Mineral Content and Biomechanical Properties of Lumbar Vertebrae. Uno Lundgren Tryckeri A.B., Götenborg, 1977.

45. Jaworski, Z.F.G.: Lamellar bone turnover system and its effector organ. Calc. Tissue Int. 36, S46, 1984.

46. Jaworski, Z.F.G., Liskova-Kiar, M., and Uhthoff, H.: Effect of long term immobilization on the pattern of bone loss in older dogs. J. Bone Joint Surg. 62B, 104, 1980.

47. Jaworski, Z.F.G., Meunier, P., and Frost, H.M.: Observations on two types of resorption cavities in human lamellar cortical bone. Clin. Orthop. 83, 279, 1972.

48. Jee, W.S.S.: The skeletal tissues. In, Histology, 5th ed. Ed: Weiss, L.; Elsevier Biomedical, New York, 1983. pp 200-255.

49. Jett, S., Wu, K., and Frost, H.M.: Tetracycline-based histological measurement of cortical-endosteal bone formation in normal and osteoporotic ribs. Henry Ford Hosp. Med. J. 15, 325, 1967.

50. Johnson, L.C.: Morphologic analysis in pathology. The kinetics of disease and general biology of bone. In, Bone Biodynamics. Ed: Frost, H.M.; Little Brown and Co., Boston, 1964. pp 543-654.

51. Johnson, M.W.: Behavior of fluid in stressed bone and cellular stimulation. Calc. Tissue Int. 36, S72, 1984.

52. Kanis, J.A.: Treatment of osteoporotic fracture. Lancet, i:27, 1984.

53. Keshawarz, N.M., and Recker, R.R.: Expansion of medullary cavity at the expense of cortex in postmenopausal osteoporosis. J. Metab. Bone Dis. Rel. Res. 5, 223, 1984.

54. Kimmel, D.B., and Jee, W.S.S.: A quantitative histologic analysis of the growing long bone metaphysis. Calc. Tissue Int. 32, 113, 1980.

55. Landeros, O., and Frost, H.M.: A cell system in which rate and amount of protein synthesis are separately controlled. Science 145, 1323, 1964.

56. Lanyon, L.E.: Functional strain as a determinant for bone remodeling. Calc. Tissue Int. 36, S56, 1984.

57. Melsen, F., Mosekilde, L., and Kragstrup, J.: Metabolic bone diseases as evaluated by bone histomorphometry. In, Bone Histomorphometry: Techniques and Interpretation. Ed: Recker, R.R.; C.R.C. Press, Boca Raton, 1983, pp 265-284.

58. Meunier, P.J., Courpron, P., Edouard, C., Alexandre, C., Bressot, C., Lips, P., and Boyce, B.F.: Bone histomorphometry in osteoporotic states. In, Osteoporosis II. Ed: Barzel, U.S.; Grune and Stratton, New York, 1979. pp 27-47.

59. Miller, M.R., and Kasahara, M.: Observations on the innervation of human long bones. Anat. Rec. 145, 13, 1963.

60. Minaire, P.: L'Ostéoporose d'Immobilization. Données Biologiques et Histologiques Quantitatives. (Thesis) Ediprim, Lyon, 1973.

61. Nordin, B.E.C.: The application of basic science to osteoporosis. In, Bone Biodynamics. Ed: Frost, H.M.; Little Brown and Co., Boston, 1964, pp 521-542.

62. Parfitt, A.M.: The cellular basis of bone remodeling: The quantum concept reexamined in the light of recent advances in the cell biology of bone. Calc. Tissue Int. 36, S37, 1984a.

63. Parfitt, A.M.: Age-related structural changes in trabecular and cortical bone: Cellular mechanisms and biomechanical consequences. Calc. Tissue Int. 36, S123, 1984b.

64. Parfitt, A.M.: Personal communications, 1973-1984.

65. Pienkowski, D., and Pollack, S.R.: The origin of stress-generated potentials in fluid saturated bone. J. Orthop. Res. 1, 30, 1983.

66. Putschar, W.G.J.: General pathology of the musculoskeletal system. In, Handbuch der Allgemeinen Pathologie. Eds: Buchner, F., Letterer, E., and Roulet, F.: Springer-Verlag, Berlin, 1960, pp 361-488.

67. Radin, E.L.: Trabecular microfractures in response to stress: The possible mechanism of Wolff's Law. In, Orthopaedic Surgery and Traumatology. Excerpta Medica, Amsterdam, 1972, pp 59-65.

68. Rasmussen, H., and Bordier, P.: The Physiological and Cellular Basis of Metabolic Bone Disease. Williams and Wilkins, Baltimore, 1974.

69. Recker, R.R.: Personal communications, 1976-1983.

70. Reilly, D.T., and Burstein, A.H.: The mechanical properties of cortical bone. J. Bone Joint Surg. 36A, 1001, 1974.

71. Roth, H., Frost, H.M., and Villanueva, A.R.: Physical characteristics of bone. I: The existence of plastic flow *in vivo*. Henry Ford Hosp. Med. Bull. 9, 149, 1961.

72. Rubin, C.T.: Skeletal strain and significance of bone architecture. Calc. Tissue Int. 36, S11, 1984.

73. Rubin, P.: Dynamic Classification of Bone Dysplasias. Year Book Medical Publishers, Chicago, 1964.

74. Sedlin, E.: Uses of bone as a model system in the study of aging. In, Bone Biodynamics. Ed: Frost, H.M.; Little Brown and Co., Boston, 1964. pp 655-666.

75. Todd, R.C., Freeman, M.A.R., and Pirie, C.J.: Isolated trabecular fatigue fractures in the femoral head. J. Bone Joint Surg. 54B, 723, 1972.

76. Uhthoff, H.K., and Jaworski, Z.F.G.: Bone loss in response to long term immobilization. J. Bone Joint Surg. 60B, 420, 1978.

77. Urist, M.R.: Observations bearing on the problem of the osteoporoses. In, Bone as A Tissue. Eds: Rodah, H., Nicholson, J.T., and Brown, E.M., Jr.; McGraw-Hill Book Co., New York, 1960, pp 18-45,

78. Urist, M.R., DeLange, R.J., and Finerman, G.A.M.: Bone cell differentiation and growth factors. Science 220, 680, 1983.

79. Urist, M.R., MacDonald, N.S., Moss, M.J., and Skoog, W.A.: Rarefying disease of the skeleton: Observations dealing with aged and dead bone in patients with osteoporosis. In, Mechanisms of Hard Tissue Destruction. AAAS, 1963, pp 385-446.

80. Villanueva, A.R., and Frost, H.M.: Evaluation of factors determining the tissue-level haversian bone formation rate in man. J. Dent. Res. 49, 836, 1970.

81. Villanueva, A.R., Ilnicki, L., Duncan, H., and Frost, H.M.: Bone and cell dynamics in the osteoporoses: A review of measurements by tetracycline bone labelling. Clin. Orthop. 49, 163, 1966.

82. Wakamatsu, E., and Sissons, H.A.: The cancellous bone of the iliac crest. Calc. Tissue Res. 4, 147, 1969.

83. Watson, M.: Microfractures in the head of the femur. J. Bone Joint Surg. 57A, 696, 1975.

34. Weinmann, J.P., and Sicher, H.: Bone and Bones. C.V. Mosby, Co., St. Louis, 1955.

85. Wu, K., and Frost, H.M.: Bone formation in osteoporosis: Appositional rate measured by tetracycline labelling. Arch. Pathol. 88, 508, 1969.

86. Wu, K., Jett, S., and Frost, H.M.: Bone resorption rates in physiological senile and postmenopausal osteoporoses. J. Lab. Clin. Med. 69, 810, 1967.

Morphology of Bone Tissue Aging

A. DHEM and V. ROBERT

Introduction

An excellent description of the changes occurring in human compact bone due to age was presented by Amprino and Bairati in 1936. According to these authors, after 50 years of age bone destruction is no longer sufficiently compensated by bone formation and, therefore, rarefaction develops.

In all the recent publications, age-related bone loss is also interpreted as the result of an imbalance occurring in normal bone remodeling (Courpron, 1972; Frost 1981a, 1981b; Jaworski, 1981; Jaworski and Duncan, 1984; Meunier et al, 1973; Parfitt, 1981, 1982). Moreover, many investigators report a decrease of bone formation (Giroux et al, 1975; Lips et al, 1978) and osteoclastic resorption (Courpron, 1981).

To understand the mechanisms involved in bone aging, we decided to undertake a comparative study of compact bone between dog and man. It seemed to us of interest to ascertain the extent of bone loss in an animal whose longevity is about five times shorter than that of man.

Materials and Methods

The bones of 52 healthy mongrel dogs of both sexes were collected for this study. Their ages varied from 6 months to 20 years; 19 dogs were over 10 years of age. To this first group we added a second one composed of 35 adult dogs of unknown age. The weight of the animals varied from 4 to 40 kg. Furthermore, we collected approximately 100 tibial diaphyses which were removed, in equal proportion, from men and women who had died either suddenly or accidentally at ages varying from 16 to 98 years.

All the illustrations presented in this paper were taken from samples embedded in methylmethacrylate after having been dehydrated with methanol, defatted with chloroform, and cleared with toluol.

Without previous decalcification, these bones were then cut into sections, 120 µm thick, by an automatic saw (Type 32, Safag, Bienne, Switzerland). After reduction to a uniform thickness of 80 µm by manual grinding on a ground glass plate under methanol, each section was placed on a fine grain Kodak Spectroscopic plate 649-0 for microradiography, and exposed to long

Current Concepts of Bone Fragility

wavelength radiations produced by a Machlett tube (Baltograph* BF 50-20, Balteau, Liège), at 13 Kv and 18 mA. The exposure lasted 15 min and the film focus distance was 61 mm.

The measurements of the surfaces of complete transverse sections in the radius bone of dogs and of the diameter of the haversian canals in the same material have been performed with the help of a semiautomatic quantitative evaluation modular system (MOP, Kontron, München, West Germany).

Results

Microradiography, which adds the degree of calcification of the structures to the histologic picture, is necessary to understand all the aspects observed in bone tissue aging (Dhem, 1970, 1973; Lacroix and Dhem, 1967).

Aging of compact bone in the dog

The process of haversian bone remodeling in dogs, estimated by counting both resorption cavities and depositing osteons in complete transverse diaphyseal sections of the radius, diminishes markedly between the end of the growth period and 4 years of age. This confirms the observations of Marotti (1964), and Amprino and Marotti (1964).

After 4 years of age and until the end of life, haversian bone remodeling remains extremely low. Expressed as a percentage of the total number of haversian canals present in a transverse section, the depositing osteons never exceed 0.5%. Moreover, after 8 years of age, the number of osteons still increases but at a lower rate. Indeed, from this age on, bone formation generally takes place in preexisting haversian canals leading to the production of osteons with two concentric parts (type T in Fig. 3).

As to quantitative measurements, the direct measure of the diaphyseal wall thickness indicates that it is proportional to the surface of the transverse section and that it is independent of age (Piret and Mohimont, 1975).

In assessing the amount of endosteal cortical bone loss due to endosteal resorption, we determined, as suggested by Garn and Poznanski (1970), the percentage of the surface occupied by bone tissue with respect to the total surface of the section (Fig. 1). For this study, the animals were divided into three groups: 1) less than 10 years of age; 2) more than 10 years of age; and 3) unknown ages. The results indicate no significant differences at a 1% level among these three groups.

The intracortical porosity was determined by measuring in percent the evolution of haversian canals whose diameter is less than 24 microns (Fig. 2).

Up to 9 years of age, the percentage is of the order of 90%. It is 92.9 ± 2.5% in animals of unknown age. Porosity appears at 9 years of age. The percentage of narrow haversian canals diminishes but varies considerably from one animal to another. In some very old animals, the narrow haversian canal percentage is less than 50% whereas it is still in the order of 80% in others of the same age.

---

* Gift of the Fonds National de la Recherche Scientifique, Brussels.

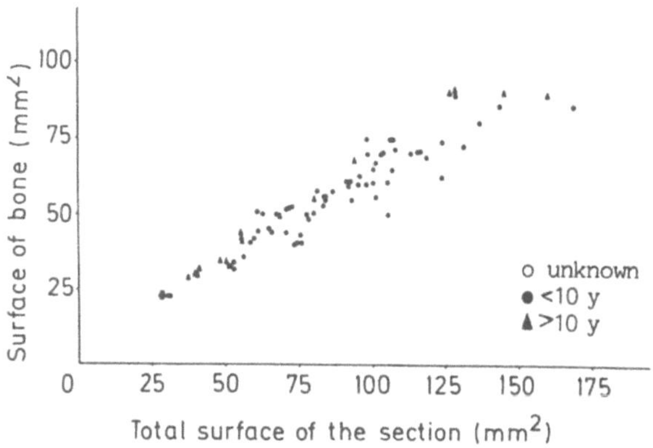

Fig. 1. Complete transverse sections of the midshaft of dog radii. Relation between bone surface and the total section surface.

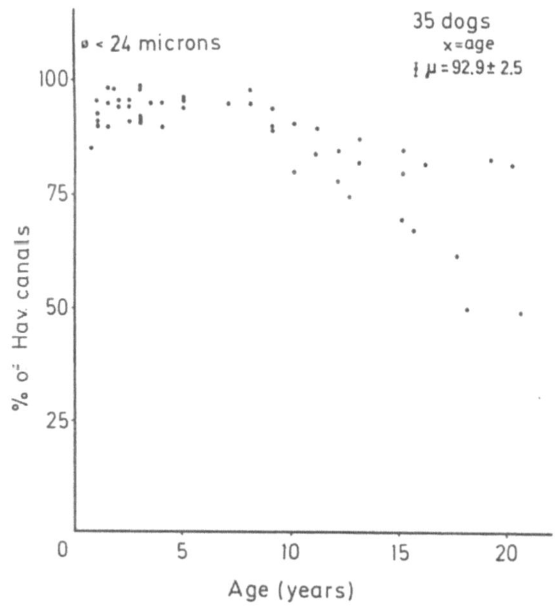

Fig. 2. Percentages of haversian canals with a diameter less than 24 microns as a function of the dogs' ages.

A microradiographic examination can elucidate these differences (Fig. 3). When the porosity is extensive, the type "W" osteons predominate. When a low porosity is observed, more than 30% of the osteons are of type "T". The latter possesses two different concentric calcified portions centred on the same haversian canal. The difference in calcification is not always as evident as shown in Figure 3, but the existence of a cementing line between the two portions makes the identification of this type of osteon easy.

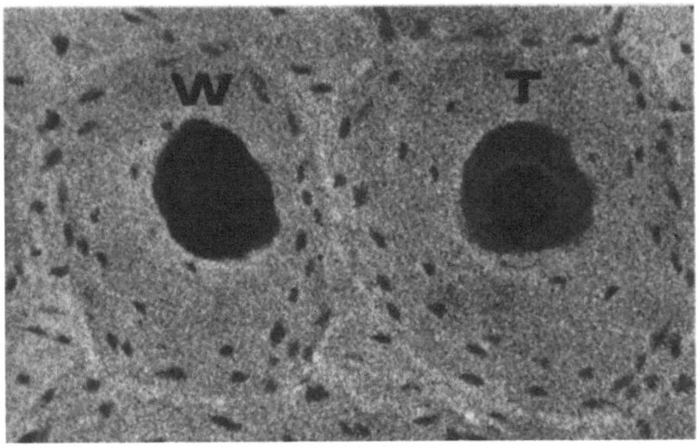

Fig. 3. Microradiograph of a transverse section in the radial diaphysis of a 17 year old dog (x 348). W: osteon with a wide haversian canal. T: osteon with two concentric portions

The type "W" osteon is fully calcified and its haversian canal is often more irregular than that depicted in Figure 3, resembling a resorption cavity, though not containing osteoclasts (Dhem and Piret, 1975).

Aging of compact bone in man

In a recent publication (Dhem, 1980), we showed by means of microradiography that the structural modifications occurring with age in human compact bone are far more complex than a simple acquisition of osteons with wide haversian canals and that they result in an important differentiation of the osteon population.

These structural modifications do not originate in an alteration of haversian bone remodelling. The latter, as in the dog, occurs sparsely once growth has ended (Lacroix and Dhem, 1967). With age, the osteon diameter tends to diminish (Amprino and Bairati, 1936; Currey, 1964) and such osteons are deposited preferentially beneath the periosteum (Arnold, 1970), whereas near the medullary cavity larger than normal resorption cavities develop and their ultimate filling is incomplete.

Certain osteons have an irregular haversian canal (Fig. 4A) with a notched perimeter as in a resorption cavity. We reported their existence in 1967 (Lacroix and Dhem, 1967) without observing, as have Jaworski et al (1972), that they don't contain osteoclasts.

In other osteons (Fig. 4B), the haversian canal is bordered by a hypercalcified ring partially buried beneath a crescent-shaped deposit.

As seen in Figure 4C, a delineated hypermineralized ring is present in the osteon at a short distance from the haversian canal. The staining of the network of osteocyte canaliculi establishes that this ring is not a cementing line (Dhem, 1980). Furthermore, it has never been observed around a new deposit. In contrast, hypermineralization of the lamellae situated within the ring is not rare (Fig. 4D).

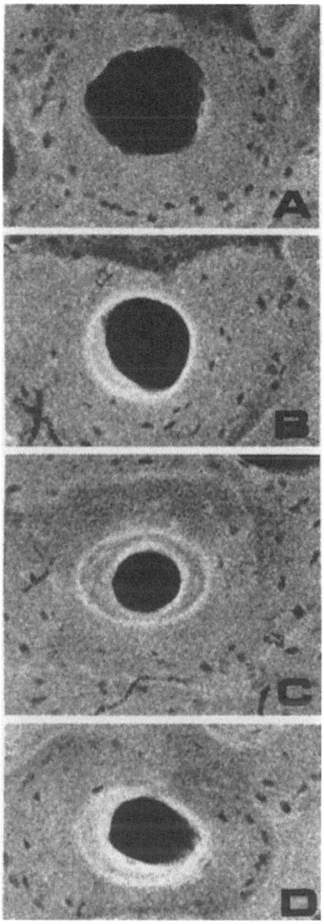

Fig. 4. Microradiographic aspects of four osteons in a transverse section of the tibia of an 80 year old man (x 310).

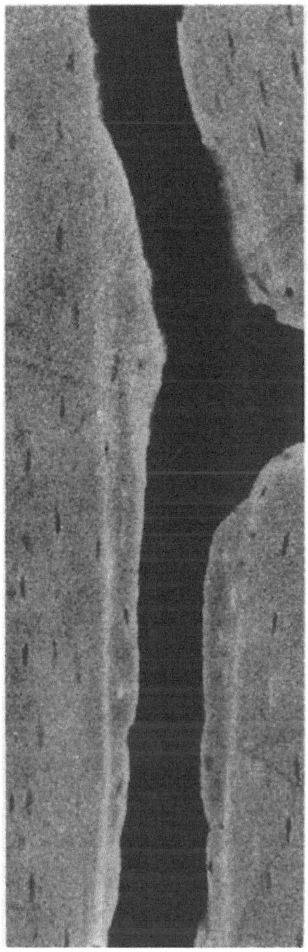

Fig. 5. Microradiograph of a longitudinal section in the diaphyseal wall of the tibia of a 68 year old man (x 310).

Each of the aspects observed in the transverse sections (Fig. 4), including the osteocytic lacuna filled with a hypermineralized deposit, can be found only in one longitudinally-sectioned haversian canal (Fig. 5).

Discussion

It can be concluded from our observations that age-related bone loss never attains in old dogs the magnitude known in man.

No expansion of the bone marrow cavity has been observed (Fig. 1).

According to Frost (1964), the progressive bone loss existing in man at the endosteal surface of the diaphysis has to be related to a continuous bone formation at the periosteal surface. However, since no difference is observed between the values measured in dogs less than ten years of age and older ones, it may suggest that the absence of bone loss leading to an expansion of bone marrow cavity could be related to the longevity of the dog and, consequently, to structural age.

Concerning intracortical porosity, estimated by the percentage of haversian canals with a diameter of more than 24 microns (Fig. 2), it exists in some animals and not in others. The absence of porosity is not sex linked. Godina (1947) mentioned that it preferentially affects large animals. Our observations could not confirm this finding.

As to the morphologic aspect, the intracortical porosity corresponds to an accumulation of osteons with large haversian canals (W in Fig. 3), often irregular, resembling that of a resorption cavity.

Boring of the haversian canals, which we carried out in the same material (Dhem, 1965), permits, however, observation of several differences between irregular haversian canals and actual resorption cavities. The latter are bored very rapidly and the reconstruction process follows immediately in the wake of the destruction process. Observed in transverse sections, they seem disposed at random, without respect for preexisting structures, and they rarely open into a haversian canal.

Direct examination of the sections, after surface staining with methylene blue, did not reveal the presence of osteoclasts (Dhem and Piret, 1975). It also permitted us to state that what resembles a Howship lacuna in microradiograph is often merely an open osteocytic lacuna.

Finally, the rapidity of osteoclastic resorption is not compatible with the fact that the percentage of osteons with large haversian canals increases only slowly with age. The same applies to the haversian canal diameter (Dhem and Robert, in press).

To explain all these observations, we propose the hypothesis that the hypercalcified ring which appears at the end of osteon deposition is not stable but dynamic. The hypercalcification would involve a destruction of the subjacent ground substance, and affecting one lamella after another would lead to a slow widening of the haversian canal.

A weak intracortical porosity corresponds to a type T osteon (Fig. 3) accumulation. It is to be noted that the latter is rarely observed before 4 years of age. The possibility exists, therefore, in certain old dogs to fill large haversian canals. According to Jaworski (1984), this reconstruction would be linked to the existence of a "coupling-factor". Perhaps the different porosities observed in old animals of the same age simply suggests differences in cellular capacity.

The osteon in Figure 4A is similar to that observed in the dog (W in Fig. 3). It probably has the same origin and consequently would explain the absence of osteoclasts in the haversian canal mentioned by Jaworski et al (1972).

The better lamellar organization, as seen under polarized light, of ground substance in man as compared to the dog (Ponlot, 1960) would explain why a hypercalcified ring, regular in its form, appears at a short distance from a haversian canal (Fig. 4C). The progress in calcification at the level of the most central osteon lamellae (Fig. 4D) is accompanied by an alteration and a disappearance of the ground substance as revealed by Foot's silver staining (Dhem, 1980).

Finally, since all the processes presented in Figure 4 appear in a single longitudinally-sectioned osteon (Fig. 5), we suggest that they correspond in reality to a particular destructive mechanism of bone tissue which we propose be called "delitescence" by analogy with that which occurs in a dehydrating crystal or by analogy with the way in which stones are divided following the direction of the layers which constitute them (Dhem, 1970; 1973; 1980; Lacroix and Dhem, 1967).

This interpretation agrees with the recently described physicochemical alterations occurring in collagen fibers with age (Struck, 1984).

References

1. Amprino, R. and Bairati, A.: Processi di ricostruzione e di riassorbimento nella sostanza compatta delle ossa dell'uomo. Z. Zellforsch. 24, 439, 1936.
2. Amprino, R. and Marotti, G.: A topographic quantitative study of bone formation and reconstruction. In, Bone and Tooth, Ed: Blackwood, H.J.J., Pergamon Press, Oxford, 1964. pp 21-33.
3. Arnold, J.S.: Focal excessive endosteal resorption in aging and senile osteoporosis. In, Osteoporosis, Ed: Barzel, U.S., Grune and Stratton, New York, London, 1970. pp 80-100.
4. Courpron, P.: Données histologiques quantitatives sur le vieillissement osseux humain. Thesis, University of Lyon, 1972.
5. Courpron, P.: Bone tissue mechanisms underlying osteoporoses. Orthop. Clin. North Am. 12,513, 1981.
6. Currey, J.D.: Some effects of ageing in human haversian systems. J. Anat. 98, 69, 1964.
7. Dhem, A.: Le forage des canaux de Havers. Rev. Chir. orthop. 51, 583, 1965.
8. Dhem, A.: Microradiographic study of ageing of compact bone in man. In, Symposium Ossium, Eds: Jelliffe, A.M. and Strickland, B., E. & S. Livingstone, Edinburgh, London, 1970. pp 289-291.
9. Dhem, A.: Les mécanismes de destruction du tissu osseux. Acta orthop. Belg. 39, 423, 1973.
10. Dhem, A.: Étude histologique et microradiographique des manifestations biologiques propres au tissu osseux compact. Bull. Acad. roy. Méd. Belg. 135, 368, 1980.
11. Dhem, A. and Piret, N.: Remarques à propos de la résorption ostéoclastique. Bull. Assoc. Anat. 59, 157, 1975.
12. Dhem, A. and Robert, V.: In press.
13. Frost, H.M.: Dynamics of bone remodelling. In, Bone Biodynamics, Ed: Frost, H.M., Little, Brown and Co., Boston, 1964. pp 315-333.
14. Frost, H.M.: The evolution of pathophysiologic knowledge of osteoporoses. Orthop. Clin. North Am. 12, 475, 1981a.

15. Frost, H.M.: Osteoporosis: Quo vadis? Orthop. Clin. North Am. 12, 683, 1981b.

16. Garn, S.M. and Poznanski, A.K.: Transient and irreversible bone losses. In, Osteoporosis, Ed: Barzel, U.S., Grune and Stratton, New York, London, 1970. pp 114-122.

17. Giroux, J.M., Courpron, P., and Meunier, P.: Histomorphométrie de l'ostéopénie physiologique sénile. Monographie du Laboratoire de Recherches sur l'Histodynamique osseuse, Lyon, 1975.

18. Godina, G.: Transformazioni strutturali durante l'accrescimento delle ossa lunghe in cani di differente mole somatica. Arch. Anat. 52, 161, 1947.

19. Jaworski, Z.F.G.: Physiology and pathology of bone remodelling. Cellular basis of bone structure in health and in osteoporosis. Orthop. Clin. North Am. 12, 485, 1981.

20. Jaworski, Z.F.G.: Coupling of bone formation to bone resorption: A broader view. Calcif. Tissue Int. 36, 531, 1984.

21. Jaworski, Z.F.G. and Duncan, H.: Osteoporosis. In, Clinical Medicine, Ed: Spittel, J.A., Jr., vol. 4, Harper & Row Publishers, Philadelphia, 1984. pp 1-18.

22. Jaworski, Z.F.G., Meunier, P., and Frost, H.M.: Observations on two types of resorption cavities in human lamellar cortical bone. Clin. Orthop. 83, 279, 1972.

23. Lacroix, P. and Dhem, A.: Le vieillissement des os. Étude microradiographique de l'os compact. Acta orthop. Belg. 33, 745, 1967.

24. Lips, P., Courpron, P., and Meunier, P.J.: Mean wall thickness of trabecular bone packets in the human iliac crest: Changes with age. Calcif. Tiss. Res. 26, 13, 1978.

25. Marotti, G.: Quantitative studies on bone reconstruction. Acta Anat. 52, 291, 1964.

26. Meunier, P.J., Courpron, P., Edouard, C., Bernard, J., Bringuier, J., and Vignon, G.: Physiological senile involution and pathological rarefaction of bone. Quantitative and comparative histological data. Clin. Endocrinol. Metab. 2, 239, 1973.

27. Parfitt, A.M.: Bone remodeling in the pathogenesis of osteoporosis. Med. Times 109, 80, 1981.

28. Parfitt, A.M.: The contribution of bone histology to understanding the pathogenesis and improving the management of osteoporosis. Clin. Invest. Med. 5, 163, 1982.

29. Piret, N. and Mohimont, C.: Étude morphométrique de la diaphyse radiale du chien. Bull. Assoc. Anat. 59, 247, 1975.

30. Ponlot, R.: Le radiocalcium dans l'étude des os. Thesis, University of Louvain, Masson, Paris, 1960.

31. Struck, H.: Mögliche Ursachen der Altersveränderung des Kollagenstoffwechsels? Z. Gerontol. 17, 85, 1984.

Biomechanical Compensatory Mechanisms for Age-Related Changes in Cortical Bone

W. C. HAYES and C. B. RUFF

Introduction

Age changes in bone mineral mass, volume and density in the human skeleton have been the subject of intensive investigation over the past 25 years. Changes with age in the histologic and mechanical properties of bone have also been studied by many investigators. The general picture emerging from these studies is a progressive net loss of bone mass with aging, beginning in the fifth decade and proceeding at a faster rate among women. Concurrent with this overall loss of bone is the change in bone material properties (Burstein et al, 1976), resulting in a bone tissue of reduced strength and modulus as described above. The major clinical consequence of these skeletal changes is an age-related increase in fracture incidence.

One structural variable that is not often considered in studies of skeletal aging is the global geometry of cortical bone. However, the geometrical distribution of bone tissue, together with its material properties, is critical in determining the structural strength and rigidity of the whole bone. The results of radiogram-metric studies suggest that some geometric remodeling of long bone cortices occurs with aging. In particular, subperiosteal apposition of bone has been observed to occur concurrently with endosteal absorption. This remodeling of the diaphysis to a larger diameter may serve a mechanical compensatory function by increasing the moment of inertia as the cortex thins with aging.

An additional motivation for improved data on long bone cross-sectional geometry is for normalization of photon absorptiometric measurements. Since its initial description, photon absorptiometry has become one of the most widely used techniques for assessing bone mineral content (BMC) of the skeleton *in vivo* (Colbert and Bachtell, 1981; Magess, 1983). Many investigators have demonstrated an inverse relationship between BMC, or BMC divided by scan width (BW), usually measured in the radius, and previous or subsequent fracture incidence. However, while significant differences in mean BMC values in groups with and without fractures have been demonstrated, these studies invariably also indicate a large overlap in values between the two groups. Thus, photon absorptiometry appears to be of limited value in distinguishing on an individual basis between high- and low-fracture risk patients. One reason for this inability to distinguish between fracture and nonfracture populations may result from inherent limitations and assumptions involved in photon absorptiometry. BMC provides a summative mineral content across an entire bone scan path. As such, it is appropriate for monitoring

Current Concepts of Bone Fragility

sequential changes in total bone mineral at the scan site in individual patients.

To compare BMC values in different individuals, however, some kind of skeletal size standardization must be carried out. Although several more sophisticated techniques have been proposed, the most common size standardization procedure has been simply to divide BMC by total (subperiosteal) bone width across the scan path. The accuracy of bone width correcting for true bone volume, however, has not yet been tested and several studies have suggested that BW is inadequate to normalize BMC measurements for either size, sex, or age differences. A second issue concerns variation in cross-sectional geometry at different longitudinal positions in the same bone. Finally, and perhaps most important, is the assumption that the geometry of the same scan site does not vary systematically with age, gender, or other variables related to bone metabolism.

We have previously reported cross-sectional geometric data on femora and tibiae from an archeologic sample of 119 individuals from the American Southwest (Ruff and Hayes, 1982; 1983). We showed increases with aging in both subperiosteal dimensions and in areal moments of inertia. We also documented significant differences with age between cross-sectional sites and between sexes in the pattern of cortical remodelling. Recently, we also addressed certain relationships between bone cross-sectional geometry and photon absorptiometric parameters for 11 femoral and tibial sites in the same population (Ruff and Hayes, 1984). The data showed that locational, age, and sex differences in BMC are largely determined by variations in cortical area. In addition, because of differences in bone geometry, variations in bone width do not reflect variations in cortical area. Consequently, use of BW to standardize for volumetric or bone size differences produces misleading results in sex and age comparisons. These results are briefly summarized here to suggest the changes in cortical cross-sectional geometry that can occur with age and to indicate some of the difficulties involved in using bone width as a normalization parameter for photon absorptiometric studies.

Geometric Compensation for Age-Related Changes in Long Bones

A sample of femora and tibiae from 119 individuals was selected from the Pecos Pueblo archeologic collections excavated from the large late prehistoric and protohistoric site in New Mexico (Ruff and Hayes, 1982; 1983). Pelvic and cranial morphology were used to determine sex, and age estimates were based on pubic symphyseal form, functional dental wear, and endocranial suture closure. Each femur or tibia was sectiond perpendicular to its longitudinal axis at five diaphyseal sites corresponding to 20, 35, 50, 65 and 80% of the bone length, measured from the distal end. In addition, one side of the femoral neck at its minimum superior-inferior breadth was sectioned. Photographs of the cut and cross-sectional surfaces were rear projected onto an electronic digitizer and subperiosteal and endosteal parameters manually traced. Parameter point coordinates at 1 mm intervals were input into program SLICE (Nagurca and Hayes, 1980) and geometric section properties (areas, moments of inertia and their orientations) were calculated.

Changes with age and bone areas of the representating cross-section -- the femoral midshaft -- are shown in Fig. 1. In both sexes, the area of the medullary (marrow) cavity and the total area bounded by the subperiosteal (outer) bone surface increase with age. Although increases in total subperiosteal area are fairly similar in men and women (averaging 7% in men

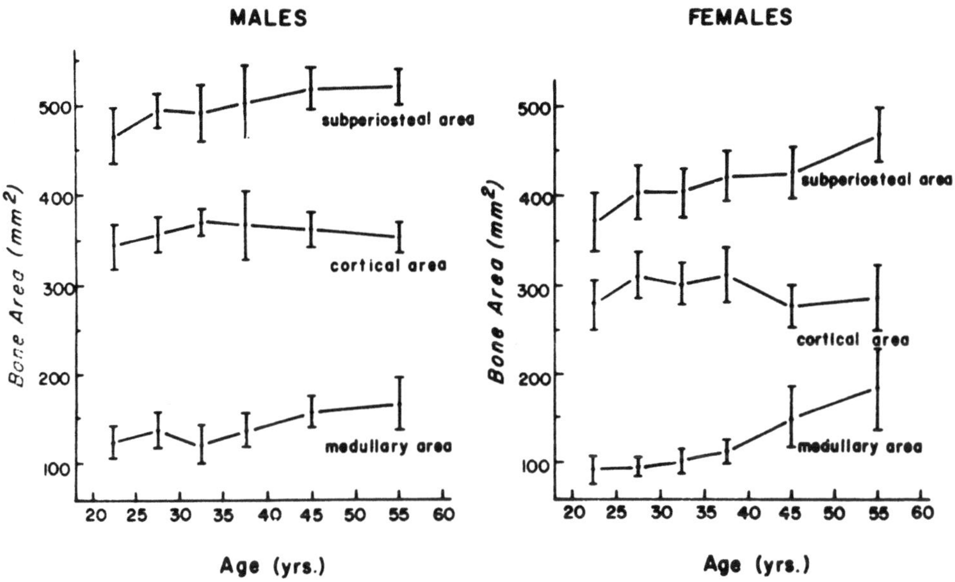

Fig. 1. Changes with age in bone areas of the femoral midshaft for the Pecos Pueblo population (Ruff and Hayes, 1983).

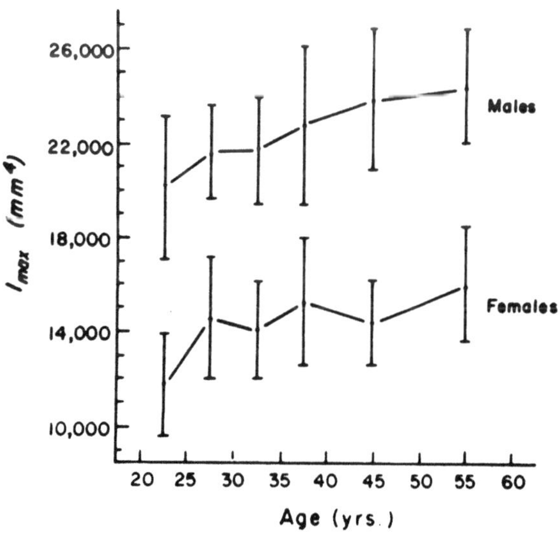

Fig. 2. Changes with age in the maximum moment of inertia of the femoral midshaft for the Pecos Pueblo population (Ruff and Hayes, 1983).

and 11% in women over all cross sections), percentage increases in medullary area are much greater in women (39% vs 19% for men over all sections). Thus, because of relatively greater endosteal absorption of bone with aging, women show a significant decline in compact cortical bone area (average 10%), whereas men show only a negligible (1%) average decrease in cortical bone area.

Figure 2 illustrates the change with age of the femoral midshaft in the maximum moment of inertia (I_{max}). For both sexes, despite age-related declines in cortical bone area, moments of inertia in femoral and tibial cross sections increase. This is due to subperiosteal expansion and progressive remodeling into a cortex of larger diameter. With more bone placed farther from the section centroid, the cross section is more efficient to resist bending and torsion. These geometric changes have consequences for properly interpreting photon absorptiometric scans and for accurately assessing fracture risk in the appendicular skeleton.

Consequences for Photon-Absorptiometry

Photon absorptiometric scans were carried out at 11 cross section locations in this same archeologic sample using a Norland Cameron I Bone Mineral Analyzer with a 3.0 mm scan beam at a scanner speed of 2 mm/sec (Ruff and Hayes, 1984). Whole bones were submerged in 6 cm of water in a plexiglass box marked with reference axes and scanned twice at each site with the average BMC and BW (bone width) recorded. Scans at two of the cross-section locations -- the femoral midshaft and the femoral neck -- were taken on all 119 individuals included in the study sample.

The variations in BMC, BW, and CA (cortical area) at the 11 femoral and tibial cross-section locations are shown in Figure 3. Both BMC and CA follow quite similar patterns of longitudinal variation in the lower limb. In both the tibia and femur, BMC and CA increase from the most distal diaphyseal section to a peak in the proximal half of the diaphysis. The only significant departures from parallelism between the two curves occur in the most proximal and distal sections where CA tends to decline more than BMC. By contrast, BW and CA do not follow similar patterns of longitudinal vari-

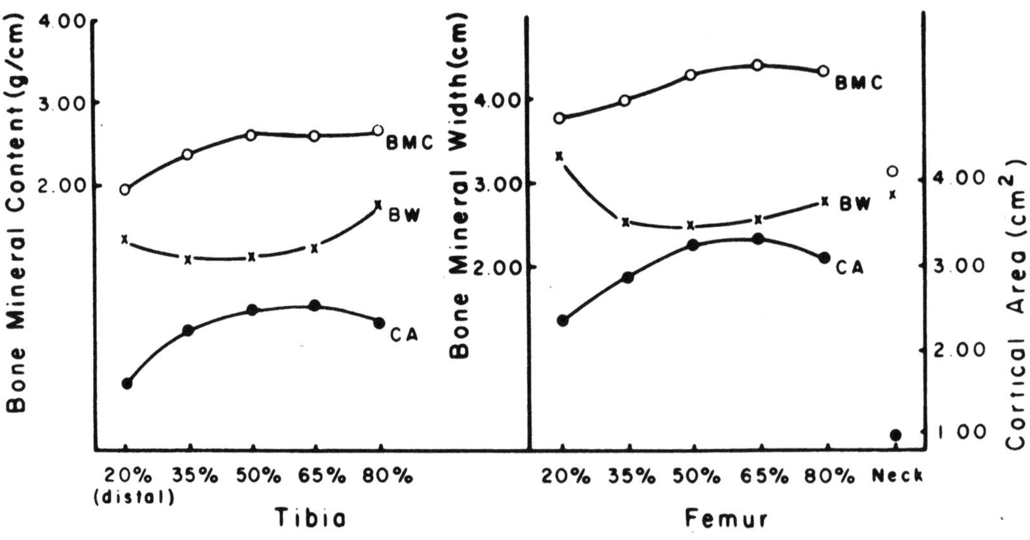

Fig. 3. Patterns of variation of bone mineral content (BMC), bone width (BW), and cortical area (CA) at eleven cross-sectional sites for the Pecos Pueblo population. BMC and CA follow similar patterns whereas BW does not adequately reflect variations in CA. (Ruff and Hayes, 1983)

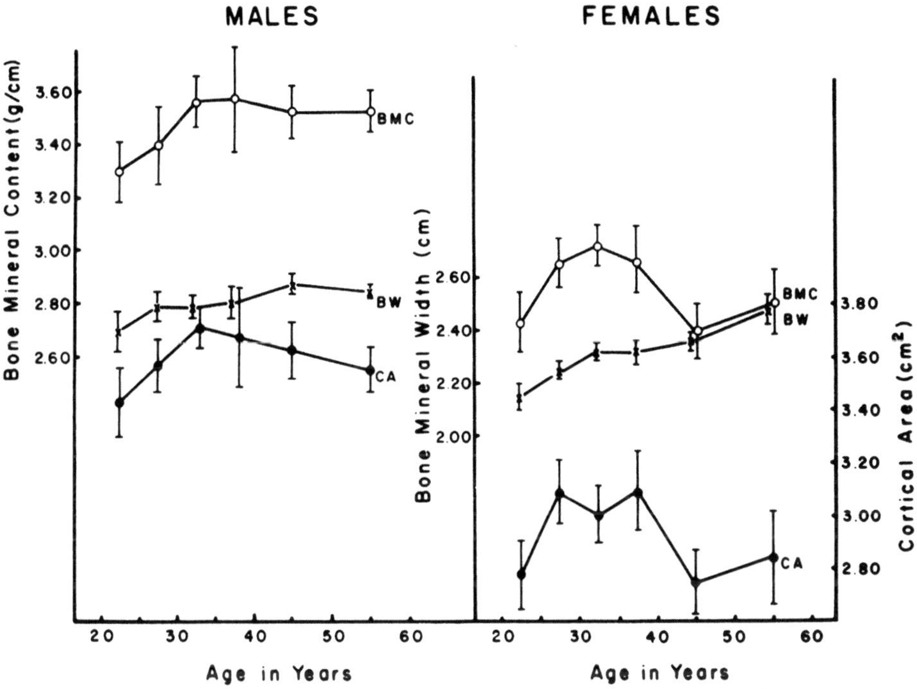

Fig. 4. Changes with age in bone mineral content (BMC), bone width (BW), and cortical area (CA) at the femoral midshaft for the Pecos Pueblo population. Age changes in BMC are parallel to those in CA but not to those in BW. (Ruff and Hayes, 1983)

ation in the lower limb. Moreover, the pattern of variation in BW is almost diametrically opposite that of CA or BMC, reaching minimum value at or near the locations of peak values in the other two properties. These differences are partly explained by the general structural arrangement of bone tissue, varying from widely flared ends and thin cortices to narrower mid-diaphyses with relatively thicker cortices.

From these results it is apparent that BW provides a relatively poor standardization for locational differences in CA in the lower limb, and that BMC/BW values cannot be assumed to reflect differences in bone mineral density at different locations. Locational differences in mean BMC/BW values (0.081 to 1.31 g/cm^2, mean 1.098 g/cm^2, coefficient of variation 5.1%) are more than twice those of BMC/CA (1.00 to 1.21 g/cm^3, mean 1.073 g/cm^3, coefficient of variation 2.4%). Age changes in these parameters are shown in Figure 4. In both men and women, BMC reaches a peak in the fourth decade, then declines much more rapidly in women. Age changes in CA are similar, following patterns almost parallel to those in BMC. Age changes in BW follow a contrasting pattern, continuously increasing throughout adulthood. The increase in BW is greater among women at the femoral midshaft location illustrated here. The effects on age analyses of dividing BMC by BW and CA are shown in Figure 5. Age changes in BMC/BW are fairly similar to those observed in BMC, with men declining only slightly in the three age groups and women declining much more rapidly. Thus, if BW is used to standardize

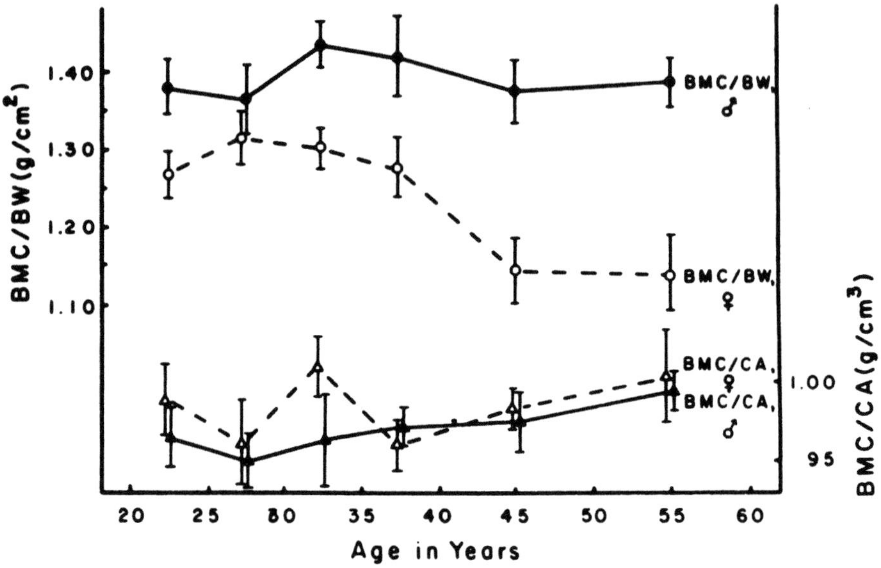

Fig. 5. Changes with age in bone mineral content (BMC) normalized to bone width (BMC/BW) and by cortical area (BMC/CA) at the femoral midshaft for the Pecos Pueblo population. The BMC/BW ratio shows a significant decline with age in women but not in men, indicating no significant change in true mineral density at the femoral midshaft. (Ruff and Hayes, 1983)

BMC for bone volume differences, it indicates a significant decline with age in mineral density for women ($F = 0.47$, $p > 0.50$). As shown in Figure 5, BMC standardized for true cortical area, however, shows no significant age trend in either sex. The almost constant BMC/CA ratio indicates that the true mineral density at the femoral midshaft changes very little throughout adulthood.

Thus, we can conclude that variation in BMC among different locations in the lower limb, men and women, and among different age groups is largely accounted for by variations in cortical bone area. We find no evidence for any significant sex or age differences in BMC standardized for true cortical area. Bone width also provides a poor estimate of bone volume differences in the lower limb. Variation in relative position of the endosteal boundary and cross-sectional shape are not reflected in a subperiosteal breadth measurement. As a consequence, standardizing BMC by BW can produce misleading results in location, sex, and age comparisons. In particular, reductions with age in BMC/BW do not indicate reduced mineral density, but rather reduced cortical area relative to cortical subperiosteal area. Thus, age changes in bone mineral are mainly volumetric, not densitometric, at least through the seventh decade. Bone geometric remodeling appears to be an important part of the skeletal aging process. Variations in the type of remodeling that occur may be a significant factor in predisposing individuals to fracture and old age.

Consequences for Diaphyseal Fracture Risk

These age-related geometric changes in long bone may also be viewed as a compensatory response to the reductions in material properties that occur with age (Burstein et al, 1976). The data indicate that the tensile strength of femoral cortical bone decreases by about 2% per decade in the age range of 20 to 90 years. It would be of interest to determine whether the geometric changes shown in Figures 1 and 2 tend to compensate for this decrease by remodeling the cross section to a more efficient geometry. To explore this hypothesis, the eccentric axial loading analysis can be applied to these data (Hayes, 1985). The geometric data at the femoral midshaft for cortical area, moments of inertia, and eccentricity of the Pecos population are first substituted into the equation for bending stresses in a curved beam. Using values for both young (20-39) and old (40+) segments of the Pecos population results in a predicted increase in the resistance to bending failure at the femoral midshaft of 6% for women and 8% for men. This increase is due primarily to the age-related increases in moments of inertia associated with the expanding periosteal and endosteal surfaces. Comparing the same age groups, our data (Hayes, 1985) indicate a reduction in the tensile strength of cortical bone between the same age groups of approximately 8%. The nearly similar compensation for the reduced mechanical properties is striking.

These calculations are based on a number of simplified assumptions. These include the consideration of only longitudinal axial loads and the use of strength data from a modern sample for analyzing age-related geometric changes in the Pecos population. These changes in bone geometry are sufficient, however, to suggest a kind of biomechanical homeostatic mechanism for maintaining long bones of approximately constant strength throughout adult life. This hypothesis certainly is worth examining further using more rigorous analytic methods and geometric data from both modern and ancient populations.

References

1. Burstein, A.H., Reilly, D.T., and Martens, M.: Aging of bone tissue: Mechanical properties. J.Bone Joint Surg. 58A, 82, 1976.

2. Colbert, C., and Bachtell, R.S.: Radiographic absorptiometry (photodensitometry). In, Non-invasive Measurements of Bone Mass and Their Clinical Application. Ed, Cohn, S.H., CRC Press, Boca Raton, 1981, pp 51-84.

3. Hayes, W.C.: Basic biomechanics of the skeleton. Proc. Current Concepts of Bone Fragility in Orthopaedics and Medicine, Springer-Verlag, 1985.

4. Mazess, R.B.: Noninvasive methods for quantitating trabecular bone. In, The Osteoporotic Syndrome: Detection, Prevention and Treatment. Ed, Avioli, L.V., Grune and Stratton, New York, 1983, pp 85-114.

5. Nagurka, M.L., and Hayes, W.C.: Technical note: An interactive graphics package for calculating cross-sectional properties of complex shapes. J.Biomech. 13, 59, 1980.

6. Ruff, C.B., and Hayes, W.C.: Subperiosteal expansion and cortical remodeling of the human femur and tibia with aging. Science 217, 945, 1982.

7. Ruff, C.B., and Hayes, W.C.: Cross-sectional geometry of Pecos Pueblo femora and tibiae: A biomechanical investigation. II. Sex, age and site differences. Am.J.Phys.Anthrop. 60, 383, 1983.

8. Ruff, C.B., and Hayes, W.C.: Bone mineral content in the lower limb: Relationship to cross-sectional geometry. J.Bone Joint Surg. 66A, 1024, 1984.

Hip Fracture and Cortical Bone Density in Aging African and Caucasian Populations

L. SOLOMON

Introduction

The progressive loss of bone mass with age is a universal phenomenon, occurring in both sexes and all races from about 40 years on. It begins earlier and is ultimately more marked in women than in men; it shows a linear correlation with age and produces frank osteoporosis with skeletal failure in 30% of caucasians over 70 years of age (Exton-Smith et al, 1969a; Garn et al, 1967; Newton-John and Morgan, 1968; Nordin, 1966).

The frequent occurrence of femoral neck fractures in the elderly is attributed to this bone depletion, and the incidence of such fractures is widely used as an index of osteoporosis in the general population (Chalmers and Ho, 1970). By this measure, postclimacteric bone loss is more pronounced in caucasoid than in black peoples (Gyepes et al, 1962; Solomon, 1968). There are several possible explanations for this phenomenon, but three in particular will be considered:

1) that caucasoids generally (and, by implication, all those destined to develop osteoporosis) have a suboptimal bone mass at maturity, thus running the risk of falling below a putative fracture level after the menopause;

2) that bone mass at maturity is similar in all populations but that some lose bone faster than others after the menopause; or

3) that postclimacteric bone loss slows down or ceases after a few years in some but continues into old age in others.

Ideally, these hypotheses should be tested in longitudinal studies of pupulation subsets. So far, this has proved to be impractical. This paper describes a cross-sectional study of fracture incidence and bone density in black and white populations living in the same urban environment.

Methods

Fracture surveys were conducted in the Johannesburg Metropolitan area over three years. All hospitals and orthopedic surgeons in the area were covered and every patient with a fracture of the femur proximal to the lesser trochanter was included in the study. The population at risk was determined from census figures. Fracture incidence was calculated as the rate for 100,000 of the population per annum.

Current Concepts of Bone Fragility

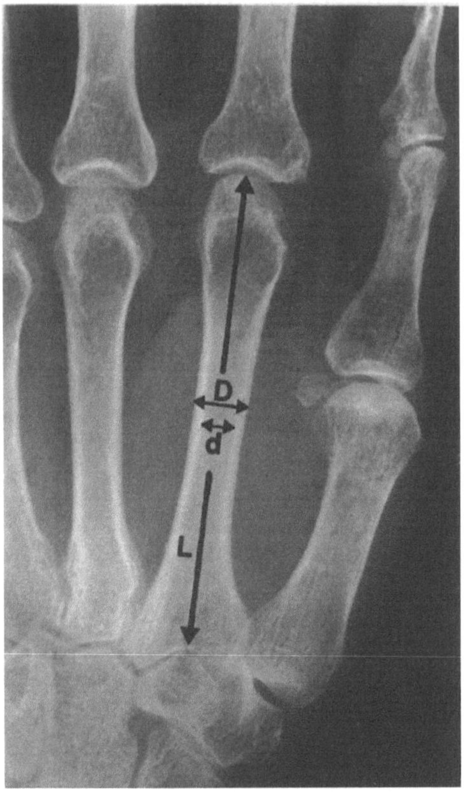

Fig. 1. Measurements made on radiograph of second metacarpus.

Bone status was assessed in two stable suburban communities, one black and one caucasian. In this true random survey, 950 blacks and 782 caucasians were examined and bone measurements were carried out on standard postero-anterior radiographs of the hands. Taking the midpoint of the second metacarpus as the reference site, the outer diameter (D) and the medullary diameter (d) were measured with a direct-reading needle-tipped Vernier micrometer (Fig. 1). The following indices were calculated, taking the mean for the right and left second metacarpi in each case:

1) Cortical thickness = D - d

2) Cortical cross-sectional area = $\frac{\pi}{4}(D^2-d^2)$ or by convention simply D^2-d^2. This is the area index which corresponds to cross-sectional bone mass (Exton-Smith et al, 1969b).

3) The ratio of cortical area to total cross-sectional area = $\frac{D^2-d^2}{D^2}$.

   This ratio index corrects for differences in skeletal size in different population groups and has been shown to have a smaller variance in normal populations than either cortical thickness or cortical area (Nordin et al, 1970).

Mean values at quinquennial intervals were plotted to show the pattern of change throughout the age range.

Results

The age and sex specific incidence of femoral neck fractures in the two communities is shown in Fig. 2. There is a striking rise in the fracture rate in caucasian women from the age of 60 on and, similarly, in caucasian men from the age of 70 on. The black population (over a million) had only four to six femoral neck fractures per annum, and even these were usually caused by severe injuries; they occurred mostly after the age of 70.

Bone density is most closely represented by the ratio index. In the caucasian population it increases rapidly throughout the period of growth to reach a maximum during the third decade in both sexes (Fig. 3). During this time and for some years after, mean values are greater in women than in men. Between 30 and 50 years of age, the proportion of cortical bone falls slightly. At about 50 years of age, the female pattern changes abruptly, and the amount of cortical bone falls progressively by a mean of about 9% per decade. In men, bone density diminishes much less rapidly --

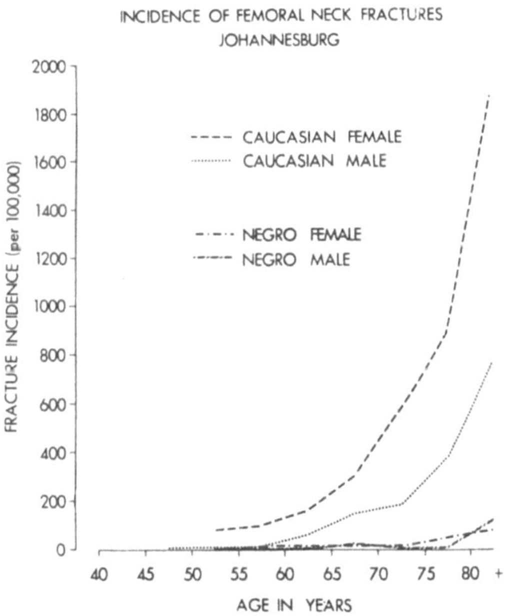

Fig. 2. Age and sex specific incidence of femoral neck frac tures in blacks and caucasians.

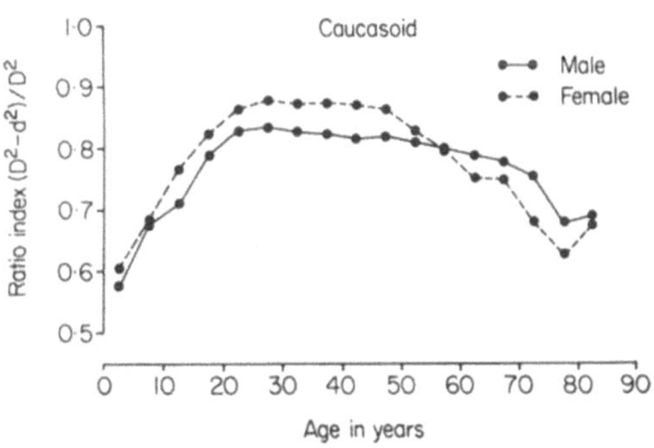

Fig. 3. Age-related pattern of metacarpal cortical density in caucasians.

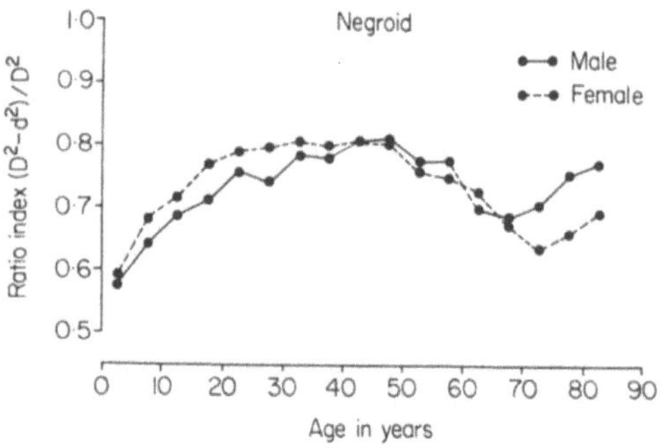

Fig. 4. Age-related pattern of metacarpal cortical density in blacks.

about 4% per decade -- up to 70 years of age; thereafter the rate of bone depletion is the same as that in women.

In blacks, the pattern of change is similar (Fig. 4), but there are important differences in detail. The early increase in bone density is slower than in caucasians and the maximum level is reached only at the end of the fourth decade. Optimal values are, if anything, lower than those of caucasians. From 50 years on, mean skeletal density again shows a steady fall, although the rate of decrease is less than that of caucasians -- 6% per decade in women and 3% in men. Moreover, from the age of 70 on the ratio index plateaus out in both women and men.

Discussion

Avioli's (1977) definition of osteoporosis as "a reduction in bone mass below that which normally characterizes the skeleton for the age, sex and race of an individual" does not allow for the possibility that entire groups (by sex or race) may be osteoporotic in comparison with others. It might be more useful to employ some other term (osteopenia ?) to describe an abnormal reduction in bone mass in an individual member of a group and to regard osteoporosis as a pathologic state leading to actual skeletal failure.

This study emphasizes the complexity of the relationship between cortical bone density and osteoporotic skeletal failure. Absolute values for the ratio index were lower in blacks than in caucasians throughout the age range, yet the femoral neck fracture rate was 20 times greater in caucasians than in blacks. Others have shown that vertebral osteoporosis is also much more common in caucasians than in South African blacks (Dent et al, 1968).

Three hypothetical explanations for the extraordinary difference in fracture rates were examined. The one most commonly espoused is that bone mass in old age is largely determined by the volume of bone at maturity (Newton-John and Morgan, 1968). There was no evidence for this in this study.

This focuses attention on the other explanations. Looking at the pattern of change rather than the absolute values, two interesting facts emerge: postmenopausal bone loss is both more rapid and more persistent in caucasians than in blacks, with a total bone loss of 30% in white women and 21% in black women. This is reflected most markedly in the rapid increase in metacarpal medullary width (Fig. 5 and 6) which, in turn, must be a measure of endosteal resorption after the menopause.

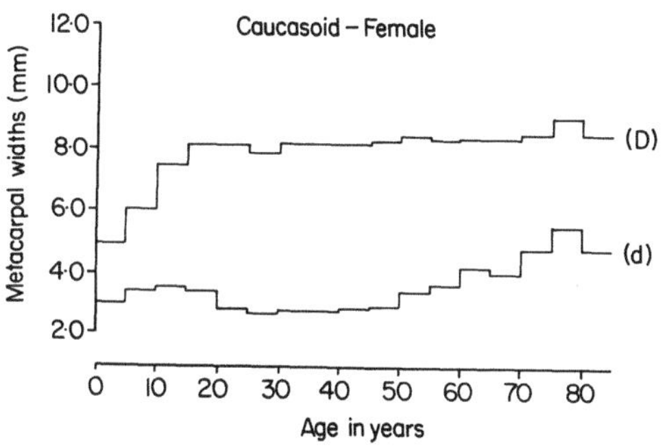

Fig. 5. Age-related change in metacarpal width (D) and medullary width (d) in caucasian women.

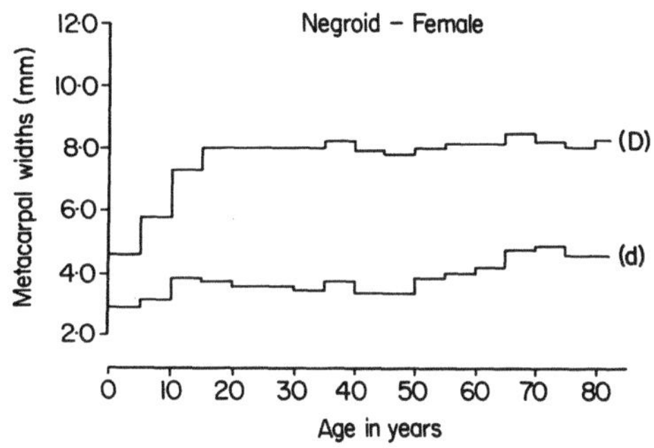

Fig. 6. Age-related change in metacarpal width (D) and medullary width (d) in black women.

Investigators at the Mayo Clinic (Riggs, 1984; Riggs et al, 1982) have presented evidence that involutional osteoporosis comprises at least two distinct syndromes: type I osteoporosis, that occurs soon after the menopause, is associated with mainly trabecular bone loss (vertebral and forearm fractures) and is due to estrogen deficiency and accelerated bone loss; and type II, that occurs much later (after 70 years), involves a steady loss of both cortical and trabecular bone and leads to both vertebral and hip fractures. They suggest that the type II syndrome is due to impaired synthesis of 1,25 $(OH)_2D$, leading to decreased calcium absorption and secondary hyperparathyroidism; a similar disorder occurs in a small proportion of type I patients and these may constitute a third (type III) syndrome.

Viewed against this model, the current study indicates that both types of defect may be less common in blacks than in caucasians. Fractures of the vertebrae and distal radius do occur in blacks but no detailed figures are available. However, the slower rate of postmenopausal bone loss in the black population may be evidence of extraovarian estrogen activity. Equally significant, the rate of bone loss is slower in blacks than in whites over 70 years of age, and this may reflect important differences in vitamin D metabolism.

Whether these comparatively small differences could account for the extraordinary differences in fracture rates remains highly questionable. How, for instance, does one explain the almost total absence of femoral fractures in that considerable segment of the black population whose bone density values fall below the 25th percentile of the caucasian group?

A new hypothesis emerges from these studies: differences in fracture rate in groups with similar bone mass could be explained by differences in the rate of bone turnover -- for the same given mass, a slower turnover rate will predispose to cumulative trabecular fracture because of the tardy renewal of tissue. As yet no comparison of turnover rate has been made in osteoporotic individuals with and those without postmenopausal skeletal failure.

References

1. Avioli, L.V.: Osteoporosis: pathogenesis and therapy. In, Metabolic Bone Disease. Eds: Avioli, L.V. and Krane, S.M. Academic Press, New York, 1977, p 307.
2. Chalmers, J., and Ho, K.C.: Geographical variations in senile osteoporosis. J. Bone Joint Surg. 52B, 667, 1970.
3. Dent, C.E., Engelbrecht, H.E., and Godfrey, R.C.: Osteoporosis of lumbar vertebrae and calcification of abdominal aorta in women living in Durban. Brit.Med.J. iv, 76, 1968.
4. Exton-Smith, A.N., Millard, P.H., Payne, P.R., and Wheeler, E.F.: Pattern of development and loss of bone with age. Lancet ii, 1154, 1969a.
5. Exton-Smith, A.N., Millard, P.H., Payne, P.R., and Wheeler, E.F.: Method for measuring quantity of bone. Lancet ii, 1153, 1969b.
6. Garn, S.M., Rohmann, C.G., and Wagner, B.: Bone loss as a general phenomenon in man. Fed.Proc. 26, 1729, 1967.
7. Gyepes, M., Mellins, H.Z., and Katz, I.: The low incidence of fracture of the hip in the Negro. JAMA 181, 1073, 1962.
8. Newton-John, H.F., and Morgan, D.B.: Osteoporosis: disease or senescence? Lancet i, 232, 1968.
9. Nordin, B.E.C.: International patterns of osteoporosis. Clin.Orthop. 45, 17, 1966.
10. Nordin, B.E.C., Young, M.M., Bulusu, L. and Horsman, A.: Osteoporosis re-examined. In, Osteoporosis. Ed.: Barzel, U.S. Grune and Stratton, New York, 1970, pp 47-67.
11. Riggs, B.L.: Abnormal vitamin D metabolism in involutional osteoporosis. In, Proc. Copenhagen International Symposium on Osteoporosis. Ed: Christiansen, C. et al. Glostrup Hospital, Denmark, 1984. pp 743-750.
12. Riggs, B.L., Wahner, H.W., Seeman, E., Offord, K.P., Dunn, W.L., Mazess, R.B., Johnson, K.A., and Melton, L.J. III: Changes in bone mineral density of the proximal femur and spine with aging. J.Clin. Invest. 70, 716, 1982.
13. Solomon, L.: Osteoporosis and fracture of the femoral neck in the South African Bantu. J. Bone Joint Surg. 50B, 2, 1968.

Hip Fracture: A Disease and an Accident

L. J. Melton III and B. L. Riggs

Introduction

It has long been debated whether hip fractures are best thought of as disease, ie, osteoporosis, or accident. Most investigators believe that age-related bone loss accounts for the rise in hip fracture incidence among the elderly (Consensus Conference 1984), and it has even been suggested that, as a result of osteoporosis, hip fractures can occur without a fall (Reeves, 1977; Smith, 1953). Others claim that osteoporosis has little etiologic relationship to hip fracture risk (Aitken, 1984; Cummings, 1985; Evans et al, 1981; Wicks et al, 1982) and that other determinants such as risk factors for falls are all important (Aitken, 1984; Wicks et al, 1982). We believe, however, that both osteoporosis and trauma are important in the production of hip fractures and that neither alone can completely account for the rise in hip fracture incidence with age. This point of view is based on the evidence outlined below.

Reduced Bone Density Concept

The theoretical fracture threshold has been estimated to lie 2.5 standard deviations (SD) below the mean bone density of young women (Newton-John and Morgan, 1970). Empirically, this prediction has been borne out, with 90% of both cervical and intertrochanteric hip fractures occurring in women with cervical and intertrochanteric bone density values of 0.95 g/cm^2 and 0.92 g/cm^2, respectively (Riggs et al, 1982). These figures lie 2.4 SD and 2.2 SD below the respective means for normal women 30 years of age.

Newton-John and Morgan (1970) hypothesized that the age-related rise in fracture incidence was due to progressively greater proportions of women falling below the fracture threshold as age increased. Our population-based studies in Rochester, Minnesota do, indeed, show that the proportion of women with cervical or intertrochanteric bone mineral density (BMD) below 1.0 g/cm^2, as measured by dual photon absorptiometry (Riggs et al, 1982), rises with age (Fig. 1). Moreover, these curves have the same sigmoidal shape predicted by Newton-John and Morgan (1970).

Could this age-related change in the proportion of women below the fracture threshold completely account for the rise in hip fracture incidence rates with age? If so, we should be able to eliminate this effect by recalculating the rates to include in the population at risk only those women in each

Current Concepts of Bone Fragility

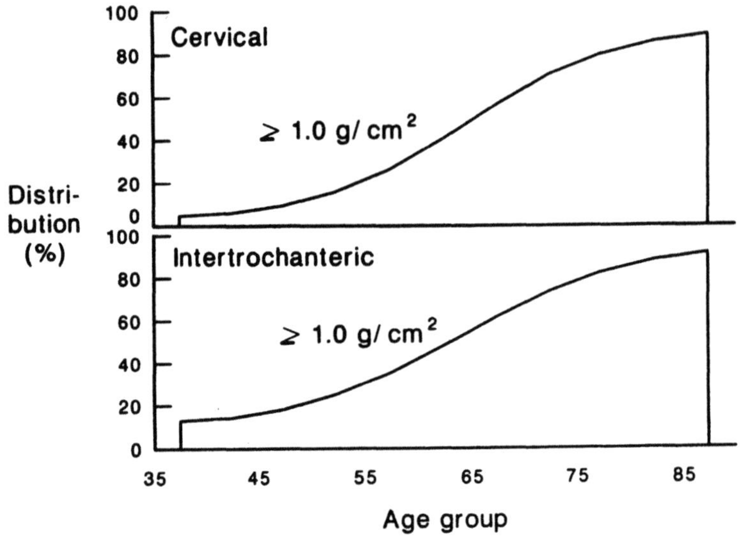

Fig. 1. Proportion (%) of Rochester, Minnesota women, by age with cervical and intertrochanteric bone mineral density ≧1.0 g/cm² and ≦1.0 g/cm². (With permission of J.Clin.Invest.)

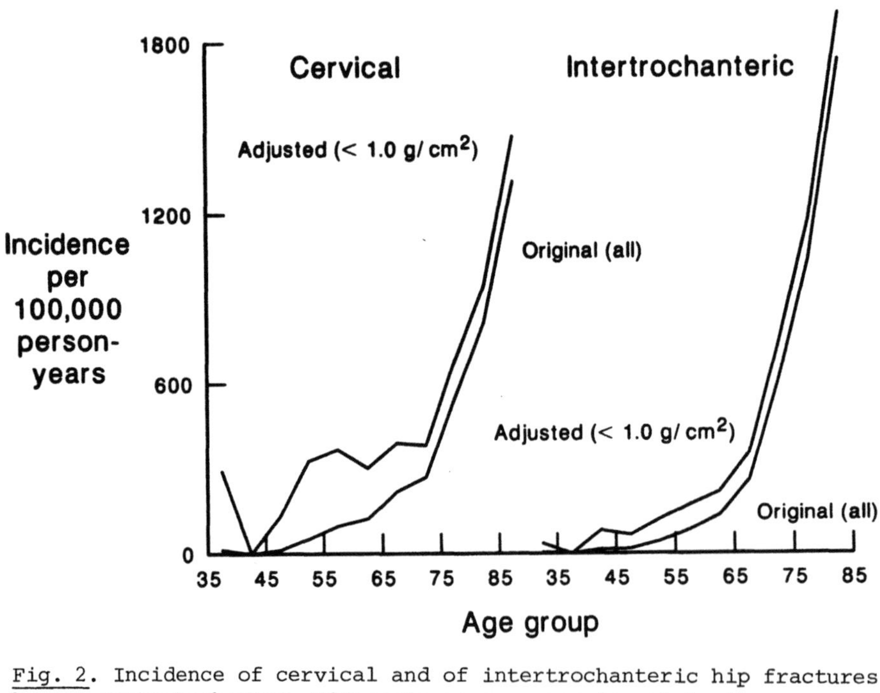

Fig. 2. Incidence of cervical and of intertrochanteric hip fractures by age among Rochester, Minnesota women, assuming that all women are at risk (original) or that only those women are at risk who have cervical or intertrochanteric femoral bone mineral density <1.0 g/cm² (adjusted). (With permission of J.Clin.Invest.)

age-group with femoral BMD <1.0 g/cm². The original estimates of hip fracture incidence require no information about BMD levels and assume that all women are at risk (Fig. 2). The basic formula used is the following:

$$\text{Incidence}(\text{age-group}_i) = \frac{\text{Number of newly diagnosed hip fractures among Rochester women in age-group}_i \text{ during the study period}}{\text{Number of person-years at risk among all Rochester women in age-group}_i \text{ during the study period}} \times 100{,}000$$

The adjusted rates, also shown in Figure 2, assume that all observed hip fractures are in women with BMD <1.0 g/cm² and, further, that the appropriate denominator in each age-group is that proportion of the total who have cervical or intertrochanteric BMD <1.0 g/cm² as estimated from a recent population-based random sample of Rochester women. It is clear from examining the figure that this adjustment procedure left the shape of the age-specific incidence curve largely unchanged. Thus, even within the population at risk with femoral BMD <1.0 g/cm², hip fracture incidence rates rise with age.

Trauma Concept

Consequently, other age-related factors, in addition to changes in the proportion of women with BMD <1.0 g/cm², must also be important in the etiology of fractures. One such factor may be falls: either an increased frequency of falls or increased traumatic energy in the falls (Melton and Riggs, 1985a). Falls alone are not a sufficient cause of these fractures either, however, as indicated by epidemiologic data showing that most falls, even among the elderly, do not result in significant injury. Rodstein (1964) found that only 1.4% of falls in a nursing home resulted in a major injury. The proportion found by Ashley and coworkers (1977) in a home for the aged was greater at 17.5%, but only eight femur fractures were observed in 651 falls. Others have reported similar results (Baker and Harvey, 1985; Berry et al, 1981; Sehested and Severin-Nielsen, 1977).

Conclusion

What then determines the occurrence of fractures? As already reported (Melton and Riggs, 1985b), the incidence of proximal femur fractures was negligible among Rochester women 35 years old and over who had bone density levels greater than 1.0 g/cm². However, the gradient of fracture risk increased with decreasing bone density below the 1.0 g/cm² level. Based on these and other risk estimates (Cann et al, 1985; Iskrant and Smith, 1969; Jensen et al, 1983), it seems reasonable to conclude that bone loss (≈ osteoporosis) is a necessary, if not sufficient, cause of the important age-related fractures. Likewise, trauma, usually in the form of a simple fall, is also a necessary but rarely a sufficient cause of limb fractures in the elderly. Together, falls and reduced skeletal resistance to trauma are thus shown to be important determinants of fracture risk. Hip fractures are, therefore, both an accident and a disease.

Acknowledgements

The authors would like to thank Miss Mary Ramaker for help in preparing the manuscript.

This work was supported in part by research grants AM-27065 and AM-30582 from the National Institutes of Health.

References

1. Aitken, J.M.: Relevance of osteoporosis in women with fractures of the femoral neck. Br. Med. J. 288, 597, 1984.
2. Ashley, M.J., Gryfe, C.I., and Amies, A.: A longitudinal study of falls in an elderly population. II. Some circumstances of falling. Age Ageing 6, 211, 1977.
3. Baker, S.P., and Harvey, A.H.: Fall injuries in the elderly. Symposium on Falls in the Elderly: Biological and Behavioral Aspects. Clin. Geriatr. Med. 1, 1985,
4. Berry, G., Fisher, R.H., and Lang, S.: Detrimental incidents, including falls, in an elderly institutional population. J. Am. Geriatr. Soc. 29, 322, 1981.
5. Cann, C.E., Genant, H.K., Kolb, F.O., and Ettinger, B.: Quantitative computed tomography for prediction of vertebral fracture risk. Bone 6, 1, 1985.
6. Consensus Conference - Osteoporosis. J.A.M.A. 252, 799, 1984.
7. Cummings, S.R.: Are patients with hip fractures more osteoporotic? Review of the evidence. Am. J. Med. 78, 487, 1985.
8. Evans, R.A., Ashwell, J.R., and Dunstan, C.R.: Lack of metabolic bone disease in patients with fracture of the femoral neck. Aust. NZ J. Med. 11, 158, 1981.
9. Iskrant, A.P., and Smith, R.W. Jr.: Osteoporosis in women 45 years and over related to subsequent fractures. Public Health Rep. 84, 33, 1969.
10. Jensen, G.F., Christiansen, C., Boesen, J., Hegadüs, V., Transbøl, I.: Relationship between bone mineral content and frequency of postmenopausal fractures. Acta Med. Scand. 213, 61, 1983.
11. Melton, L.J., and Riggs, B.L.: Risk factors for injury after a fall. Symposium on Falls in the Elderly: Biological and Behavioral Aspects. Clin. Geriatr. Med. 1, 1, 1985a.
12. Melton, L.J., and Riggs, B.L.: Impaired bone strength and fracture pattern at different skeletal sites: In, Current Concepts of Bone Fragility in Orthopaedics and Medicine. Eds: Uhthoff, H.-K. and Stahl, E., Springer-Verlag, 1985b.
13. Newton-John, H.F., and Morgan, D.B.: The loss of bone with age, osteoporosis and fractures. Clin. Orthop. 71, 229, 1970.
14. Reeves, B.: What comes first, the fracture or the fall? A study of subcapital fractures. J. Bone Joint Surg. 59B, 375, 1977.

15. Riggs, B.L., Wahner, H.W., Seeman, E., Offord, K.P., Dunn, W.L., Mazess, R.B., Johnson, K.A., and Melton, L.J. III: Changes in bone mineral density of the proximal femur and spine with aging: Differences between the postmenopausal and senile osteoporosis syndromes. J. Clin. Invest. 70, 716, 1982.

16. Rodstein, M.: Accidents among the aged: Incidence, causes, and prevention. J. Chronic Dis. 17, 515, 1964.

17. Sehested, P., and Severin-Nielsen, T.: Falls by hospitalized elderly patients: Causes, prevention. Geriatrics 32, 101, 1977.

18. Smith, L.D.: Hip fractures: The role of muscle contraction or intrinsic forces in the causation of fractures of the femoral neck. J. Bone Joint Surg. 35A, 367, 1953.

19. Wicks, M., Garrett, R., Vernon-Roberts, B., and Fazzalari, N.: Absence of metabolic bone disease in the proximal femur in patients with fracture of the femoral neck. J. Bone Joint Surg. 64B, 319, 1982.

Economic and Social Burden of Osteoporosis

S. NAROD and R. A. SPASOFF

Introduction

With the aging of our population, health problems like osteoporosis are assuming greater importance. We can assess osteoporosis by means of suitable diagnostic instruments. Radiographs are considered inadequate for this purpose as they may not detect any abnormality until bone loss approaches 30% (Consensus Conference, 1984). Dual photon absorptiometry has been recently used by Melton (1985) to estimate the distribution of vertebral mineral density. To our knowledge, this technique has not yet been applied to any Canadian population.

To assess the economic and social impact of osteoporosis, we must focus on its major clinical effects, ie, fractures. We will first present Canadian data for several fractures, and illustrate their use to estimate the economic and social burden from the disease.

Data Sources

Statistics Canada routinely collects data on deaths from all causes (Statistics Canada, 1984), hospital separations from acute care hospitals (Statistics Canada, 1982a), and surgical procedures performed (Statistics Canada, 1982b). We have examined the data for fractures of the radius, humerus, and hip. Patients with fractures of the spine are so irregularly hospitalized that hospital data are not meaningful. Similarly, hospital data will greatly underestimate the incidence rates for fractures of the humerus and wrist. Almost all hip fractures will be admitted to hospital, but because there may be multiple admissions for a single fracture, hospital separation data (which consider each individual admission) may overestimate the actual incidence rates. Since most femoral neck fractures receive a single corrective procedure, we believe that the data for surgical procedures best estimate the incidence of hip fractures in Canada.

In addition, we reviewed the charts of all patients discharged from the Ottawa Civic Hospital with a primary diagnosis of fracture of the neck of the femur between May 1, 1983 and April 30, 1984. Patients under the age of 65, those who had evidence of other underlying bone disease, and those who had suffered moderate to severe trauma (invariably motor vehicle accidents) were excluded.

Current Concepts of Bone Fragility

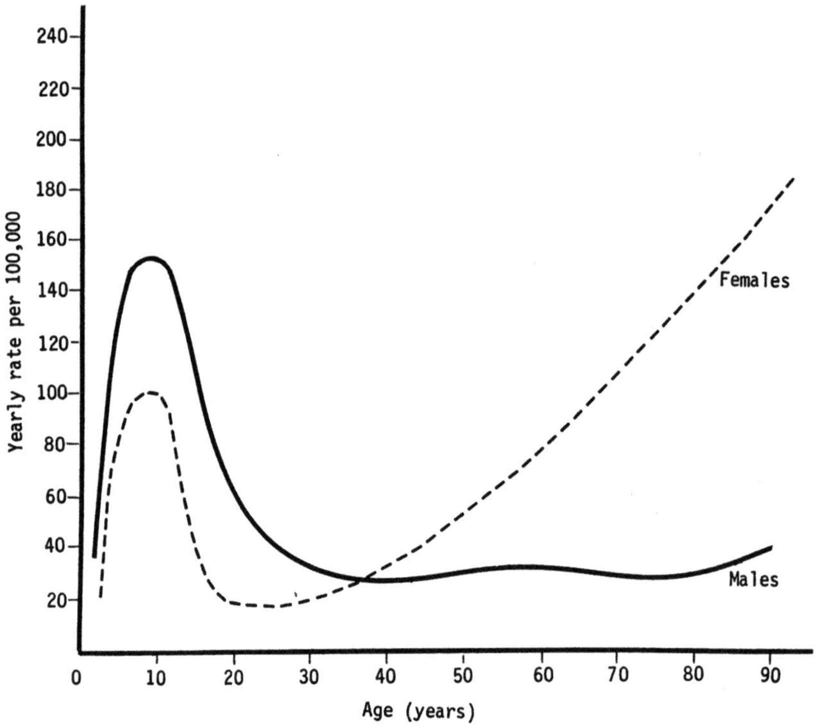

Fig. 1. Fractures of radius/ulna. Hospital separations, Canada 1980-1981.

Demographic projections were borrowed from the Woods Gordon report on the Impact of Demographic Change on the Health Care System, prepared for the Task Force on the Allocation of Health Care Resources in 1984 (Woods Gordon, 1984). The median projections used here assume constant fertility and mortality, with a net migration of 80,000 per year (lower than at present).

Morbidity

Although hospitalization reports for wrist fractures underestimate the total number of such fractures, a characteristic pattern for those fractures emerges (Fig. 1). We see a bimodal distribution, the first peak representing the traumatic fractures of youth, and the later increase -- seen only in women -- representing the effects of postmenopausal bone loss. This is the pattern described as postmenopausal or Type I osteoporosis (Riggs and Melton, 1983), with fractures beginning to increase with the menopause and therefore becoming frequent in women only. It is characterized by accelerated loss primarily of trabecular bone. The levelling off of the rate after the age of 65, described by Riggs and Melton, is not seen in the Canadian data. This may be due to an increased tendency to hospitalize with advancing age, but were this the case we would expect to see the effect in the curve for men as well.

Fractures of the humerus (not illustrated) demonstrate a similar bimodal pattern, becoming more common in women after age 45. Thereafter, the fracture rate doubles approximately every ten years.

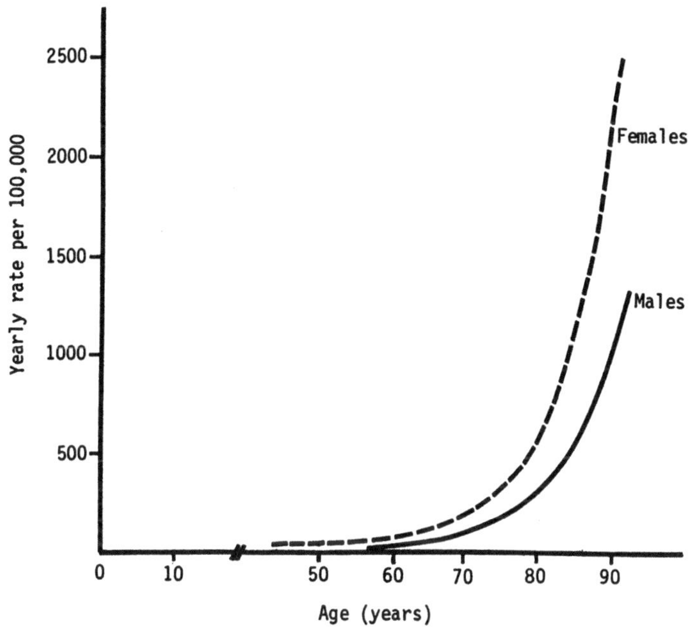

Fig. 2. Fractures of neck of femur. Surgical procedures, Canada 1980-81.

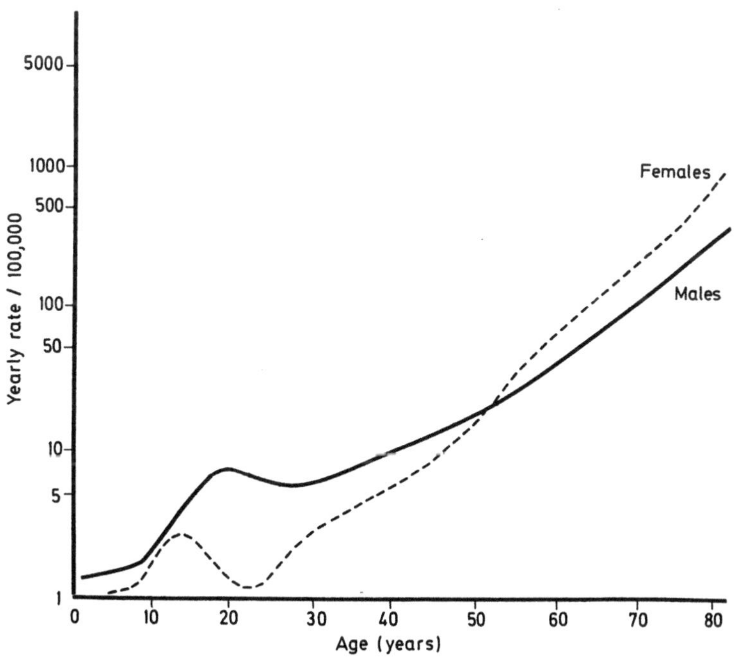

Fig. 3. Fractures of neck of femur. Surgical procedures, Canada 1980-81.

The effect of aging is most pronounced on fractures of the hip (Fig. 2). This senile or Type II osteoporosis is believed to result with age from the linear loss of both cortical and trabecular bone. The rarity of these fractures before 70 years of age is quite distinct from the pattern for Colles fractures of the wrist, and supports the idea that the two have separate origins. When we examine the logarithmically-transformed version of the same data (Fig. 3), we see the risk beginning much earlier, around age 30, and doubling approximately every five years thereafter. From these figures we have calculated that 13% of Canadian women will suffer from a fractured hip by age 85.

The incidence of hip fractures in Canada approximates that of the northern European countries and Israel (Matkovic et al, 1980)(Fig. 4; Table I). The United States figure is surprisingly higher than our Canadian estimate, a discrepancy difficult to explain. The United States rates are based on the experience in Rochester, Minnesota from 1965 to 1974 (Gallagher et al, 1980), whereas the Canadian data are based on national hospitalization records for the year 1981. Since no reports have been published to show that the hip fracture rate is declining in North America, secular change is an unlikely explanation for the difference. Age and sex effects have been removed by standardization. The populations of Rochester and Canada are both predominantly caucasian, so that racial differences cannot explain the discrepancy. The Rochester study excluded trauma victims. We were unable to do this with the Canadian data base, but the net effect of this discrepancy in methods would be to reduce the difference between the Canadian and United States

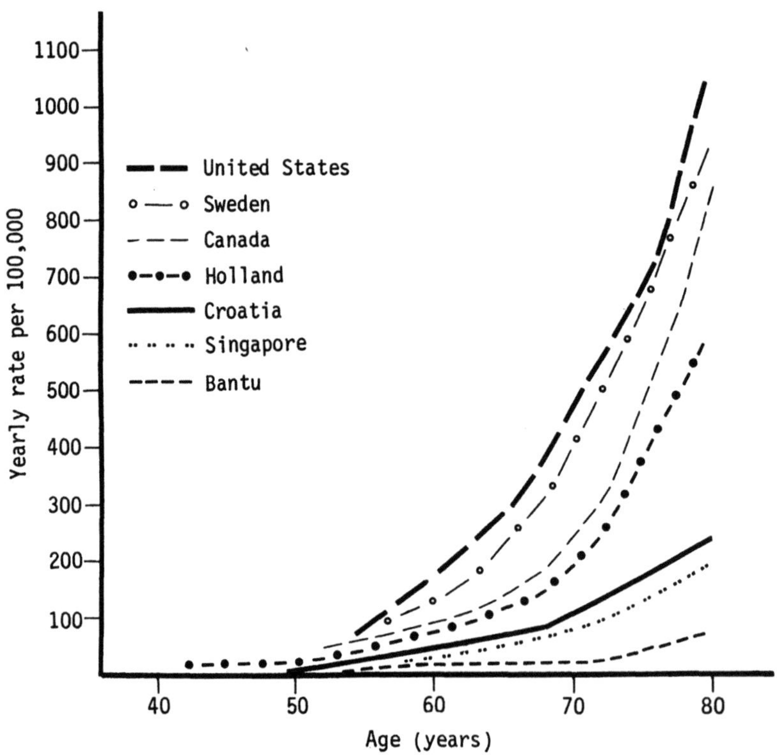

Fig. 4. Fractures of hip. Age-specific incidence for seven countries.

Table I. Age-adjusted* annual incidence of fractures per 100,000

Location	Male	Female
United States	42.9	124.5
Malmo	32.5	105.5
Canada	32.7	89.8
Jerusalem	35.8	82.4
Finland	25.6	61.5
Holland	23.9	54.6
Hong Kong	23.4	39.2
Yugoslavia	16.7	22.4
Singapore	24.0	18.9
Bantu	4.9	6.2

* Adjusted to 1977 United States population

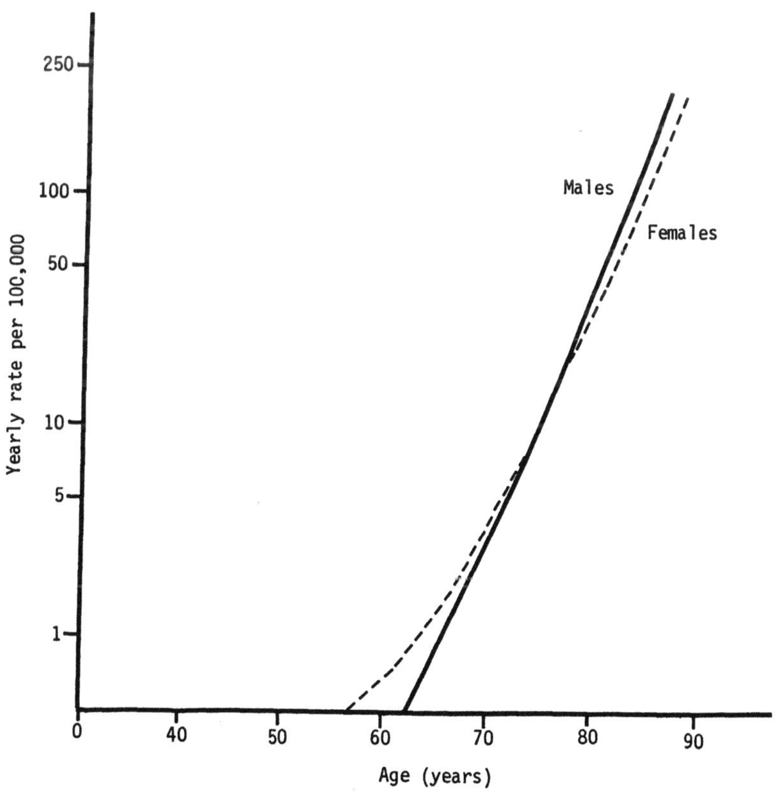

Fig. 5. Fractures of neck of femur. Mortality rate, Canada 1981-82

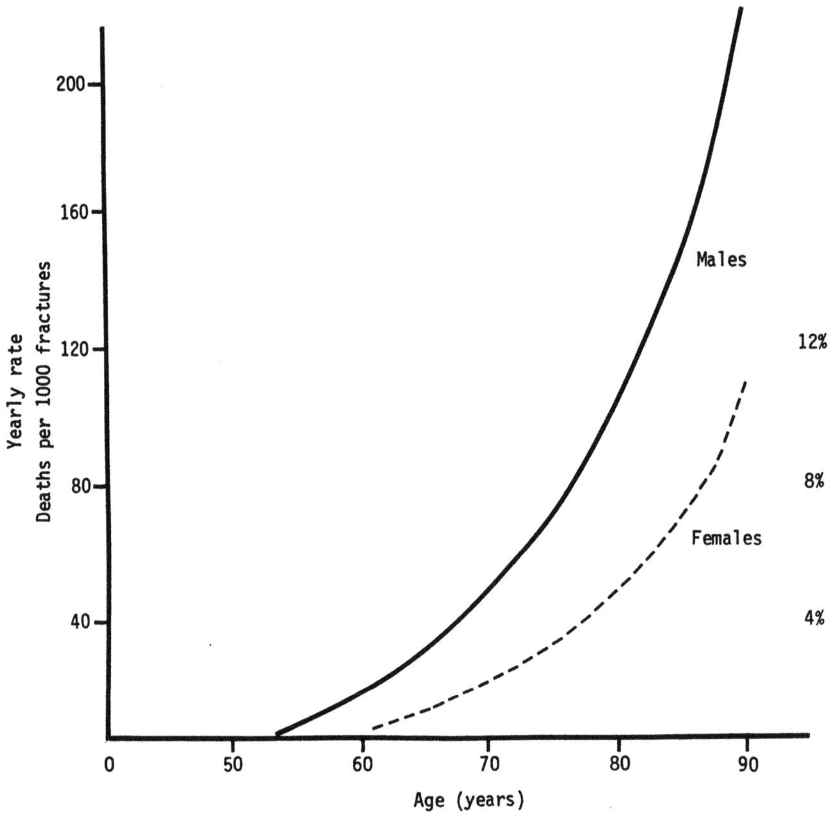

Fig. 6. Fractures of neck of femur. Case fatality rate, Canada 1980-81.

Table II. Taxonomy of the economic burden of ill health

A. Direct costs

1. Personal health care
   a) hospital costs
   b) nonhospital medical care costs
   c) other costs

2. Nonpersonal, public health care costs

3. Education

4. Research

B. Indirect costs

1. Mortality

2. Morbidity
   a) treated (institutional)
   b) untreated

Source: Adapted from Fraser, R.D., Spasoff, R.A. and Prime, M.: An Estimate of the Economic Burden of Ill-health, Ontario Council of Health, 1976 rates. It may be that the high rates of fracture discovered in Rochester cannot be qeneralized for the entire United States. Apart from racial mixture, Olmstead county residents likely differ from Americans as a whole in a number of ways, including diet, hysterectomy rates, use of estrogens, exercise, etc. Finally, the Rochester rates are based on a single community and are subject to sampling error.

Mortality

Hip fracture is the only complication of osteoporosis likely to cause death. Although commonly thought of as a problem of elderly women, the mortality rate for this fracture varies little between the sexes (Fig. 5). The incidence of fractures is higher in women than in men, but the case fatality rate is much higher in Canadian men (Fig. 6). In 1981, a man with a hip fracture was twice as likely to die as a result of complications than a woman of similar age with a similar problem.

Economic Burden

Estimates of economic burden should address direct costs and indirect costs attributable to the disease (Table II).

Direct costs

Direct costs include health care -- acute hospital care, long-term care, physicians' services and drugs -- along with certain public expenditures which are smaller and are not addressed here. Since the satisfactory data are available only for hospital costs, and since fractured hips are the only complication of osteoporosis which are regularly treated in hospital, we will focus on these fractures.

Acute hospital care costs

These are difficult to estimate in Canada because our system of hospital accounting does not identify costs associated with the care of individual patients. A conventional approach has been to multiply the average length of stay for the condition by the average per diem cost. Thus, the average length of stay for hip fractures in Canada was 30.5 days in 1981 (the last year for which data are available) and the average per diem cost for Canadian hospital was $295.00 in 1984 (Fournier, 1985), leading to an estimate of $8,998.00 for the hospital care of each hip fracture (Table III). To this

Table III. Costs* of acute care for hip fractures

Location	Year	Hospital	Physician	Total
Canada	1984	$8,998.	$ 467.	$9,465.
Kingston	1983	$4,850.	$ 450.	$5,000.
London	1983	$5,550.	$ 450.	$6,000.
Rochester	1976	$4,269.(US)	$1,203.(US)	$5,472.(US)

* Approximate

should be added the fees for surgical and anesthetic care -- $467.00 in Ontario in 1984 (Ontario Health Insurance Plan, 1984) -- for a total cost of $9,465.00 for the acute care of each fracture. Obviously, the hospital component of this figure is a crude estimate since not all days of care are of equal intensity. Knowledgable individuals have advised us that it is likely an overestimate since hip fractures are relatively inexpensive to care for.

More sophisticated costing procedures estimate the costs of individual patients' care by measuring the variable costs associated with their care (input of personnel time, supplies, etc), and allocating to them a percentage of the fixed institutional costs (eg, overhead and capital costs). We have obtained data from two recent studies in Ontario. A 1983 study at the Kingston General Hospital (Shaw, 1985) produced an estimate of just over $5,000.00 per case for combined hospital and medical care; the costs varied depending on whether fixation or hip replacement was undertaken, but the final costs for the two approaches were remarkably similar. A study at St. Joseph's Hospital in London (Bock, 1985) produced an estimate of just over $6,000.00 for the total costs of acute care for 1983. These two estimates are remarkably consistent, and confirm the suspicion that the earlier crude estimate was too high. Turning to the United States, a 1976 study from Rochester (Owen et al, 1980) estimated $5,500.00 for the costs of acute care only.

On the basis of these estimates, we consider that $6,000.00 is a reasonable estimate for the cost of acute care in Ontario in 1984.

Rehabilitation care

This is the next major component which ought to be addressed, but we lack national data for the proportion of cases who go to rehabilitation services. Although data from the Hospital Medical Records Institute indicate the immediate destination of patients discharged from participating hospitals, rehabilitation services are provided in so broad a range of facilities that the data are difficult to interpret. Review of a small sample of cases at the Ottawa Civic Hospital revealed that 13% of patients were transferred directly to rehabilitation facilities, an estimate which is close to one provided by a local physiatrist. The estimated duration of stay in Ottawa-Carleton is 40 days (Simard, 1985). The average daily cost of rehabilitation in Canada was $217.00 in 1983-84; naturally this is subject to the problems noted above regarding average costs of care, but here we have no alternatives. Of our sample, 37% of patients were transferred to some interim institutional care, whether rehabilitation or other. Although the total cost of this care is unknown, it could easily add $3,500.00 to the cost of care when the costs of physicians' services are considered (daily costs of $217.00 for hospital care plus an estimated $20.00 for physicians' services over a period of 40 days, for 37% of patients).

Long-term care

Even more imponderable is the cost of the long-term care occasioned by hip fractures. We lack information systems which will track patients through the health care system beyond rehabilitation or convalescent care, and in any case some patients soon go into care for other reasons; it is therefore difficult to determine the proportion that should be attributed to hip fractures. Of our sample, 21% went directly to a chronic care facility following discharge from a general hospital.

Total direct costs

We are finally ready to attempt an estimate of the total direct costs of hip fractures to the Canadian population. Statistics Canada data for surgical procedures suggest an incidence of 11,102 hip fractures in Canada in 1981 among persons aged 65 and over. We are prepared to ascribe all these cases to osteoporosis. At $6,000.00 per fracture, this comes to $66.6 million dollars for the total cost of acute care. When we add another $3,500.00 per case for rehabilitation and convalescent care, we come to a total of just over $100 million per year, identical (on a per capita basis) to a recent estimate of $1 billion per year for the United States (Owen et al, 1980). This works out to 0.4% of total Canadian health care costs, but is certainly an underestimate due to the exclusion of long-term care costs and to the smaller but certainly significant costs of manifestations of osteoporosis other than hip fracture.

Indirect costs

Indirect costs refer to economic effects other than health care costs, and are usually measured in terms of lost productivity due to morbidity and premature mortality. Again, we are short of data, but this time it may not matter as much since the victims of osteoporotic hip fractures are rarely in the work force. We note, however, the inability of this approach to deal adequately with retired persons and with housewives, both of whom figure prominently among the victims of osteoporosis. The effects on these patients will be considered under the heading of social impact. Another type of indirect economic impact should be counted. Many of the victims of hip fractures are women, many of whom have husbands. When such a patient becomes incapacitated and must move into an institution, chances are that her husband will be unable to care for himself and will also have to enter an institution. The amount of the resulting long-term care is unknown.

Social Impact

Here we consider all the noneconomic impacts of osteoporosis, ie, those not affecting economic productivity, but many associated manifestations of osteoporosis in addition to hip fractures. These impacts might be considered under three headings:

1) Pain and suffering - An attempt is sometimes made to place an economic value on these consequences, usually based either on court awards for similar afflictions or on subjective values placed on them by panels of raters.

2) Decreased functional ability and quality of life - We are not aware of any population data which address this question, but note that musculoskeletal complaints are the leading cause of disability in Canada (Health and Welfare Canada and Statistics Canada, 1981).

3) Loss of independence - As noted above, our information systems do not yet allow us to track the flow of patients through the health care system. The Ontario Placement Coordination Services are currently trying to develop such a system.

Table IV. Patient flow through a teaching hospital (hip fractures)

Origin	Destination*								
	Home	Home aged	Nurs. home	Chrn. hosp.	Gen. hosp.	Rehab. hosp.	Conv. home	Died	Total
Home	31	1	2	17	20	16	4	4	95
HFA	-	8	1	4	3	-	-	3	19
NH	-	-	5	3	7	2	-	5	22
CH	-	-	-	3	-	-	-	-	3
Total	31	9	8	27	30	18	4	12	139

* 20/95 = 21% of those at home entered long-term care
18/139 = 13% went directly to rehabilitation facility
52/139 = 37% went to an interim institution

Our review of the patients treated in an Ottawa teaching hospital revealed (Table IV) that of 139 patients, 9% died while in hospital, 34% returned to the same residence from which they had come, while 20% went to a more intensive level of institutional care; unfortunately, the disposition of 37% was unknown because they went to an intermediate placement such as another general hospital, a rehabilitation facility, a convalescent home, or because the institution to which they went was not coded. Of those who were living independently before the fracture, 21% went straight to institutional care and 4% died; thus, over one-quarter never went home.

Projections

The aging of our population is well known. The Woods Gordon study predicted that the proportion of the population aged 65 or older will increase from 9.7% at present to 13.0% by the year 2001 and to 18.2% by 2021. We have

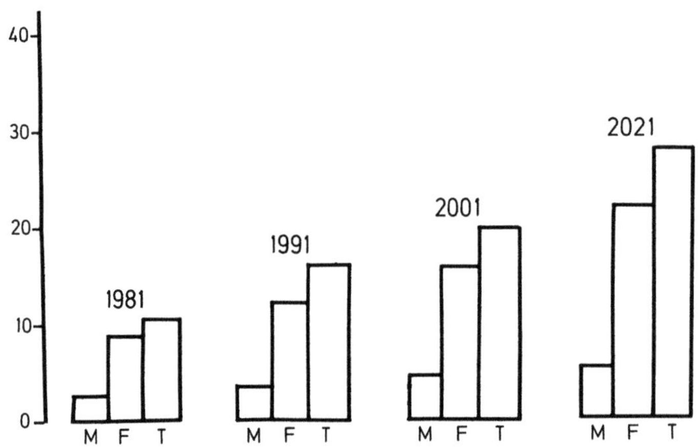

Fig. 7. Fractures of hip - projected number by year.
Canada - Totals (thousands), ages 65 and above.

applied to these figures the age-specific incidence rates displayed earlier. The results (Fig. 7) show that the number of hip fractures in older persons will almost double by the year 2001, and will increase 2.5 times by the year 2021 to about 28,000 per year, unless we are able to prevent some of this morbidity.

Summary

We have presented data drawn primarily from Canadian health statistics to provide a Canadian perspective of the social and economic burden of osteoporosis, and to show the possibilities and the limitations of routinely collected data. We have illustrated the use of these data in estimating the economic and social costs of this growing problem, especially in the elderly. Finally, we have estimated the future impact of this problem, if current patterns continue.

References

1. Bock, C.: Personal communication, 1985.
2. Consensus Conference: Osteoporosis. JAMA 252,792, 1984
3. Fournier, L.: Personal communication, 1985.
4. Gallagher, J.C., Melton, L.J., Riggs, B.L., and Bergstrath, E.: Epidemiology of fractures of the proximal femur in Rochester, Minnesota. Clin. Orthop.Rel.Res. 150, 163, 1980.
5. Health and Welfare Canada and Statistics Canada: The health of Canadians: Report of the Canada Health Survey. Statistics Canada Publication #82-538, 1981.
6. Matkovic, V., et al: Osteoporosis and epidemiology of fractures in Croatia: an international comparison. Henry Ford Hosp.Med.J. 28, 116, 1980.
7. Melton, L.J.: Strength and fracture patterns at different sites. Proc. Current Concepts of Bone Fragility in Orthopaedics and Medicine, University of Ottawa, 1985; Springer-Verlag.
8. Ontario Health Insurance Plan: Schedule of Benefits, 1984.
9. Owen, R.A., Melton, L.J., Gallagher, J.C., and Riggs, B.L.: The national cost of acute care of hip fractures associated with osteoporosis. Clin. Orthop.Rel.Res. 150, 172, 1980.
10. Riggs, B.L., and Melton, L.J.: Evidence for two distinct syndromes of involutional osteoporosis. Amer.J.Med. 75, 899, 1983.
11. Shaw, T.: Personal communication, 1985.
12. Simard, R.: Personal communication, 1985.
13. Statistics Canada: Causes of Death. Publication #84-203, Annual, 1984.
14. Statistics Canada: Hospital Morbidity. Publication #82-206, Annual, 1982a.
15. Statistics Canada: Surgical Procedures and Treatments. Publication #82-208, Annual, 1982b.
16. Woods-Gordon: Investigation of the impact of demographic change on the health care system in Canada. Task Force on the Allocation of Health Care Resources, August 1984.

Involutional Osteoporosis. Critical Evaluation of Medical Treatments

C. Anderson

Introduction

A review of the published reports on the medical treatment for involutional osteoporosis leaves the skeptical reader with a number of questions. This presentation will only deal with four of these: 1) the statistical acceptability of results obtained from these studies when the measured end point is a reduction in fracture rates; 2) the interpretation of results obtained from the application of indirect measurements to individuals at risk of losing bone or who have lost bone; 3) incomplete knowledge concerning the physiopathology of bone loss or the cellular response to pharmacologic agents; and 4) inattention to concomitant morbid conditions which contribute to an increased incidence of fractures.

Data Analysis and Discussion

1) No statistically acceptable results can be obtained from prospective double-blind trials, even when conducted on a sufficiently large population sample size at risk, if the measured end point is a reduction in fracture rates.

Since the initial manifestations of postmenopausal osteoporosis are related to events occurring in the axial skeleton, an attempt to measure a reduction in the rates of these events is sought as an index of therapeutic adequacy.

This premise is based on the fact that these events -- whether clinically manifest or not -- may occur at a constant rate. However, Kanis (1984) has reported that a careful study of the published literature suggests that these events may occur at a declining rate from the time a group of patients with the condition is observed. Furthermore, this author noted that the rate of these events occurring in the axial skeleton varied inversely with the duration of two published studies (Nordin et al, 1980; Riggs et al, 1982), whether these were treated or control patients.

Let us assume, based on a controlled clinical trial, that the following published figures are correct (Table I): the vertebral body fracture rates in normal healthy elderly women is 0.23% per 100 patient years; the vertebral body fracture rates in patients with symptomatic osteoporosis is 9.2% per 100 years; and patients with symptomatic osteoporosis have subclinical vertebral body fracture rates of 83.4% per 100 patients years. If we were

Current Concepts of Bone Fragility

Table I. Necessary sample size (test and controls) to have 90% probability of detecting a significant difference in incidence of osteoporotic fractures*

Fall in fracture frequency	Sample size for estimated incidence of		
	0.23 $p < 0.05$	9.2 $p < 0.05$	83.4 $p < 0.05$
50%	65,400	1500	38

* Using two-tailed tests of significance.
Modified from J.A. Kanis, Lancet 1, 27-33, 1984

to expect a reduction in spinal event rates of 50% between treated and control patients at a level of significance of less than 5%, we would require 65,400 patients in the first instance, 1,500 patients in the second instance, and 38 patients in the third. Anyone attempting to establish a therapeutic trial for postmenopausal osteoporosis realizes how utopic the first two figures are, while Kleerekoper (1984) has clearly indicated that after intensive recruitment of patients with pure postmenopausal osteoporosis, approximately one quarter of these will be judged to have adequately completed a controlled treatment protocol. Thus, even the latter figure is not easily achieved.

2) Most studies to date report the application of indirect measurements of bone mass/volume in individuals considered at risk of losing bone or in individuals who have lost bone.

Due to the prevalence of clinical events comprising the axial skeleton, investigators have developed a variety of procedures to measure either rates of bone loss in a susceptible population or rates of bone accretion in previously bone-depleted patients (Parfitt, 1983). The methods currently employed for measuring trabecular (vertebral body) bone include histomorphometry, photodensitometry, compton-scatter, dual-energy photon absorptiometry, and computed tomography.

In our center, gross discrepancies have been observed using histomorphometric assessment of trabecular bone in iliac crest bone biopsies and dual-energy photon absorptiometry of the spine. Until further studies are carried out to elucidate intermethodologic correlations, the real significance of the particular measurement employed will always be disputed. For example, does trabecular bone volume and behavior at the iliac crest actually reflect volume and behavior of vertebral trabecular bone? Do radiologic methods actually measure bone volume or only bone mineral? The implications of these questions bear greatly on the course of any proposed treatment of the bone-depleted patient (Fig. 1 and 2).

3) Current knowledge is incomplete as to the pathophysiology of bone loss or the cellular responses to pharmacologic agents.

Figure 3 reflects currently accepted changes in bone volume from birth to senescence. During the growth period, the skeleton is modelled and remodeled until all epiphyseal growth plates disappear. Then follows a pro-

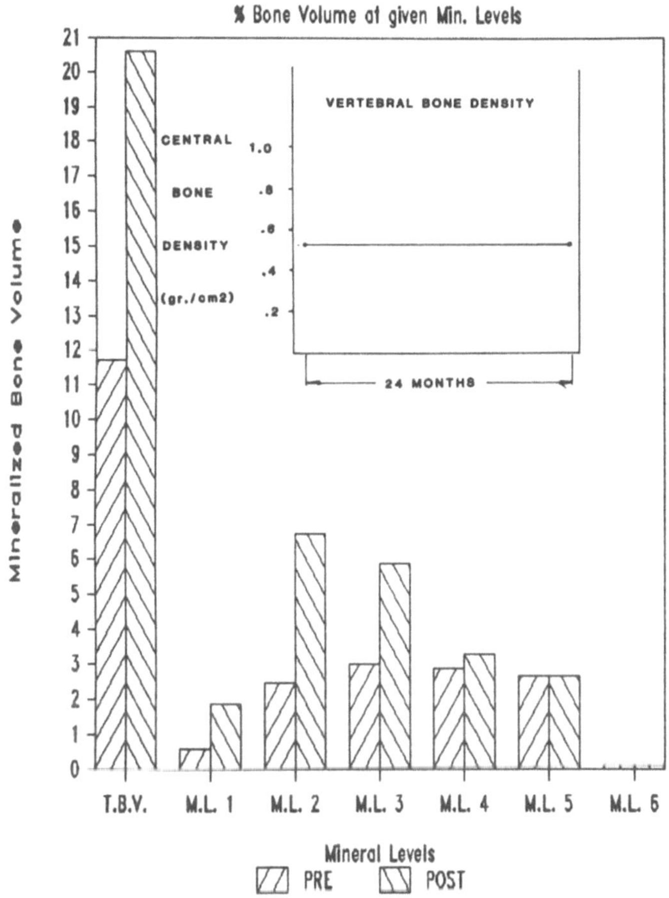

Fig. 1. Discrepancies between results of measurements of trabecular bone volume/mass by histomorphometric analyses of two transiliac crest bone biopsies and two dual beam photon absorptiometric readings of the spine. The patient had postmenopausal osteoporosis and had undergone eight cycles of coherence therapy for osteoporosis (Anderson et al, 1984). By histomorphometric analysis of iliac crest trabecular bone the patient's total bone volume increased significantly. Repeat dual photon absorptiometric scan after completion of therapy showed no change. Quantitative radiodensitometric analysis of $100 \pm 5\mu$ thick sections of iliac crest trabecular bone showed a preponderance of bone which was not fully mineralized in the posttreatment specimen when compared to the pretreatment specimen.

longed period where, in both sexes, the biomechanical compatibility of the skeleton is affected by a supracellular series of events which depend on the activity of bone remodeling units. It is widely believed that approximately 0.7% of the skeletal volume is lost per year as a result of bone re-

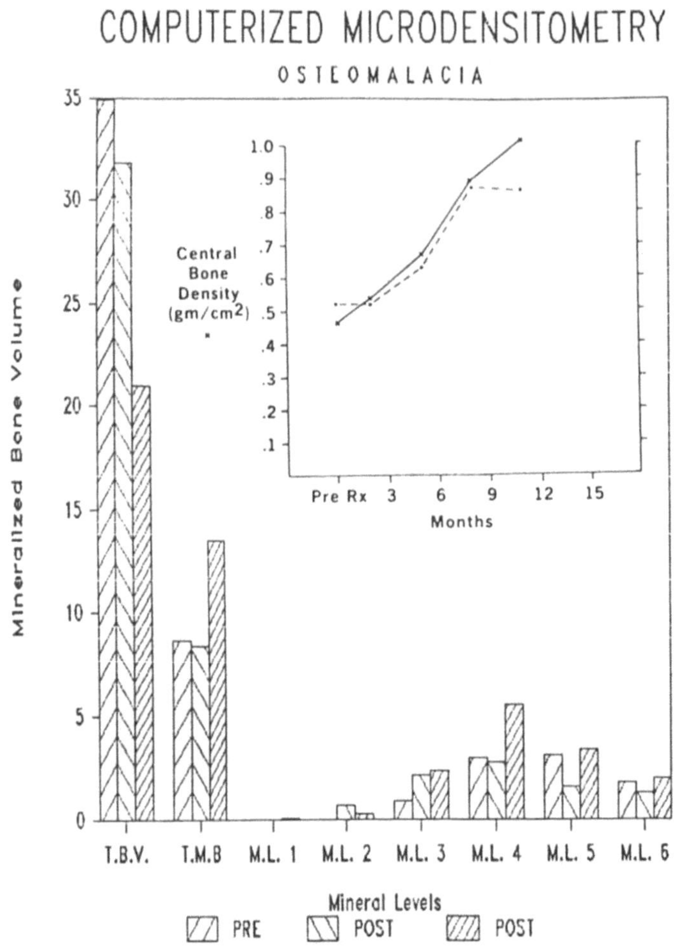

Fig. 2. Discrepancies between results of measurements of trabecular bone volume/mass by histomorphometric analyses of three transiliac crest bone biopsies and five dual beam photon absorptiometric readings of the spine. The patient had severe osteomalacia and was treated for 18 months with calcium and vitamin D. The trabecular total bone volume (TBV) decreased, the trabecular total mineralized bone (TMB) increased but the increase was mainly due to domains of bone which show varying degrees of mineralization relative to previous biopsies.

modeling. Yet, in women, skeletal biomechanical competence is altered because, beginning at or around the menopause, the annual skeletal loss of volume increases to approximately 2.5% per year. This accelerated loss of skeletal volume in women lasts from between 10 to 15 years, after which bone remodeling slows down and the rate of loss is said to become similar to that of men. Both sexes then continue to lose skeletal volume equally but, by this time, women manifest greater skeletal osteopenia.

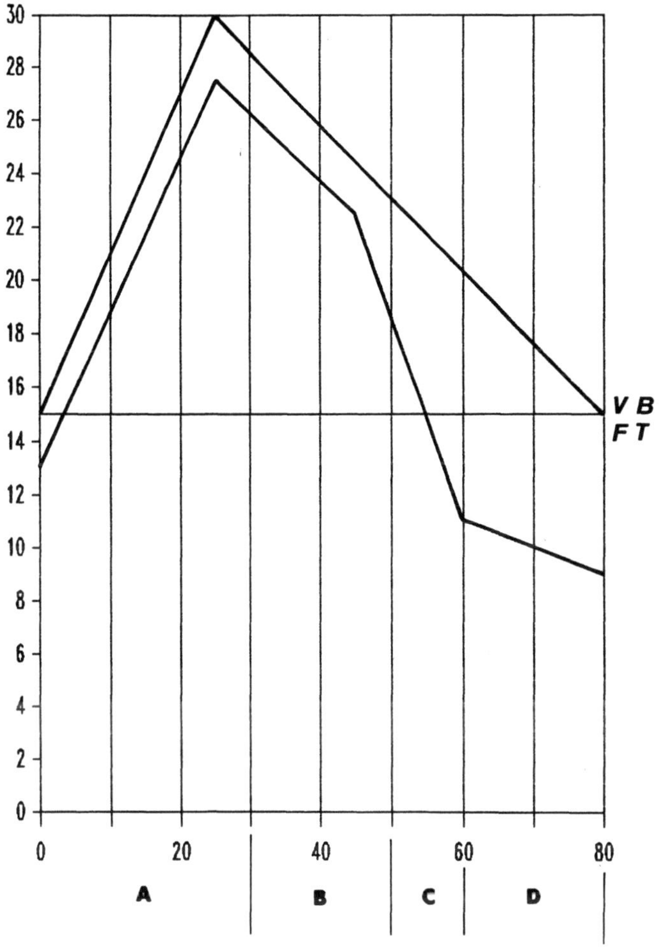

Fig. 3. Schematic representation of bone mass/volume in relation to different ages: A) growth period; B) adulthood; C) postmenopausal phase; D) senescence.

In essence, net skeletal volume balance depends on the multicellular events which govern bone replacement. Some of these are:

i) *Activation* - an accepted yet causally unknown minimal excitatory stimulus which triggers the activity of variable numbers of remodeling centers on all bone surfaces.

ii) *Resorption* - a temporary process of focal bone removal, its action being governed by the number of osteoclasts, and the intensity and duration of their activity.

iii) *Reversal phase* (referred to as coupling) - the phase during which osteoclasts are replaced by nondescript mononuclear cells; these will eventually either turn into osteoblasts or signal the differentiation of other osteoprogenitor cells at the site of resorption into osteoblasts.

iv) Assuming that coupling is a constant phenomenon which follows bone resorption, the *formation phase* becomes established. This being a temporary process of focal bone accretion, its action is governed by the number of osteoblasts, the intensity and life-span of these cells' bone matrix-forming capacity, and the capability of these cells to mineralize that bone matrix. Thus, a new bone structural unit is formed which is a) young, b) theoretically reflects the need for a different stress/load-related architecture at that site, and c) theoretically provides the requirements of mineral homeostasis.

An important and underemphasized concept of bone remodeling activity is the generation of the bone remodeling space, ie, the volume of the skeleton where bone is being resorbed or formed as a result of the activities of combined remodeling units at any time (Jaworski, 1981). The more units being activated to remodel bone, the larger the remodeling space, the greater the skeletal radiolucency, and the lesser the skeletal radiodensity, and vice versa. Therapeutic efforts which decrease or eliminate the activation of new bone remodeling units may not interfere with those units activated before the start of therapy. These preexisting units might then proceed to completion of their activity giving rise to a decrease in the remodeling space and an increase in radiodensity of the skeleton. Actually, although the radiologic investigations may show an increase in bone mass, skeletal volume may not increase (Fig. 4).

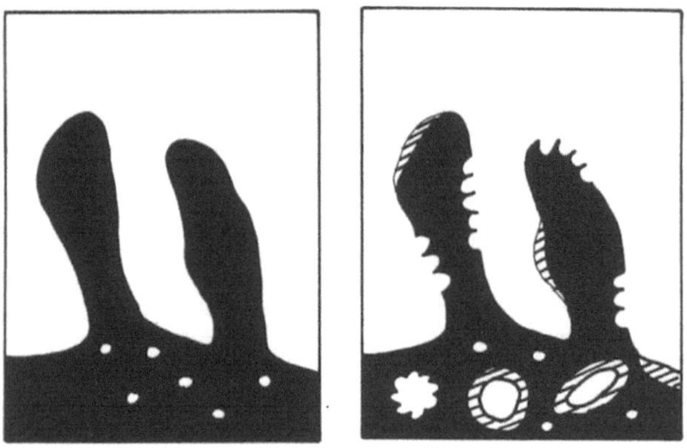

Fig. 4. This diagram is an exaggerated attempt to demonstrate the architectural changes which could occur in the same geographic area of bone. The subsequent effects on bone remodeling space, radiolucency and radiodensity should be apparent. On the right side, there are numerous areas of bone resorption and bone formation with an increase in the bone remodeling space. On the left side, there is no bone remodeling activity and the bone remodeling space is absent.

From data available in the medical literature and from data collected during our laboratory studies of the effects of continued treatment of spayed dams with various substances, we have produced a table depicting our understanding of events which govern the behavior of the trabecular bone remodeling unit in the vertebral body (Table II). It will be seen that there is a general loose relationship between net volume balance and the bone remodeling space. This relationship elucidates the differences in net volume bal-

Table II. Theories as to different components of basic multicellular unit of bone remodeling activity during aging phases and response to treatment

	Phases				Medication						
	A	B	C	D	PTH	CT	Est	Prog	Ca	D_3	Fl
Activation	H	N	H	D	H	D	N	H	D	H	H
Resorption	H	N	H	L	H	D	D	H	D	H	D
Osteoclast #	H	N	H	L	H	D	D	D	D	H	D
Volume resorbed	H	N	H	L	H	D	H	H	D	H	H
Duration of resorption	N	N	L	LL	D	D	L	L	L	D	L
Coupling	N	N	D	D	?	?	D	D	?	?	D
Formation	H	N	D	D	H	D	D	H	N	H	N
Osteoblast #	H	N	D	D	H	D	N	H	N	H	N
Volume matrix formed	H	N	D	D	H	D	N	H	D	H	N
Volume matrix mineralized	N	N	N	N	D	N	N	D	N	H	N
Duration of formation	N	N	L	LL	D	N	D	N	N	D	N
Half-life of B.S.U.	N	L	L	LL	D	L	L	L	L	D	L
Net volume balance	I	D	DD	D	DD	S	S	D	S	D	I
Remodeling space	I	N	I	I	I	D	D	D	D	I	I

ance and explains how this may be dependent on the different activities of the components of the remodeling units and their effect on the bone remodeling space. With the exception of fluoride (Eriksen et al, 1984; Meunier et al, 1984; Singh and Jolly, 1970), which appears to preferentially stimulate activity on endosteal and periosteal bone envelopes, thus increasing skeletal volume, calcitonin (Chesnut, 1984; Chesnut et al, 1983; Minaire et al, 1984), estrogens (Christiansen, 1984; Eisinger et al, 1984; Hart et al, 1984; Lindsay, 1984) and calcium prevent blone loss, while parathyroid hormone (PTH) (Kleerekoper et al, 1983; Raisz, 1983; Reeve et al, 1984), progestogens, and vitamin D metabolites (Gallagher, 1984) do not. Whether the former prevent bone loss by themselves or through indirect mechanisms is not clear. It is interesting to note that the bone remodeling space is decreased after treatment with calcitonin, estrogen, progestogens and calcium. This observation substantiates the increases in bone mass reported by numerous investigators who have used these substances in the treatment of postmenopausal osteoporosis, especially when instituted during the immediate postmenopausal years when remodeling activity is high and the remodeling space is large.

4) It is known that most patients with involutional osteoporosis have concomitant morbid conditions which contribute to the increase in fracture rates.

A logical sequela to advances in preventive medicine was the recognition by Albright in 1947 that postmenopausal osteoporosis is a significantly morbid process. If public health records of fracture incidence in elderly women in the western world adequately reflect the incidence of osteopenia, and if we are to believe population epidemiologists who state that by the turn of the century the elderly of our population will increase significantly, preventative measures to retain bone mass will have to be instituted or orthopedists will face a major task.

Yet, at the present time, osteopenia is only one of the contributors to fracture morbidity in the elderly. Specialists in various fields of medicine frequently see osteopenic patients with predisposing conditions leading to repeated trauma, falls and fractures. Yet, little time or effort is usually directed to correct or minimize these conditions.

A study by Gryfe et al (1977) showed that the incidence of falls in individuals of both sexes over the age of 65 is 66.8% per year, and that the fall-rate not only increases with age but that increase was more prevalent in women than in men. He reported that 17.5% of these falls resulted in a fracture of one type or another. Furthermore, fracture falls, resulting ultimately in complications leading to death, occurred at the end of a "cluster" of successive falls.

The clinical factors related to falls in an elderly population in New Zealand was reported by Campbell et al (1981). These authors reported that "pattern-falls" (ie, falls with minimal environmental upset) were often associated with impaired balance and postural instability, functional motor abnormalities and impaired mobility, poor vision, transient ischemic attacks, as well as chronic brain syndrome.

Brocklehurst et al (1978) reported that while 75% of falls in the elderly occur in the home, about one-quarter of them could be attributed to transient cerebral ischemia; one-fifth of the falls could be attributed to impaired blood pressure reflexes when rising out of a chair or bed, poor vision and impaired mobility associated with arthritis. Furthermore, they stated that in approximately one-fifth of femoral neck fractures, these elderly patients were on therapeutic doses of barbiturates to induce sleep at night.

It is obvious, therefore, that many constellations of factors contribute to fractures in the elderly. It is unfortunate that these falling-fracturing patients are not treated more aggressively with physiotherapy and rehabilitation as well as for osteopenia. Indeed, it would be interesting to find out just how much the reported osteopenia-related fracture rates can be altered with a more integral form of treatment.

Summary

Some of the problems associated with successful treatment for postmenopausal osteoporosis have been reviewed. These include statistical inadequacy of reported therapeutic modalities, methodologic and physiopathologic uncertainties, as well as associated morbid conditions leading to fractures.

The best treatment of potentially osteoporotic patients is prevention of bone loss combined with ancillary measures to overcome the physical limitations of the elderly population.

Acknowledgements

Acknowledgement of support for research is extended to the Medical Research Council of Canada, the Procter and Gamble Company, the Canadian Geriatrics Research Society on behalf of the Energy and Chemical Workers Union, the University Hospital Research Trust Fund and the University of Western Ontario.

References

1. Albright, F.: Osteoporosis. Ann. Int. Med. 27, 861, 1947.

2. Anderson, C., Cape, R.D.T., Crilly, R.G., Hodsman, A.B., and Wolfe, B.M.J.: Preliminary observations on a form of coherence therapy for osteoporosis. Calc. Tiss. Int. 36, 341, 1984.

3. Brocklehurst, J.C., Exton-Smith, A.N., Lempert-Barber, S.M., Hunt, L.P., and Palmer, M.K.: Fracture of the femur in old age: A 2-centre study of associated clinical factors and the cause of the fall. Age and Ageing 7, 7, 1978.

4. Campbell, A.J., Reinken, J., Allan, B.C., and Martinez, G.S.: Falls in old age: A study of frequency and related clinical factors. Age and Aging 10, 264, 1981.

5. Chesnutt III, C.H.: Synthetic salmon calcitonin diphosphonates, and anabolic steroids in the treatment of postmenopausal osteoporosis. In, Osteoporosis 2, Copenhagen International Symposium on Osteoporosis, June 3-8, 1984, pp 549-555.

6. Chesnut III, C.H., Baylink, D.Y., Gruber, H.E., Ivey, Y., Matthews, M., Nelp, W.B., and Sisom, K.: Anabolic steroids and calcitonin in the treatment of postmenopausal osteoporosis. In, Clinical Disorders of Bone and Mineral Metabolism. Excerpta Medica, 1983, pp 355-359.

7. Christiansen, C.: Prophylactic treatment for age-related bone loss in women. In, Osteoporosis 2, Copenhagen International Symposium on Osteoporosis, June 3-8, 1984, pp 587-593.

8. Eisinger, Y., Laponche, A.M., and Duaniche, Y.: Trabecular bone mass in postmenopausal osteoporosis - effect of various hormonal treatments. In, Osteoporosis 2, Copenhagen International Symposium on Osteoporosis, June 3-8, 1984, pp 657-658.

9. Eriksen, E.F., Mosekilde, L., and Melsen, F.: Effect of sodium fluoride, calcium phosphate and vitamin D_2 for 5 years on bone balance and remodeling in osteoporotics. In, Osteoporosis 2, Copenhagen International Symposium on Osteoporosis, June 3-8, 1984, pp 659-661.

10. Gallagher, Y.C.: The role of vitamin D in the treatment of postmenopausal osteoporosis. In, Osteoporosis 2, Copenhagen International Symposium on Osteoporosis, June 3-8, 1984, pp 755-761.

11. Gryfe, C.I., Amies, A., and Ashley, M.J.: A longitudinal study of falls in an elderly population: I. Incidence and morbidity. Age and Ageing 6, 201, 1977.

12. Hart, D.M., Abdalla, H., Clarke, D., and Lindsay, R.: Preservation of bone mass in postmenopausal women during therapy with estrogen and progestogens. In, Osteoporosis 2, Copenhagen International Symposium on Osteoporosis, June 3-8, 1984, pp 697-699.

13. Jaworski, Z.F.G.: Physiology and pathology of bone remodeling. Orthop. Clin. North Am. 12, 485, 1981.

14. Kanis, J.R.: Treatment of osteoporotic fracture. Lancet 1, 27, 1984.

15. Kleerekoper, M.: Problems associated with the execution of a clinical trial for osteoporosis. Workshop on the Coherence Therapy for Osteoporosis. University of Western Ontario, London, Ontario, Canada, Feb. 10-11, 1984.

16. Kleerekoper, M., Villanueva, A.R., Mathews, C.H.E., Rao, D.S., Pumo, B. and Parfitt, A.M.: PTH mediated bone loss in primary and secondary hyperparathyroidism. In, Clinical Disorders of Bone and Mineral Metabolism. Excerpta Medica, 1983, pp 200-203.

17. Lindsay, R.: Treatment of osteoporosis with antiresorptive drugs - estrogen, progestins and calcium. In, Osteoporosis 2, Copenhagen International Symposium on Osteoporosis, June 3-8, 1984, pp 557-562.

18. Meunier, P.J., Galus, K., Brianson, D., Reeve, J., Podbesek, R., Edouard, C., Arlot, M., Charhon, S., Delmas, P., Benevise, B., Valentin, A., and Chapuy, M.C.: Treatment of primary osteoporosis with drugs that increase bone formation: Sodium fluoride, LPTH1-34, ADFR concept. In, Osteoporosis 2, Copenhagen International Symposium on Osteoporosis, June 3-8, 1984, pp 595-602.

19. Minaire, E., Meunier, P.J., Depassio, Y., Pilonchery, G., and Caulin, F.: Treatment of active osteoporosis with calcitonin. In, Osteoporosis 2, Copenhagen International Symposium on Osteoporosis, June 3-8, 1984, pp 613-615.

20. Nordin, B.E.C., Heyburn, P.J., and Peacock, M.: Osteoporosis and osteomalacia. Clin. Endocrinol. Metab. 9, 177, 1980.

21. Parfitt, A.M.: Assessment of trabecular bone status - Introduction. In, Clinical Disorders of Bone and Mineral Metabolism. Excerpta Medica, 1983, pp 27-29.

22. Raisz, L.G.: Mechanisms of parathyroid hormone mediated bone loss. In, Clinical Disorders of Bone and Mineral Metabolism. Excerpta Medica, 1983, pp 196-199.

23. Reeve, Y., Podbesek, R.D., Price, T.R., Arlot, M., Bartlett, C., Deacon, A.C., Edouard, C., Green, Y.R., Hesp, R., Hulme, P., Katz, D., Tellez, M., Zanelli, G.D., Zanelli, Y.M., and Meunier, P.J.: Studies of a "short-cycle" ADFR regimen using parathyroid peptide LPTH 1-34 in idiopathic osteoporosis and in a dog model. In, Osteoporosis 2, Copenhagen International Symposium on Osteoporosis, June 3-8. 1984. pp 567-573.

24. Riggs, B.L., Seeman, E., Hodgson, S.F., Taves, D.L., and O'Fallon, W.M.: Effect of the fluoride/calcium regimen on vertebral fracture occurrence in postmenopausal osteoporosis. N. Engl. J. Med. 306, 446, 1982.

25. Singh, A. and Jolly, S.S.: Chronic toxic effects on the skeleton. In, World Health Organization No. 59, Fluoride and Human Health, 1970. pp. 239-244.

Repetitive Loading to Prevent Osteoporosis in the Vertebral Column

D. B. BURR, R. B. MARTIN, S. LEFEVER, N. FRANKLIN, and G. THOMPSON

Introduction

"It is the question of the kind of functional stimulus which is effective and the manner of its action that remains as the most obscure problem in skeletogenesis." This statement was made in 1936 by P.D.F. Murray, and again in an introduction to a paper by Glucksmann (1938) dealing with the effects of pressure on the orientation of bone structure. This statement can, with equal applicability, be repeated today about the signals for bone modeling and remodeling. There is no doubt that increased exercise leads to increased bone mass and structural strength; this has been demonstrated repeatedly (Dalen and Olsson, 1974; Krolner et al, 1983; Martin et al, 1981; Nilsson and Westlin, 1971; Saville et al, 1969; Smith, 1973; Smith et al, 1981a; 1981b; Woo et al, 1981).

The real question is not whether exercise is effective in reducing loss of skeletal mass -- it clearly has some effect -- but in defining an appropriate treatment to prevent such losses. It is known that the intensity of exercise is important to the induction of osteogenic activity (Booth and Gould, 1975; Smith et al, 1981a) but what this may mean specifically in terms of the loading environment is not certain. It may be enlightening to solve the puzzle, and to expose the effective functional stimuli for bone remodeling, by analyzing why some exercise prescriptions apparently are not effective. The results of such failed experiments often are not reported, but may be more helpful than the results of experiments that worked.

It has been known for years that static or noncyclic loads are less effective than dynamic ones to stimulate bone formation (Hert et al, 1969; 1971; 1972; Liskova, 1965; Liskova and Hert, 1971). The importance of dynamic loads has recently been reaffirmed (Lanyon and Rubin, 1984). Loads applied statically for two months did not prevent bone loss either endosteally or intracortically, but dynamic loading at equivalent peak strain magnitudes increased net bone formation periosteally.

Since static loads are ineffective for increasing net bone formation, some aspect of the impulse, or the way the impulse is delivered, must be an important signal which can initiate the remodeling process. Possible factors might be frequency, the duration of loading, or the strain rate.

The effects of frequency on skeletal remodeling have not been investigated. The range of frequencies applied to bone during routine human endeavors is

Current Concepts of Bone Fragility

so small that it is unlikely that frequency can be a major factor under normal loading conditions.

The duration of loading may influence the amount of bone formation, although Rubin and Lanyon (1984) recently reported that 36 cycles per day (cpd) at physiologic strain magnitudes (2,000 microstrain) was just as effective in stimulating new bone formation as 1800 cpd at the same magnitudes. This suggests that the duration of loading may provide the switch -- the ON-OFF mechanism -- eventually leading to increased bone mass. It does not indicate whether 36 cpd applied for longer periods (ie, more days) will increase the effectiveness of the loading regimen. The six-week loading period used by Rubin and Lanyon (1984) is a relatively short time in which to see significant increases in bone mass. Longer periods might ultimately produce more bone formation, but may not increase the rate at which it is formed. Moreover, adaptive remodeling is phasic; the initial response may be a rapid but transient one. Uhthoff and Jaworski (1978; Jaworski et al, 1980) found that bone loss in immobilized dogs occurred in two stages, and that the more permanent bone loss did not begin until the dogs were immobilized for 12 weeks.

Our own laboratory analyses have shown that even short periods of impact loading are highly effective in promoting increased surface bone apposition (Radin et al, 1984). Rabbits whose lower limbs were exposed to 50 ms impact loads (2400 cycles per day at 1.5x body weight) showed significant new bone formation after only three weeks. Moreover, the bone responds differently to a 50 ms impact load than to a 500 ms impact load, even though the manner in which the load is applied and the amount of load are equivalent. Significantly increased bone mass was found in the calcaneus after only three weeks of a 50 ms load (40 min/day), while no increase was found even after six weeks of a 500 ms load.

Exercises which do not impart an impulse load are not effective at increasing bone mass. The effects on bone formation of a variety of exercise programs have been investigated with inconsistent results. In some cases, bone mass is increased with exercise while in other cases bone mass decreases or remains unchanged. A closer examination of these programs reveals an interesting fact: exercise programs in which the load is applied at lower rates appear consistently less effective than exercise programs in which the load is applied at higher rates. For example, racquet sports in which highly

The strain rate, in combination with the strain magnitude, may provide the signal which controls the amount and rate of bone formation (Goodship et al, 1979; Lanyon et al, 1982). It has been suggested that impact loading, which is associated with high strain rates, may be more beneficial to the skeleton than other forms of exercise (Tipton, 1983). It is possible that loading associated with higher strain rates will increase the effectiveness of any exercise program (Lanyon, 1981), and this may be the reason that vigorous exercise is more beneficial than less vigorous exercise. O'Connor et al (1982) demonstrated persuasively that the rate of change in strain was a highly significant factor causing increased bone formation. They suggested that some relationship exists between strain magnitude and strain rate which allows the skeleton to perceive a stimulus only if both the magnitude and rate are above a threshold level. This is consistent with reports of the effectiveness of dynamic loads (Lanyon and Rubin, 1984). O'Connor et al (1982) also suggest that if bone is strain-rate dependent, it may be possible to stimulate remodeling or reduce loss by smaller amounts of high strain rate loading for shorter durations.

impulsive loads are applied to the skeleton are consistently effective in stimulating net bone formation in both the appendicular and axial skeletons (Jacobsen et al, 1984; Jones et al, 1977; Lewis, 1971; Montoye et al, 1980). Swimming is effective for the appendicular skeleton, but less so for the axial skeleton (Jacobsen et al, 1984; Nilsson and Westlin, 1971). Walking is less effective than running (Brewer et al, 1983; Dalen and Olsson, 1974; Martin et al, 1981; White et al, 1984; Williams et al, 1984; Woo et al, 1981). Static compression or other nonimpulsive forms of bed exercise are less effective than impact loads (Hantmann et al, 1973; Schneider et al, 1975), even in otherwise immobilized patients (Vogel, cited in Williams, 1984). Other ballistic sorts of exercises (eg, throwing) also have significant positive effects on skeletal mass (King et al, 1969; Watson, 1973).

All of this information leads us to believe that the rate at which the load is applied is a crucial variable in preventing or reversing osteoporotic changes. The duration of loading required to cause net bone formation appears to be relatively low if the load is applied impulsively. Therefore, we asked the questions:

1) Can a 50 ms impulsive load applied through the lower extremity, as in walking or running, alter bone balance in the vertebral column?

2) Will 50 ms impulsive loads applied for short durations directly through the axial skeleton prevent the loss of bone mass in the vertebral column of sedentary animals?

Material and Methods

Experiment 1

Six skeletally mature female white New Zealand rabbits weighing 3.5 - 5.0 kg, were divided equally into control (CG) and experimental EG) groups. The

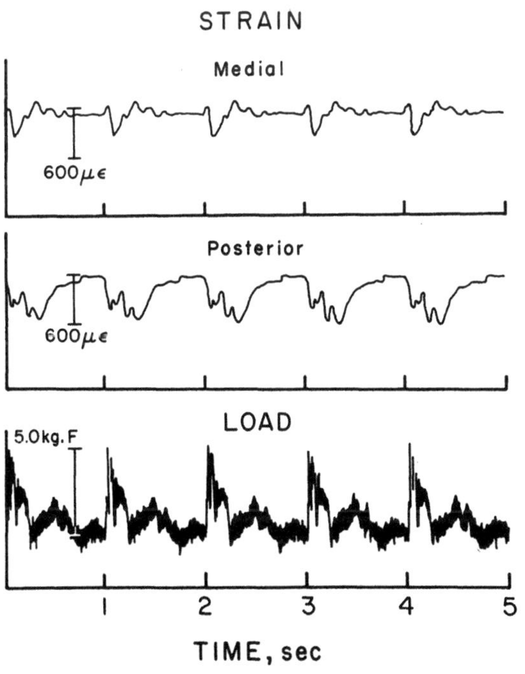

Fig. 1. Tibial strain and load recordings when loads were applied to the hindlimb of rabbits. Strains were recorded on medial and posterior surfaces of the tibia using uniaxial strain gages, oriented with respect to the long axis of the tibia.

right hind leg of each animal in the EG was held in maximum extension and impulse loaded (50 ms) to 1-1/2x body weight for 1200 cycles/day (cpd) at 1 Hz for three weeks (Fig. 1). The apparatus used to load the animals has been described (Radin et al, 1973); it uses the rabbit's own weight to provide an inertial load similar in some respects to that produced in human walking. Strains were measured on the medial and posterior aspects of the tibia at midshaft in two rabbits, using uniaxial strain gages (BLH Electronics, EA-13-125AD-120); strains 400 - 600 microstrain were measured during the loading period (Fig. 1). The strain-gaged animals were not used for the histomorphometric portion of the study. The CG was sham-loaded in the apparatus. Except for the loading period, the animals were left unrestrained in their cages. All animals received a standard diet ad libitum.

Each rabbit was labeled with tetracycline (30 mg/kg) at the end of weeks 2 and 3. Two days after the final label, the animals were killed and undemineralized complete cross-sections were prepared of the L6, L1, T12, T1 and C7 vertebrae. The sections were stained with tetrachrome and examined microscopically under UV light. The amount of bone formation on periosteal, endosteal and haversian surfaces, and the amount of intratrabecular resorption were compared for experimental and control groups using Mann-Whitney U tests.

Experiment 2

Eight skeletally-mature female white New Zealand rabbits were randomly assigned to EG and CG, which were made sedentary by housing them in small cages which severely restricted movement. A 50 ms impulse load was applied to the pelvis of each rabbit in the EG at 1-1/2x body weight for 1000 cpd at 2 Hz for four weeks.

The axial loading apparatus and load-time curve are shown in Fig. 2. Each rabbit was positioned prone in the apparatus with its neck and shoulders restrained by a yoke which was free to slide along a pair of bars parallel to the spine. The pelvic girdle was similarly restrained by straps to a platform which was also able to slide along the bars. The pelvis platform was a methylmethacrylate mold of the rabbit's ischial tuberosities. A load transducer was connected to the mold and to a dual channel Gould Brush 220 chart recorder to monitor the load applied to the pelvis. The forelegs and hindlegs were unrestrained. The animals were not tranquilized, but were acclimated to the apparatus for one week.

The CG were sham-loaded by putting them into the loading apparatus but not applying load.

Each rabbit was labeled with tetracycline intramuscularly at the beginning of weeks 1 and 2 and with DCAF (20 mg/kg) at the end of weeks 3 and 4). At the end of week 4, the animals were killed and undemineralized complete cross-sections were prepared of L7, L4, L5, and C7 vertebrae. The sections were stained with tetrachrome and viewed microscopically using UV light. The amount of bone formation and resorption (at 100 x) and the rate of bone apposition (at 562.5 x) were assessed stereologically. We used a correction to weight single and double labeling, based on Frost's (1980) work on label escape error and data from Schwartz and Recker (1982):

$$L = (DL + SL/2)/Area$$

where DL and SL are double-labeled and single-labeled surfaces, respectively.

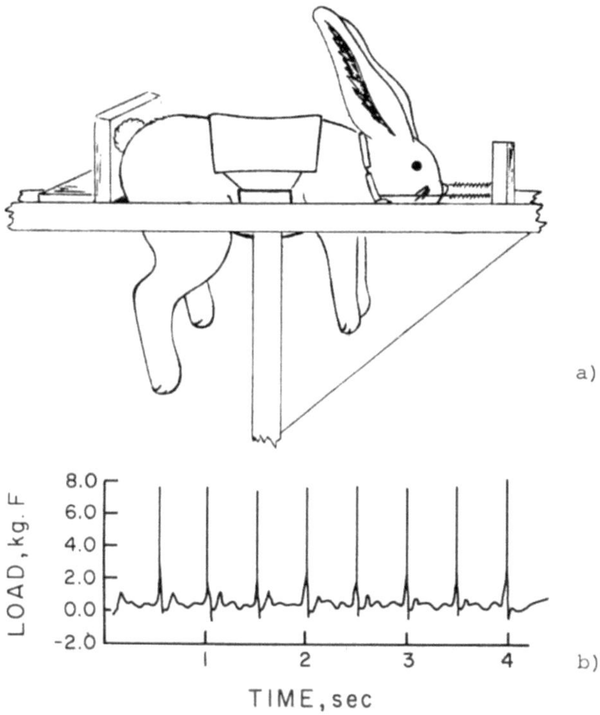

Fig. 2. a) The apparatus used to apply impulse axial load to the rabbit vertebral column. b) Load-time curve for impulse axial loading. Negative values denote tension on the load cell after the impulse load is applied.

The EG and CG were compared using randomization tests for paired samples and Mann-Whitney U tests for independent samples.

Results

Impulse loads applied to the lower extremity did not stimulate increased net bone formation on endosteal and periosteal vertebral surfaces, but, in fact, there was a slight tendency for loading to inhibit net formation on these surfaces (Fig. 3). The differences between the EG and CG were small and not statistically significant, but were consistent across all vertebrae (except in L1 where there was no difference at all). Lower extremity impulse loads, however, did cause a general increase in osteonal remodeling in all vertebrae studied. Examination of the vertebral column at five levels showed nearly twice as much osteonal labeling in the EG as in the CG at all levels (Fig. 4).

The importance of these results resides in two significant observations. First, the vertebral column apparently responds to loads applied through the lower extremity, even when the loads are relatively small and the strains are trivial (ie, below the minimum effective strain, or MES

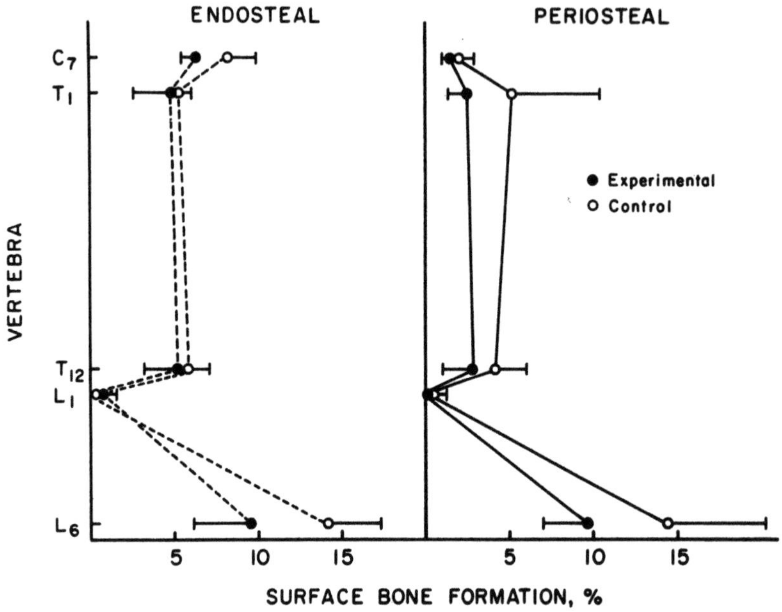

Fig. 3. Percent bone formation on endosteal and periosteal surfaces of rabbit vertebrae, measured by tetracycline labeling. Loads applied to the rabbit hindlimb slightly inhibit surface bone formation in the vertebrae.

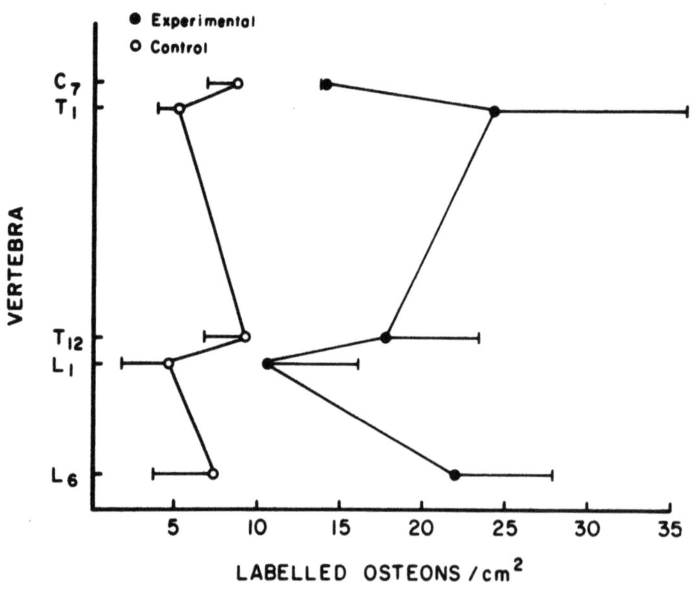

Fig. 4. Osteonal bone formation in vertebrae of rabbits exposed to hindlimb impulse loads. Loads applied to the rabbit hindlimb cause an increase in osteonal remodeling in the vertebrae.

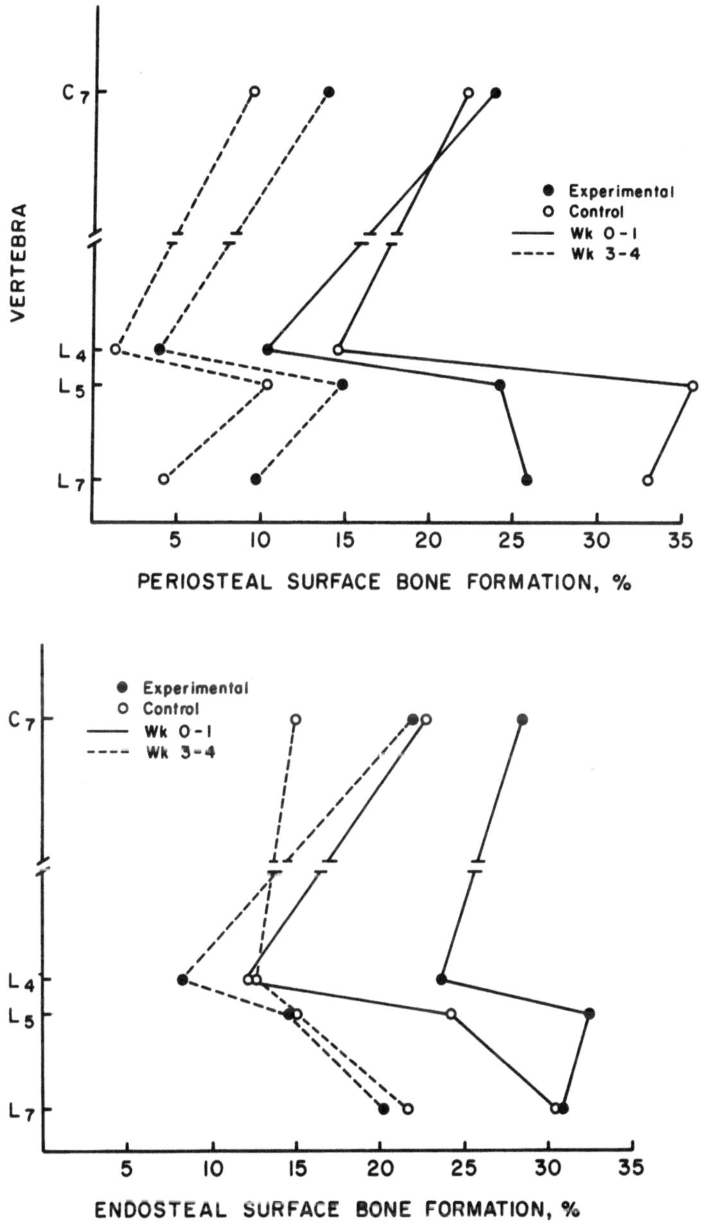

Fig. 5. Percent bone formation on periosteal and endosteal surfaces of vertebrae of sedentary rabbits exposed to impulse axial loads. Measurements made at the beginning (wk 0-1) and the end (wk 3-4) of the loading experiment. Surface bone formation was reduced in both loaded (experimental) and sedentary control animals. In the loaded animals, reductions in bone formation on periosteal surfaces were consistently less than those in sedentary animals, while reductions in bone formation on endosteal surfaces were consistently greater in the loaded animals.

(Frost, 1983)), if the load is rapidly applied. The doubling of osteonal bone formation is evidence of some bone response. The second observation is that remodeling on periosteal and endosteal surfaces is not stimulated by impulse loading of the lower extremity, but appears slightly inhibited. This inhibition is subtle, but its effect over time could be to slow the loss of bone on endosteal surfaces.

The reasons for the different results on endosteal/periosteal surfaces compared with those on haversian surfaces are not clear. It raises the possibility that the different bone envelopes are somehow independently controlled by their different local conditions, eg, strain, marrow, periosteum or other nonsystemic factors. This suggestion is consistent with other data on bone responses to altered mechanical environments (Goodship et al, 1979; Jaworski et al, 1980; Lanyon et al, 1982; Uhthoff and Jaworski, 1978).

Application of loads directly to the vertebral column for short periods slowed but did not prevent bone loss in sedentary individuals. In both EG and CG, bone formation decreased on both periosteal and endosteal surfaces over the four week experiment, but the total surface bone formation was greater in the EG than the CG after four weeks. The reduction in periosteal surface bone formation in the EG was consistently less than the reduction on periosteal surfaces of the CG (Fig. 5). On endosteal surfaces, bone formation in the EG was depressed below that of the control animals in all vertebrae except C7. (The reason for the difference in C7 could be that the animals were not fully immobilized; the head and neck were not constrained but were free to move.) Axial loading for 1000 cpd, therefore, did not fully prevent the reductions in bone formation observed in the sedentary animals, but clearly had some effect on skeletal remodeling. We believe that this

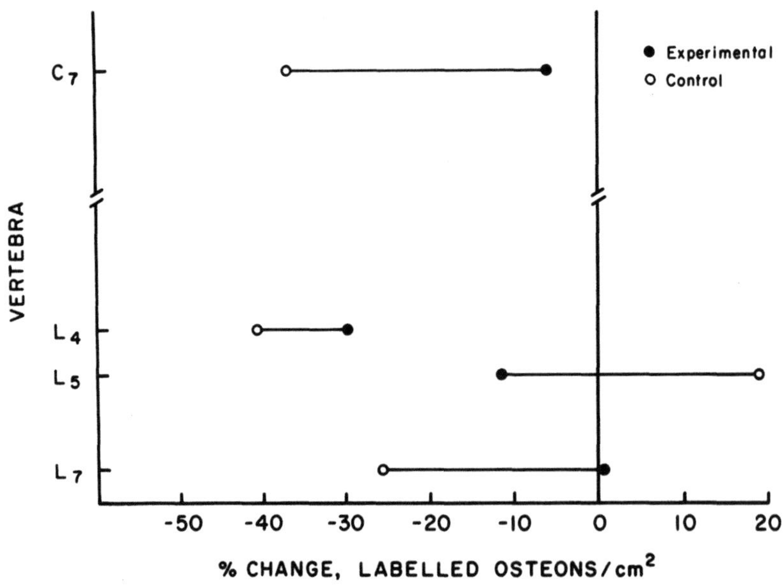

Fig. 6. Osteonal bone formation in vertebrae of sedentary rabbits exposed to impulse axial loads. In general, osteonal bone formation was reduced by 25-40% in the sedentary control animals, but only by about 10% in the loaded animals. The L5 vertebra was an exception.

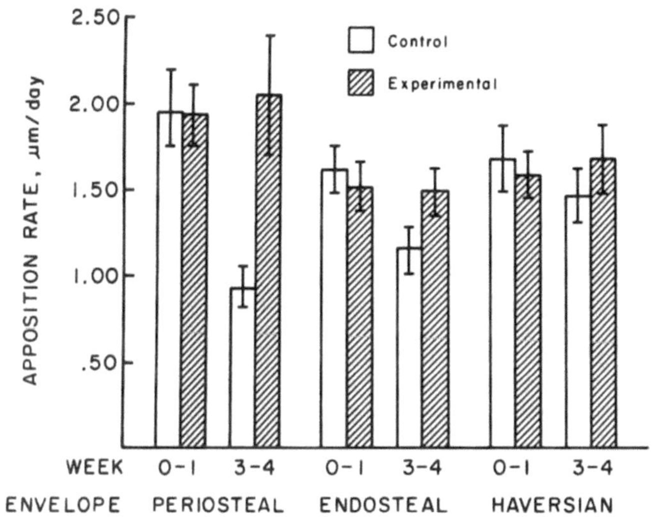

Fig. 7. Bone apposition rate in vertebrae of sedentary rabbits exposed to impulse axial loads. Data for L4, L5, and L7 vertebrae are combined. Over the 4-week experimental period, bone apposition rate declined significantly ($p < .05$) in the sedentary animals, but apposition rate did not decline and was normal in the loaded animals.

effect, in which the reduction of periosteal new bone formation is minimized and in which loss of bone endosteally is inhibited, would in the long run retard the loss of bone mass.

Figure 6 shows the change in osteonal labeling over the four week experimental period. Overall, there were reductions in osteonal labeling in both the EG and the CG. However, with the exception of the L5 vertebra, the reduction in osteonal labeling was much more severe in the sedentary, non-loaded animals than in the loaded animals. This suggests that loading had some effect on preventing the reduction in osteonal bone formation observed in purely sedentary animals.

Inactivity caused a significant slowing of bone apposition in the CG (Fig. 7). After four weeks, apposition rate on all bone envelopes had significantly declined in every control animal ($P < .05$). Axial loading prevented any reduction in bone apposition rate on periosteal and endosteal surfaces; apposition rate did not change at all in the experimental animals.

This reaffirms that impulse loads can alter bone remodeling even when the magnitude of the loads is small and the loading duration is short. The data are also consistent with the idea that impulse loads can inhibit remodeling on endosteal surfaces where the tendency is towards net bone loss. The effects of these alterations in the remodeling process would, in the long run, be sufficient to retard bone loss, particularly in sedentary individuals, and would have beneficial effects on the skeletal system by inhibiting the activation of new remodeling sites, allowing conservation of existing bone mass.

Discussion

These changes are most interesting in light of Frost's recent suggestions about enabling factors for bone modeling and remodeling. Frost (1985) suggests that strains above some threshold value will inhibit remodeling and retard bone loss. The effects of inhibited remodeling on periosteal and endosteal surfaces will be to slow endosteal bone loss and to slow periosteal bone gain. The observable morphologic effect of these will be a reduction of surface labeling when observed at times greater than σ_r, the time required to complete the initial resorption phase, after the start of the loading. In nonsedentary animals, impulse loading was associated with reduced tetracycline labeling on both periosteal and endosteal surfaces, in accordance with this theory. If increased load stimulated the remodeling function, it is difficult to see how these results could be explained, since after three weeks of loading we should have observed an increase in the amount of surface label. Of course, the differences between experimental animals and controls are small, and a larger study could result in different findings. However, the results were consistent for all vertebral levels, suggesting that the data are credible.

Inhibiting the tendency to remove bone adjacent to marrow will conserve trabecular bone until a new equilibrium with the strain environment has been reached. From this standpoint, we suggest that hindlimb impulse loading will, over a period of time, eventually lead to increased bone mass in the vertebral column, although mass was not increased during our three-week loading experiment (and we would have been surprised should we have found differently).

Frost (1985) suggests that immobilization increases activation frequency of new remodeling units, leading to increased loss of bone endosteally. We observed a reduction of surface label on both periosteal and endosteal surfaces over the four-week experimental period in sedentary animals. Equally important, we also observed significantly decreased formation rates in sedentary animals. These changes are typical of those found in disuse osteoporosis in which remodeling is activated, but the rate at which bone forms is reduced. These changes lead to decreased bone mass.

When axial loads are applied to the vertebral column for 1000 cpd, however, remodeling on the trabecular endosteal surfaces of vertebrae was decreased more than in the sedentary animals, while that on periosteal surfaces was decreased less. Perhaps more important is that loading prevented the decreases in bone formation rate observed in the sedentary animals. This, together with the inhibition of remodeling endosteally and the less depressed periosteal formation, would tend to conserve bone mass. It is important to point out that net bone loss would still occur, and that the small amount of loading applied in these experiments is not sufficient to completely prevent this loss. It is significant, however, that such small amounts of loading do apparently have an impact on skeletal remodeling, causing some alteration in the amount of surface bone formation and having a well-defined and significant effect on apposition rate. If the loads are increased somewhat, made more impulsive, or applied over a period of months rather than weeks, these data would suggest that the skeletal system should respond in ways which would conserve bone mass, and which would have a long-term positive effect on bone balance.

Conclusion

The following conclusions may be drawn from these experiments. Some of these conclusions are firmly supported by the data, while others must be offered for the time being as unproven hypotheses.

In nonsedentary animals, impulse loads 1-1/2 x body weight applied to the lower extremity:

1) do not significantly increase the amount of periosteal or endosteal new bone formation in the vertebral column -- in fact, there is a slight inhibition of remodeling;

2) cause a significant increase in osteonal remodeling.

In sedentary animals, impulse loads 1-1/2 x body weight applied axially:

1) suffice to prevent decreased bone apposition rate in the vertebral column;

2) slow the reduction of bone formation on periosteal and haversian envelopes in the vertebrae, but appear to inhibit bone remodeling on endosteal surfaces;

3) may, over a period of months, retard the loss of bone mass caused by inactivity.

All in all, in both sedentary and nonsedentary animals, impulse loads will affect skeletal remodeling in the vertebral column even when the magnitude of the loads is small. The effects of the loading on the different bone envelopes, however, appear to be independently controlled by their different local environments. This suggests that the rate of load application interacts with the magnitude of the load and other local factors to cause the skeletal system to adapt in different ways to altered mechanical environments.

Summary

The rate at which loads are applied to the skeleton may be an important variable which interacts with strain magnitude to alter the amount and rate of bone modeling and remodeling at any given time. The duration of loading required to simulate bone formation is relatively low if the loads are applied impulsively. In separate experiments, 50 millisecond impulse loads (1.5 x body weight) were applied either to the hindlimb or directly to the vertebral column for 1000-12000 cycles per day. Fluorochrome labels were used to monitor bone formation in lumbar, thoracic and cervical vertebrae during the three- to four-week experiments. Impulse loads applied to the hindlimb did not stimulate increased bone formation on trabecular or periosteal vertebral surfaces, but did cause osteonal bone formation to double. Loads applied directly to the vertebral column did not prevent loss in otherwise sedentary animals. When compared to completely sedentary animals, however, bone formation in the loaded animals was reduced less on periosteal and haversian envelopes, while remodeling may have been inhibited on trabecular endosteal surfaces.

These effects on the different bone envelopes suggest that loading is independently controlled by their different local environments. In addition, impulse loading prevented the reduced rate of bone formation found in sedentary animals. These results indicate that impulse loads will affect skeletal remodeling in the vertebral column, even when the magnitude of the load is small, provided the load is impulsive. This effect is significant enough to retard, but not prevent, bone loss when loads are applied for only 1000 cycles per day.

Acknowledgements

The authors wish to thank Beth Edgar and Louise Fragale for their help and expertise in preparation of histologic specimens, and Nina Clovis for her contributions to the histomorphometric analysis of vertebrae.

References

1. Booth, F.W., and Gould, E.W.: Effects of training and disuse on connective tissue. In, Exercise and Sports Science Reviews. Ed: Keough, J.F., Academic Press, New York, 1975, pp 83-112.

2. Brewer, V., Meyer, B.M., Keele, M.S., Upton, S.J., and Hagan, R.D.: Role of exercise in prevention of involutional bone loss. Med.Sci. Sport Exer. 15, 445, 1983.

3. Dalen, N., and Olsson, K.C.: Bone mineral content and physical activity. Acta Orthop.Scand. 45, 170, 1974.

4. Farkas, : Personal communication.

5. Frost, H.M.: Bone histomorphometry: Correction of the labeling "escape error." Metab.Bone Dis.Rel.Res. 25, 167, 1980.

6. Frost, H.M.: A determinant of bone architecture. The minimum effective strain. Clin.Orthop. 175, 286, 1983.

7. Frost, H.M.: MES communications. Unpublished manuscripts, 1985.

8. Frost, H.M.: Osteogenesis imperfecta: The set point proposal (A possible causative mechanism). Clin.Orthop. (in press)

9. Glucksmann, A.: Studies on bone mechanics in vitro. I. Influence of pressure on orientation of structure. Anat.Rec. 72, 97, 1938.

10. Goodship, A.E., Lanyon, L.E., and McFie, H.: Functional adaptation of bone to increased stress. J. Bone Joint Surg. 61A: 539, 1979.

11. Hantmann, D.A., Vogel, J.M., Donaldson, C.L., Friedman, R., Goldmsith, R.S., and Hulley, S.B.: Attempts to prevent disuse osteoporosis by treatment with calcitonin, longitudinal compression and supplementary calcium and phosphate. J.Clin.Endocrinol.Metab. 36, 845, 1973.

12. Hert, J., Liskova, M., and Landregot, B.: Influence of long-term continuous bending on the bone. Folia Morphol.(Prague) 17, 389, 1969.

13. Hert, J., Liskova, M., and Landa, J.: Reaction of bone to mechanical factors. Part 1. Continuous and intermittent stressing of rabbit tibia. Folia Morphol.(Prague) 19, 290, 1971.

14. Hert, J., Pribylova, E., and Liskova, M.: Reaction of bone to mechanical stimuli. Part 3: Microstructure of compact bone of rabbit tibia after intermittent loading. Acta Anat. 82, 218, 1972.

15. Jacobson, P.C., Beaver, W., Grubb, S.A., Taft, T.N., and Talmage, R.V.: Bone density in women: College athletes and older athletic women. J. Orthop.Res. 2, 328, 1984.

16. Jaworski, Z.F.G., Liskova-Kiar, M., and Uhthoff, H.-K.: Effect of long-term immobilisation on the pattern of bone loss in older dogs. J. Bone Joint Surg. 62B, 104, 1980.

17. Jones, H.H., Priest, J.D., Hayes, W.C., Tichenor, C.C., and Nagel, D.A.: Humeral hypertrophy in response to exercise. J. Bone Joint Surg. 59A, 204, 1977.

18. King, J.W., Brelsford, H.J., and Tullos, H.S.: Analysis of the pitching arm of the professional baseball pitcher. Clin.Orthop. 67, 116, 1969.

19. Krolner, B., Toft, B., Nielsen, S.P., and Tondevold, E.: Physical exercise as prophylaxis against involutional vertebral bone loss: A controlled trial. Clin.Sci. 64, 541, 1983.

20. Lanyon, L.E.: Osteoporosis and mechanically related bone remodeling. In, Osteoporosis. Proc. Int.Symp., Jerusalem Osteoporosis Center. Eds: Menczel, J., Robin, G.C., Makin, M., and Steinberg, R. John Wiley and Sons, Chichester, 1981, pp 148-156.

21. Lanyon, L.E., and Rubin, C.T.: Static vs dynamic loads as an influence on bone remodelling. J.Biomech. 17, 897, 1984.

22. Lanyon, L.E., Goodship, A.E., Pye, C.J., and MacFie, J.H.: Mechanically adaptive bone remodelling. J.Biomech. 15, 141, 1982.

23. Lewis, C.W.D.: Who's for tennis? New Zealand Med.J. 74, 21, 1971.

24. Liskova, M.: The thickness changes of the long bone after experimental stressing during growth. (Czech.) Plzen.Lek.Sborn. 25, 95, 1965.

25. Liskova, M., and Hert, J.: Reaction of bone to mechanical factors. Part 2. Periosteal and endosteal bone apposition in the rabbit tibia due to intermittent stressing. Folia Morphol.(Prague) 19, 301, 1971.

26. Martin, R.K., Albright, J.P., Clarke, W.R., and Niffenegger, J.A.: Load-carrying effects on the adult beagle tibia. Med.Sci.Sport Exer. 13, 343, 1981.

27. Montoye, H.J., Smith, E.L., Fardon, D.F., and Howley, E.T.: Bone mineral in senior tennis players. Scand.J.Sports Sci. 2, 26, 1980.

28. Murray, P.D.F.: Bones. University Press, Cambridge, 1936.

29. Nilsson, B.E., and Westlin, N.E.: Bone density in athletes. Clin. Orthop. 77, 179, 1971.

30. O'Connor, J.A., Lanyon, L.E., and MacFie, H.: The influence of strain rate on adaptive bone remodelling. J.Biomech. 15, 767, 1982.

31. Radin, E.L., Parker, H.G., Pugh, J.W., Steinberg, R.S., Paul, I.L., and Rose, R.M.: Response of joints to impact loading. III. Relationship between trabecular microfractures and cartilage degeneration. J.Biomech. 6, 51, 1973.

32. Radin, E.L., Martin, R.B., Burr, D.B., Caterson, B., Boyd, R.D., and Goodwin, C.: Effects of mechanical loading on the tissues of the rabbit knee. J.Orthop.Res. 2, 221, 1984.

33. Rubin, C.T., and Lanyon, L.E.: Regulation of bone formation by applied dynamic loads. J. Bone Joint Surg. 66A, 397, 1984.

34. Saville, P.D., and Whyte, M.P.: Muscle and bone hypertrophy. Positive effect of running exercise in the rat. Clin.Orthop. 65, 81, 1969.

35. Schneider, V.S., Hulley, S.B., and Donaldson, C.L.: Prevention of bone mineral changes induced by bed rest: Modification by static compression simulating weight. Report of the USPHS Hospital of San Francisco. (NASA-CR-141453), 1975.

36. Schwartz, M.P., and Recker, R.R.: The label escape error: Determination of the active bone-forming surface in histologic sections of bone measured by tetracycline double labels. Metab.Bone Rel.Res. 4, 237, 1982.

37. Smith, E.L.: The effects of physical activity on bone in the aged. In, International Conference on Bone Mineral Measurement. Ed: Mazess, R.B., DHEW Pub. No. (NIH) 75-683, Washington, DC. 1973, pp 397-405.

38. Smith, E.L., Jr., Reddan, W., and Smith, P.E.: Physical activity and calcium modalities for bone mineral increase in aged women. Med.Sci. Sport Exer. 13, 60, 1981a.

39. Smith, E.L. Jr., Smith, P.E., and Munns, K.A.: Physical activity: A modality for bone mineral increase in aging women. In, Osteoporosis. Proc. Int.Symposium, Jerusalem Osteoporosis Center, Eds: Menczel, J., Robin, G.C., Makin, M., Steinberg, R., John Wiley and Sons, Chichester, 1981b.

40. Tipton, C.M.: Considerations for exercise prescriptions in future space flights. Med.Sci.Sport Exer. 15, 441, 1983.

41. Uhthoff, H.K., and Jaworski, Z.F.G.: Bone loss in response to long-term immobilisation. J. Bone Joint Surg. 60B, 420, 1978.

42. Watson, R.C.: Bone growth and physical activity in young males. In, International Conference on Bone Mineral Measurement. Ed.: Mazess, R.B., DHEW Pub. No. (NIH) 75-683, Washington, D.C., 1973. pp 380-386.

43. White, M.K., Martin, R.B., Yeater, R.A., Butcher, R.L., and Radin, E.L.: The effects of exercise on the bones of postmenopausal women. Int. Orthop. (SICOT) 7, 209, 1984.

44. Williams, J.A., Wagner, J., Wasnich, R., and Heilbrum, L.: The effect of long-distance running upon appendicular bone mineral content. Med. Sci.Sport Exer. 16, 223, 1984.

45. Woo, SL-Y., Kuei, S.C., Amiel, D., Gomez, M.A., Hayes, W.C., White, F.C., and Akeson, W.H.: The effect of prolonged training on the properties of long bone: A study of Wolff's Law. J.Bone Joint Surg. 63A: 780, 1981.

Orthopedic Management of Osteoporosis: Effects of Nutrition and Exercise on the Skeleton

J. M. LANE, J. H. HEALEY, V. J. VIGORITA, and J. R. WERNTZ

Introduction

Broadly defined, osteoporosis is that condition of the skeleton in which a loss of bone mass is usually evident radiographically by diffuse rarefaction (osteopenia) or clinically by a fracture. This loss can be caused by any defect in the biochemical makeup of the major constituents of bone: collagen, mineral, or proliferative disorders of the marrow. Known defects in collagen, classically seen in the osteoporotic states of scurvy and osteogenesis imperfecta, are rare disorders. Known defects or alterations in mineral availability lead to osteomalacia. Mostly, however, osteoporosis is seen in patients with no obvious attributive biochemical defect. Here, the key may be an alteration in cellular activity -- whether decreased osteoblastic activity, increased resorptive activity, or asynchrony of these phases -- that results in a net loss of bone. Neoplastic conditions in the marrow, such as multiple myeloma, hyperplastic marrow disorders, sickle cell disease and thalassemia, constitute additional entities. However, the most common cause of osteoporosis is an idiopathic or poorly understood age-related phenomenon in which collagen, mineral, or marrow-related diseases have not been identified.

Osteoporosis is of great clinical significance when one considers the magnitude of the problem. By the eighth decade of life, roughly 50% of women will develop spinal compression fractures (Iskrant, 1968) and at age 60, a significant number will have had a distal forearm (Colles') fracture. Osteoporosis has been shown in the elderly to be the underlying cause of most hip fractures which result in significant morbidity and mortality (40-70% in 1-2 years). The cost in medical terms is in the billions of dollars (Avioli, 1981).

Definition

Osteopenia in adults is characterized radiographically by attenuation of the horizontal trabecular pattern, and clinically by wedge fractures of the thoracic spine and crush fractures of the lumbar spine (Fig. 1). Under this general heading are incorporated many disease processes including osteomalacia, osteopenia, endocrinopathies, marrow-packing disorders, and idiopathic osteoporosis (Lane and Vigorita, 1983; 1985). (Table I)

Current Concepts of Bone Fragility

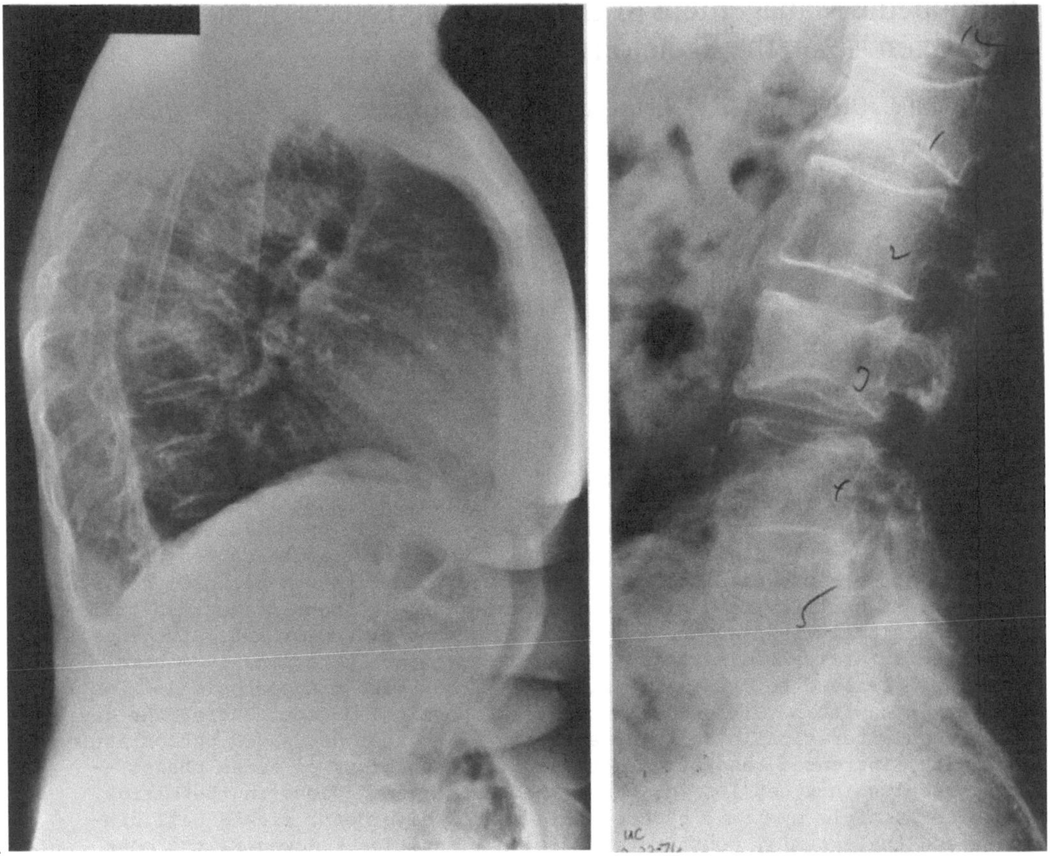

a b

Fig. 1. Lateral radiographs of osteoporotic spine. a) Thoracic spine demonstrating osteopenia, thinning of end plates, and wedge fractures at apex of kyphosis in an osteoporotic woman. b) Lumbar spine illustrating "cod fish" crush fractures of L1, L3 and L4. Note the partial wedging of L1 and full wedging of T12 at the biomechanical transition and between the thoracic and lumbar spine in a small alcoholic osteoporotic patient.

Osteoporosis occurs most characteristically in postmenopausal white women who are over 65 years old, approximating 15% of that population. Although most patients with osteoporosis have been inappropriately defined as senile, suggesting a poor understanding of this age-related phenomenon, there are known contributory factors of subgroups, such as association with postmenopausal estrogen deficiency, alcohol intake, immobilization, and specific metabolic disorders such as Cushing's disease. In fact, in the series of Avioli et al, 8% of the patients with osteoporosis had frank osteomalacia (Avioli et al, 1979), a distinct clinicopathologic entity (Table II).

Osteomalacia, a failure to mineralize the organic matrix, is seen classically in rickets, but more commonly in adult nutritional deficiencies, malabsorption syndromes, and aberrant states of vitamin D metabolism. Defects in calcium and phosphorus metabolism per se, as well as inborn errors of

Table I. Causes of systemic osteopenia

1.	Endocrine estrogen deficiency (postmenopausal) hypogonadism hyperparathyroidism hyperthyroidism acromegaly? diabetes mellitus (juvenile)
2.	Glucocorticoid-related Cushing's (endogenous) iatrogenic (exogenous)
3.	Malnutrition
4.	Mineral disturbance osteomalacia (see Table II)
5.	Collagen disturbance scurvy osteogenesis imperfecta homocystinuria
6.	Hematologic sickle cell anemia thalassemia
7.	Neoplastic myeloma leukemia lymphoma
8.	Mechanical disuse, immobilization
9.	Idiopathic osteoporosis juvenile age-related

metabolism such as hypophosphatasia (Weinstein and Whyte, 1981), also play a role. Commonly-used drugs like phenytoin sodium which disrupts vitamin D homeostasis (Dent et al, 1970) and phosphate-binding antacids such as aluminum hydroxide, may produce significant osteomalacia when used excessively Moser, 1974). Pathologically, there is a marked increase in unmineralized bone or osteoid, and usually a demonstrable decrease in the rate of mineralization as shown by tetracycline labeling. Although clinical radiographs may demonstrate normodensity or osteopenia, bone scans typically show so-called hot spots at the sites of stress microfractures (Looser's or Milkman's fractures) (Fig. 2). Milder degrees of osteomalacia have been identified in as many as 35% of patients with hip fractures (Jenkins et al, 1973). In addition to a high prevalence of osteoporosis, studies at The Hospital for Special Surgery in New York and the Massachusetts General Hospital have revealed osteomalacia as the underlying disorder in as many as 25% of the hip fractures in the elderly (Anonymous, 1983; Doppelt, 1984; Scileppi et al, 1981). Numerous series have also identified a subgroup termed hyperosteoidosis among osteopenic populations, which is characterized by increased

Table II. Clinical-pathologic differences between osteoporosis and osteomalacia

	Osteomalacia	Osteoporosis
Definition	Undermineralized bone	Decreased amount of bone
Symptoms	Generalized musculoskeletal	Localized to fracture sites
Radiographic features	Pseudofractures and Looser lines, frank fractures	Osteopenia, frank fractures
Calcium	Low to normal	Normal
Phosphate	Low to normal	Normal
Alk. phosphatase	High	Normal
Parathyroid hormone	High or normal	Normal or mildly increased
Pathology	Increased osteoid (the nonmineralized component of bone	Thin and discontinuous
Tetracycline labels	Indistinct, smudged	Discrete
Calcification rate	Decreased	Normal

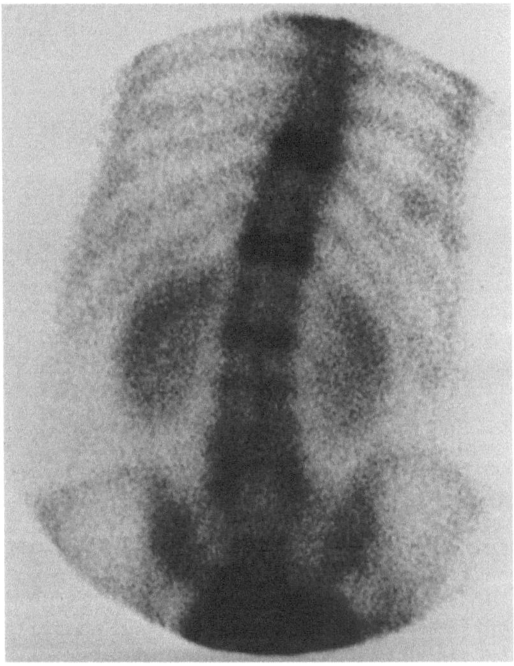

Fig. 2. Technetium^{99} diphosphonate bone scan of the spine. This illustration demonstrates the mild scoliosis and numerous active fractures. The two thoracic fractures are recent and the upper lumbar fracture is 1-1/2 years old. All fractures over 2 years are no longer bone scan positive.

amounts of unmineralized bone, but a lesser amount than that seen in osteomalacia (Parfitt et al, 1979).

Endocrinopathies can also give rise to osteopenia (Melson and Mosekilde, 1978). Common endocrine dysfunctions associated with osteopenia include hyperthyroidism, hyperparathyroidism, and hypersteroidism. In hyperthyroidism and hyperparathyroidism there is increased osteoblast and osteoclast activity but the net effect is bone loss. The role of steroids in the etiology of osteopenia is unclear (Gallagher et al, 1973), although corticosteroid-induced osteoporosis during the treatment of asthma and rheumatoid arthritis is clinically documented. Consequent to the malabsorption of calcium in hypersteroidism, induced states of secondary hyperparathyroidism may account for significant bone loss. In addition, the sometimes observed hypercalciuria may be the result of impaired renal tubular reabsorption of calcium, a situation which is clinically reversible by hydrochlorthiazide therapy (Minaire, et al, 1974).

Although poorly understood, *marrow-packing disorders* also give rise to osteopenia. Thalassemia, multiple myeloma, and leukemia characteristically expand the marrow cavity at the expense of trabecular bone. This view may be simplistic, however. Morphologic observations have shown iron deposition at the mineralization front in trabecular bone in thalassemia (Gratwick et al, 1978), and neoplastic conditions may be associated with the production of bone resorbing factors or osteoclast-activating factors (Raisz et al, 1975). Age-related lymphoid hyperplasia of the bone marrow may be a contributing etiologic factor, as suggested by radiographic data showing a diffuse radiolucent appearance of untreated lymphoproliferative disorders such as lymphomas and chronic lymphocytic leukemia (Vigorita et al, 1983).

Pathophysiology

Excluding conditions such as malabsorption, liver, and renal disease, inadequate sunlight, alcoholism, and steroid therapy, all of which may contribute significantly to aberrant bone metabolism, there remains a large group of patients who suffer from severe loss of bone mass. Although bone mass decreases with age (Meunier et al, 1973), a phenomenon that is poorly under-

Table III. Significant risk factors in the development of osteoporosis

Inactive lifestyle
Early or surgically-induced menopause
Low dietary calcium intake
Steroid medication
Low weight, small build
Caucasian
Family history
Scoliosis
Northwestern European background
Blond or red hair
Bruises easily
Freckles
Hypermobility
Poor teeth

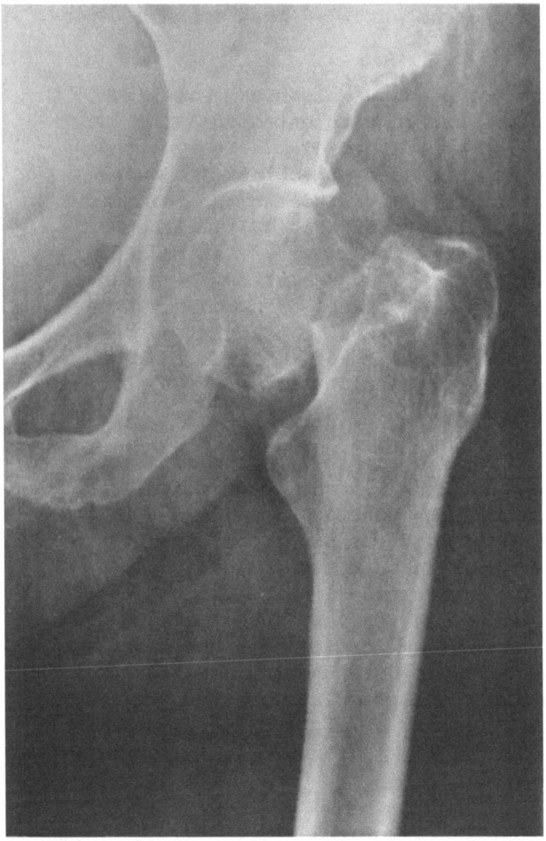

Fig. 3. Femoral neck fracture and relationship to metabolic bone disease status.

a) Typical AP radiograph of a displaced femoral neck fracture in a 72 year old woman.

b) Transilial bone biopsy (Von Kossa stain) of normal cortical/trabecular bone in a patient with a femoral neck fracture. There is increased cortical porosity but cortical and trabecular volume are within normal values for peer related women.

a

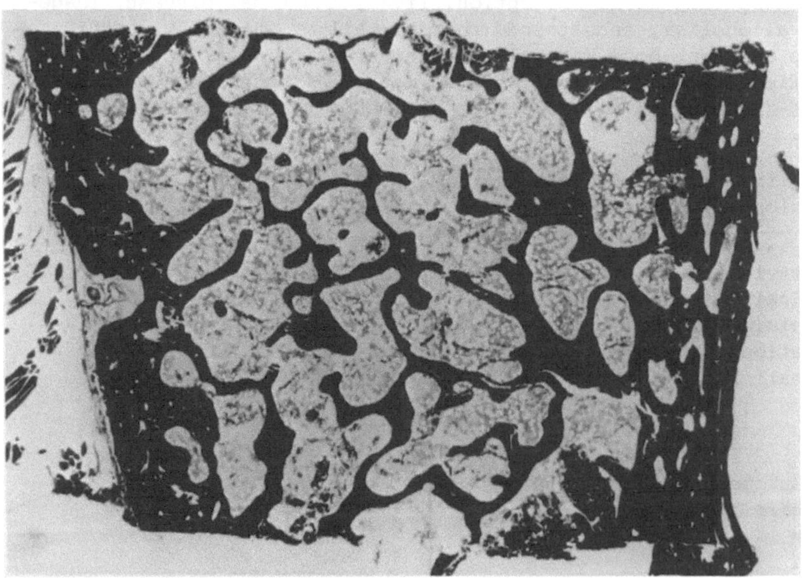

b

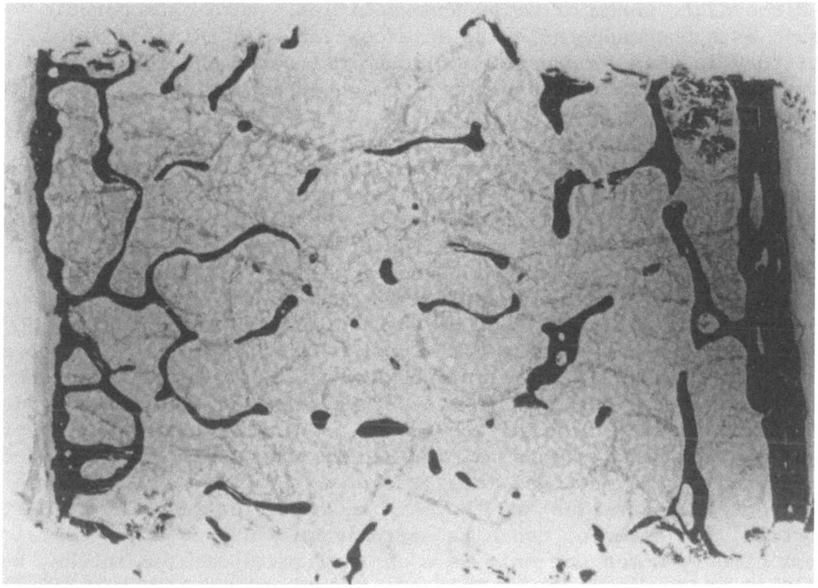

3c) Transilial bone biopsy (Von Kossa stain of osteoporotic woman with a femoral neck fracture demonstrating decreased cortical, trabecular and total bone volume.

stood, genetic and environmental factors seem to play a significant role in the initiation of debilitating osteoporosis. Women have a greater incidence of osteoporosis than men. White women, particularly of northwestern European background, have a much higher incidence than those of Mediterranean descent. Only rarely do black women have clinically evident osteoporosis. It is more commonly found in women with a slender build than those who are obese. A fair complexion, freckles, blond hair, hypermobility, and scoliosis are all associated characteristics (Lane and Vigorita, 1983; 1985) (Table III). The cause of idiopathic osteoporosis of the young remains unknown (Smith, 1980).

Orthopedic risk factors relate primarily to spinal deformity and hyperlaxity but not to osteoarthritis. In a carefully matched series comparing patients with osteoarthritis to osteoporosis at The Hospital for Special Surgery, no concordance between the groups was observed. There appeared to be a normal prevalence of osteoarthritis in the osteoporotic group. In contrast, scoliosis was a dominant risk factor (Fig. 2). Only 15% of the osteoarthritic patients had scoliosis compared with 58% of the osteoporotic. Of those with scoliosis, 76% had osteoporosis (Healey and Lane, 1985; Healey et al, 1985). Hip fractures are usually pathologic and indicate significant underlying metabolic bone disease, as shown in 60-70% of patients in a Hospital for Special Surgery study (Scileppi et al, 1981) (Fig. 3).

In defining the pathophysiology of osteoporosis, careful balance studies have indicated an increased level of urinary calcium in the initial stages that correlates well with the increased bone resorption. In fact, 15% of the patients in one study had an increased immunoassay of parathyroid hormone (Riggs et al, 1973). However, most patients at the time of clinical diagnosis have no discernible serum or urine abnormalities. Rare osteoporotic conditions such as hypophosphatasia are an exception. In this condition, a familial history is usually present and subnormal serum and leukocyte alkaline phosphatase and increased urinary phosphoethanolamine are found (Weinstein and Whyte, 1981).

Nutrition has been suggested as a key element in the initiation of osteoporosis (Gallagher and Riggs, 1978). Specifically, poor calcium intake has been identified in a significantly higher percentage of patients with osteoporosis than in the general population (Birge et al, 1967; Markovic et al, 1979). Young children require 400 to 700 mg of calcium per day; growing adolescents, 1300 mg/day; premenopausal women, 800 mg/day; pregnant women, 1500 mg/day; and lactating women, 2000 mg/day. Goldsmith and Johnston (1975), in a large survey of patients on the West Coast of the United States, showed that women who have breast fed their infants have less bone mass than those who have not. Most of the patients in that study, however, had not had adequate calcium supplementation during the breast-feeding period. A study of postmenopausal calcium requirements has indirectly suggested that 1500 mg of calcium is required to prevent bone loss (Recker et al, 1977). Dairy products and leafy green vegetables are the main source of calcium in the diet; one dairy portion, for example, contains approximately 250 mg of elemental calcium. Most elderly women not only have an inadequate calcium intake, but also have poor adaptation to a low calcium diet. Recent studies have suggested that the deficient production of 1,25-dihydroxy vitamin D in osteoporotic patients accounts for their inability to respond to the deficient calcium intake (Slovik et al, 1981). Subclinical lactase deficiency may further contribute to the problem. Chronic calcium deficiency has been implicated in increasing hip fracture rates. In Yugoslavia, among the elderly, the hip fracture incidence is threefold higher in low calcium areas compared with regions with high dietary calcium intake.

Bone cells respond to mechanical stimulus. Exercise is mediated to bone cells probably via biophysical signals such as bioelectricity. These physical stimuli may directly affect the cell maintenance of target bone cells. Several investigators have demonstrated production of cyclic AMP following stimulation of osteoblasts. Impact-loading exercises have been demonstrated to cause bone accretion in young menstruating women, diminish bone loss in the postmenopausal population (0.5% vs 2%) bone loss/year in exercised versus sedate postmenopausal women), and protect the anorexic individual from acquired osteoporosis (Drinkwater et al, 1984; Jacobson et al, 1984; Rigotti et al, 1984; Smith et al, 1981).

Since bone loss is closely associated to the menopause, estrogen has long been implicated in the pathogenesis of osteoporosis. When one considers that the graafian follicle, corpus luteum, and ovarian stromal cells are all involved in estrogen production, either directly or through peripheral metabolism elsewhere in the body, the ovary constitutes a significant source of estrogen. Meema et al (1975) have shown that following the onset of menopause bone loss increases irrespective of the age at which the menopause occurs. Consequently, patients whose menopause occurs 10 years earlier than is common will have significantly advanced bone loss thereafter. Although most women have decreased estrogen levels following the menopause, only 20% of all postmenopausal women have more than a fourfold decrease. However, most postmenopausal women have estrogen levels below those of men. Estrogen, therefore, has been identified as a key factor controlling bone function. This can be seen not only in primary estrogen-deficiency states, but also in antiestrogen metabolic conditions such as hyperprolactinemia (Klibanski et al, 1980). To date, however, no direct receptors for the various forms of known estrogens have been identified on bone cell surfaces. The effect, therefore, must be considered secondary. Current theories suggest that estrogen has an antagonistic effect on bone resorbing hormones such as parathyroid hormone and possibly a direct effect in the gastrointestinal absorption and excretion of calcium and phosphorus perhaps via enhanced metabolism of vitamin D. A clinical observation is of relevance here: obesity, an unusual finding among osteoporotics, is known to be associated with increased levels of estrogen and decreased urinary calcium. Recent studies suggest that estrogen directly stimulates the release of endogenous calcitonin, a hormone whose principal action is to inhibit bone resorption (Chesnut et al, 1980; Deftos et al, 1981; Hammond et al, 1979; Tiegs et al, 1985).

Osteoporosis does not develop in all postmenopausal women but both men and women lose bone mass with age. After closure of the physes, bones continue to change their anatomic dimensions by gradually increasing the periosteal and endosteal diameters. At the menopause in women, and only gradually in elderly men, the endosteal diameter increases more rapidly than the periosteal diameter, leading to a net loss of cortical bone. Within this framework, further loss of both cortical and trabecular bone seems to lead to a high risk of fracture in approximately 15% of postmenopausal women. A high rate of wedge and crush fractures of the vertebral bodies has been noted in a French population of patients whose transiliac trabecular volume was less than 11% (Courpron et al, 1977). Fifty percent of the patients with such fractures of the vertebrae at The Hospital for Special Surgery were found to have an iliac trabecular bone volume of 15% or less, and only rarely do individuals with an iliac trabecular bone volume of more than 25% suffer vertebral crush fractures.

The belief that there is a morphologic homogeneity in nonosteomalacic adult osteoporosis is no longer justified (Avioli et al, 1979). Based on iliac bone morphology, it can be seen that certain disorders are characterized by particular histologic changes. Broadly speaking, classic age-related or involutional osteoporosis usually shows marked decrease in bone volume with little evidence of osteoblast and osteoclast activity. However, in some of these patients, and in most patients with active steroid osteoporosis and subclinical hyperparathyroidism, there are marked increases in osteoclastic numbers and both active and inactive resorption surfaces. The latter condition is referred to as a high-turnover osteoporosis. In others, the predominant picture is that of increased osteoid or hyperosteoidosis. These are distinct from frank osteomalacia in both extent and degree of osteoid, and in the presence of relatively normal calcification rates. Meunier et al (1979), studying iliac biopsies in a large osteoporotic population, found that 10% of the patients with collapsed vertebrae and low trabecular bone volume had high bone remodeling rates; 33% had depressed osteoblastic activity; and 57% had pathologic findings that were indistinguishable histologically and dynamically from those in nonosteoporotic senile subjects with physiologic diminution of bone volume.

Clinical Presentation and Diagnosis

Osteopenia will be detected by physicians incidentally on a skeletal radiograph or in a new fracture. The most commonly associated fractures (Fig. 1 and 3) include Colles' fractures of the wrist, rib fractures, thoracic spinal wedge fractures, lumbar spinal crush fractures and hip fractures. Spinal fractures result in foreshortening of the thoracic pelvic distance

Table IV. Fractured hips -- incidence abnormalities in histomorphometry*

	Women	Men
Increased osteoid (≧ 3% trabecular osteoid volume)	33%	27%
Moderate osteopenia (≦ 15% trabecular bone volume)	28%	45%
Increased bone resorption (incr. 2 x active osteoclast surfaces)	35%	30%

* Some patients had more than one defect.

and kyphoscoliosis. Most vertebral fractures occur at the apex of the thoracic convexity and at the junction of the thoracic-lumbar spine. The hip fracture rate increases with age and approximates 1% per year in individuals over 75 years of age. Within this group, a study at the New York Hospital demonstrated a 60-70% incidence of significant metabolic bone disease evenly spread between marked osteoporosis, hyperosteoidosis, and augmented bone resorption (Table IV)(Fig. 3). Patients with less than 15% trabecular volume had a significantly greater risk of displaced fracture and a 40% chance of union compared with an 85-90% union rate in patients with normal bone mass (Scileppi et al, 1981).

It is important to note that as much as 30% of the bone mass can be removed from a vertebral body before osteopenia can be positively identified radiographically. All remarks about osteopenia, as identified in the prior discussion, do not clearly differentiate osteoporosis from osteomalacia, endocrine dysfunction, neoplastic or hyperplastic marrow-packing conditions.

Diagnostic tools have been developed to help in the differentiation and quantitation of osteopenia; these may be divided into invasive and non-invasive techniques.

Invasive techniques center on diagnostic studies specifically directed toward identifying endocrine dysfunction, calcium balance, malabsorption, liver and renal function, and marrow status. Preliminary screening laboratory studies, as used by the Metabolic Bone Disease Unit at the Hospital for Special Surgery, are directed at identifying significant metabolic dysfunction. Studies of the levels of serum calcium, phosphorus, alkaline phosphatase, and 24-hour urinary calcium, creatinine, and hydroxyproline are aimed at determining mineral and collagen-turnover disorders. Renal function is evaluated by tests of creatinine clearance and blood urea nitrogen. Endocrine functions that are regularly studied include plasma cortisol (for evaluation of adrenal status), 25-hydroxyvitamin D and 1,25-dihydroxyvitamin D (to evaluate vitamin D cascade), midposition parathyroid hormone (to evaluate the parathyroid gland), T3 and T4 (to evaluate the thyroid gland), and glucose (to test for diabetes mellitus). Studies of hematopoietic function include tests for levels of total protein, albumin (to evaluate liver function), serum protein electrophoresis, Bence Jones proteins, blood count, and sedimentation rate. Second-level studies that are directed toward more specific disorders, such as malabsorption, are only performed if clearly indicated by history, physical examination, preliminary laboratory data, or bone biopsy.

The most critical invasive study is the transiliac bone biopsy, obtained from an area 2 cm posterior and 2 cm caudad to the superior anterior iliac spine. The area is infiltrated with a local anesthetic and the biopsy is taken by a cutting needle with the diameter of at least 5 mm. This is now well established internationally as the standard site from which to obtain pathologic specimens. Furthermore, numerous investigators have demonstrated that the transiliac bone biopsy is a reliable procedure for indicating general skeletal disease (Villaneuva et al, 1977). The other merits of the biopsy are a very low complication rate and the presence of hematopoietic tissue for analysis. Double labeling of the skeleton by the administration of two oral doses of tetracycline (oxytetracycline 250 mg t i d, and demeclocycline 300 mg b i d), 10 to 14 days apart, allows meaningful interpretation of bone dynamics, the distance between the two autofluorescent markers in the tissue permitting determination of the rate of accretion of bone (Frost, 1969). Differentiation of mineralized and unmineralized components of bone necessitates special undecalcified processing using plastic embedding procedures. Undecalcified specimens can be analyzed for cortical and trabecular bone area, osteoid area, and a variety of variables such as bone formation, based on methods established by Frost (1969). Current methods use optical drawing tubes integrated with a computer. Bone morphometry enables the diagnostician to quantitate the amount of bone loss, classify it as active or inactive, and determine the relative defects in bone mineralization. Examination of undecalcified bone biopsy is the only technique that determines the degree of unmineralized bone (Hruska et al, 1978).

Noninvasive techniques to determine the degree of osteopenia have been used to quantitate bone mass and to follow its status during various modes of treatment. The use of radiography, using the femoral trabecular pattern as an index of osteoporosis, has been reported by Singh et al (1972) and is relatively sensitive in identifying patients with osteoporosis in the general population. However, there is a broad overlap in the degrees of osteoporosis and only a moderate correlation between the femoral trabecular index and bone density. While radiographic morphometry uses the measurements of cortical thickness in relation to its width as a measure of density, radiographic photodensitometry attempts to estimate bone mass by measuring the optical density of the radiograph in which the relative exposure of bone images on radiographs presumably reflects proportionally the mass of bone. While the former technique suffers from measurement imprecision, the data from the latter technique may not compensate adequately for factors such as soft tissue thickness. The technique of single photon absorptiometry uses monoenergetic radiation passed across the bone, with the changes in beam intensity recorded by a nuclear counting instrument. This method is currently used widely since it is accurate, has a high degree of reproducibility, and has been successful in predicting bone mass (Mazess, 1971). However, the degree of correlation is dependent on the anatomic site. Techniques utilizing two monoenergetic radionuclides (dual photon absorptiometry) are currently also in vogue (Wilson and Madsen, 1972). This new method can study the axial spine as well as extremity skeleton. Continuing problems of interpretation center around the standardization of techniques, variation in anatomic site, and interference of marrow components. Nevertheless, serial examinations may be of considerable assistance in following the osteoporotic patient. Radionuclide uptake (Genant et al, 1974), Compton scattering (Garnett et al, 1973), neutron activation of calcium (Cohn et al, 1974), and computerized tomography (Cann et al, 1980) are still in the experimental stage.

Treatment

The treatment of osteoporosis is still not consistently satisfactory (Lane and Vigorita, 1983). Part of the problem is clinical diversity and morphologic heterogeneity of osteopenic disorders. Decreased mechanical stress, as seen in disuse and immobilization, most dramatically in astronauts in space flight, is related to increased bone resorption (Minaire et al, 1974). Thus, physical activity may be of benefit even in the relatively inactive lifestyles of most aging persons. Conservative management of the symptomatic patient should always include a comprehensive general rehabilitation program emphasizing spine extension and abdominal strengthening exercises.

Replacement calcium, even in patients with osteoporosis due to calcium deficiency, does not lead to increased bone mass, although it is somewhat successful in halting bone loss. Studies of carefully screened populations have suggested, however, that calcium, estrogen, vitamin D, and sodium fluoride in various combinations may play a role in the treatment of osteoporosis (Aloia et al, 1982; Briancon and Meunier, 1981; Gallagher and Riggs, 1978; Jowsey et al, 1972; Meema et al, 1975; Recker et al, 1977; Riggs et al, 1982). Recker et al (1977) in studies of perimenopausal women demonstrated that either conjugated estrogen (0.625 mg/day) or elemental calcium (1.5 g/day) led to a dramatic decrease in the usual postmenopausal rate of bone loss. These and other studies, however, have usually been carried out for only three to six years following the menopause, but prolonged effect after eight years has not been demonstrated in preliminary studies. Similar studies with 20 to 30-year follow-ups have not yet been completed, so we do not know if such a regimen will provide continued protection. Estrogen administration initiated six years after the menopause has had only a marginal effect on reducing late bone loss (Riggs et al, 1982). Estrogen appears to be most effective in prophylaxis during early menopause. Dosages of conjugated equine estrogen (0.625 mg/day) or ethinyl estradiol (20 mg/day) are reportedly effective. Calcium is also most effective in early postmenopausal women. Milk, cheese, ice cream, and other sources of calcium should be encouraged. However, oral calcium supplementation may be required to augment intake to 1.5 g of elemental calcium per day. Calcium carbonate, lactate, and gluconate are in current use. High-dose calcium may lead to constipation and may also be contraindicated in patients with a history of renal calculus. Urinary calcium should be maintained at 100 to 250 mg per 24 hours when adequate calcium supplementation has been achieved.

Recent studies suggest that estrogen supplementation, even in small doses, results in up to a ninefold increase in the risk of uterine cancer as well as stroke and thrombosis. Therefore, unless the patient is observed carefully for abnormalities such as uterine bleeding, estrogen supplementation may be hazardous. It is preferably given to women with premature menopause and should be ideally initiated within three years of the menopause. Progesterone 10 mg (day 15-25) appears to significantly limit uterine endometrial cancer associated with estrogen supplementation and is recommended by these authors.

Vitamin D supplementation of more than 10,000 IU/day is unwarranted unless osteomalacia has been identified by bone biopsy. In light of the potentially deleterious effects of estrogen, we recommend the use of only calcium and physiologic vitamin D without estrogen except in individuals who have had a recent premature menopause. However, when estrogen is necessary, the safest regimen appears to be interrupted estrogen therapy with the cyclical addition of a synthetic progestin (Hammond et al, 1979). The administration

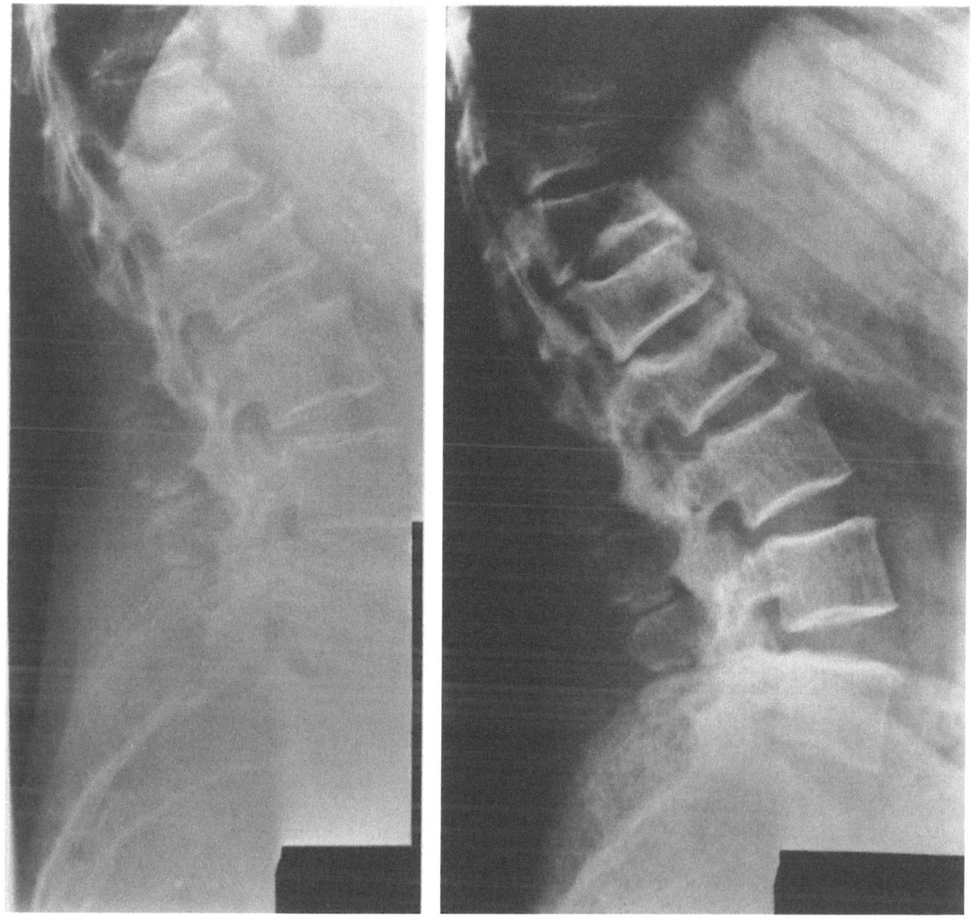

Fig. 4. The lateral lumbar radiographs of an osteoporotic woman with multiple fractures. a) Pretreatment status demonstrating multiple fractures, osteopenia, and narrowed end plates. b) 26 months after treatment with 1500 mg elemental calcium, 400 units vitamin D, and 1 mg/kg NaF. The patient's spine shows no new fractures, significant bone accretion, thickening of the end plates, and hypertrophy of the trabecular pattern.

of estrogen, calcium, and vitamin D will not lead to bone accretion, but should delay the usual physiologic resorption of bone in a postmenopausal woman.

Sodium fluoride, given orally in a dosage of 1 mg/kg of body weight per day, corrected for creatinine clearance (dose decreased by percentage of decreased creatinine clearance), leads to increased bone accretion (Briancon and Meunier, 1981; Jowsey et al, 1972) and a decreased fracture rate (Minaire et al, 1974). At the Hospital for Special Surgery (Lane et al, 1984), trabecular bone volume is increased by 20% per year and cortical bone by 10% per year at this dosage level when administered with daily supplemental elemental calcium (1500 mg) and low-dose vitamin D (400 IU). Fluoritic bone

Table V. Algorithm for investigation of vertebral crush fractures

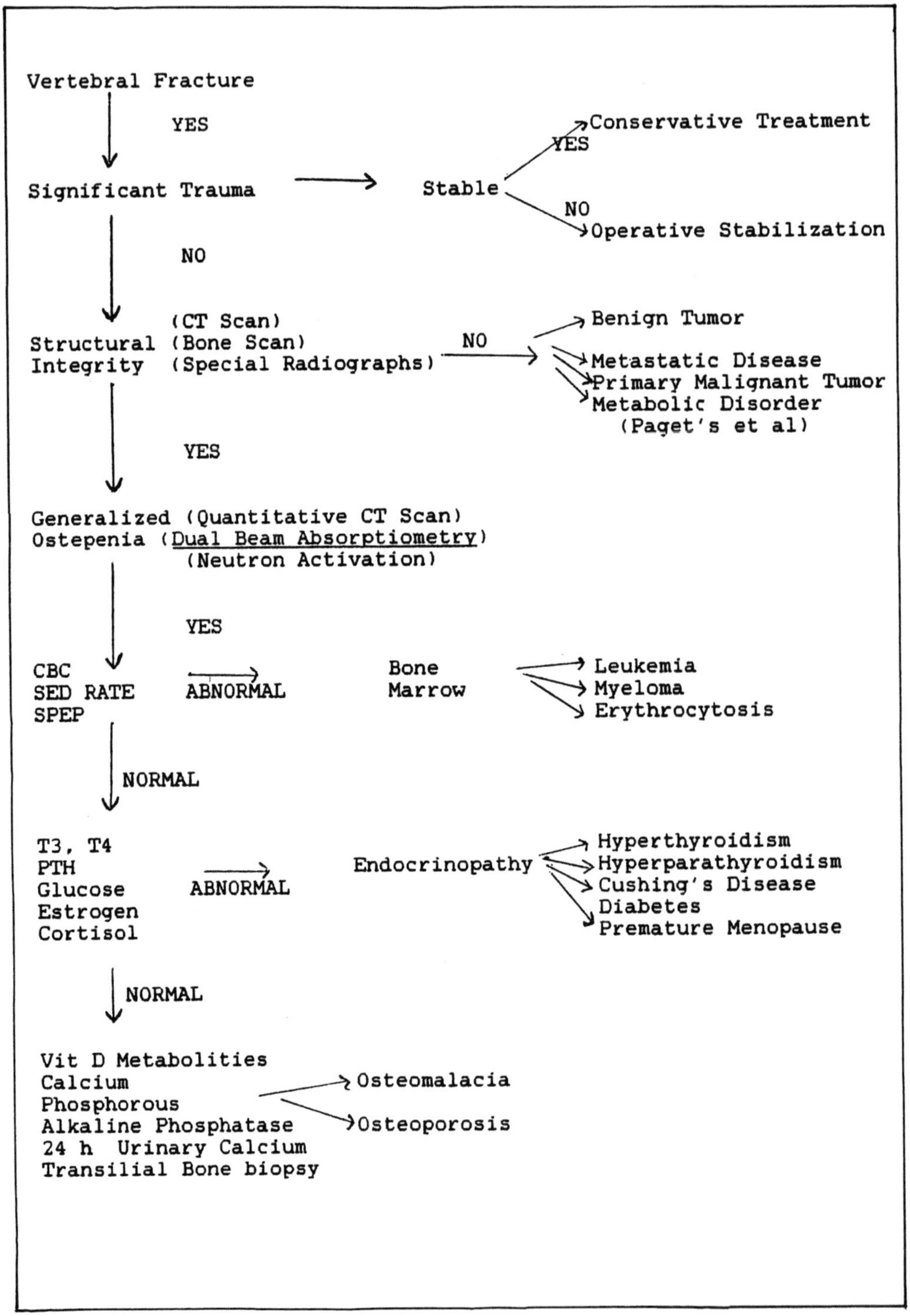

accretion can be recognized by an increased number of osteocytes, slightly enlarged lacunae, and pericellular basophilia (Mazess, 1971). In this population, 66% had no fractures after the onset of therapy and in over 90% of the patients no more fractures developed in the vertebral spine after 18 months of therapy (Fig. 4). Hip fracture rate was not influenced during the first two years of treatment and then demonstrated a trend toward a lower rate thereafter (not statistically significant).

Long-term therapeutic schedules have yet to be determined. One guide is to give sodium fluoride, calcium, and vitamin D for at least two years and continue treatment until yearly spinal bone scans are normal for one year. Thereafter, the calcium supplement should be maintained. Sodium fluoride given in the absence of supplemental calcium is hazardous. While increasing bone mass, unopposed sodium fluoride may lead to considerable increase in the unmineralized bone component (hyperosteoidosis) and even to pronounced secondary hyperparathyroidism. The side effects of sodium fluoride include nausea, indigestion, and transient arthralgias of the feet and ankles. Other agents now under experimental protocols include diphosphonates, calcitonin, parathormone, vitamin D metabolites, and anabolic steroids such as stanozolol (Chesnut et al, 1980; Gruber et al, 1984; Makin et al, 1981). These agents have been used to exploit experimental evidence showing decreased bone resorption (with diphosphonates and calcitonin), increased bone turnover (with parathormone), increased calcium absorption (with vitamin D metabolites), and increased bone formation (with stanozolol).

Patients with acute fractures secondary to osteopenic bone require modified treatment. At the time of fracture, the physician should recognize the possibility of underlying metabolic bone disease and appropriate diagnostic studies should be initiated (Table V). All osteoporotic patients should be placed on 1500 mg elemental calcium and 400-800 units of vitamin D, since dietary calcium is the predominate source of calcium for fracture repair. Following spinal fractures, immobilization with bracing should be limited to the period required to regain ambulation; thereafter, braces only bypass the spine and encourage further loss of vertebral bone mass. General conditioning and impact-loading activities significantly prevent further bone loss.

The physician should evaluate osteoporotic patients, and identify and document the risk factors (Table III). Where possible, underlying causes of osteopenia should be corrected. For example, a thin young woman with surgically-induced menopause (bilateral oophorectomy) and a poor dietary calcium history is at significant risk for developing osteoporosis. Calcium replacement is warranted. In addition, carefully monitored estrogen replacement with regular Pap smears to detect endometrial atypia should be considered. An elderly woman with symptomatic spinal crush fractures, progressive loss of height, a family history of osteoporosis, and a relatively inactive lifestyle may require sodium fluoride, for bone accretion, and a regular exercise program.

REFERENCES

1. Aloia, J.F., Zanzi, I., Vaswani, A., Ellis, K., and Conn, S.H.: Combination therapy for osteoporosis with estrogen, fluoride, and calcium. J.Am.Geriat.Soc. 30, 13, 1982.

2. Anonymous: Bone biopsies of fractured hips often reveal osteomalacia. Med.World News, Apr. 25, 1983, pp 73-75.

3. Avioli, L.V.: Postmenopausal osteoporosis: Prevention vs cure. Fed. Proc. 40, 2418, 1981.

4. Avioli, L.V., Baran, D.T., Whyte, M.P., and Teitelbaum, S.L.: The biochemical and skeletal heterogeneity of 'postmenopausal osteoporosis'. In, Osteoporosis II. Ed: Barzel, U.S.; Grune and Stratton, New York, 1979, pp 49-64.

5. Birge, S.J., Jr., Keutmann, H.T., Cuatrecasas, P., and Whedon, G.D.: Osteoporosis, intestinal lactase deficiency and low dietary calcium intake. New Engl.J.Med. 276, 445, 1967.

6. Briancon, D., and Meunier, P.J.: Treatment of osteoporosis with fluoride, calcium, and vitamin D. Orthop.Clin.North Am. 12, 629, 1981.

7. Cann, C.E., Genant, H.K., Ettinger, B., and Gordan, G.S.: Spinal mineral loss in oophorectomized women: Determination by quantitative computed tomography. JAMA 224, 2056, 1980.

8. Chesnut, C.H., III, Baylink, D.J., Sisom, K., Nelp, W.B., and Roos, B.A.: Basal plasma immunoreactive calcitonin in postmenopausal osteoporosis. Metabolism 29, 559, 1980.

9. Cohn, S.H., Ellis, K.J., Wallach, S., Zanzi, I., Atkins, H.L., and Aloia, J.F.: Absolute and relative deficit in total-skeletal calcium and radial bone mineral in osteoporosis. J.Nucl.Med. 15, 428, 1974.

10. Courpron, P., Meunier, P., Bressot, C., and Giroux, J.M.: Amount of bone in iliac crest biopsy. In, Bone Histomorphometry. Ed: Meunier, P.J. Armour Montague, Paris, 1977, pp 39-53.

11. Deftos, L.J., Weisman, M.H., Williams, G.W., et al: Influence of age and sex on plasma calcitonin in human beings. New Engl.J.Med. 302, 1351, 1981.

12. Dent, C.E., Richens, A., Rowe, D.J.F., and Stamp, T.C.B.: Osteomalacia with long-term anticonvulsant therapy in epilepsy. Br.Med.J. 4, 69, 1970.

13. Doppelt, S.H.: Vitamin D, rickets, and osteomalacia. Orthop.Clin. North Am. 15, 671, 1984.

14. Drinkwater, B.L., Nelson, K., Chesnut, C.H., Bremner, W.J., Shainholtz, S., and Southworth, M.B.: Bone mineral content of amenorrheic and eumenorrheic athletes. New Engl.J.Med. 311, 277, 1984.

15. Frost, H.M.: Tetracycline-based histological analysis of bone remodeling. Calcif.Tiss.Res. 3, 211, 1969.

16. Gallagher, J.C. and Riggs, B.L.: Current concepts in nutrition: Nutrition and bone disease. New Engl.J.Med. 298, 193, 1978.

17. Gallagher, J.C., Aaron, J., Horsman, A., Wilkinson, R., and Nordin, B.E.C.: Corticosteroid osteoporosis. Clin.Endocrinol.Metab. 2, 355, 1973.

18. Garnett, E.S., Kennett, T.J., Kenyon, D.B., and Webber, D.E.: A photon scattering technique for the measurement of absolute bone density in man. Radiology 106, 209, 1973.

19. Genant, H.K., Bautovich, G.J., Singh, M., Lathrop, K.A., and Harper, P.V.: Bone seeking radionuclides: An in-vivo study of factors affecting skeletal uptake. Radiology 113, 373, 1974.

20. Goldsmith, N.F. and Johnston, J.L.: Bone mineral effects of oral contraceptives, pregnancy, and lactation. J.Bone Joint Surg. 57A, 657, 1975.

21. Gratwick, G.M., Bullough, P.G., Bohne, W.H.O., Markenson, A.L., and Peterson, C.M.: Thalassemic osteoarthropathy. Ann.Intern.Med. 88, 494, 1978.

22. Gruber, H.E., Ivey, J.L., Baylink, D.J., Matthews, M., Nelp, W.B., Sison, K., and Chesnut, C.H., III: Long-term calcitonin therapy in postmenopausal osteoporosis. Metabolism 33, 295, 1984.

23. Hammond, C.B., Jelovsek, F.R., Lee, K.L., Creasman, W.T., and Parker, R.T.: Effects of long-term estrogen replacement therapy. II. Neoplasia. Am.J.Obstet.Gynecol. 133, 525, 1979.

24. Healey, J.H. and Lane, J.M.: Structural scoliosis in osteoporotic women. Clin.Orthop.Rel.Res. 195, 216, 1985.

25. Healey, J.H., Vigorita, V.J., and Lane, J.M.: The coexistence and characteristics of osteoarthritis and osteoporosis. J.Bone Joint Surg. 67A, 586, 1985.

26. Hruska, K.A., Teitelbaum, S.L., Koppelman, R., Richardson, C.A., Miller, P., Debman, J., Martin, K., and Slatopolsky, E.: The predictability of the histological features of uremic bone disease by noninvasive techniques. Metab.Bone Dis.Rel.Res. 1, 39, 1978.

27. Iskrant, A.P.: The etiology of hip fractures in females. Am.J.Public Health 58, 485, 1968.

28. Jacobson, P.C., Beaver, S.A., Grubb, T., Taft, T.N., and Talmage, R.V.: Bone density in women athletes and older athletic women. J.Orthop.Res. 2, 328, 1984.

29. Jenkins, D.H.R., Roberts, J.G., Webster, D., and Williams, E.O.: Osteomalacia in elderly patients with fracture of the femoral neck. A clinico-pathologic study. J.Bone Joint Surg. 55B, 575, 1973.

30. Jowsey, J., Riggs, B.L., Kelly, P.J. and Hoffman, D.L.: Effect of combined therapy with sodium fluoride, vitamin D and calcium in osteoporosis. Am.J.Med. 53, 43, 1972.

31. Klibanski, A., Neer, R.M., Beitins, I.Z., Ridgway, E.C., Zervas, N.T., and McArthur, J.W.: Decreased bone density in hyperprolactinemic women. New Engl.J.Med. 303, 1511, 1980.

32. Lane, J.M. and Vigorita, V.J.: Current concepts of osteoporosis. J. Bone Joint Surg. 65A, 274, 1983.

33. Lane, J.M. and Vigorita, V.J.: Osteoporosis. Orthop.Clin.North Am. 15, 711, 1985.

34. Lane, J.M., Healey, J.H., Schwartz, E., Vigorita, V.J., Schneider, R., Einhorn, T.A., Suda, M., Falls, M., and Robbins, W.: Treatment of osteoporosis with sodium fluoride and calcium: Effects upon vertebral fracture incidence and bone histomorphometry. Orthop.Clin.North Am. 15, 729, 1984.

35. Makin, M., Menczel, J., Robin, G., Barzel, W.S., Better, O., Edelstein, S., Harell, A., Kidroni, G., Liberman, U.A., Popovitzer, M.M., and Weinreb, A.: International Symposium on Osteoporosis. Hebrew University of Jerusalem, 1981.

36. Markovic, V., Kostial, K., Simonovic, I., Buzina, R., Brodarec, A., and Nordin, D.E.C.: Bone status and fracture rates in two regions of Yugosalvia. Am.J.Clin.Nutr. 32, 540, 1979.

37. Mazess, R.B.: Estimation of bone and skeletal weight by direct phonton absorptiometry. Invest.Radiol. 6, 52, 1971.

38. Meema, S., Bunker, M.L., and Meema, H.E.: Preventive effect of estrogen on postmenopausal bone loss: A follow-up study. Arch.Intern.Med. 135, 1436, 1975.

39. Melsen, F. and Mosekilde, L.: Dynamic studies of trabecular bone formation and osteoid maturation in normal and certain pathological conditions. Metab.Bone Dis.Rel.Res. 1. 45, 1978.

40. Meunier, P., Courpron, P., Edouard, C., Bernard, J., Brignuier, J. and Vignon, G: Physiological senile involution and pathological rarefaction of bone. Quantification and comparative histological data. Clin. Endocrinol.Metab. 2, 239, 1973.

41. Meunier, P.J., Courpron, P., Edouard, C., Alexander, C., Bressot, C., Lips, P., and Boyce, B.F.: Bone histomorphometry in osteoporotic states. In, Osteoporosis II. Ed: Barzel, U.S., Grune and Stratton, New York, 1979, pp 27-47.

42. Minaire, P., Meunier, P., Edouard, C., Bernard, J., Coupron, P., and Bourret, J.: Quantitative histological data on disuse osteoporosis. Comparison with biological data. Calcif.Tiss.Res. 17, 57, 1974.

43. Moser, C.R. and Fessel, W.J.: Rheumatic manifestations of hypophosphatemia. Arch.Intern.Med. 134, 674, 1974.

44. Parfitt, A.M., Oliver, I., and Villaneuva, A.R.: Bone histology in metabolic bone disease: The diagnostic value of bone biopsy. Orthop. Clin.North Am. 10, 329, 1979.

45. Raisz, L.G., Luben, R.A., Mundy, G.R., Dietrich, J.W., Horton, J.E., and Trummel, C.L.: Effect of osteoclast activating factor from human leukocytes on bone metabolism. J.Clin.Invest. 56, 408, 1975.

46. Recker, R.R., Saville, P.D., and Heaney, R.P.: Effect of estrogens and calcium carbonate on bone loss in postmenopausal women. Ann.Intern. Med. 87, 649, 1977.

47. Riggs, B.L., Arnaud, C.D., Jowsey, J., Goldsmith, R.S., and Kelly, P.R.: Parathyroid function in primary osteoporosis. J.Clin.Invest. 52, 181, 1973.

48. Riggs, B.L., Seeman, E., Hodgson, S.F., Traves, D.R., and O'Fallon, W.M.: Effect of the fluoride/calcium regimen on vertebral fracture occurrence in postmenopausal osteoporosis: Comparison with conventional therapy. New Engl.J.Med. 306, 446, 1982.

49. Rigotti, N.A., Nussbaum, S.R., Herzog, D.B., and Neer, R.M.: Osteoporosis in women with anorexia nervosa. New Engl.J.Med. 311, 1601, 1984.

50. Scileppi, K.P., Stulberg, B.N., Vigorita, V.J., Lane, J.M., Vossburg, R., and Arnold, W.D.: Bone histomorphometry in femoral neck fractures. Surg.Forum 32, 543, 1981.

51. Singh, M., Riggs, B.L., Beabout, J.W., and Jowsey, J.: Femoral trabecular pattern index for evaluation of spinal osteoporosis. Ann. Intern.Med. 77, 63, 1972.

52. Slovik, D.M., Adams, J.S., Neer, R.M., Holick, M.R., and Potts, J.T., Jr.: Deficient production of 1,25 dihydroxyvitamin D in elderly osteoporotic patients. New Engl.J.Med. 305, 372, 1981.

53. Smith, E.M., Jr., Reddan, W., and Smith P.E.: Physical activity and calcium modalities for bone mineral increases in aged women. Med.Sci. Sports Exerc. 13, 60, 1981.

54. Smith, R.: Idiopathic osteoporosis in the young. J.Bone Joint Surg. 62B, 417, 1980.

55. Tiegs, R.D., Body, J.J., Heinz, W.W., Barta, J., Riggs, B.L., and Health, H., III: Calcitonin secretion in postmenopausal osteoporosis. New Engl.J.Med. 312, 1097, 1985.

56. Vigorita, V.J. and Suda, M.K.: The microscopic morphology of fluoride-induced bone. Clin.Orthop. 172, 274, 1983.

57. Vigorita, V.J., Suda, M.K., and Lane, J.M.: Marked osteoporosis with idiopathic lymphoid hyperplasia of the marrow: A report of three cases. Arch.Pathol.Lab.Med. 107, 276, 1983.

58. Villaneuva, A.R., Parfitt, A.M., and Duncan, H.: Comparison of haversian bone dynamics between 11th rib and iliac trephine biopsies. In, Bone Histomorphometry. Ed: Meunier, P.J., Armour Montague, Paris, 1977, pp 75-78.

59. Weinstein, R.S., and Whyte, M.P.: Heterogeneity of adult hypophosphatasia: Report of severe and mild cases. Arch.Intern.Med. 141, 727, 1981.

60. Wilson, C.R., and Madsen, M.: Dichromatic absorptiometry of vertebral bone mineral content. Invest.Radiol. 12, 180, 1972.

Subject Index

MIX
Papier aus verantwortungsvollen Quellen
Paper from responsible sources
FSC® C105338

If you have any concerns about our products,
you can contact us on
ProductSafety@springernature.com

In case Publisher is established outside the EU,
the EU authorized representative is:
Springer Nature Customer Service Center GmbH
Europaplatz 3, 69115 Heidelberg, Germany

Printed by Libri Plureos GmbH
in Hamburg, Germany